Essentials in Ophthalmology

Series Editor
Arun D. Singh, Cleveland Clinic Foundation, Cole Eye Institute
Cleveland, OH, USA

Essentials in Ophthalmology aims to promote the rapid and efficient transfer of medical research into clinical practice. It is published in four volumes per year. Covering new developments and innovations in all fields of clinical ophthalmology, it provides the clinician with a review and summary of recent research and its implications for clinical practice. Each volume is focused on a clinically relevant topic and explains how research results impact diagnostics, treatment options and procedures as well as patient management.

The reader-friendly volumes are highly structured with core messages, summaries, tables, diagrams and illustrations and are written by internationally well-known experts in the field. A volume editor supervises the authors in his/her field of expertise in order to ensure that each volume provides cutting-edge information most relevant and useful for clinical ophthalmologists. Contributions to the series are peer reviewed by an editorial board.

Jorge L. Alió • Jorge L. Alió del Barrio
Editors

Modern Keratoplasty

Surgical Techniques and Indications

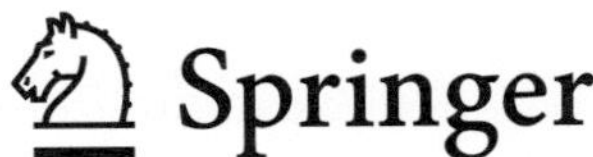 Springer

Editors
Jorge L. Alió
Vissum Miranza
Miguel Hernández University
Alicante, Spain

Jorge L. Alió del Barrio
Vissum Miranza
Miguel Hernández University
Alicante, Spain

ISSN 1612-3212   ISSN 2196-890X   (electronic)
Essentials in Ophthalmology
ISBN 978-3-031-32410-9   ISBN 978-3-031-32408-6   (eBook)
https://doi.org/10.1007/978-3-031-32408-6

This Springer imprint is published by the registered company Springer Nature Switzerland AG
The registered company address is: Gewerbestrasse 11, 6330 Cham, Switzerland

Preface

Over the last two decades, corneal surgery has experienced major and highly significant changes.

In the recent past, most of the cases that required a corneal graft were the subject of penetrating keratoplasty as the only repeatable, reliable, and effective corneal grafting surgical technique. Only in few anecdotical cases were lamellar techniques used. Such lamellar techniques, introduced some time ago by advanced corneal surgeons who anticipated their clinical value, were performed with an incomplete knowledge about the surgical anatomy of the cornea, its optics, and using inadequate instrumentation. With this background, such lamellar techniques were simply an art that was seldom practiced and only by a few talented surgeons, but with questionable clinical outcomes.

However, the mind of the human being never stops and this indeed also applies to corneal surgeons. The conceptualization of corneal surgical innovations based on improvements in the level of knowledge of corneal anatomy and its surgical management, the development of instruments such as femtosecond laser, and the general introduction of corneal topography, tomography, and high-resolution anterior segment OCT have led to a completely new perspective on corneal grafting that has been modified by the creation of highly precise, highly refined, and sophisticated surgical techniques that have evolved into the different corneal lamellar techniques that are in practice today.

Parallel to this, and alongside the continuous improvement in the outcomes of modern penetrating and lamellar corneal transplantation techniques (DALK, DSAEK, DMEK, and others), and the impressive improvement in eye banking techniques and more advanced knowledge of the immunological processes that govern the local immune response at the cornea and ocular surface, it is clear that with this alone, we are not able to treat and overcome corneal blindness. Today, it has become evident that we need to develop new and radically different methods to alleviate and treat corneal blindness. This is why, slowly but surely, corneal regeneration procedures are becoming a new promising group of techniques to restore the transparency and health condition of the diseased ocular surface, stroma, and endothelium. Based on this perspective, in this book we have tried to include all that is known at this moment, based on evidence, about corneal transplantation techniques, as practiced by modern corneal surgeons.

Corneal surgery has become today a highly specialized discipline in ophthalmology. It not only requires a high level of education in both clinical and basic sciences, but also an extremely high level of surgical training in surgeries that are not frequent and should be carefully selected and performed to be successful. It requires good knowledge about anatomy but also about immunology and a comprehensive approach to the treatment of ocular surface diseases. Globally speaking, corneal surgery today is a highly specialized, highly technified, and highly qualified subspeciality that demands properly trained eye surgeons to accomplish successful outcomes in the treatment of corneal blinding diseases.

While editing this book, we have envisaged a future, in which cell biologists, pharmacologists, and bioengineers may all intervene in corneal surgery, increasing its capability and efficiency in the treatment of corneal diseases. Throughout the chapters of this book, we aim to integrate all this new surgical, clinical, and basic knowledge into what is today the modern practice of keratoplasty and what is going to be developed to implement corneal surgery in the coming years. The term *Modern Keratoplasty* really addresses this concept and fundamentals that, as understood by the authors, corneal surgery will further evolve in the coming years for a better treatment of corneal disease and corneal blindness.

Alicante, Spain   Jorge L. Alio
Alicante, Spain   Jorge L. Alio del Barrio

Preface

Sight is God's most precious gift to mankind; cherish it, preserve it, donate it (HSD).

After cataract, corneal blindness is the commonest cause of curable sight loss. It is not surprising therefore that attempts to replace the cornea are part of recorded ancient medical history. The concept and the idea of rendering an opaque cornea clear or by replacing the cornea preceded the actual procedure by several years. Donor tissue was the first challenge to confront the early surgeons and it seems natural that they resorted to animal donor tissue, heralding the early phase of xenogeneic corneal grafts, refining techniques from animal to animal corneas before applying them for animal to human corneas. Porcine cornea was reportedly the first tissue used in a xenograft to the human eye followed by rabbit corneal tissue. Elegant accounts of the history and prehistoric considerations are in the published literature by Charles McGhee, Chad Rostrom, Gabriel Van Rij, and Satish Srinivasan [1–4].

The year 2005 was significant in that it represented the completion of a century of successful full-thickness or penetrating keratoplasty (PK). Today we live in an era where a new drug or procedure is introduced, developed, practiced, and rendered obsolete, in its components or entirely, within a professional career, more than once. Such is the pace of "progress." The progress of PK was not linear. The challenges, complications, and failures of PK compared less favorably with lamellar keratoplasty (LK) but visual outcomes of successful grafts were better with PK, leading to fluctuating popularity of one over the other.

The advent of topical anesthesia (cocaine), improvements, innovations, and inventions in instrumentation, suture material and microsurgical techniques, eye banking, the operating microscope, and not least the realization of the existence of the endothelium and its importance in the physiology of corneal transparency constituted major landmarks on the path to successful PK. Things that we today take for granted did not happen overnight. They were the product of the cumulative research and efforts of numerous individuals, institutions, and industry.

Despite a century and a score years of success, PK was plagued by major problems that defied resolution. Immune-mediated graft rejection and failure, suture-related complications including severe infection, induced astigmatism from unpredictable and irregular scarring along the circumference of the graft-host junction, which remained forever weak and prone to rupture with even trivial trauma, with devastating consequences, are long recognized and remain today as major issues. However, Hope, that translated to viable solutions to some but not all of the above issues, came from revisiting old principles with advances in knowledge and modern technology. PK gave way to LK.

Lamellar keratoplasty is today the norm where indicated and where possible. The key principles of LK are "replacing like for like," which applies to all LK, and the "thinner the better" that applies primarily to endothelial keratoplasty (EK). The initial techniques introduced by Gerrit Melles and Francis Price [5–7] for both anterior lamellar keratoplasty and EK were manual and crude compared to modern techniques, but were game changing and the start of a revolution in corneal transplantation. The near like-for-like replacement in anterior lamellar keratoplasty came from Mohammed Anwar's big bubble technique for deep anterior lamellar (DALK) [8]. This was initially proposed as a Descemet's membrane baring technique but with the discovery of the pre-Descemet's layer (Dua's layer, PDL/DL) [9] it became obvious that in over 80% of cases of DALK by the big bubble technique the host PDL/DL was retained (the type 1 big bubble); hence it was not a true like-for-like replacement but nevertheless a desirable outcome as it conferred extra strength to the eye and posed fewer intraoperative risks. Knowledge of the PDL/DL improved understanding of DALK (type 1, type 2, and mixed bubbles) and made the operation safer. The cleavage plane offered by the PDL/DL enabled successful completion of DALK even when air injection produced a very small or no big bubble. DALK by any technique (air bubble, visco bubble, or manual dissection) confers two main advantages, a stronger eye compared to PK and retention of the healthy host endothelium, obviating the risk of endothelial rejection and associated graft failure [10]. The disadvantages of suture-related complications, induced astigmatism, and delayed visual recovery associated with PK, however, remain. The recent innovation of Bowman's membrane transplant, by Melles' group [11], represents the thinnest anterior lamellar transplant, which both strengthens and flattens the cornea in keratoconus eyes. A similar outcome has been demonstrated by stromal lenticule transplantation.

Descemet's stripping endothelial keratoplasty (DSEK) was the novel EK procedure that heralded a paradigm shift in corneal transplantation. Manual preparation of donor lenticules was rapidly replaced by automated keratomes, adding Descemet's stripping automated endothelial keratoplasty (DSAEK) to the nomenclature. These procedures did away with the need for sutures, eliminated induced astigmatism, led to rapid visual recovery, and as a bonus, reduced the risk of endothelial rejection, probably related to reduced antigen load (there is no epithelium and the posterior stroma has fewer keratocytes and considerably fewer antigen-presenting dendritic cells), and reduced inflammation due to absence of sutures. However, the final thickness and contour assumed by the transplanted lenticule (thick and more curved at the periphery) caused a hyperopic refractive change with patients often attaining no better than 6/12 or 6/9 vision. The realization that thinner donor lenticules apposed better to the posterior curvature of the recipient cornea and gave better visual outcomes was the driver to create thinner donor lenticules and the evolution of the technique of ultra-thin (UT) DSAEK, pioneered by Massimo Busin [12].

Pre-Descemet's endothelial keratoplasty (PDEK) wherein the donor transplant tissue consisting of the PDL/DL, Descemet's membrane, and endothelium, obtained by creating a type 1 big bubble in the donor cornea, was proposed and demonstrated ex vivo by Harminder Dua [9, 13], first intentionally performed by Amar Agarwal (others had inadvertently performed this thinking that they were performing Descemet's membrane endothelial keratoplasty [DMEK]—see below) and reported by Agarwal and Dua [14], can be regarded as the thinnest UT-DSAEK. PDEK gives visual outcomes similar to DMEK but has the advantage of being technically less challenging and provides the option of obtaining tissue from very young donors including infants.

Some of these innovations occurred contemporaneously rather than chronologically. Maintaining his indelible stamp on EK, Melles introduced the technique of Descemet's membrane endothelial keratoplasty (DMEK), the ultimate in like-for-like replacement [15]. It has all the advantages of any EK procedure with considerable refinement on size of the entry wound and a significantly better visual outcome. It is technically challenging both in terms of harvesting donor Descemet's membrane for transplantation and unscrolling, centration, and attachment in the recipient eye. Young donors have thinner Descemet's membrane which scrolls tightly, making them less suitable for DMEK. The support and tamponade afforded by the PDL/DL makes use of young donor tissue a viable option for PDEK as a type 1 big bubble can be produced in a cornea of any age. Nevertheless, DMEK is the gold standard procedure in EK. DMEK and PDEK, unlike DSAEK and UT-DSAEK, do not require expensive equipment (automated keratomes) with expensive maintenance costs. Growing experience, education, and training will make these procedures more accessible to surgeons globally.

This pace of progress has occurred at a price. As with any innovation that offers a potential of better outcomes, there is a learning curve for the first generations of surgeons who take it on and for the patients who they take on. Success is built on some or more failures. Donor tissue wastage occurs as harvesting techniques are refined and standardized, and failed grafts lead to repeat grafts. Eye banks struggle to keep pace with surgical innovations and surgeon's demands compounded by global donor tissue shortage, augmented by the pandemic. However, the worst is probably behind us. Eye banks have taken on the challenge of providing pre-cut DSAEK tissue, pre-prepared (pre-stained, pre-stamped, and pre-loaded) DMEK and PDEK tissue, easing the pressure on surgeons.

The imminent future offers the exciting prospect of endothelial cell transplantation, pioneered by Shigeru Kinoshita [16]. The introduction of cultured endothelial cells into the anterior chamber through a paracentesis port is the simplest of all techniques. The face-down position that the patient has to adopt to allow the injected cells to gravitate to the back of the cornea is probably more inconvenient, but the results, as demonstrated by ongoing studies, are as good as any. A taster of this concept is seen in the techniques of Descemet's stripping only (DSO) and Descemetorhexis without endothelial keratoplasty (DWEK), wherein the guttata bearing central Descemet's membrane (in Fuchs' endothelial keratoplasty) is peeled off and the surrounding endothelial cells encouraged to migrate on to the surface thus exposed, restoring sight and function.

The story of corneal transplantation will not be complete without jumping from the back to the front of the cornea and penning a few words on corneal epithelial regeneration and limbal stem cell transplantation. Much of this went through an equally exciting period of innovation and discovery, but is now old hat. Auto limbal grafts, cadaver allo limbal grafts, and living related allo limbal grafts, with their variations and subtle nuances, are well established and practiced procedures. Ex vivo expansion of sheets of limbal, conjunctival, and oral mucosal epithelial cells on substrates such as fibrin and amnion is also well established and practiced. Systemic immunosuppression, with all its implications in terms of drug toxicity and monitoring, constitutes the biggest challenge with allografts. Autografts give excellent results, driving developments in the exploration of the use of autologous mesenchymal stem cells from sources such as liver, bone marrow, and dental pulp and from other sources such as the umbilical cord and embryonic tissue.

The holy grail of a synthetic and/or tissue engineered cornea, complete from epithelium to endothelium, is running the roller coaster of promise and not living up to the promise. To learn all about modern keratoplasty, and the past and future of keratoplasty, Jorge Alio's book on "Modern Keratoplasty" is a must read.

Nottingham, UK   Harminder S. Dua

References

1. Crawford AZ, Patel DV, McGhee CNJ. A brief history of corneal transplantation: from ancient to modern. Oman J Ophthalmol. 2013;6(Suppl 1):S12–7.
2. Rostron CK. The history of corneal transplantation. In: Hakim NS, Papalois VE, editors. History of organ and cell transplantation; 2003. p. 274–92. https://doi.org/10.1142/9781848160057_0013.
3. Gabriël van Rij G, van Dooren BTH. The history of corneal transplantation. In: Hjortdal J, editor. Corneal transplantation. Cham: Springer International Publishing; 2016. p. 1–8. https://doi.org/10.1007/978-3-319-24052-7_1.
4. Srinivasan S. Evolution and revolution in corneal transplant surgery. J Cataract Refract Surg. 2021;47(7):837–8.
5. Melles GR, Lander F, Rietveld FJ, Remeijer L, Beekhuis WH, Binder PS. A new surgical technique for deep stromal, anterior lamellar keratoplasty. Br J Ophthalmol. 1999;83(3):327–33.
6. Melles GRJ. Landmark study on descemet stripping with endothelial keratoplasty: where has it led us? J Cataract Refract Surg. 2021;47(5):561–2.
7. Price FW Jr, Price MO. Descemet's stripping with endothelial keratoplasty in 200 eyes: early challenges and techniques to enhance donor adherence. J Cataract Refract Surg. 2006;32(3):411–8.
8. Anwar M, Teichmann KD. Big-bubble technique to bare Descemet's membrane in anterior lamellar keratoplasty. J Cataract Refract Surg. 2002;28(3):398–403.
9. Dua HS, Faraj LA, Said DG, Gray T, Lowe J. Human corneal anatomy redefined: a novel pre-Descemet's layer (Dua's layer). Ophthalmology. 2013;120(9):1778–85.
10. Dua HS, Freitas R, Mohammed I, Ting DSJ, Said DG. The pre-descemet's layer (Dua's layer, also known as the Dua-Fine layer and the pre-posterior limiting lamina layer): discovery, characterisation, clinical and surgical applications, and the controversy. Prog Retin Eye Res:101161. https://doi.org/10.1016/j.preteyeres.2022.101161.

11. van Dijk K, Liarakos VS, Parker J, Ham L, Lie JT, Groeneveld-van Beek EA, Melles GR. Bowman layer transplantation to reduce and stabilize progressive, advanced keratoconus. Ophthalmology. 2015;122(5):909–17.
12. Busin M, Madi S, Santorum P, Scorcia V, Beltz J. Ultrathin descemet's stripping automated endothelial keratoplasty with the microkeratome double-pass technique: two-year outcomes. Ophthalmology. 2013;120(6):1186–94.
13. Dua HS, Faraj LA, Said DG. Dua's layer: discovery, characteristics, clinical applications, controversy and potential relevance to glaucoma. Exp Rev Ophthalmol. 2015;10:531–47.
14. Agarwal A, Dua HS, Narang P, et al. Pre-descemet's endothelial keratoplasty (PDEK). Br J Ophthalmol. 2014;98:1181–5.
15. Dapena I, Ham L, Droutsas K, van Dijk K, Moutsouris K, Melles GR. Learning curve in descemet's membrane endothelial keratoplasty: first series of 135 consecutive cases. Ophthalmology. 2011;118(11):2147–54.
16. Numa K, Imai K, Ueno M, Kitazawa K, Tanaka H, Bush JD, Teramukai S, Okumura N, Koizumi N, Hamuro J, Sotozono C, Kinoshita S. Five-year follow-up of first 11 patients undergoing injection of cultured corneal endothelial cells for corneal endothelial failure. Ophthalmology. 2021;128(4):504–14.

Acknowledgments

We, the editors Jorge Alio and Jorge Alio del Barrio, wish to express our gratitude to all the authors who have contributed to this book for their dedication and talent. Only with their expertise, experience, and generosity can an endeavor like this be possible. Many thanks to all.

Jorge L. Alio
Jorge L. Alio del Barrio

Contents

Introduction: Current Status of Modern Corneal Transplantation—Success, Failures and Turning Points

1

Jorge L. Alió, Dominika Wróbel-Dudzińska, and Tomasz Żarnowski

Key Points

- Corneal keratoplasty is a broad term that includes all the numerous methods of surgery to improve sight, relieve pain and treat severe infection or corneal damage. The indications for transplantation have changed with the development of surgical techniques and equipment and the possibility of performing not only full-thickness but also partial-thickness grafts.
- The success of modern keratoplasty should be analyzed from an anatomical perspective (graft survival) and functional results (refractive outcomes and regularity of the cornea).
- In this chapter, we present a complete review of the main complications and risk factors that determine the success and failure rate of corneal grafts.

J. L. Alió (✉)
Vissum Miranza, Miguel Hernández University, Alicante, Spain
e-mail: jlalio@vissum.com

D. Wróbel-Dudzińska · T. Żarnowski
Department of Diagnostics and Microsurgery of Glaucoma, Medical University of Lublin, Lublin, Poland

Introduction

Corneal diseases are reported to be the second leading cause of reversible blindness worldwide [1]. The only effective treatment for this ailment is a corneal graft, considered the most successful organ transplantation in the human body [2]. The reasons for such success are mainly based on the fact that the cornea is an immunologically privileged tissue due to the absence of blood and lymphatic vessels, the blood-eye barrier, the presence of immunomodulatory factors in aqueous humor, the relative paucity of mature antigen-presenting cells (APCs), and good intraocular penetration of topical steroids.

The indication for corneal graft surgery as a solution for cornea-related visual handicaps and blindness has changed over time. Haziness and corneal scaring due to infection were the first indication of corneal keratoplasty. Over time, keratoconus, Fuchs endothelial dystrophy and bullous keratopathy, graft failure after a previous keratoplasty have now become the main indications [3].

Corneal transplant is classified as **therapeutic** or tectonic (when removing an infective cornea resistant to treatment, or affected by an impending or already established perforation, or severe trauma with corneal tissue loss) and **visual-optical** (to restore corneal clarity and improve vision). **Cosmetic indications** in severely distorted blind eyes are also performed in cases

J. L. Alió, J. L. A. del Barrio (eds.), *Modern Keratoplasty*, Essentials in Ophthalmology, https://doi.org/10.1007/978-3-031-32408-6_1

1

when the goal is to remove scars or corneal haze, which is mainly an esthetic defect.

According to research by the World Health Organization (WHO), corneal disease is one of the most common causes of vision deterioration and blindness worldwide, in both adults and children [4]. The Vision Share Consortium of Eye Banks in the USA estimates that the number of patients with corneal diseases exceeds ten million. Each year, injuries and ulceration of the cornea cause blindness in 1.5–2 million people. However, in many cases, it is possible to transplant the cornea, the organ with the highest success rate.

Modern Modalities of Corneal Transplantations

Depending on the amount of corneal thickness tissue to exchange, corneal transplants can be divided into:

1. *Penetrating,* in which a fragment of the full-thickness cornea is replaced,
2. *Lamellar,* where only the affected part of the cornea is exchanged.

Penetrating Keratoplasty (PK) full-thickness corneal transplantation is still the gold standard treatment for opaque or morphologically abnormal corneas due to infections or immunological diseases and profound corneal defects due to stromal scarring with posterior corneal involvement and corneal ulcerations or perforations and injuries [5].

According to Alio et al., the main causes for PK are combined endothelial and stromal diseases like chronic pseudophakic bullous keratopathy in 31.5% of cases, followed by keratoconus and ectatic cornea disorders in 11.6% and cornea scarring in 10.4% [6].

The risk of expulsive hemorrhage and vitreous body outflow that may happen during open-sky surgery, prolonged visual rehabilitation, high astigmatism, unpredictable refractive outcome, secondary glaucoma, and a higher risk of graft rejection prompted ophthalmologists to search for new techniques consisting of replacing only the affected and damaged part of the cornea, constituting the basis of lamellar keratoplasty. The new methods not only maintain eyeball integrity but also provide the opportunity of avoiding complications associated to open-sky surgery and lead to a lower rate of graft rejection due to less tissue being transplanted. This has been possible due to a better understanding of the corneal anatomy, advanced surgical techniques, instruments, microscopes and medications.

Deep Anterior Lamellar Keratoplasty (DALK) was developed to avoid the complications of PK [7, 8]. According to the literature, its current main surgical indications are for keratoconus or corneal ectasia (keratoglobus, pellucid marginal degeneration) in 51.3 % of cases, followed by herpetic or other infectious keratitis (bacterial, fungal and parasitic) in 18.9% with opacities located in the deep stroma, chronic inflammation with stromal scarring and stromal dystrophies (granular, lattice) [9].

There are a variety of surgical techniques to perform DALK including manual dissection, manual dissection supported by air [8] or viscoelastic [10], or big bubble technique [11] or assisted by femtosecond laser [12].

Nowadays, we can offer customized treatment consisting of focused surgeries. Furthermore, due to advanced equipment, for example, femtosecond laser, we can perform perfect cuts that provide more regular sealing, better and faster healing and less irregular astigmatism, thus leading to better refractive outcomes. Consequently, lamellar procedures have replaced penetrating keratoplasty.

In comparison to PKP, the incidence of graft rejection is lower (due to the absence of the endothelial rejection), DALK also has superior biomechanical properties, may end in reduced induction of higher-order aberrations, visual rehabilitation is faster, and the risk of intra- and postoperative complications is significantly reduced. However, DALK has a difficult learning curve and is more technically demanding. It is worth bearing in mind that, sometimes irregularities in the interface or double anterior chamber may appear. Nonetheless, the number of procedures has increased over the last years. DALK has apparently better long-term anatomical survival rates (85–98% at 5 years) [6].

Posterior lamellar keratoplasty techniques aim to remove the Descemet membrane and endothelium followed by their replacement from the donor of either Descemet and endothelium alone (**DMEK**) or with posterior stroma remains (**DSAEK**). The main causes for endothelial keratoplasty (**EK**) are posterior corneal dystrophies—endothelial dystrophy including Fuchs endothelial dystrophy (FED) in 58.3% of cases, pseudophakic bullous keratopathy (PBK) in 30.6% [7] and previous graft failure in 16.5% [6], iridocorneal endothelial syndrome (ICE) or other causes of endothelial dysfunction due to trauma, foreign body or age.

The advantages of EK are lower corneal postoperative astigmatism due to the absence of sutures, and suture-related problems such as infiltrates and astigmatism, and thus a faster visual rehabilitation and a lower rejection rate. Unfortunately, graft dislocation may happen, and primary graft failure. Moreover, this technique requires special technical equipment (e.g., a microkeratome to prepare the donor tissue). The advantages of DMEK over DSAEK are faster visual rehabilitation and a lower graft rejection rate due to the thinner graft (no stromal tissue), but it is demanding for the surgeon and associated with a higher rate of rebubbling. However, it has been reported that endothelial keratoplasty (EK) survival increases over time at the same time as surgeon and center experience. It is worth bearing in mind that a hyperopic shift of approximately 0.8–1.5 D [13] is observed in DSAEK depending on the lenticule thickness that is transplanted.

According to recent studies, DMEK is definitely a better option than DSAEK in terms of visual outcomes achieved with a faster visual recovery and improved graft survival [14].

Currently, with the improvements in corneal transplantation surgical techniques and improvements in corneal banking, supplying more and better corneal donor material, the number of cor-neal transplants has increased in the last 30 years, which is undoubtedly related to the development of microsurgery, the use of nonabsorbable sutures, the introduction of better antibiotics and corticosteroids, wider immunology knowledge, as well as the introduction of tissue preservation/banking procedures (previously, it was necessary to immediately transplant tissues after donation). As a result, the range of indications for corneal transplants has also expanded, which was initially limited to hopeless cases.

According to the European Cornea and Cell Transplantation Registry (**ECCTR), the cornea is the most frequently transplanted intact tissue, with over 180,000 transplants performed annually worldwide** [15]. As it was stated in the Eye Bank Association of America Report of 2020, the total number of corneal grafts was 66,278. This figure decreased from 85,601 in comparison to the previous year. There were 15,402 penetrating keratoplasties (PK) performed (a decrease of 11.6%), while endothelial keratoplasty (EK) numbers decreased by 14.9% to 26,095. In 2019, the number of penetrating keratoplasty grafts performed was 17,409 grafts and 30,650 endothelial keratoplasty grafts due to a 23% increase in DMEK procedures. Regrafting was needed in 12.8% of cases (PK in 18.5%, ALK in 3.6% and EK in 9.9%) [16].

The ECCTR estimated that about 30,000 corneal transplantations are performed annually in Europe. But the total number of registered keratoplasties was 12,913 in 2019. Sixteen percent of these were regrafting procedures [15].

As reported by the NHS transplant registry, there were 4580 corneas transplants performed per million population in the UK from 1s April 2019 to 31 March 2020. According to the indication, there were 32% transplants for FED, 15.8% for PBK, 18.7% for regrafts, 16.9% for others, 8.9% for keratoconus and 7.8% for infectious. PK grafts accounted for 30.3% of transplants in 2020–2021, 29.4% of the grafts were DSAEK and 29.1% were DMEK and 7% were anterior lamellar keratoplasty [17].

In 2020, Canadian eye banks distributed 3786 corneas for surgical use, 1327 corneas for DSAEK ad 937 for DMEK and 845 for

PK. Results relating to ocular tissues in 2020 showed reduced numbers compared to 2019, with a 25% decrease in the number of overall donors, which correlated to a 16% decrease in ocular tissue produced and released for transplant during 2020 [18].

As reported by the Australian Corneal Graft Registry 2020 Annual Report, there were 40,864 registered corneal grafts. Twenty-three percent of them failed [19].

Success, Failures and Complications of Modern Corneal Transplants

Corneal transplantation is the most common, widely practiced and most successful form of solid-tissue transplantation in the human body due to the immune-privileged condition of the eye.

The success of modern keratoplasty techniques should be analyzed both from the anatomical perspective (graft survival) and the functional result of the transplant, which involves not only how transparent the tissue grafted is but also how regular the resulting cornea surface is and the refractive outcome, which is frequently unacceptable for an adequate visual rehabilitation leading to binocularity problems.

Concerning anatomical success, the overall first-year survival rate of all types of corneal grafts appears to be as high as 91%. Unfortunately, the long-term reality is that the overall **anatomical success** rate diminishes to 63.7–83% in PKP, 85–98% in DALK and 79.4–96% in EK at 5 years and only 62% of PKP grafts are functional at 10 years [20]. These results are very impressive in comparison to other solid-tissue transplant outcomes, but are still far away from the successful outcomes of most of the modern ophthalmic surgical techniques such as cataract surgery, refractive surgery or retinal detachment procedures [21]. This is especially true when factors such as the level of corneal irregularity or final refractive outcome are taken into consideration to further qualify the **functional success** of a cor-

neal graft procedure. We shall analyze in detail these outcome considerations later in this chapter.

Complications of Corneal Transplants That Affect the Outcome

Despite the new surgical techniques and equipment, better pre- and postoperative treatment and diagnostics methods, there is still a risk of complications. They vary somewhat between the different types of corneal transplants, especially intraoperative complications. In PKP and DALK, suture-related problems (breaking or loosening sutures, exposure, vascularization, infection, immune infiltrates) and wound dehiscence may occur. As stated in the literature, persistent epithelial defects range from 0% to 77.2% in PKP during active inflammation [22]. Filamentary keratitis is also common after PKP. In addition, elevated intraocular pressure, glaucoma, pupillary block, Urrets-Zavalia syndrome, synechias, postoperative inflammation/infection, even endophthalmitis, unpredictable refractive outcome and anisometropia, cataract formation may happen in all types of corneal grafts.

The most common complication during DALK is perforation of the Descemet membrane, which may occur in approximately 10–39.2% of cases, especially at the beginning of the learning curve of the surgeon [23]. After surgery pseudo-anterior chamber or double anterior chambers may appear. Endothelial keratoplasty is also technically demanding, and we can encounter graft dislocation or irregular graft profile, detachment problems or even residual host Descemet membrane, interface haze, potentially significant loss of donor endothelial cells during the surgery and in pseudophakic eyes opacification of the hydrophilic acrylic lens.

Corneal graft failure is another significant problem characterized by the difficulty of restoration of the visual function without any accompanying diseases. Thus, corneal transplant survival rates vary according to the primary corneal disease.

The long-term success of corneal graft depends on the cause of the corneal damage, surgical technique used, the expertise of the surgeon, the possibility of organ rejection and other factors that we are still unaware of. If we wish to improve our outcomes in corneal transplantation, we need to know the anatomical and functional reasons for failures.

Graft Failure Modalities

Generalizing corneal graft failure can be classified as

1. *Anatomical failure*: defined as an irreversible decrease in graft transparency despite the correct treatment.
2. *Functional failure*: consisting of unsatisfactory visual acuity due to irregular cornea with astigmatism, high order abberations (HOA) or inadequate refractive outcomes that limit the binocularity outcome. The pre-existing ocular morbidities or complications that happen at the postoperative, especially glaucoma, may also limit the visual outcome.

Ad. 1. Frequency and Main Causes of Corneal Graft Anatomical Failure

1. Primary graft failure (PGF) which happens when the graft presents edema from the first postoperative day and transparency does not recover within 3 months. It might be the result of donor endothelial cell dysfunction, incorrect tissue preservation or surgical trauma during the harvesting or transplantation process.
2. Secondary graft failure (SGF) occurs when a previously transparent graft becomes obscure with deterioration of vision.
   (a) Immunological rejection: when an immune reaction occurs, causing graft decompensation.
   (b) Nonrejection causes: unclassifiable in any of the other two categories.
   - endothelial decompensation without rejection
   - IOP elevation/glaucoma
   - diseases of the ocular surface, especially limbal stem cell deficiency, dry eye disease
   - recurrence of the primary disease, herpetic disease
   - wound dehiscence/hypotony and trauma
3. Morphological graft failure involves poor visual function but with clear transparent graft (severe irregular astigmatism).

Anatomical Failure in the Different Types of Corneal Grafts

Anatomical failure is defined as an outcome that limits corneal transparency leading to lack of functional recovery concerning the preoperative condition in terms of gains in best corrected visual acuity (BCVA). According to the literature, the 5-year survival graft rate ranges from 63.7 to 83% for PK, 90 to 98% for DALK and 79.4 to 96% in EK and 30 to 66% for PK regrafts [6].

Penetrating Keratoplasty

As reported by Alio et al., the main reason for graft failure in primary PK was 16.4% PGF (primary graft failure), 28.2% immunological rejection, 17.8% surface disease and 17.3% late endothelial decompensation. In PK regraft, 34% of the graft failure was due to immunological rejection, 18.5% to ocular surface disease and 17.3% to endothelial decompensation [7].

Wiliams et al. observed graft failure in 28% due to allograft rejection, 20% to late endothelial failure, 11% due to infection, 5% glaucoma, 3% PGF and 34% due to others [20]. According to

Roozbahani, the most common complication after therapeutic PK, was cataract, which appeared in 81.8% of phakic eyes, followed by 47.1%, graft failure and 45.1% secondary glaucoma 9.8% of cases developed infection, 7.84% had a persistent corneal epithelial defect and unfortunately in almost 4% of patients evisceration was performed [24].

Deep Anterior Lamellar Keratoplasty

The review study of Williams et al. showed a DALK PGF rate of 12%. Other causes of graft failure were: 18% infection, 12% scaring, 5% late endothelial failure, 43% others, and 9% poor functional performance due to astigmatism [20]. In accordance with Alio, in the DALK population, the main reason for graft failure was in 37.8% of cases due to ocular surface diseases such as limbal stem cell deficiency, infectious keratitis, persistent epithelial defect and keratolysis [7].

Endothelial Keratoplasty

According to the Spanish study, the main reason for failure in EK was 31.9% endothelial decompensation without rejection in DSAEK and 15.4% in DMEK, PGF was the main cause of failure in 64.1% of failed DMEKs and 23.2% of failed DSAEKs [7].

A large study about DSEK reported that the causes of graft failure were: in 32% of cases late endothelial failure, 28% PGF, 13% allograft rejection, 3% infection and 24% others [20]. Researchers from USA revealed that in FED with DSEK the leading cause of the graft failure was: in 29% of cases PGF, 19% late endothelial graft failure, 6% allograft rejection and 43% unsatisfactory vision. In DMEK procedure, PGF was 66%, late endothelial failure 20%, allograft rejection 2% and unsatisfactory vision 7% [25]. The main reason for failure in the Birbal study about DMEK was 67.4% graft

detachment, 30.5% late endothelial failure and 2.1% PGF [26]. Aboshiha et al. compared differential survival of penetrating and lamellar transplants in the management of failed corneal grafts performed due to keratoconus or FED and PBK; they showed that the most common cause of failure of the first graft was endothelial decompensation in 36.4% of cases, irreversible rejection in 20.6% and primary graft failure in 15% [27].

To sum up, in DSEK PGF ranged from 0 to 29%, graft rejection from 0–45.4%, respectively, to DMEK PGF varied from 0 to 12.5%, SGF from 0 to 6% and graft rejection from 0.8 to 5% [23].

Ad. 2

One of the main but underestimated reasons for functional graft failure is poor visual acuity. The refractive outcomes of the corneal transplant are determined by many factors such as tissue distribution of the donor graft, suturing technique and healing at the graft–host junction.

Functional Outcomes of Corneal Graft Procedures

Many times, it is the functional outcome, rather than the anatomical one, that is the real limitation of the outcome of anatomically successful corneal grafts. The reasons are the uncontrollable astigmatic outcome, the induction of high levels of regular and irregular astigmatism and the frequent induction of anisometropia incompatible with adequate binocularity. Such refractive issues are usually overlooked in most of the reports about the clinical success of corneal grafts but in real practice happen much more frequently than anatomical failures in such a way that today they constitute probably one of the main reasons for corneal graft failure, especially in PKP and DALK surgeries.

The functional outcome of corneal grafts should be estimated including the following data:

1. Subjective: UCVA, BCVA, refractive outcome, refractive binocularity compared to the fellow eye and level of anisometropia
2. Objective:
   (a) Ocular surface stability and tear film dynamics and corneal irregularities induce irregular astigmatism, corneal anterior and posterior higher-order aberrations (HOAs), corneal forward and backward light scattering, pupil decentration or abnormalities.
   (b) Level of corneal irregular astigmatism, HOA and level of anisometropia when the refractive outcome is compared to that of the fellow eye.
   (c) Vision-related quality of life analysis, which measures the impact that the outcome of the surgery has induced on the patient's daily life. This parameter is very seldomly investigated and reported in studies about the outcomes of corneal graft procedures.

All these variables lead to poor functional vision. Thus, there are only a few studies reporting the functional outcomes of PK performed as a therapeutic or tectonic procedure and their visual acuity prognosis is poor. The achieved BCVA was 20/276 in the Roozbahani study and 20/100, according to Krysik [24, 28]. Such poor visual acuity results should be classified as a complete functional failure.

The tables (Tables 1.1 and 1.2) below show the distribution of BCVA according to the indication for the surgery and procedures performed. To sum up, 51–69% of corneal transplant procedures should be classified as functional failures due to the low visual acuity achieved.

Unfortunately, the BCVA achieved in many cases is not satisfactory. As stated in the Australian Corneal Graft Registry (ACGR) 2020, although visual acuity improved from counting fingers to 6/12 by 1 year after the corneal graft in keratoconus patients, more than half of the recipients were still wearing spectacles. Fifty-four percent of patients after penetrating keratoplasty for keratoconus needed spectacles and 14% contact lenses. After DALK 41% used glasses and 8% used contact lenses to achieve functional visual acuity. The short-term survival of penetrating keratoplasty was very good, reaching 87% of cases, but unfortunately, excellent visual acuity was only achieved by approximately half of all the grafts. Moreover, the survival rate dropped to 46% at 15 years postoperatively [20].

The functional results were also shown in another study. There was a significant improvement between the pre- and postoperative values of visual outcomes. 65.4% of patients with DALK achieved BCVA ≥20/40 and, 66.7% with EK, 51.3% with PK. The results were better than in primary PK. DMEK showed better visual results than DSEK [6].

According to the tables above, the worst functional results were observed in PKP and the best visual acuity was achieved in the DMEK procedure. The leading type of corneal transplant with acceptable anatomical success was DALK, while PKP has the highest percentage of anatomical failure.

Table 1.1 Distribution of BCVA following corneal transplant for the most common indication for 2 years follow-up according to the European Corneal and Cell Transplantation Registry [29]

2-year postoperatively	FED (%)	KC (%)	PBK (%)	Regraft (%)	Trauma (%)	Infection (%)
Functional failure BCVA <20/32	10	12	44	44	55	43
Qualified failure BCVA <20/40	6	8	9	9	14	9
BCVA ≥20/40	84	80	47	47	31	48

Table 1.2 Distribution of BCVA according to the surgical procedure performed

Study	No of eyes and procedure	BCVA general	BCVA 6 months	BCVA 1 year	BCVA 5 years	BCVA 10 years
Feizi [30]	45 PK				$\geq$20/40 91.1%	
	54 DALK				$\geq$20/40 83.3%	
Yüksel [31]	38 DALK			$\geq$20/40 76.3%		
				$\geq$20/20 7.9%		
	38 PKP			$\geq$20/40 47.4%		
				$\geq$20/20 5.3%		
Alzahrani [32]	16 DALK			$\geq$20/40 81%		
	21 PKP			$\geq$20/40 66%		
Gadhvi [33]	338 DALK			$\geq$20/40 75.9%		
Amar [34]	31 DALK			$\geq$20/40 58%		
	16 DSAEK			$\geq$20/40 68.75%		
Dickman [35]	2725 EK		EK Fuchs 0.32 (log MAR)	EK Fuchs 0.29 (log MAR)	EK Fuchs 0.29 (log MAR)	
			EK PBK 0.58 (log MAR)	EK PBK 0.55 (log MAR)	EK PBK 0.51 (log MAR)	
	2390 PKP		PKP 0.47/0.77 (log MAR)	PKP 0.39/0.74 (log MAR)	PKP 0.32/0.70 (log MAR)	
Khattak [36]	108 DALK	20/142 (0.25 ± 0.28 log MAR)				
	99 PK	20/123 (0.28 ± 0.24)				
Birbal [26]	500 DMEK		<20/40 6%	<20/40 2.2%	<20/40 1.4%	
			$\geq$20/40 94%	$\geq$20/40 97.8%	$\geq$20/40 98.6%	
			$\geq$20/25 75.1%	$\geq$20/25 80.1%	$\geq$20/25 82.4%	
			$\geq$20/20 41.1%	$\geq$20/20 48.3%	$\geq$20/20 53.6%	
			$\geq$20/17 12.9%	$\geq$20/17 14.7%	$\geq$20/17 15.5%	
Vassiliauskaite [37]	100 DMEK			$\geq$20/40 96%	$\geq$20/40 98%	$\geq$20/40 98%
				$\geq$20/25 81%	$\geq$20/25 82%	$\geq$20/25 89%
				$\geq$20/20 (1.0)-49%	$\geq$20/20 53%	$\geq$20/20 64%
Peraza-Nieves [38]	500 DMEK		<20/40 6%			
			$\geq$20/40 94%			
			$\geq$20/25 75.1%	$\geq$20/25 1%		
			$\geq$20/20 41.1%	$\geq$20/20 49%		
			$\geq$20/17 13%	$\geq$20/18 15%		
Heinzelmann [39]	DMEK 450			$\geq$20/25 53%		
	DSEK 89			$\geq$20/25 15%		
	PKP 329			$\geq$20/25 10%		
Phillips [40]	100 DSEK		20/20 13%			
	100 DMEK		20/20 55%			
Ham [41]	250 DMEK		20/25 73%	20/25 76.8%		
			20/20 44%	20/20 44%		
Siggel [42]	120 DMEK		$\geq$20/40 92%	$\geq$20/40 88%		
			$\geq$20/25 49%	$\geq$20/25 50%		
			$\geq$20/20 20%	$\geq$20/20 22%		

(continued)

Table 1.2 (continued)

Study	No of eyes and procedure	BCVA general	BCVA 6 months	BCVA 1 year	BCVA 5 years	BCVA 10 years
Schlögl [43]	97 DMEK			≥20/40 90%	≥20/40 88%	
				≥20/25 40%	≥20/25 48%	
Weller [44]	66 DMEK					≥20/40 91%
						≥20/25 67%
Dunker [45]	29 DMEK			≥20/25 66%		
				≥20/20 24%		
	25 UT-DSAEK			≥20/25 32%		
				≥20/20 4%		
Wacker [46]	52 DSEK			≥20/25 26%	≥20/25 56%	
Weisenthal [47]	64 DSAEK				≥20/25 64%	
					≥20/20 41%	
	64 DMEK				≥20/25 73%	
					≥20/20 51%	

Anatomical Outcomes After Regraft

As reported by Srujana in his study, primary graft failure was observed in 40.6% of cases and secondary graft failure in 59.4%, mainly due to graft infection, graft rejection, secondary glaucoma and endothelial decompensation. After regrafting PGF was not observed, but graft rejection occurred in 43.8%, and secondary glaucoma was present in 59.4% [23]. The 5-year graft failure for repeated PK ranged from 34% to 70% [48].

Functional Outcomes After Regraft

The BCVA of the regrafts ranged from 20/60 to 20/600. BCVA of 20/200 or better was observed in 43.8% of cases, with 31.2% having a BCVA of 20/80 or better, 18.8% having a BCVA of 20/60 and no case with a CDVA of 20/40 or better [23]. Generalizing, a BCVA of 20/40 or better was achieved in only 4.8–43.1% of clear PK regrafts by the last follow-up visit [48].

Survival Rate of Corneal Graft

Following the ECCTR report, the overall graft survival rate was 96% at 3 months, 95% at 6 months, 93% at 1 year and 89% at 2 years post-operatively. Graft survival varied between indications and techniques performed. In the 2-year follow-up, the highest graft survival was 98% in keratoconus, followed by 94% in corneal dystrophies other than Fuchs endothelial dystrophy, 92% in FED, 82% in infectious keratitis, 82% in PBK, 82% in regraft and 80% in trauma. There was no difference observed between PK and DALK performed for keratoconus in the 2-year graft survival rate (98% vs. 99%). As far as FED is concerned, the 2-year graft survival observed was 97% in PK, 93% with DSAEK and 71% with DMEK. Statistics for PBK were as follows; 87% with PK, 81% with DSAEK and 58% with DMEK. Moreover, graft failure was observed in 4% of cases (1% due to endothelial decompensation, less than 1% due to primary graft failure, infection, endothelial rejection, recurrence of original disease and graft detachment) [30]. Total graft failure, according to ACGR, is around 22%, with 4% early graft failure and 2% due to the rest [27]. Another study showed that despite the immunosuppressive regimen in high-risk corneal transplants, graft rejection ranged from 30 to 60% and up to 70% within 10 years [21].

In the UK, 1 year graft survival after first-time corneal transplants for keratoconus was 96–98%, for FED 87–90% and PBK 85–89%. Five-year graft survival for KCN 90–94%, FED 77–82%, PBK 58–66%. The survival rate of the first-time

Table 1.3 Five-year anatomical and functional success rate [4–6, 10, 20, 24, 35]

Type of corneal transplant/outcomes	Anatomical outcome (graft survival rate) (%)	Functional outcome (BCVA ≥20/40) (%)
DALK	85	65.4
PK	63.7–83	51.3
DSAEK	79.4–96	68.75
DMEK	90–96	90–97.8

graft in low-risk patients was around 90% at 5 years [16]. Unfortunately, a reduction in success rates is observed over time [49].

According to the Singapore Corneal Transplant Study (SCTS), the overall corneal graft survival rate at 1 year was 91%, at 5 years 66.8%, at 10 years 55.4%, at 15 years 52%, and 20 years 44%. Graft survival decreased over time from 91% at 1 year to 44% at 20 years' follow-up. Allograft rejection and late endothelial failure accounted for more than 60% of graft failures [50]. Similar results were reported by the Australian Corneal Graft Registry (ACGR). After 15 years corneal graft survival rates had dropped to 46% for full-thickness grafts and 41% for lamellar grafts [21].

Table 1.3 summarizes the 5-year anatomical and functional success rates of different types of corneal grafts.

The above-mentioned results are quite good in comparison to other solid transplants, but we need to bear in mind that good anatomical results and long graft survival do not guarantee good functional outcomes, which affect the patient's quality of life. In the past, the most important aim in corneal transplantation was graft survival. Nowadays, patients are more demanding; thus, refractive outcomes such as functional/good quality of vision are now highly important. Thus, there is still much to be done on this topic.

Conclusion: Real Success Rate of Modern Corneal Transplantation Procedures

To conclude, despite the advanced surgical techniques, innovative equipment, the surgeon's skills, and proper pre- and postoperative treat-ment, the outcomes of corneal graft surgery still constitute a problem taking into consideration the data presented in this chapter. If anatomical success is further completed with functional outcome success, we must conclude that modern keratoplasty techniques have a wide scope and potential to be improved by the control of immunity, ocular surface, and, nowadays, more evident, the functional outcome. Overall, we can conclude from the most recently available literature that the success rate expectation of PKP has a mean of 63.7–83% anatomical and 51.3% functional success, DALK 85% anatomical and 65.4% functional success, DSAEK 79.4–96% anatomical and 68.75% functional success, and DMEK 90–96% anatomical and 90–97.8% functional success [5, 6, 10, 20, 24, 35].

Therefore, we need to optimize the anatomical and functional outcomes of modern corneal transplantation techniques, as presented in this chapter and which are related to many factors.

Better strategies should be developed in cases of immunological rejection, ocular surface inflammation and glaucoma. In addition, it is worth pointing out that only 1.5% of the worldwide demand for corneal transplants is currently fulfilled. According to another source, it has been estimated that there is only 1 corneal donor available for every 70 needed [53]. Moreover, the COVID-19 pandemic continues to significantly impact the reduction in tissue donation and graft production. The gap between organ demand and supply is a huge universal problem in transplantation. Likewise, the problem is growing in spite of efforts made in medical, educational, and social fields and mass media support. This reality has created the need for completely new therapeutic alternatives for the management of end-stage organ disease. Moreover, bearing in mind the fact that the functional outcomes of corneal transplants are not satisfactory, new research should continue in the future to aim at discovering systems and devices capable of totally replacing the traditional transplantation procedures or alternative methods that are less dependent on the availability of allogeneic tissue and new solutions based on modern approaches such as advanced therapies and stem cell corneal regeneration, bioengineered artificial corneas, the development of natural corneal replacements and biosynthetic matrices for host tissue regeneration.

Take Home Notes

- In spite of corneal grafting being one of the most frequent and successful organ transplantations in the human body, there is still much to be done to improve the outcomes.
- Anatomical and functional results vary in different types of cornea graft procedures, and unfortunately, in many cases, they are far below patients' expectations and significantly affect the quality of life.
- Bearing in mind moderate outcomes, lack of the tissue and highly trained surgeons to perform this difficult and costly procedure, there is a need to develop new techniques and/or novel therapeutic approaches.

Conflict of Interest None of the authors have any conflict of interest to disclose.

References

1. Oliva MS, Schottman T, Gulati M. Turning the tide of corneal blindness. Indian J Ophthalmol. 2012;60:423–7.
2. Singh R, Gupta N, Vanathi M, Tandon R. Corneal transplantation in the modern era. Indian J Med Res. 2019;150(1):7–22. https://doi.org/10.4103/ijmr.IJMR_141_19.
3. Trevor Roper PD. The history of corneal grafting. In: Casey TA, editor. Corneal grafting. London: Butterwork; 1972. p. 1–5.
4. Pineda R. World corneal blindness. In: Colby K, Dana R, editors. Foundations of corneal disease. Cham: Springer; 2020. https://doi.org/10.1007/978-3-030-25335-6_25.
5. Patel SV. Graft survival after penetrating keratoplasty. Am J Ophthalmol. 2011;151(3):397–8. https://doi.org/10.1016/j.ajo.2010.10.006.
6. Montesel A, Alió Del Barrio JL, Yébana Rubio P, Alió JL. Corneal graft surgery: a monocentric long-term analysis. Eur J Ophthalmol. 2021;31(4):1700–8. https://doi.org/10.1177/1120672120947592. Epub 2020 Aug 5.
7. Castroviejo R. Keratoplasty in treatment of keratoconus. Arch Ophthalmol. 1949;42(6):776–800.
8. Archila EA. Deep lamellar keratoplasty dissection of host tissue with intrastromal air injection. Cornea. 1984;5(3):217–8.
9. Gómez-Benlloch A, Montesel A, Pareja-Aricò L, Mingo-Botín D, Michael R, Barraquer RI, Alió J. Causes of corneal transplant failure: a multicentric study. Acta Ophthalmol. 2021;99(6):e922–8. https://doi.org/10.1111/aos.14708. Epub 2021 Jan 9.
10. Melles GR, Rietveld FJ, Beekhuis WH, Binder PS. A technique to visualize corneal incision and lamellar dissection depth during surgery. Cornea. 1999;18:80–6.
11. Anwar M, Teichmann KD. Big-bubble technique to bare Descemet's membrane in anterior lamellar keratoplasty. J Cataract Refract Surg. 2002;28:398–403.
12. Alio JL, Abdelghany AA, Barraquer R, Hammouda LM, Sabry AM. Femtosecond laser assisted deep anterior lamellar keratoplasty outcomes and healing patterns compared to manual technique. BioMed Res Int. 2015;2015:397891. https://doi.org/10.1155/2015/397891, 6 pages.
13. Dupps WJ Jr, Qian Y, Meisler DM. Multivariate model of refractive shift in Descemet-stripping automated endothelial keratoplasty. J Cataract Refract Surg. 2008;34:578–84.
14. Singh A, Zarei-Ghanavati M, Avadhanam V, Liu C. Systematic review and meta-analysis of clinical outcomes of Descemet membrane endothelial keratoplasty versus Descemet stripping endothelial keratoplasty/Descemet stripping automated endothelial keratoplasty. Cornea. 2017;36(11):1437–43. https://doi.org/10.1097/ICO.0000000000001320.
15. https://www.google.com/url?sa=t&rct=j&q=&esrc=s&source=web&cd=&cad=rja&uact=8&ved=2ahUKEwj1q8D-wsv1AhXhkYsKHbpiBDkQFnoECBQQAQ&url=https%3A%2F%2Fec.europa.eu%2Fresearch%2Fparticipants%2Fdocuments%2FdownloadPublic%3FdocumentIds%3D080166e5c9dc9246%26appId%3DPPGMS&usg=AOvVaw1mXgu_EptMyZ-HN0ELt9vU.
16. Eye banking statistical report 2019. Eye Bank Association of America. https://restoresight.org/what-we-do/publications/statistical-report.
17. NHS. Survival rates following transplantation. [Survival rates following transplantation.] 2020. https://www.organdonation.nhs.uk/helping-you-to-decide/about-organ-donation/statistics-about-organ-donation/transplant-activity-report/.
18. https://professionaleducation.blood.ca/en/organs-and-tissues/reports/eye-and-tissue-reports-and-surveys/report-canadian-eye-and-tissue-data-1.
19. https://www.flinders.edu.au/fhmri-eye-vision/corneal-graft-registry.
20. Williams KA, Keane MC, Coffey NE, et al. The Australian corneal graft registry 2018 report. Flinders Unviersity. https://dspace.flinders.edu.au/xmlui/handle/2328/37917. Published 2018.
21. Lundström M, Manning S, Barry P, et al. The European registry of quality outcomes for cataract and

refractive surgery (EUREQUO): a database study of trends in volumes, surgical techniques and outcomes of refractive surgery. Eye Vis. 2015;2:8. https://doi.org/10.1186/s40662-015-0019-1.

22. Wan S, Cheng J, Dong Y, Xie L. Epithelial defects after penetrating keratoplasty in infectious keratitis: an analysis of characteristics and risk factors. PLoS One. 2018;13(11):e0208163. https://doi.org/10.1371/journal.pone.0208163. Published 2018 Nov 28.

23. Alió Del Barrio JL, Bhogal M, Ang M, Ziaei M, Robbie S, Montesel A, Gore DM, Mehta JS, Alió JL. Corneal transplantation after failed grafts: options and outcomes. Surv Ophthalmol. 2021;66(1):20–40. https://doi.org/10.1016/j.survophthal.2020.10.003. Epub 2020 Oct 14.

24. Roozbahani M, Hammersmith KM, Nagra PK, Ma JF, Rapuano CJ. Therapeutic penetrating keratoplasty: a retrospective review. Eye Contact Lens. 2018;44(Suppl 2):S433–41. https://doi.org/10.1097/ICL.0000000000000522.

25. Price DA, Kelley M, Price FW Jr, Price MO. Five-year graft survival of Descemet membrane endothelial keratoplasty (EK) versus Descemet stripping EK and the effect of donor sex matching. Ophthalmology. 2018;125(10):1508–14. https://doi.org/10.1016/j.ophtha.2018.03.050. Epub 2018 May 3.

26. Birbal RS, Ni Dhubhghaill S, Bourgonje VJA, et al. Five-year graft survival and clinical outcomes of 500 consecutive cases after Descemet membrane endothelial keratoplasty. Cornea. 2020;39(3):290–7.

27. Aboshiha J, Jones MNA, Hopkinson CL, Larkin DFP. Differential survival of penetrating and lamellar transplants in management of failed corneal grafts. JAMA Ophthalmol. 2018;136(8):859–65. https://doi.org/10.1001/jamaophthalmol.2018.1515. PMID: 29931227; PMCID: PMC6142952.

28. Krysik K, Wroblewska-Czajka E, Lyssek-Boron A, Wylegala EA, Dobrowolski D. Total penetrating keratoplasty: indications, therapeutic approach, and long-term follow-up. J Ophthalmol. 2018;2018:9580292. https://doi.org/10.1155/2018/9580292. PMID: 29850220; PMCID: PMC5933013.

29. Dunker SL, Armitage WJ, Armitage M, Brocato L, Figueiredo FC, Heemskerk MBA, Hjortdal J, Jones GLA, Konijn C, Nuijts RMMA, Lundström M, Dickman MM. Outcomes of corneal transplantation in Europe: report by the European Cornea and Cell Transplantation Registry. J Cataract Refract Surg. 2021;47(6):780–5. https://doi.org/10.1097/j.jcrs.0000000000000520.

30. Feizi S, Javadi MA, Karimian F, Abolhosseini M, Moshtaghion SM, Naderi A, Esfandiari H. Penetrating keratoplasty versus deep anterior lamellar keratoplasty in children and adolescents with keratoconus. Am J Ophthalmol. 2021;226:13–21. https://doi.org/10.1016/j.ajo.2021.01.010. Epub 2021 Jan 30.

31. Yüksel B, Kandemir B, Uzunel UD, Çelik O, Ceylan S, Küsbeci T. Comparison of visual and topographic outcomes of deep-anterior lamellar keratoplasty and penetrating keratoplasty in keratoconus. Int J Ophthalmol. 2017;10(3):385–90. https://doi.org/10.18240/ijo.2017.03.10. Published 2017 Mar 18.

32. Alzahrani K, Dardin SF, Carley F, Brahma A, Morley D, Hillarby MC. Corneal clarity measurements in patients with keratoconus undergoing either penetrating or deep anterior lamellar keratoplasty. Clin Ophthalmol. 2018;12:577–85.

33. Gadhvi KA, Romano V, Fernández-Vega Cueto L, Aiello F, Day AC, Allan BD. Deep anterior lamellar keratoplasty for keratoconus: multisurgeon results. Am J Ophthalmol. 2019;201:54–62. https://doi.org/10.1016/j.ajo.2019.01.022. Epub 2019 Feb 2.

34. Amar SP, Sinha R, Kalra N, Agarwal T, Sharma N, Titiyal JS. Demographic and clinical profile, surgical outcome, and quality of life in patients who underwent bilateral lamellar corneal grafts. Indian J Ophthalmol. 2021;69(7):1747–52. https://doi.org/10.4103/ijo.IJO_3194_20. PMID: 34146020; PMCID: PMC8374770.

35. Dickman MM, Peeters JM, van den Biggelaar FJ, Ambergen TA, van Dongen MC, Kruit PJ, Nuijts RM. Changing practice patterns and long-term outcomes of endothelial versus penetrating keratoplasty: a Prospective Dutch Registry Study. Am J Ophthalmol. 2016;170:133–42. https://doi.org/10.1016/j.ajo.2016.07.024. Epub 2016 Aug 4.

36. Khattak A, Nakhli FR, Al-Arfaj KM, Cheema AA. Comparison of outcomes and complications of deep anterior lamellar keratoplasty and penetrating keratoplasty performed in a large group of patients with keratoconus. Int Ophthalmol. 2018;38(3):985–92. https://doi.org/10.1007/s10792-017-0548-9. Epub 2017 May 22.

37. Vasiliauskaitė I, Oellerich S, Ham L, Dapena I, Baydoun L, van Dijk K, Melles GRJ. Descemet membrane endothelial keratoplasty: ten-year graft survival and clinical outcomes. Am J Ophthalmol. 2020;217:114–20. https://doi.org/10.1016/j.ajo.2020.04.005. Epub 2020 Apr 10.

38. Peraza-Nieves J, Baydoun L, Dapena I, Ilyas A, Frank LE, Luceri S, Ham L, Oellerich S, Melles GRJ. Two-year clinical outcome of 500 consecutive cases undergoing Descemet membrane endothelial keratoplasty. Cornea. 2017;36(6):655–60. https://doi.org/10.1097/ICO.0000000000001176.

39. Heinzelmann S, Böhringer D, Eberwein P, Reinhard T, Maier P. Outcomes of Descemet membrane endothelial keratoplasty, Descemet stripping automated endothelial keratoplasty and penetrating keratoplasty from a single centre study. Graefes Arch Clin Exp Ophthalmol. 2016;254(3):515–22. https://doi.org/10.1007/s00417-015-3248-z. Epub 2016 Jan 7.

40. Phillips PM, Phillips LJ, Muthappan V, Maloney CM, Carver CN. Experienced DSAEK surgeon's transition to DMEK: outcomes comparing the last 100 DSAEK surgeries with the first 100 DMEK surgeries exclusively using previously published techniques. Cornea. 2017;36(3):275–9. https://doi.org/10.1097/ICO.0000000000001069.

41. Ham L, Dapena I, Liarakos VS, et al. Midterm results of Descemet membrane endothelial keratoplasty: 4 to 7 years clinical outcome. Am J Ophthalmol. 2016;171:113–21.
42. Siggel R, Adler W, Stanzel TP, Cursiefen C, Heindl LM. Bilateral Descemet membrane endothelial keratoplasty: analysis of clinical outcome in first and fellow eye. Cornea. 2016;35(6):772–7. https://doi.org/10.1097/ICO.0000000000000811.
43. Schlögl A, Tourtas T, Kruse FE, Weller JM. Long-term clinical outcome after Descemet membrane endothelial keratoplasty. Am J Ophthalmol. 2016;169:218–26. https://doi.org/10.1016/j.ajo.2016.07.002. Epub 2016 Jul 15.
44. Weller JM, Kruse FE, Tourtas T. Descemet membrane endothelial keratoplasty: analysis of clinical outcomes of patients with 8-10 years follow-up. Int Ophthalmol. 2022;42(6):1789–98. https://doi.org/10.1007/s10792-021-02176-3.
45. Dunker SL, Dickman MM, Wisse RPL, Nobacht S, Wijdh RHJ, Bartels MC, Tang ML, van den Biggelaar FJHM, Kruit PJ, Nuijts RMMA. Descemet membrane endothelial keratoplasty versus ultrathin Descemet stripping automated endothelial keratoplasty: a multicenter randomized controlled clinical trial. Ophthalmology. 2020;127(9):1152–9. https://doi.org/10.1016/j.ophtha.2020.02.029. Epub 2020 Mar 2.
46. Wacker K, Baratz KH, Maguire LJ, McLaren JW, Patel SV. Descemet stripping endothelial keratoplasty for Fuchs' endothelial corneal dystrophy: five-year results of a prospective study. Ophthalmology. 2016;123(1):154–60. https://doi.org/10.1016/j.ophtha.2015.09.023. Epub 2015 Oct 17.
47. Weisenthal RW, Yin HY, Jarstad AR, Wang D, Verdier DD. Long-term outcomes in fellow eyes comparing DSAEK and DMEK for treatment of Fuchs corneal dystrophy. Am J Ophthalmol. 2022;233:216–26. https://doi.org/10.1016/j.ajo.2021.06.013. Epub 2021 Jun 19.
48. Armitage WJ, Goodchild C, Griffin MD, Gunn DJ, Hjortdal J, Lohan P, et al. High-risk corneal transplantation: recent developments and future possibilities. Transplantation. 2019;103:2468–78. https://doi.org/10.1097/TP.0000000000002938.
49. Anshu A, Li L, Htoon HM, de Benito-Llopis L, Shuang LS, Singh MJ, et al. Long-term review of penetrating keratoplasty: a 20-year review in Asian eyes. Am J Ophthalmol. 2020;224:254–66. https://doi.org/10.1016/j.ajo.2020.10.014.
50. Gain P, Jullienne R, He Z, Aldossary M, Acquart S, Cognasse F, Thuret G. Global survey of corneal transplantation and eye banking. JAMA Ophthalmol. 2016;134(2):167–73. https://doi.org/10.1001/jamaophthalmol.2015.4776.

Suggested Reading

Srujana D, Kaur M, Urkude J, Rathi A, Sharma N, Titiyal JS. Long-term functional and anatomic outcomes of repeat graft after optically failed therapeutic keratoplasty. Am J Ophthalmol. 2018;189:166–75. https://doi.org/10.1016/j.ajo.2018.03.011. Epub 2018 Mar 14.

Part I

Preparing the Patient

Modern Eye Banking: Preservation, Type of Tissues, and Selection

2

Loïc Hamon, Loay Daas, Adrien Quintin, Tarek Safi, Isabel Weinstein, and Berthold Seitz

Key Points

- In present times, the role of eye banks has evolved beyond simply storing corneas.
- Continuous improvement of preservation techniques extends storage time and provides better tissue quality.
- The increasing number of keratoplasty techniques and the high demand for "ready-to-use" tissue is challenging eye banks to improve and develop new preparation techniques.
- Besides necessary examinations, new approaches to tissue analysis in eye banks—such as the sterile donor tomography—allow a better selection of corneal tissues.
- These new challenges in tissue preservation, preparation and selection are propelling eye banks into the era of "modern eye banking.".

L. Hamon (✉) · L. Daas · I. Weinstein · B. Seitz
Department of Ophthalmology, Saarland University Medical Center (UKS), Homburg, Germany

Klaus Faber Center for Corneal Diseases, Saarland University Medical Center, Homburg, Germany

LIONS Eye Bank Saar-Lor-Lux, Trier/Westpfalz, Saarland University Medical Center,
Homburg, Germany
e-mail: loic.hamon@uks.eu; loay.daas@uks.eu;
isabel.weinstein@uks.eu; berthold.seitz@uks.eu

A. Quintin · T. Safi
Department of Ophthalmology, Saarland University Medical Center (UKS), Homburg, Germany
e-mail: adrien.quintin@uks.eu; tarek.safi@uks.eu

Introduction

Since the first penetrating keratoplasty (PKP) was performed by Eduard Zirm in 1905 [1], the number of keratoplasties has inexorably increased worldwide [2]. According to the German keratoplasty register [3], 8912 keratoplasties were performed in 2020 in Germany (Fig. 2.1). In order to meet this need, it is necessary to work with specialized and organized structures more than ever. **Eye banks** fulfill this role.

In the past, the role of eye banks was limited to collection, storage and evaluation of the tissues prior to transplantation. The technique of keratoplasties has constantly evolved over the years with the purpose to minimize immune reactions [4] and to reduce postoperative astigmatism [5]. These improvements include new trephination techniques, for example, the femtosecond [6] and the excimer laser-assisted trephination [7], new suture techniques, for example, the double running cross-stitch suture [8, 9] and the development of new lamellar techniques, for example, the Descemet Membrane Endothelial Keratoplasty (DMEK) [10, 11] or the Deep Anterior Lamellar Keratoplasty (DALK) [12]. Eye banks have followed this evolution toward **modern keratoplasty**, extending their role to the (pre-)selection and preparation of tissues for surgeons, entering a new Era of **modern eye banking**.

© The Author(s), under exclusive license to Springer Nature Switzerland AG 2023
J. L. Alió, J. L. A. del Barrio (eds.), *Modern Keratoplasty*, Essentials in Ophthalmology,
https://doi.org/10.1007/978-3-031-32408-6_2

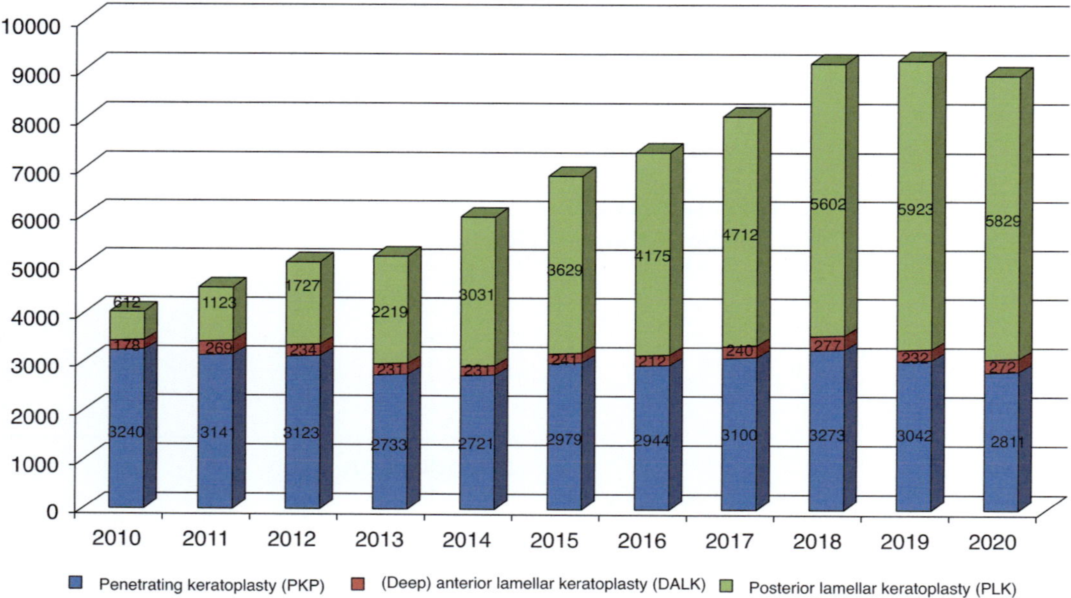

Fig. 2.1 Keratoplasties in Germany. Until 2013 dominated by penetrating keratoplasties (PKP), posterior lamellar keratoplasties and particularly DMEK has experienced a substantial expansion in Germany, representing 65.4% of 8912 keratoplasties in 2020. (*Source: The German Keratoplasty Registry listed in Homburg/Saar since 2006*)

Donor's Screening and Tissue Collection

Corneal transplantation safety is widely dependent upon clinical donor selection. The risk of donor-to-host disease transmission through corneas has been a major concern since the beginning of keratoplasty. Regarding the first known case of donor-to-host retinoblastoma transmission in 1939 [13] or the well-established cases of Creutzfeldt-Jakob and rabies transmissions in the 1970s [14], with lethal consequences for the recipients, many diseases have been proven or assumed to be transmissible from donor to recipient via corneal transplantation. The epidemic of acquired immune deficiency syndrome (AIDS) in the 1980s, as late stage of the human immunodeficiency virus (HIV), brought a major change in general awareness of transmissible diseases [15]. In order to minimize this risk, careful donor selection is necessary. Regulatory agencies such as the European Eye Bank Organization (EEBA) and the Eye Bank Association of America (EBAA) are continuously working to minimize this risk with well-documented and broadly accepted regulations in the field. A list of contraindications for corneal donation (Table 2.1) and new testing to exclude potentially transmissible diseases are regularly adapted and updated. However, these tests have a cost (financial, but also false positivity that could discard transplantable corneas) and the decision to implement or exclude new tests must be based on scientific evidence [17].

If the donor has no contraindications, the eye bank staff can proceed with the collection of the donor corneas [18]. There are, in principle, two ways to collect donor corneas:

Table 2.1 Contraindications for corneal donation [16]

Unknown cause of death

History of a disease of unknown etiology

Donors with following malignant diseases:
- Retinoblastoma
- Hematologic neoplasm (leukemia, lymphoma, myeloma)
- Malignant tumor of the anterior segment of the eye (such as conjunctival intraepithelial neoplasia, squamous cell carcinoma, malignant melanoma, metastasis)

Risk of transmission caused by prions:
- Creutzfeldt-Jakob disease or variant Creutzfeldt-Jakob disease
- History of rapid progressive dementia or degenerative neurological disease such as Alzheimer's disease, multiple sclerosis, amyotrophic lateral sclerosis
- Recipients of hormone-derived from human pituitary gland (before 1987)
- Recipient of graft of cornea, dura matter or sclera

Uncontrolled systemic infection:
- Bacterial disease
- Systemic viral diseases such as rabies
- Fungal or parasitic infection

Exception for septicemia, if the cornea is stored in organ culture media to allow detection of any bacterial contamination of the tissue

History or clinical evidence of human immunodeficiency virus (HIV) or acquired immunodeficiency syndrome (AIDS)

Acute or chronic hepatitis B, hepatitis C and/or human T-lymphotropic virus (HTLV) I/II

History of chronic systemic autoimmune and/or inflammatory disease that could impact the quality of collected tissue

Donors from or have traveled in zones with high-risk for epidemical diseases (in accordance with the European Centre of Disease Control):
- Zika virus
- New coronavirus (2019-nCoV)
- Ebola virus

Ingestion or exposure to substances such as cyanide, lead, mercury, gold

Recent history of vaccination with a live attenuated virus

Transplantation with xenografts

Behaviors or presence on the donor's body of physical signs implying a risk of transmissible disease(s) such as bruises, lacerations, etc.

1. **Whole globe collection** is a simple and quick method of collecting donor tissue. The collection of the "whole eye globe" can be performed in the morgue, in a refrigerated room or at the donor's bed, depending on the possible collection process. The globe is brought forward (pulled) with an instrument and the optic nerve is cut with scissors. It must then be prepared at the eye bank for the surgery. An advantage of this method is that it saves time during the collection process. Another advantage is the removal—at the same time—of scleral tissue allowing other types of surgery such as sclerocorneoplasty [19] or scleral patches [20]. The symbolism of the removal of the eye (as a whole "organ") is unfortunately perceived as "intrusive" by donor's relatives, which may lead to a higher rate of donation refusal.

2. **Corneoscleral explantation** (15 mm disc) is a more expensive alternative regarding time and resources. It is performed in the same way as an ophthalmic surgical procedure, in sterile conditions and using surgical equipment (Fig. 2.2). After conjunctival dissection, and the corneoscleral disc is removed using a 15 mm diameter round hand-trephine. An exactly concentric trephination is important in order to guarantee that the graft can be optimally processed later on. After corneal collection, plastic shells are applied for aesthetic reconstruction and the eyelids are tightly closed. The deceased will not show any aesthetic restrictions. This method of procurement, although more complex, has a much higher acceptance rate by the donors' relatives [22, 23]. The corneoscleral disc is also already cut, avoiding further manipulations in the eye bank prior to preservation.

After collection, the whole globes or corneas are taken to the eye bank, where they are preserved, examined and prepared for surgical purposes.

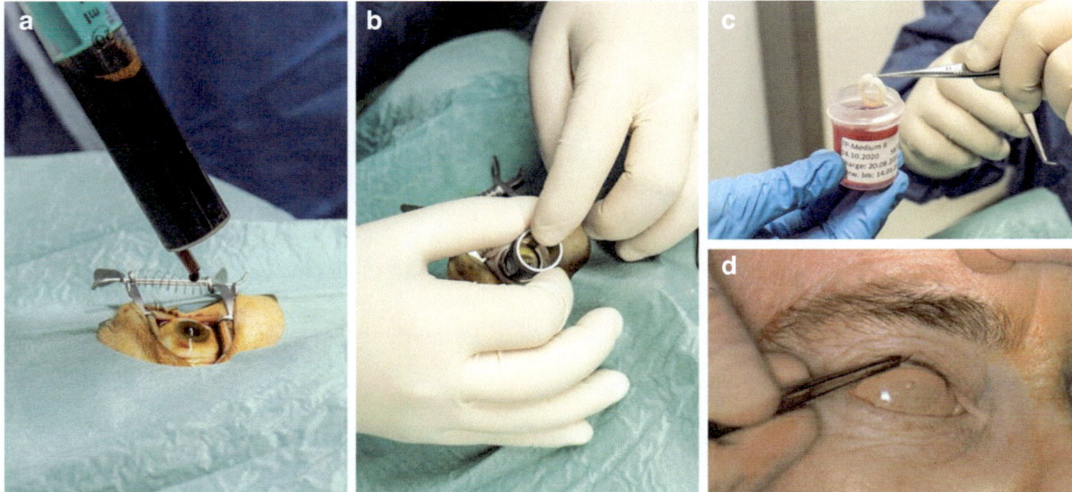

Fig. 2.2 Cornea procurement—corneoscleral technique. The material for corneal removal is prepared in a sterile manner. Eye bank staff need to wash and sterilize themselves like for intraocular surgery. (**a**) Povidone-iodine 1.25% is applied slowly 5 min before trephination, in order to minimize potential contamination [21]. (**b**) Trephination is performed with a 15 mm diameter round trephine. An exactly concentric trephination is important in order to guarantee that the graft can be optimally processed later on. (**c**) After trephination, the corneoscleral disc is placed in a container with *organ culture medium II* (also called *transport medium*). (**d**) A plastic disc is inserted in the place of the trephined corneoscleral disc. The eyelids are closed and glued or sutured. Thus, there is no evidence of the procedure for the relatives

Preservation Techniques

Moist Chamber Preservation

Introduced in 1935 [24], the conservation of whole globes in moist chambers directly after enucleation was the only preservation technique until the 1960s. The explanted globes were stored in an airtight container. The air was humidified through a wet gauze placed in the container. Containers were stored at low temperatures (4–8°C) or alternatively put on ice [25] until surgery. This uncomplicated method allowed the preservation of the globe for up to 2–3 days [26]. However, the sterility of the tissue could not be ensured and the restricted storage period did not leave enough time for sufficient quality control by the eye banks. Nowadays, this technique has been replaced by more advanced alternatives but still remains used in certain developing countries where the implementation of more expensive methods is problematic.

Cryopreservation

Cryopreservation has long been a goal in the field of eye banking, promising a very long preservation period and a lower risk for tissue infections. The first protocols for cryopreservation were developed in the 1960s [27, 28]. In 1981, Sperling [29] also developed a technique for cryopreservation of corneas kept under organ culture conditions, then frozen. Nevertheless, despite all attempts, cryopreservation protocols for human corneas were not able to provide tissues with the endothelial qualities required to ensure a transplantable cornea [30, 31]. To date, donor corneas cannot reliably be frozen.

With the beginning of the worldwide COVID-19 pandemic in 2019 [32], some eye banks have experienced difficulties in finding viable donors. This disturbance in the constancy of cornea procurement has led to a renewed interest in cryopreservation techniques [33] and new protocols may emerge. Nevertheless, the absence of active viral structural proteins in SARS-CoV-2 positive donor corneas [34] and the negligible risk of transmission after proper donor selection [35] should allow a return to normal donation in the very near future.

Hypothermic Storage

This storage technique at 2–8 °C was developed by McCarey and Kaufman in 1974 [36]. The original McCarey–Kaufman (M–K) medium consisted of tissue culture medium TC-199, dextran (an osmotic agent preventing corneal swelling), bicarbonate and antibiotics (penicillin/streptomycin) and claimed a storage period of up to 10 days. Other solutions introduced later, such as the modified M–K medium [37], K-sol [38] or the very popular Optisol (GS) [39], claimed better storage capabilities and an extended storage period of 14–16 days [40].

Hypothermic storage is by far the most widely used preservation technique for corneoscleral discs in North America [41]. Donor corneoscleral discs are stored in flat cylindrical containers, allowing morphological inspection with the slit-lamp and endothelium inspection by specular microscopy, both under sterile conditions if using special fixation devices. As the appearance of the endothelial cells vary with temperature, an examination at room temperature is recommended. Degenerative changes are not rare during hypothermic storage and may lead to severe endothelial cell loss. The low temperature drastically reduces the metabolic process of the corneas, according to the Arrhenius relation. Wound healing is, therefore, not possible, and tissue damage may progress [42].

The technique of hypothermic storage is simple and does not require expensive equipment. Donor corneas are also directly available for corneal surgery. Compared to organ culture, storage time appears shorter, but more recent storage solutions nonetheless allow for scheduled surgery.

Organ Culture Preservation

The organ culture technique aims at the long-term preservation of the isolated human cornea under simulated physiological conditions. Summerlin et al. first investigated this storage method in vitro in 1973 [43]. In 1976, this method was adapted by Doughman et al. to be used for eye banking [44]. Since Sperling popularized this preservation method in Europe, corneal graft preservation is mostly done by organ culture on this side of the Atlantic [45]. This technique was also (re)introduced in the USA as "Minnesota system corneal preservation" [46] but has not supplanted hypothermic storage in North America.

The corneas are suspended in a cell culture container filled with an organ culture medium (modified Minimal Essential Medium—MEM, so-called *medium I*) and supplemented with fetal or newborn calf serum (2–10%), antibiotics and antimycotics (Fig. 2.3). Cell culture containers are stored at 30–37 °C for a maximum recommended period of 28 days, with medium renewal after 7–14 days, depending on the organ culture medium composition. Some eye banks have investigated storage periods of up to 48 days [47], but this practice is largely not recommended [2]. At the beginning of the culture period, corneas are kept in quarantine while microbiological testing is carried out in accordance with current standards [48, 49]. The *medium I* being isotonic, the organ-cultured cornea swells to twice its normal thickness during storage [50]. Before penetrating keratoplasty can be performed, the organ-cultured cornea has to be transferred from *medium I* into another hypertonic organ culture medium (so-called *medium II*) for stromal deswelling, containing a macromolecule, mostly dextran T500, with concentrations varying from 4 to 8% between eye banks [45]. The dextran cannot, due to technical limitations, be added to the isotonic *medium I* [51]. Deswelling time in *medium II* is usually between 1 and 7 days. Nevertheless, the proven toxicity of dextran on endothelial cells [52, 53] imposes a deswelling time as short as possible, as the cornea can—in

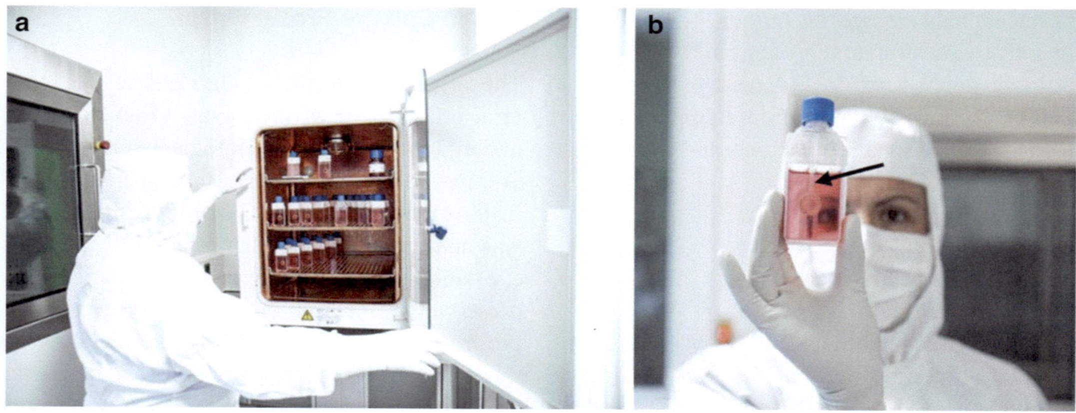

Fig. 2.3 Organ-cultured corneas in cell culture flasks. (**a**) Organ-cultured corneas are stored at +34 °C in an incubator up to 28 days. (**b**) In cell culture flask, corneoscleral discs are maintained vertically on a plastic holder (*arrow*)

theory—already be implanted after only 12 h of deswelling [54, 55]. This process of deswelling is not necessary prior to DMEK.

Organ culture offers many advantages compared to hypothermic storage, such as the control of pathogen contamination during the storage time [56], a longer storage time [45] and better endothelial vitality [57]. To permit these possibilities, the organ culture procedure is more complicated and more expensive than hypothermic storage and requires well-equipped facilities.

Type of Tissues

In recent years, a marked trend toward lamellar surgery instead of PKP has been observed [58]. Anterior or posterior lamellar surgeries have advantages in terms of visual rehabilitation and immune response rate. Nevertheless, PKP still has an important place for certain indications and in case of complicated surgery with a more uncertain prognosis [59]. This multiplicity of techniques encourages eye banks to adapt and vary their procedures for graft preparation and storage in order to meet this increasing demand.

Penetrating Keratoplasty

The penetrating keratoplasty (PKP) consists of a transplantation of all the layers of the cornea and represented the only feasible keratoplasty until the end 1950s [60]. Before transplantation, the preserved corneas, previously transferred into *medium II* for deswelling (in case of organ culture) [35, 54], must be appropriately dimensioned in order to match the recipient's bed.

The type of trephination has a major impact on the correct placement of the first four or eight cardinal sutures [61, 62] and, thus on the postoperative astigmatism. Recipient trephination can be mechanical or nonmechanical. Conventional mechanical trephination is always associated with deformation of the recipient corneal tissue, including deformation of the incised edges, with irregular cut surfaces related to the axial and radial forces induced by the use of the trephine [62, 63]. Nonmechanical trephination includes femtosecond or excimer laser cutting techniques. Significant improvement in postoperative astigmatism can be achieved using the Homburg/Erlangen technique of nonmechanical excimer laser trephination [7, 64, 65]. This induces significantly lower corneal astigmatism, more regular topography, and, thus, ultimately, better vision [7, 64].

For each keratoplasty, the diameter of the graft should be individualized according to the specificities of the patient. This diameter is determined before the surgery for each patient. Each graft should be as large as possible (for optical reasons) and as small as necessary (for immunological reasons) [62, 66, 67]. Excessive oversizing or undersizing of the graft relative to the recipient bed should be avoided to prevent distension or retraction of the peripheral donor tissue.

Mechanical or nonmechanical trephination of the graft is usually performed in the operating room by the surgeon. The role of eye banks prior to PKP is limited to providing a corneoscleral disc of the best possible quality.

Anterior Lamellar Keratoplasties

Stromal corneal pathologies and keratoconus are typical indications for anterior lamellar keratoplasty. In these cases, **deep anterior lamellar keratoplasty (DALK)** has become an increasingly popular alternative compared to PKP [68].

In this procedure, the recipient's corneal stroma is totally excised, leaving only the endothelium and the Descemet membrane, with or without pre-Descemet's layer [69]. To dissociate the posterior stroma of the endothelial layer, several techniques have been proposed. A popular technique is the "big bubble technique" by Anwar et al. [70]. Descemet's membrane and endothelium of the previously trephined donor cornea are removed in a second step. The donor and recipient trephination is usually performed manually. Still, it can also be performed with an excimer laser, thus combining the advantages in terms of visual rehabilitation and immunological "protection" of a DALK [71] and the advantages in terms of graft regularity and low astigmatism of an excimer-PKP for the patient [5]. The donor's full-thickness stroma is then positioned against the recipient's Descemet membrane and sutured using standard techniques as for PKP [68].

A major advantage of DALK is the absence of allograft endothelial immune reaction, as donor endothelium is not transplanted. Moreover, tissue preserved in the eye bank but presenting insufficient endothelial cells for PKP or posterior lamellar surgery may still be selected and prepared for DALK. This allows greater flexibility in tissue management and allocation for eye banks.

Posterior Lamellar Keratoplasties

Posterior lamellar keratoplasty techniques have steadily improved over the past 20 years, allowing faster visual recovery and triggering fewer immune reactions compared to PKP due to the use of very thin grafts [72]. Indications for posterior lamellar keratoplasty include all diseases of the corneal endothelium. Patients with Fuchs' endothelial corneal dystrophy (FECD) represent by far the largest group. Other endothelial diseases include congenital hereditary endothelial dystrophy (CHED), posterior polymorphous corneal dystrophy (PPCD), herpetic endothelitis or buphthalmus [58].

Descemet membrane endothelial keratoplasty (DMEK) is becoming increasingly popular internationally and especially in Europe and can now also be used in difficult conditions of the anterior segment of the eye [10, 58]. In DMEK, only the Descemet membrane and the corneal endothelium are transplanted. The transplant is prepared prior to DMEK, with a risk of membrane rupture that may cause graft loss [73]. Several techniques for DMEK donor preparation have been described, such as direct peeling with microkeratome [74], the submerged corneas using backgrounds away (SCUBA) method, where the cornea is submerged in Optisol, balanced salt solution (BSS) or organ culture medium to reduce surface tension during the preparation [75] or pneumatic dissection [76]. The use of artificial anterior chambers with aspiration or pressurization also proves to be useful in facilitating the dissection [77]. Following dissection, the Descemet membrane with corneal endothelium is prepared in order to be injected into the anterior chamber by the surgeon in place of the previously removed recipient's affected endothelium (descemetorhexis) [11].

Descemet's stripping automated endothelial keratoplasty (DSAEK) is one of the most performed "endothelial keratoplasties" in North America [73]. The technique consists of the removal of endothelial tissue from the recipient and to implant a donor posterior lenticle (<200 µm) composed of posterior stroma + Descemet membrane + endothelium. Many factors contribute to visual outcomes following DSAEK, which are generally poorer after DMEK [78], including the presence of a stromal interface (stroma-to-stroma contact) and techniques to prepare the donor lenticules [73]. For these reasons, the amount of DMEK (97.3% in the year 2020) outweighed by far the number of DSAEK in the past years in Germany [3].

The donor lenticle can be prepared mechanically using a microkeratome for intrastromal cutting in corneal preparation, achieving a lenticle thickness under 200 µm. The femtosecond laser-prepared lenticle has been explored to improve lenticule uniformity, unfortunately resulting in rougher stromal beds and increased irregularity, without providing expected visual results [79]. Nowadays, ultra-thin lenticules (<130 µm) are preferred and used for so-called **ultra-thin DSAEK (UT-DSAEK)** [58]. To achieve this thinness, donor corneas undergo two passes with a microkeratome, first with a thicker and second with a thinner pass [73]. Ultra-thin tissue can also be prepared using low-pulse energy, high-frequency femtosecond laser [80].

Prestripped, Precut and Preloaded Tissues in Eye Banks

Advances in the field of eye banking have resulted in the preparation and validation of prepared tissues suitable for elective procedures [81]. Eye banks have therefore started preparing precut and preloaded tissues for (UT-)DSAEK [82] and prestripped and preloaded tissues for DMEK [83, 84].

The use of prestripped tissues offers advantages, such as the guaranteed immediate availability of the graft, gain of time and reduced surgical complexity of the DMEK or DSAEK surgery [85–87]. Nevertheless, recent studies have shown severe endothelial cell loss after prestripping compared to nonpre-stripped DMEK-tissues preserved in *organ culture medium I*, with endothelial cell loss reaching up to 23% for prestripped corneas versus 4% for nonpre-stripped corneas after 5 days of storage [88, 89]. Prestripped tissues have also shown decreased adhesion forces and elastic modulus, which may contribute to increased re-bubbling rates, compared to nonpre-stripped tissues [90].

Preloaded DMEK tissues are generally prestripped and then preloaded in a transport cartridge in order to be injected by the surgeon [91], comparable to a preloaded intraocular lens (IOL) in cataract surgery. In recent years, several non-touch DMEK preloading techniques have been developed [91, 92]. These techniques induce less endothelial cell loss than previous preloading techniques, with comparable cell loss as prestripped tissues, and demonstrate the practicality of preparing injectable endothelial membranes [93]. Nevertheless, the preparation of prestripped and preloaded membranes must be performed in accredited and experienced eye banks [85, 94] and the use of preloaded tissues should be limited to centers without on-site eye banks or prompt availability of nonstripped tissues. A preparation (stripping and nontouch loading) immediately before surgery by an experienced surgeon should ensure the optimum viability of the tissue. However, prestripped tissues preserved in *medium I* (without dextran) [52, 95] for 1 day, with a mean endothelial cell loss of 4.1% [96], represent a reasonable compromise between tissue quality and organizational constraints [11].

Concerning (UT-)DSAEK, precut tissues provided similar visual and refractive outcomes as nonpre-cut tissues [97]. In addition, re-bubbling rates were also similar for precut and nonpre-cut transplants [98]. Donor endothelial cell loss from 6 to 12 months was also comparable after both techniques [97]. However, laboratory data on the biomechanics of DSAEK grafts suggests that surgeon-cut DSAEK grafts present higher elastic modulus and adhesion force compared to eye bank-prepared DSAEK grafts [99].

Outcomes for using preloaded tissues for DMEK and (UT-)DSAEK were also compared in the literature. Romano et al. showed a significantly higher visual acuity but also, unfortunately, a higher rate of re-bubbling for prestripped + preloaded DMEK, compared to precut + prestripped UT-DSAEK [100].

Amniotic Membrane and Scleral Patches

Beside corneas, eye banks can also collect, preserve and prepare alternative tissues such as amniotic membrane (the innermost layer of a fetal membrane) or scleral tissues.

The **amniotic membrane** can be used, in regards to its advantageous biological and immunological properties [101], as a biological bandage (amniotic membrane patch [AMT]) for the treatment of nonhealing corneal ulcers or to support physiological wound-healing [102]. Small- or medium-sized perforations, leaking descemetoceles, and corneal melting may be treated with AMT as tectonic surgery, if donor cornea is not available [103].

Procurements of amniotic membrane are realized under strict aseptic conditions after elective cesarean section [104]. In the eye bank, the amniotic membrane is rinsed from blood remnants and small segments are prepared and then cut into multiple pieces of different dimensions (e.g., 2×2, 5×5 or 10×10 mm) [103]. After preparation, these pieces are conserved using cryopreservation at -75 to -85 °C [102] or lyophilization [105]. Prior to surgery, patches are warmed at room temperature and/or rehydrated.

Scleral tissue can also be prepared in eye banks for tectonic purposes, for example, in case of necrotic scleritis. The outside of the globe is carefully cleaned and all other tissues must be removed [106]. The sclera can then be stored dry or in 95% ethanol for at least 1 year until transplantation [107].

Tissue Selection

Before cultured corneas can be transplanted, they have to fulfill certain quality criteria in accordance with current international and/or national standards [16, 108]. These standards vary according to the type of transplantation (PKP, anterior or posterior lamellar keratoplasty) and the elective or urgent nature of the surgery. Besides necessary examinations, new approaches to tissue analysis have been developed in recent years, allowing an even better quality of transplanted corneas from modern eye banks.

Microbiological Testing

In case of hypothermic storage, microbiological testing with samples of the storage solution is generally not performed, as the storage time is too short to receive the results before keratoplasty [45]. Moreover, the number of contaminating microbes should be low and not grow at this temperature after proper decontamination during retrieval [21] and before storage. Supplemented antibiotics have a low effect during hypothermic storage but become active in the eye after keratoplasty as the body temperature recovers [109]. Although the rate of keratitis or endophthalmitis post-keratoplasty is very low [110], cases of graft-related infections—mostly fungal—have been described [111].

In case of organ culture, microbiological testing of the medium sample is realized during a quarantine period at the beginning of the culture process [48, 49]. The microbiological safety of donor corneas is obtained by discarding contaminated tissues prior to keratoplasty [112]. The contamination rate widely varies between eye banks [45] and can be reduced through strict adherence to a quality management system (QMS) [113].

Morphological Examination: Slit-Lamp Biomicroscopy

Slit-lamp biomicroscopy has been a fundamental method of tissue evaluation since the first instituted criteria for eye bank certification [114]. The technique has not changed in the past several decades and remains the gold standard for determining surgical suitability. Slit-lamp biomicroscopy allows an evaluation of all layers of the cornea from both anterior and posterior perspectives, using different magnifications and illumination techniques, including direct illumination, retro-illumination, specular reflection, and sclerotic scatter, to focus on different layers [114].

The examination is performed under sterile conditions and remains very simple. In case of hypothermic storage, the cylindrical storage plates are put on a fixation device mounted on the slit lamp. In case of organ culture, the cell culture flasks are fixed on a horizontal support positioned in place of the chin rest.

Donor corneas are usually examined at the beginning of the preservation period to exclude a morphological anomaly. The corneas that have passed this screening will be analyzed under specular microscopy. A cornea presenting a scar can still be used for an emergency keratoplasty, DSAEK, DMEK or—depending on the donor's consent—for research projects. Donor corneas are mostly re-examined with a slit lamp at the end of the preservation period for definitive tissue validation for patient's allocation.

Endothelial Evaluation: Inverted Light or Specular Microscopy

The evaluation of the endothelial cell layer is of major importance to ensure tissue viability. Indeed, a too low endothelial cell density (ECD) before keratoplasty is associated with postoperative graft failure [115]. Endothelial cell loss occurs during the keratoplasty and continues after the surgery [116]. Up to 70% endothelial cell loss has been observed after 20 years [117]. Considering these facts, endothelial microscopy using light or specular microscopes was added in the early 2000s in eye bank protocols for tissue evaluation. According to European standards, a minimum ECD of 2000 cells/mm^2 is needed for penetrating or posterior lamellar keratoplasty in order to ensure long-term graft survival [2]. A minimum ECD between 1000

and 2000 cells/mm^2 is advised for anterior lamellar keratoplasty or for emergency/tectonic surgery, but no minimum ECD is officially required [118]. Corneas with ECD lower than 2000 cells/mm^2 and corneas with endothelial cell loss of more than 25% during cultivation have to be discarded for elective penetrating or posterior lamellar surgery.

Two other parameters are important for assessing endothelial viability: morphology and vitality of the endothelial cells. Corneas with considerable polymegethism or pleomorphism have reduced functional reserves and an increased incidence of postoperative graft failure [119]. Therefore, corneas with large central multicellular necrosis, distinct endothelial cell necrosis, fold-associated endothelial cell necrosis, grouped endothelial cell necrosis affecting more than 10% of the total endothelial cell area, pronounced polymegethism, pronounced pleomorphism, pronounced granulation/vacuolization or cornea guttata (CG) also need to be discarded [2].

Inverted light microscopy is the first-choice technique for organ-cultured corneas. The endothelial cells are visualized by swelling the intracellular space using a hypotonic solution allowing endothelial layer inspection regardless of the corneal hydration [120]. Intracellular border swelling disappears after a couple of minutes. Application of vital stains such as trypan blue may help to discriminate dead or necrotic cells [120]. To evaluate donor cornea endothelium, inverted light microscopy should be performed in the center, in the four paracentral/midperipheral quadrants and in the periphery of the donor cornea [121] (Fig. 2.4).

Specular microscopy can also be used and is the first-choice if using hypothermic storage. The images generated are similar to in vivo specular microscopy images performed on patients pre- and postoperatively. In contrast to inverted light microscopy, specular microscopy is usually restricted to the center of the cornea, and visualized areas are relatively small because of a microscope-related fixed magnification. However, this technique does not require osmotic stimulation of the endothelial cells. Thus, the donor cornea can remain in its cylindrical plate,

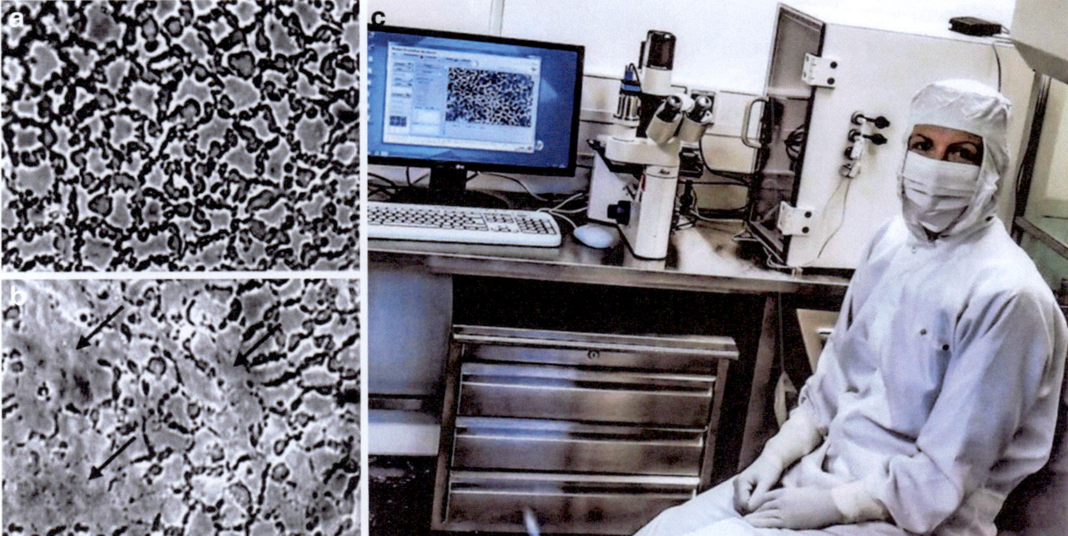

Fig. 2.4 Evaluation of corneal endothelium vitality. The evaluation is performed with an inverted light microscope under sterile conditions in the eye bank. (**a**) Zone presenting healthy endothelial cells. The use of hypotonic solution to better perceive the intracellular spaces and thus differentiate the endothelial cells gives this with spiculated aspect of cell membranes. (**b**) Another endothelial area with zones presenting necrosis (*arrows*). (**c**) A member of the eye bank staff performing endothelial cell count

avoiding manipulations and associated endothelial cell loss [121].

After each endothelial evaluation, findings should be documented in detail, preferably together with corresponding endothelial images. Specific software for light or specular microscopes can help to determine parameters describing the endothelial mosaic in terms of variation in cell shape and percentage of hexagonal cells in addition to the assessment of the cell density [45].

Sterile Donor Tomography

Any corneal microsurgeon who performs keratoplasties may have inadvertently transplanted a donor cornea with (subclinical) keratoconus or with prior keratorefractive surgery, typically resulting in significant postoperative refractive disadvantages for the patient [122–125]. Given the increasing number of performed keratorefractive procedures in recent decades, eye banks will soon have to deal more intensively with the problem of identifying donor corneas with abnormal refraction. Indeed, donor tissues with prior keratorefractive surgery or with pre-existing "refraction-affecting" pathologies cannot always be reliably recognized by slit-lamp examination alone. By means of illustration, previous studies demonstrated a false negative rate of 3.4–50.0% for the identification of post-LASIK (laser-assisted in situ keratomileusis) donor corneas, depending on whether detection was based on slit-lamp examination, clinical history, or a combination of both [126–128]. Therefore, many authors have highlighted the need for improved screening of donor corneas in order to avoid refractive surprises after keratoplasty [129–132]. Among the methods that have been proposed through the years as refractive screening devices for corneal tissues in the eye bank, several authors have focused on the potential role of donor tomography [131, 133, 134]. A limitation of these devices was the difficulty of performing a tomographic measurement without having to remove the corneoscleral disc from its container, i.e., in a sterile manner, due to the flat interfaces of the container.

Our department succeeded, in collaboration with our Institute of Experimental Ophthalmology, in enabling and approving a new concept to topographically measure donor corneal tissues in their sterile cell culture flask to detect potential curvature and/or thickness deviation such as keratoconus, prior refractive surgery or high astigmatism [135–137].

Since 2018, 1061 donor corneas (Klaus Faber Center for Corneal Diseases incl. LIONS Eye Bank Saar-Lor-Lux, Trier/Westpfalz, in Homburg/Saar) have been routinely measured preoperatively using the swept-source anterior segment optical coherence tomograph (AS-OCT) CASIA 2 (Tomey Corp., Nagoya, Japan). Because this device uses a central wavelength of $\lambda = 1310$ nm and allows a penetration depth of up to 13 mm in vivo [138], measurements of donor corneas are possible, achieving a lateral range of up to about 7 mm diameter, essentially constrained by the tissue holder [139]. This technique enables a sterile assessment and excludes potential measurement-related contamination of tissues within their sealed cell culture flask, which is mounted on the chin rest of the AS-OCT in a holder previously constructed by a three-dimensional (3D) printer (Ultimaker 2 Go, Ultimaker B.V., Geldermalsen, The Netherlands) (Fig. 2.5). In order to allow reliable measurements of corneal tissues, preoperative donor tomography was performed >12 h after transferring them into medium II (hypertonic medium enriched with 6% dextran T500), i.e., after >12 h of deswelling [54, 55]. During measurement, a raster scan is performed from the posterior surface of the donor cornea, generating a 3D volume data set and achieving a depth resolution of 5.621 μm/voxel in an aqueous medium and a lateral resolution of 6 μm/voxel [137]. Subsequently, the measured raw data were imported into MATLAB (MathWorks Inc., Natick, Massachusetts, USA) and preprocessed to extract artifacts due to flask

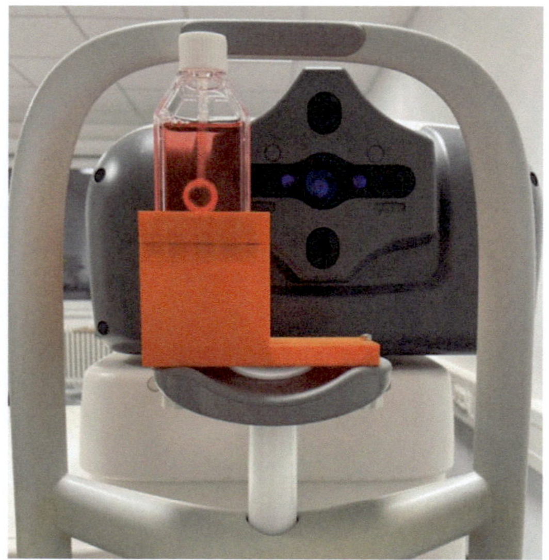

Fig. 2.5 Sterile donor tomography in the eye bank. Preoperative measurements of donor corneas are performed using the anterior segment optical coherence tomography (AS-OCT) in a sterile manner through their cell culture flask, mounted on the chin rest of the AS-OCT in a holder previously constructed using a three-dimensional printer

wall and tissue holder, remove background noise, adjust the contrast size, reduce the brightness of the central reflex and to detect the edge of the anterior and posterior surfaces of the donor cornea [135, 137]. Considering the different displacement of the apex of each sample from the zero point of the coordinate system in space, the translation, rotation and 3D tilt of samples were taken into account [137], thus not influencing the calculation of the donor corneas' keratometry. Subsequently, a spherocylindrical surface model was adapted with raytracing and, ultimately, various geometric features such as the central corneal thickness (measured at the apex) and the anterior and posterior radii of curvature at the steep and flat meridian were determined, from which the refractive power was calculated (Table 2.2).

Table 2.2 Result values of sterile donor tomography in the eye bank

			n = 1061 donor corneas	
			Mean $(\bar{x}) \pm$ SD	Range (min.–max.)
Refractive power (D)	Anterior surface	Steep	50.5 ± 2.0	45.4–62.0
		Flat	48.9 ± 1.5	42.7–56.1
	Posterior surface	Steep	−6.2 ± 0.3	−7.5 to −5.3
		Flat	−5.9 ± 0.3	−6.9 to −5.0
Central corneal thickness (µm)			612 ± 81	379–1029

Refractive power and pachymetry of the 1061 donor corneas were measured in their cell culture flask
$\bar{x}$ = mean; SD = standard deviation; min. = minimum; max. = maximum

To avoid postoperative refractive surprises after keratoplasty, donor corneas whose refractive power deviates too much from the mean are discarded for penetrating or anterior lamellar keratoplasty. In Homburg/Saar, we have so far set the threshold at curvature deviations of more than $\bar{x}$ (mean) ± 3 standard deviations (eminence-based) [140, 141] (status February 2022: donor corneas with a total refractive power of <39.9 and >47.8 D). Those donor tissues may, however, still be suitable for posterior lamellar keratoplasty, such as DMEK or DSAEK. Furthermore, in the future, sterile donor tomography could enable: (1) the harmonization of donor and recipient tomography [142, 143], which could potentially minimize persistent residual astigmatism after suture removal for a particular donor-recipient pair; and (2) the improvement of the IOL power calculation in a classical triple procedure by means of regression analysis between pre- and postoperative total refractive power of donor corneal tissues [144]. These projects are currently under research, as well as (a) the reliability [55] and (b) the validity of donor tomography by means of available keratometric measurements during the donor's lifetime, or alternatively using histological reprocessing of unused corneal tissues to detect evidence of keratorefractive myo-pia correction or keratoconus in respectively remarkably flat and steep donor corneas.

Detection of Cornea Guttata in the Eye Bank

Cornea guttata (CG) was first described in 1921 by Vogt as a clinical finding characterized by droplet-like changes on the posterior surface of the cornea detected using the slit-lamp examination [145, 146]. CG is formed by the accumulation of basement membrane and deposition of collagen and fibril fibers resulting in endothelial excrescences disrupting the endothelial mosaic [147]. Since the endothelial layer regulates the inflow of aqueous humor into the stroma through an active transport pump, the presence of CG leads to the loss of endothelial cells and interferes with the function of the endothelial layer to keep a transparent cornea [149, 148]. Although, in many cases, CG is considered an isolated finding without clinical significance, in many other cases, the disease progresses to become clinically significant; at that point, the disease entity is called Fuchs' endothelial corneal dystrophy (FECD). As the disease progresses, the endothelial layer can no longer maintain the transparency of the cornea resulting in corneal edema and visual loss [150–152]. The prevalence of CG varies in the literature and increase with increasing age reaching up to 11% in one study [153, 154]. CG usually appears centrally and spreads peripherally as the disease progresses and can be clinically detected by its "beaten metal" appearance on the slit-lamp biomicroscopy [155]. Using specular microscopy as a diagnostic method, CG can be objectively detected and quantified [156].

Unfortunately, the detection of CG in donor corneas is not as simple as in living patients. On one side, the visualization of CG in the swollen donor corneas stored in their culture medium clinically using the slit lamp is extremely difficult and, in most cases, not possible. On the other side, its detection using the inverted light microscopy in the eye banks is neither simple nor standardized. Therefore, in order to assess the prevalence and severity of cornea guttata in donor corneas, two large-scale studies analyzed the prevalence and clinical significance of cornea guttata in 1758 patients after PKP and 664 patients after DMEK [157, 158]. These studies showed a CG prevalence of 14.9% after PKP and 18.7% after DMEK, of which 13.6% and 16.9% represented a low-grade CG without clinical significancy, respectively, whereas 1.3% and 1.9% showed high-grade CG, respectively. Only high-grade CG showed a significant negative impact on clinical parameters such as visual acuity and central corneal thickness. In total, around 13% and 8% of the whole population studied underwent a progression from either a healthy corneal transplant to one having CG, or from a transplant with low-grade CG to high-grade CG after PKP and DMEK, respectively. These results highlight the importance of detecting CG in donor corneas in the eye bank, especially high-grade CG, to prevent the transplantation of such diseased corneas.

In order to characterize the features of CG seen under the inverted light microscope used in the eye banks, a large retrospective study aimed to establish semi-quantitative morphological criteria for the detection of CG in donor corneas [59, 141]. This study included 262 patients who underwent keratoplasties. These patients were classified according to the postoperative CG grade whereafter their corresponding 1582 preoperative endothelial pictures taken by an inverted light microscope were analyzed. The results of this study showed that three morphological criteria correlated with the presence of cornea guttata. Those are the presence of less than 50% of the cells in an endothelial picture having a hexagonal or a circular shape, the presence of cell membrane defects and interruptions and the presence of a small thickening of the cell membrane "blebs."

Artificial intelligence has been a hot topic in recent years and has greatly contributed to the improvement of diagnostic techniques in the field of ophthalmology [159]. Artificial intelligence can also be used in the field of eye banking for the (semi-)automated detection of CG in specular microscopy images. Such a project is currently under development at the Klaus Faber Center for Corneal Diseases, incl. LIONS Eye Bank Saar-Lor-Lux, Trier/Westpfalz, in collaboration with the German Research Center for Artificial Intelligence (DFKI). The programmed machine learning algorithms based on complex neural networks allow automated endothelial cell count as well as the detection of abnormalities in specular microscopy images, including areas of necrosis and the presence of GC (Fig. 2.6). This emerging technology should greatly contribute to improving the cornea selection for eye banks.

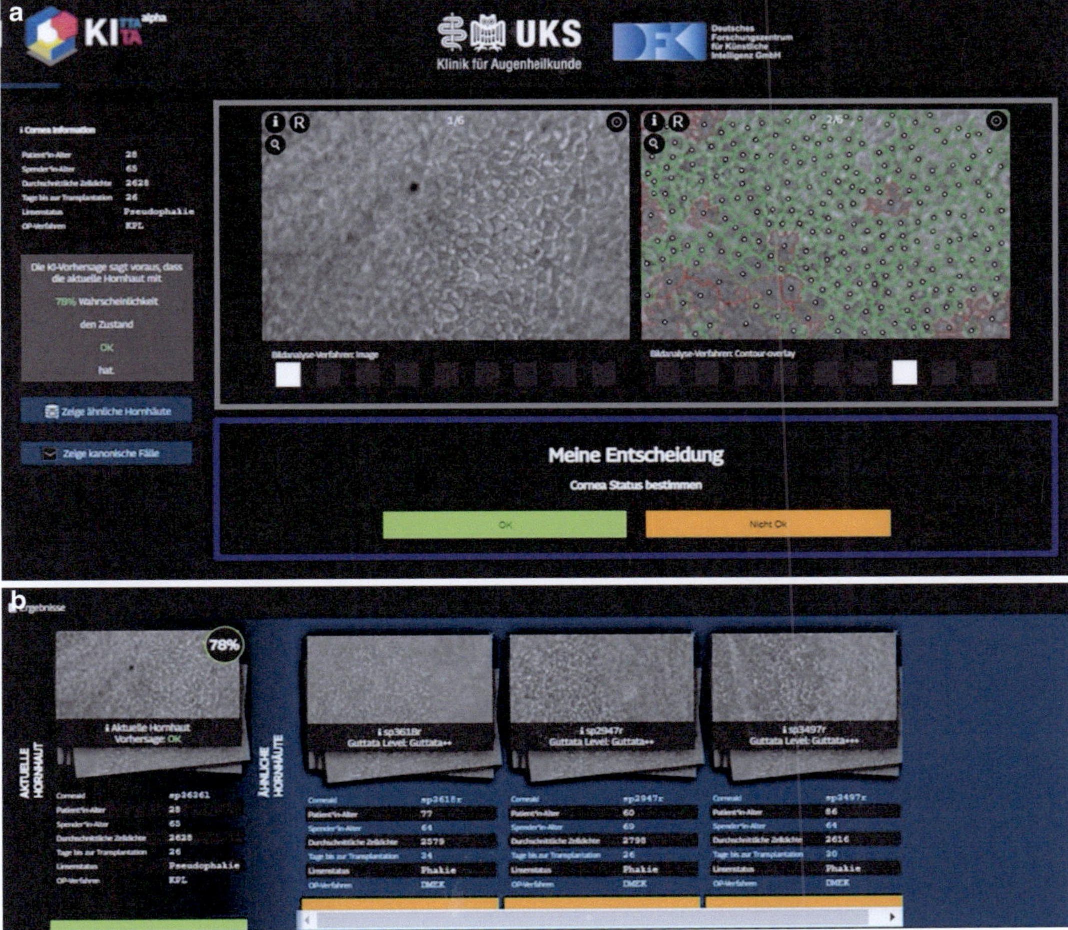

Fig. 2.6 Automated detection of cornea guttata (CG) in the eye bank using artificial intelligence (AI). Kittool: decision support tool for the detection of CG integrating two components: (**a**) Graphical analytic tools, whereby endothelial cells are processed to generate several cell representations such as "honeycomb" representation for an enhanced visualization of the endothelial layer. (**b**) Machine learning classifiers including Case-Based Reasoning (CBR) for AI-based support enable automated CG detection in the eye bank by comparison with previous endothelial cell images with known postoperative classification of the graft endothelium after keratoplasty

Benefits of a Highly-Structured Quality Management System (QMS) by Example of the LIONS Eye Bank Saar-Lor-Lux, Trier/Westpfalz

A quality management system (QMS) is an essential component of a highly functioning eye bank to ensure a maximum level of quality and safety of human tissues [160]. While a number of different quality management systems can be used, the ISO (International Organization for Standardization) 9001:2015 standard can be adopted for the entire process from donation to transplantation. This standard follows a process-oriented approach with the goal of continuous improvement. The quality management system is based on the principle of good practice and provides defined instructions and standard operating procedures (SOPs) for every step of the donation-transplantation process and documentation and processing of data.

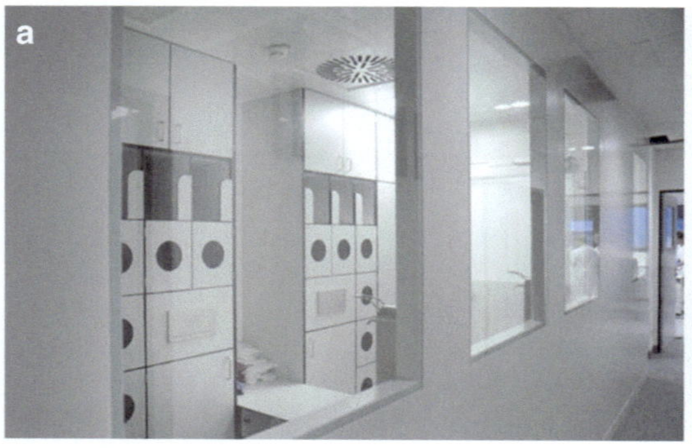 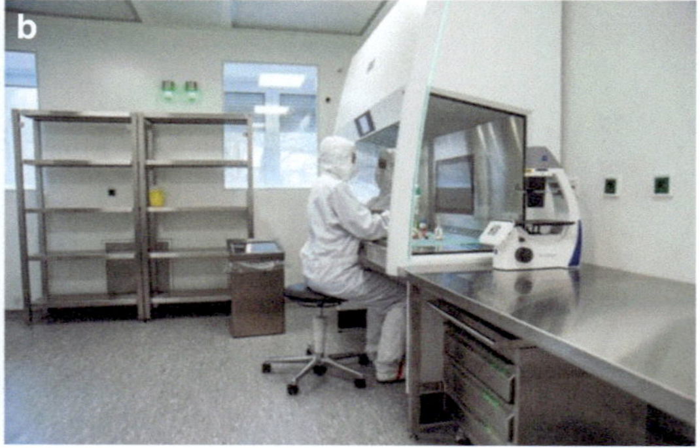

Fig. 2.7 Sterile room in the Klaus Faber Center for Cornea Diseases, incl. LIONS Eye Bank Saar–Lor–Lux, Trier/Westpfalz. (**a**) Decontamination corridor. The staff dresses in several steps through this corridor (cleanroom grades D and C) before arriving in the clean rooms grade B according to ISO Cleanroom Standards for the manufacture of Sterile Medicinal Products. (**b**) A staff member sterilely dressed, renewing the organ culture medium of organ-cultured corneas under maximum sterile conditions, under laminar flow (grade A)

The eye bank is bound by the laws, technical norms, guidelines and legislative frameworks of its country which give guiding values to the process of corneal donation, handling of the donor tissue within the eye bank, transport of tissues and transplantation [2, 108]. The eye bank must be located in a suitable facility and equipped with the necessary technical apparatus, instruments and materials. The Klaus Faber Center for Corneal Diseases (KFZH) including the LIONS Eye Bank Saar-Lor-Lux, Trier/Westpfalz for example, which was newly founded in 2019, provides a class A clean room and all facilities which sets the highest quality standard for the cultivation work-flow (Fig. 2.7).

Managing human resources is an essential part of a well-functioning eye bank. The staff must successfully complete initial basic training and necessary refresher courses and demonstrate essential knowledge in order to carry out the expected tasks. Before retrieving human corneas, personnel must be sufficiently trained and be familiar with the necessary documentation regarding the consent of the donor family, donor selection criteria, contraindications, and the proper techniques for harvesting the cornea and reconstruction of the eye.

Upon arrival at the eye bank, an identification code -is assigned to the corneal tissue. The tissue is quarantined and serologic and microbiologic examinations [21] in accordance with state regulations as well as slit-lamp examinations and evaluations of the endothelial cell density (ECD) and morphology are performed before the tissue can be declared suitable for transplantation [161]. The traceability of the donor and the recipient must be ensured and documented throughout the entire process. In addition, the LIONS Eye Bank Saar-Lor-Lux, Trier/Westpfalz routinely uses sterile donor tomography to further improve the quality of the donor tissue and avoid transplanting tissues with curvature abnormalities [140].

Written instructions should be available as a documental architecture that can easily be accessed and kept up-to-date for the entire process. Instructions need to be shared with and followed by the personnel of the eye bank as well as interested external parties. Each document should provide detailed instructions. These need to be written, authenticated, approved and distributed. In the event of changes to the organization, new legislative requirements, new medical-scientific knowledge or changes in the process, the documents need to be updated.

Internal and external audits need to be held regularly in order to monitor, maintain and improve the quality management system and obtain national and international accreditations. Furthermore, the eye bank should continuously monitor and analyze data to ensure continuous performance improvement. Hereby, tissue quality can constantly be increased and the number of discarded tissues due to quality concerns can be diminished [113].

Future Perspectives

The number of active eye banks has decreased drastically in recent years [162]. The global activity is refocused on large structures with more resources, allowing optimal conditions of preservation as well as a better selection and preparation of tissues. These large structures, in charge of the "production" of tissues for external institutions, are developing "ready-to-use" tissues to facilitate transport and use [91]. This trend is expected to grow in the future due to its economic and logistical advantages. Nevertheless, these practices tend to transform eye banks into "market places" for surgeons, a development that presents risks of unequal access to "good quality" tissue for small institutions and their patients and breaks the link between patients, surgeons and eye banks.

Advances in preservation processes are being developed, with—for example—the active storage machine (ASM), a device where corneas are conserved in banks of "storage plates" (Fig. 2.8), allowing almost physiological conditions of electrolytic medium and pressure for donor corneas [163, 164].

In terms of selection techniques, new methods of tissue analysis such as high-resolution two-photon imaging provide information about the cells metabolic state and structural organization of the stroma, with subcellular resolution [165]. The rise of artificial intelligence and convolutional neural networks should enable automation and better efficiency of tissue selection processes in eye banking.

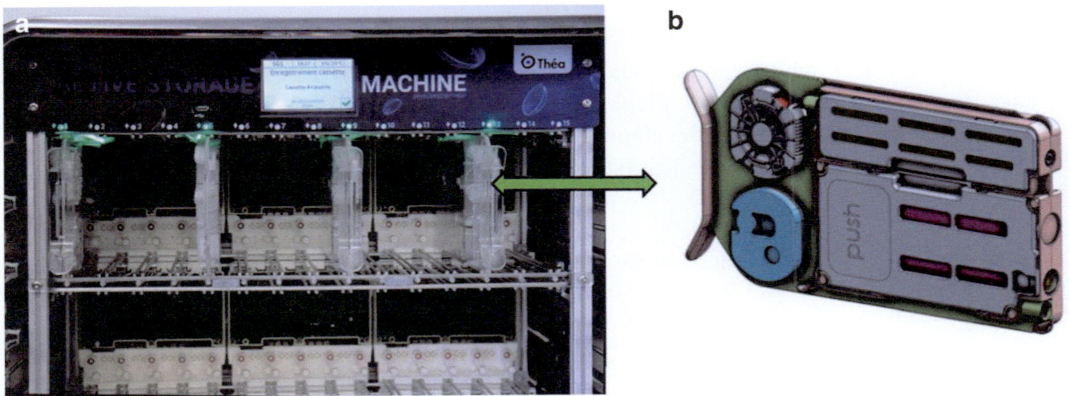

Fig. 2.8 Active Storage Machine (ASM). (**a**) Docking station with monitoring system for modular bioreactors fitted into slots. (**b**) "Bioreactor." The cornea, located in the heart of the bioreactor, separates the endothelial and epithelial chambers. The endothelial chamber is filled with culture medium (containing red phenol as pH indicator) from a tank. Fluid is circulated by a peristaltic pump driven by a pressure sensor, a solenoid valve and a microcontroller. The pressure inside the endothelial chamber is kept at 21.5 mmHg. Used medium is removed to a waste compartment. ()

Take Home Notes

- **Hypothermic storage**, simple and not expensive but allowing only short-term storage, and **organ culture**, more complex and expensive but allowing better control, longer storage and better endothelial quality, currently remain the two major storage methods in eye banks.
- The use of **prestripped** and **preloaded** tissues produced by eye banks for DMEK and DSAEK represents a valuable option for surgeons in centers without on-site eye banks or prompt availability of nonstripped tissues but should be carried out by accredited and experienced eye banks and as close as possible to the elective surgery.
- New selection techniques such as the **sterile donor tomography** or the **detection of cornea guttata** using artificial intelligence allow a better selection and allocation of tissues in the eye bank in order to avoid transplanting tissues with curvature or morphological abnormalities.
- A well-designed **quality management system** is essential to ensure the quality and safety of corneal tissue and to face the multiple new challenges of modern eye banking.
- Improvement of existing techniques and new advances for tissue preservation, preparation and selection promises **further developments** in the field of eye banking in the near future.

Acknowledgments The authors thank Prof. Dr. Gilles Thuret, the team of CHU Saint-Etienne (France) and SINCLER company for their contribution to the section concerning the "active storage machine (ASM)" and the availability of Fig. 2.8.

The authors thank Ms. Christina Turner (director's assistant and in charge of the publication and education pool, Department of Ophthalmology, Saarland University Medical Center (UKS), Homburg/Saar, Germany) who reviewed the first draft of the manuscript and ensured a correct English language.

Funding Funding/Support: No funding or grant support.

Conflicts of Interest The following authors have **no financial disclosures** and **no conflict of interest**: Loïc Hamon, Loay Daas, Adrien Quintin, Tarek Safi, Isabel Weinstein, and Berthold Seitz.

The authors attest that they meet the current ICMJE criteria for authorship.

References

1. Zirm E. [A successful total keratoplasty]. Albrecht Von Graefes Arch Klin Exp Ophthalmol. 1906;64:580–93.
2. European Eye Bank Association (EEBA). Technical guidelines for ocular tissue (TGOT). Venice: EEBA; 2020. https://www.eeba.eu/files/pdf/EEBA_Technical_Guidelines_for_Ocular_Tissue_Revision11.pdf. Accessed 22 Feb 2022.
3. Flockerzi E, Maier P, Böhringer D, Reinshagen H, Kruse F, Cursiefen C, Reinhard T, Geerling G, Torun N, Seitz B, All German Keratoplasty Registry Contributors. Trends in corneal transplantation from 2001 to 2016 in Germany; a report of the DOG-section cornea and its keratoplasty registry. Am J Ophthalmol. 2018;188:91–8. https://doi.org/10.1016/j.ajo.2018.01.018.
4. Molter Y, Milioti G, Langenbucher A, Seitz B. [Appearance, recurrence and prognosis of immunological graft rejection after penetrating keratoplasty]. Ophthalmologe. 2020;117:548–56. https://doi.org/10.1007/s00347-019-00975-9.
5. Seitz B, Langenbucher A, Naumann GO. [Perspectives of excimer laser-assisted keratoplasty]. Ophthalmologe. 2011;108:817–24. https://doi.org/10.1007/s00347-011-2333-x.
6. Holzer MP, Rabsilber TM, Auffarth GU. Penetrating keratoplasty using femtosecond laser. Am J Ophthalmol. 2007;143:524–6. https://doi.org/10.1016/j.ajo.2006.08.029.
7. Seitz B, Langenbucher A, Kus MM, Küchle M, Naumann GOH. Nonmechanical corneal trephination with the excimer laser improves outcome after penetrating keratoplasty. Ophthalmology. 1999;106:1156–65.
8. Hoffmann F. [Suture technique for perforating keratoplasty]. Klin Monatsbl Augenheilkd. 1976;169:584–90.
9. Suffo S, Seitz B, Daas L. [The Homburg cross-stitch marker for double-running sutures in penetrating keratoplasty]. Klin Monbl Augenheilkd. 2021;238:808–14. https://doi.org/10.1055/a-1275-0807.
10. Melles GR. Descemet membrane endothelial keratoplasty (DMEK). Cornea. 2006;25:987–90. https://doi.org/10.1097/01.ico.0000248385.16896.34.
11. Seitz B, Daas L, Flockerzi E, Suffo S. [Descemet membrane endothelial keratoplasty DMEK - Donor and recipient step by step]. Ophthalmologe. 2020;117:811–28. https://doi.org/10.1007/s00347-020-01134-1.
12. Luengo-Gimeno F, Tan DT, Mehta JS. Evolution of deep anterior lamellar keratoplasty (DALK).

Ocul Surf. 2011;9:98–110. https://doi.org/10.1016/s1542-0124(11)70017-9.

13. Hata B. The development of glioma in the eye to which the cornea of a patient, who suffered from glioma, was transplanted. Acta Soc Ophthalmol Jpn. 1939;43:1763–7.

14. Armitage WJ, Tullo AB, Ironside JW. Risk of Creutzfeldt-Jakob disease transmission by ocular surgery and tissue transplantation. Eye. 2009;23:1926–30.

15. Caron MJ, Wilson R. Review of the risk of HIV infection through corneal transplantation in the United States. J Am Optom Assoc. 1994;65:173–8.

16. European Eye Bank Association. Minimum Medical Standards (MMS). Venice: EEBA; 2020. https://www.eeba.eu/files/pdf/EEBA%20Minimum%20Medical%20Standards%20Revision%205%20Final.pdf. Accessed 24 Feb 2022.

17. Heim A, Wagner D, Rothämel T, Hartman U, Flik J, Verhagen W. Evaluation of serological screening of cadaveric sera for donor selection for corneal transplantation. J Med Virol. 1999;58:291–5.

18. Martin C, Tschernig T, Hamon L, Daas L, Seitz B. Corneae from body donors in anatomy department: valuable use for clinical transplantation and experimental research. BMC Ophthalmol. 2020;13(20):284. https://doi.org/10.1186/s12886-020-01546-2.

19. Serfözö A, Suffo S, Viestenz A, Seitz B, Daas L. [Central sclerocorneoplasty à chaud in bacterial superinfected mycotic keratitis confirmed by confocal microscopy at the base of recurrent herpetic keratitis]. Klin Monbl Augenheilkd. 2021;239(10):1245–7. https://doi.org/10.1055/a-1386-5229.

20. Sangwan VS, Jain V, Gupta P. Structural and functional outcome of scleral patch graft. Eye. 2007;21:930–05.

21. Li S, Bischoff M, Schirra F, Langenbucher A, Ong M, Halfmann A, Herrmann M, Seitz B. [Correlation between microbial growth in conjunctival swabs of corneal donors and contamination of organ culture media]. Ophthalmologe 2014;111:553–9.

22. Lawlor M, Kerridge I, Ankeny R, Dobbins TA, Billson F. Specific unwillingness to donate eyes: the impact of disfigurement, knowledge and procurement on corneal donation. Am J Transplant. 2010;10:657–63. https://doi.org/10.1111/j.1600-6143.2009.02986.x.

23. Wykrota AA, Weinstein I, Hamon L, Daas L, Flockerzi E, Suffo S, Seitz B. Approval rates for corneal donation and the origin of donor tissue for transplantation at a university-based tertiary referral center with corneal subspecialization hosting a LIONS Eye Bank. BMC Ophthalmol. 2022;22:17. https://doi.org/10.1186/s12886-022-02248-7.

24. Filatov VP. Transplantation of the cornea. Arch Opthalmol. 1935;13:321–47.

25. Bourne WM. Corneal preservation. In: Kaufman HE, Barron BA, Waltman SR, Mc Donald MB, editors. The cornea. Oxford: Butterworth-Heinemann; 1988. p. 713–24.

26. Basu PK, Hasany SM, Ranadive NS, Chipman M. Damage to corneal endothelium cells by lysosomal enzymes in stored human eyes. Can J Ophthalmol. 1980;15:137–40.

27. Capella JA, Kaufman HE, Robbins JE. Preservation of viable corneal tissue. Arch Ophthalmol. 1965;74:669–73. https://doi.org/10.1001/archopht.1965.00970040671015. PMID: 5891917.

28. O'Neill P, Mueller FO, Trevor-Roper PD. On the preservation of corneae at -196 degrees C for full-thickness homografts in man and dog. Br J Ophthalmol. 1967;51:13–30. https://doi.org/10.1136/bjo.51.1.13.

29. Sperling S. Cryopreservation of human cadaver corneas regenerated at 31 degrees C in a modified tissue culture medium. Acta Ophthalmol (Copenh). 1981;59(1):142–4148. http://doi.org/10.1111/j.1755-3768.1981.tb06722.x.

30. European Directorate for the Quality of Medicines and Healthcare (EDQM). Guide to the quality and safety of tissues and cells for human application, vol. 2. Strasbourg: Council of Europe; 2017. p. 185–95.

31. Rodríguez-Fernández S, Álvarez-Portela M, Rendal-Vázquez E, Piñeiro-Ramil M, Sanjurjo-Rodríguez C, Castro-Viñuelas R, Sánchez-Ibáñez J, Fuentes-Boquete I, Díaz-Prado S. Analysis of cryopreservation protocols and their harmful effects on the endothelial integrity of human corneas. Int J Mol Sci. 2021;22:12564. https://doi.org/10.3390/ijms222212564.

32. Tsang HF, Chan LWC, Cho WCS, Yu ACS, Yim AKY, Chan AKC, Ng LPW, Wong YKE, Pei XM, Li MJW, Wong SC. An update on COVID-19 pandemic: the epidemiology, pathogenesis, prevention and treatment strategies. Expert Rev Anti Infect Ther. 2021;19:877–88. https://doi.org/10.1080/14787210.2021.1863146.

33. Chaurasia S, Das S, Roy A. A review of long-term corneal preservation techniques: relevance and renewed interests in the COVID-19 era. Indian J Ophthalmol. 2020;68:1357–63. https://doi.org/10.4103/ijo.IJO_1505_20.

34. Casagrande M, Fitzek A, Spitzer MS, Püschel K, Glatzel M, Krasemann S, Nörz D, Lütgehetmann M, Pfefferle S, Schultheiss M. Presence of SARS-CoV-2 RNA in the cornea of viremic patients with COVID-19. JAMA Ophthalmol. 2021;139:383–8. https://doi.org/10.1001/jamaophthalmol.2020.6339.

35. Hamon L, Bayyoud T, Seitz B. Ocular findings in patients with COVID-19: impact on eye banking [Letter]. Clin Ophthalmol. 2021;15:2051–2. https://doi.org/10.2147/OPTH.S317378.

36. McCarey BE, Kaufman HE. Improved corneal storage. Invest Ophthalmol. 1974;13:165–73.

37. Basu PK. A review of methods for storage of cornea for keratoplasty. Indian J Ophthalmol. 1995;43:55–8.

38. Keates RH, Rabin B. Extending corneal storage with 2.5% chondroitin sulfate (K-Sol).

Ophthalmic Surg. 1988;19:817–20. https://doi.org/10.3928/0090-4481-19881101-13.

39. Lindstrom RL, Kaufman HE, Skelnik DL, Laing RA, Lass JH, Musch DC, Trousdale MD, Reinhart WJ, Burris TE, Sugar A, Davis RM, Hirokawa K, Smith T, Gordon JF. Optisol corneal storage medium. Am J Ophthalmol. 1992;114:345–56.

40. Steinemann TL, Kaufmann HE, Lindstrom RL, Beuerman RW, Varnell ED. Intermediate-term storage media (K-Sol, Dexsol, Optisol). In: Brightbill FS, editor. Corneal surgery. St Louis: Mosby; 1993. p. 609–13.

41. Moshirfar M, Odayar VS, McCabe SE, Ronquillo YC. Corneal donation: current guidelines and future direction. Clin Ophthalmol. 2021;15:2963–73. https://doi.org/10.2147/OPTH.S284617.

42. Armitage WJ. Preservation of human cornea. Transfus Med Hemother. 2011;38:143–7. https://doi.org/10.1159/000326632.

43. Summerlin WT, Miller GE, Harris JE, Good RA. The organ-cultured cornea: an in vitro study. Invest Ophthalmol. 1973;12:176–80.

44. Doughman DJ, Harris JE, Schmitt MK. Penetrating keratoplasty using 37 C organ cultured cornea. Trans Sect Ophthalmol Am Acad Ophthalmol Otolaryngol. 1976;81:778–93.

45. Pels E, Beele H, Claerhout I. Eye bank issues: II. Preservation techniques: warm versus cold storage. Int Ophthalmol. 2008;28:155–63. https://doi.org/10.1007/s10792-007-9086-1.

46. Lindstrom RL, Doughman DJ, Skelnik DL, Mindrup EA. Minnesota system corneal preservation. Br J Ophthalmol. 1986;70:47–54. https://doi.org/10.1136/bjo.70.1.47.

47. Frueh BE, Böhnke M. Corneal grafting of donor tissue preserved for longer than 4 weeks in organ-culture medium. Cornea. 1995;14:463–6.

48. Thuret G, Carricajo A, Chiquet C, Vautrin AC, Celle N, Boureille M, Acquart S, Aubert G, Maugery J, Gain P. Sensitivity and rapidity of blood culture bottles in the detection of cornea organ culture media contamination by bacteria and fungi. Br J Ophthalmol. 2002;86:1422–7. https://doi.org/10.1136/bjo.86.12.1422.

49. Thuret G, Carricajo A, Vautrin AC, Raberin H, Acquart S, Garraud O, Gain P, Aubert G. Efficiency of blood culture bottles for the fungal sterility testing of corneal organ culture media. Br J Ophthalmol. 2005;89:586–90. https://doi.org/10.1136/bjo.2004.053439.

50. Müller LJ, Pels E, Vrensen GF. The effects of organ-culture on the density of keratocytes and collagen fibers in human corneas. Cornea. 2001;20:86–95.

51. Sperling S. Human corneal epithelium in organ culture. The influence of temperature and medium of incubation. Acta Ophthalmol. 1979;57:269–76.

52. Abdin AD, Daas L, Pattmöller M, Suffo S, Langenbucher A, Seitz B. Negative impact of dextran in organ culture media for pre-stripped tissue

preservation on DMEK (Descemet membrane endothelial keratoplasty) outcome. Graefes Arch Clin Exp Ophthalmol. 2018;256:213–5.

53. Spelsberg H, Reinhard T, Sundmacher R. [Epithelial damage of corneal grafts after prolonged storage in dextran-containing organ culture medium – a prospective study]. Klin Monbl Augenheilkd. 2002;219:417–21.

54. Hamon L, Daas L, Mäurer S, Weinstein I, Quintin A, Schulz K, Langenbucher A, Seitz B. Thickness and curvature changes of human corneal grafts in dextran-containing organ culture medium before keratoplasty. Cornea. 2021;40:733–40. https://doi.org/10.1097/ICO.0000000000002543.

55. Hamon L, Quintin A, Mäurer S, Weinstein I, Langenbucher A, Seitz B, Daas L. Reliability and efficiency of corneal thickness measurements using sterile donor tomography in the eye bank. Cell Tissue Bank. 2022;23(4):695–706. https://doi.org/10.1007/s10561-021-09980-2.

56. Borderie VM, Laroche L. Microbiologic study of organ-cultured donor corneas. Transplantation. 1998;66:120–3.

57. Thuret G, Chiquet C, Bernal F, et al. Prospective, randomized, clinical and endothelial evaluation of 2 storage times for cornea donor tissue in organ culture at 31 degrees C. Arch Ophthalmol. 2003;121:442–50.

58. Bachmann B, Schaub F, Cursiefen C. [Treatment of corneal endothelial disorders by DMEK and UT-DSAEK. Indications, complications, results and follow-up]. Ophthalmologe. 2016;113:196–203. https://doi.org/10.1007/s00347-016-0221-0.

59. Seitz B, Daas L, Hamon L, Fraenkel D, Szentmàry N, Langenbucher A, Suffo S. La kératoplastie transfixiante. In: Thuret G, Muraine M, Gain P, editors. L'endothélium cornéen. Paris: Elsevier-Masson; 2021. p. 121–5.

60. Hallerman W. [Some remarks on keratoplasty]. Klin Monatsbl Augenheilkd. 1959;135:252–9.

61. Olson RJ. Modulation of postkeratoplasty astigmatism by surgical and suturing techniques. Int Ophthalmol Clin. 1983;23:137–51.

62. Seitz B, Langenbucher A, Naumann GOH. Trephination in penetrating keratoplasty. In: Reinhard T, Larkin F, editors. Essentials in ophthalmology - corneal and external eye disease. Berlin: Springer; 2006. p. 123–52.

63. Naumann GOH. Part II: corneal transplantation in anterior segment diseases. The Bowman Lecture (Number 56) 1994. Eye. 1995;9:395–421.

64. Seitz B, Hager T, Langenbucher A, Naumann GOH. Reconsidering sequential double running suture removal after penetrating keratoplasty – a prospective randomized study comparing excimer laser and motor trephination. Cornea. 2018;37:301–6.

65. Seitz B, Daas L, Milioti G, Szentmàry N, Langenbucher A, Suffo S. [Excimer laser-assisted penetrating keratoplasty: on 1 July 2019 excimer laser penetrating keratoplasty celebrates its 30th

anniversary - Video article]. Ophthalmologe. 2019;116:1221–30. https://doi.org/10.1007/s00347-019-00990-w.

66. Seitz B, Langenbucher A, Zagrada D, Budde W, Kus MM. [Corneal dimensions in various types of corneal dystrophies and their effect on penetrating keratoplasty] Klin Monatsbl Augenheilkd. 2000;217:152–8.

67. Seitz B, Langenbucher A, Küchle M, Naumann GOH. Impact of graft diameter on corneal power and the regularity of postkeratoplasty astigmatism before and after suture removal. Ophthalmology. 2003;110:2162–7.

68. Muraine M, Toubeau D, Gueudry J, Brasseur G. Impact of new lamellar techniques of keratoplasty on eye bank activity. Graefes Arch Clin Exp Ophthalmol. 2007;245:32–8. https://doi.org/10.1007/s00417-006-0390-7.

69. Dua HS, Faraj LA, Said DG, Gray T, Lowe J. Human corneal anatomy redifined. A novel pre-Descemet's layer (Dua's layer). Ophthalmology. 2013;120:1778–85. https://doi.org/10.1016/j.ophtha.2013.01.018.

70. Anwar M, Teichmann KD. Big-bubble technique to bare Descemet's membrane in anterior lamellar keratoplasty. J Cataract Refract Surg. 2002;28:398–403.

71. Daas L, Hamon L, Ardjomand N, Safi T, Seitz B. [Excimer laser-assisted DALK: a case report from the Homburg Keratoconus Center (HKC)]. Ophthalmologe. 2021;118:1245–8. https://doi.org/10.1007/s00347-021-01342-3.

72. Anshu A, Price MO, Price FW Jr. Risk of corneal transplant rejection significantly reduced with Descemet's membrane endothelial keratoplasty. Ophthalmology. 2012;119:536–40.

73. Boynton GE, Woodward MA. Eye-bank preparation of endothelial tissue. Curr Opin Ophthalmol. 2014;25:319–24. https://doi.org/10.1097/ICU.0000000000000060.

74. Yoeruek E, Bartz-Schmidt KU. Novel surgical instruments facilitating Descemet membrane dissection. Cornea. 2013;32:523–6. https://doi.org/10.1097/ICO.0b013e3182588ae9.

75. Price MO, Giebel AW, Fairchild KM, Price FW Jr. Descemet's membrane endothelial keratoplasty: prospective multicenter study of visual and refractive outcomes and endothelial survival. Ophthalmology. 2009;116:2361–8. https://doi.org/10.1016/j.ophtha.2009.07.010.

76. Venzano D, Pagani P, Randazzo N, Cabiddu F, Traverso CE. Descemet membrane air-bubble separation in donor corneas. J Cataract Refract Surg. 2010;36:2022–7.

77. Muraine M, Gueudry J, He Z, Piselli S, Lefevre S, Toubeau D. Novel technique for the preparation of corneal grafts for descemet membrane endothelial keratoplasty. Am J Ophthalmol. 2013;156:851–9. https://doi.org/10.1016/j.ajo.2013.05.041.

78. Tourtas T, Laaser K, Bachmann BO, Cursiefen C, Kruse FE. Descemet membrane endothelial keratoplasty versus Descemet stripping automated endothelial keratoplasty. Am J Ophthalmol. 2012;153:1082–1090.e1082.

79. Vetter JM, Butsch C, Faust M, Schmidtmann I, Hoffmann EM, Sekundo W, Pfeiffer N. Irregularity of the posterior corneal surface after curved interface femtosecond laser-assisted versus microkeratome-assisted Descemet stripping automated endothelial keratoplasty. Cornea. 2013;32:118–24. https://doi.org/10.1097/ICO.0b013e31826ae2d8.

80. Phillips PM, Phillips LJ, Saad HA, Terry MA, Stolz DB, Stoeger C, Franks J, Davis-Boozer D. "Ultrathin" DSAEK tissue prepared with a low-pulse energy, high-frequency femtosecond laser. Cornea. 2013;32:81–6. https://doi.org/10.1097/ICO.0b013e31825c72dc.

81. Parekh M, Ruzza A, Steger B, Willoughby CE, Rehman S, Ferrari S, Ponzin D, Kaye SB, Romano V. Cross-country transportation efficacy and clinical outcomes of preloaded large-diameter ultra-thin Descemet stripping automated endothelial keratoplasty grafts. Cornea. 2019;38:30–4. https://doi.org/10.1097/ICO.0000000000001777.

82. Bielefeld V, Vabres B, Baud'huin M, Lebranchu P, Le Meur G, Orignac I. [UT-DSAEK using grafts provided by a tissue bank, a one-year follow-up study of 79 grafts]. J Fr Ophtalmol. 2021;44:176–88. https://doi.org/10.1016/j.jfo.2020.04.060.

83. Newman LR, DeMill DL, Zeidenweber DA, Mayko ZM, Bauer AJ, Tran KD, Straiko MD, Terry MA. Preloaded Descemet membrane endothelial keratoplasty donor tissue: surgical technique and early clinical results. Cornea. 2018;37:981–6. https://doi.org/10.1097/ICO.0000000000001646.

84. Ruzza A, Salvalaio G, Bruni A, et al. Banking of donor tissues for Descemet stripping automated endothelial keratoplasty. Cornea. 2013;32:70–5. https://doi.org/10.1097/ICO.0b013e31825e8442.

85. Martin AI, Devasahayam R, Hodge C, Cooper S, Sutton GL. Analysis of the learning curve for pre-cut corneal specimens in preparation for lamellar transplantation: a prospective, single-centre, consecutive case series prepared at the Lions New South Wales Eye Bank. Clin Exp Ophthalmol. 2017;45:689–94.

86. Marty AS, Burillon C, Desanlis A, et al. Validation of an endothelial roll preparation for Descemet membrane endothelial keratoplasty by a cornea bank using "no touch" dissection technique. Cell Tissue Bank. 2016;17:225–32.

87. Terry MA, Straiko MD, Veldman PB, et al. Standardized DMEK technique: reducing complications using pre-stripped tissue, novel glass injector, and sulfur hexafluoride (SF6) gas. Cornea. 2015;34:845–52.

88. Safi T, Daas L, Kiefer GL, Sharma M, Ndiaye A, Deru M, Alexandersson J, Seitz B. Semi-quantitative criteria in the eye bank that correlate with cornea guttata in donor corneas. Klin Monbl Augenheilkd. 2021;238:680–7.

89. Safi T, Seitz B, Berg K, Schulz K, Langenbucher A, Daas L. Reproducibility of non-invasive endothelial cell loss assessment of the pre-stripped DMEK roll after preparation and storage. Am J Ophthalmol. 2021;221:17–26. https://doi.org/10.1016/j.ajo.2020.08.001.

90. Romano V, Parekh M, Kazaili A, Steger B, Akhtar R, Ferrari S, Kaye SB, Levis HJ. Eye bank versus surgeon prepared Descemet stripping automated endothelial keratoplasty tissues: influence on adhesion force in a pilot study. Indian J Ophthalmol. 2022;70:523–8. https://doi.org/10.4103/ijo.IJO_3637_20.

91. Rickmann A, Wahl S, Hofmann N, Knakowski J, Haus A, Börgel M, Szurman P. Comparison of pre-loaded grafts for Descemet membrane endothelial keratoplasty (DMEK) in a novel preloaded transport cartridge compared to conventional precut grafts. Cell Tissue Bank. 2020;21:205–13. https://doi.org/10.1007/s10561-020-09814-7.

92. Ighani M, Dzhaber D, Jain S, De Rojas JO, Eghrari AO. Techniques, outcomes, and complications of preloaded, trifolded Descemet Membrane Endothelial Keratoplasty using the DMEK EndoGlide. Cornea. 2021;40:669–74. https://doi.org/10.1097/ICO.0000000000002648.

93. Català P, Vermeulen W, Rademakers T, van den Bogaerdt A, Kruijt PJ, Nuijts RMMA, LaPointe VLS, Dickman MM. Transport and preservation comparison of preloaded and prestripped-only DMEK grafts. Cornea. 2020;39:1407–14. https://doi.org/10.1097/ICO.0000000000002391.

94. Terry MA. Precut tissue for descemet stripping automated endothelial keratoplasty: complications are from technique, not tissue. Cornea. 2008;27:627–9. https://doi.org/10.1097/QAI.0b013e3181775e55.

95. Menzel-Severing J, Walter P, Plum WJ, Kruse FE, Salla S. Assessment of corneal endothelium during continued organ culture of pre-stripped human donor tissue for DMEK surgery. Curr Eye Res. 2018;43:1439–44.

96. Bayyoud T, Röck D, Hofmann J, Bartz-Schmidt KU, Yoeruek E. [Precut technique for Descemet's membrane endothelial keratoplasty, preparation and storage in organ culture]. Klin Monbl Augenheilkd. 2012;229:621–3.

97. Terry MA, Shamie N, Chen ES, Phillips PM, Hoar KL, Friend DJ. Precut tissue for Descemet's stripping automated endothelial keratoplasty: vision, astigmatism, and endothelial survival. Ophthalmology. 2009;116:248–56. https://doi.org/10.1016/j.ophtha.2008.09.017.

98. Pagano L, Gadhvi KA, Coco G, Fenech M, Titley M, Levis HJ, Ruzza A, Ferrari S, Kaye SB, Parekh M, Romano V. Rebubbling rate in pre-loaded versus surgeon prepared DSAEK. Eur J Ophthalmol. 2021:11206721211014380. https://doi.org/10.1177/11206721211014380.

99. Romano V, Kazaili A, Pagano L, Gadhvi KA, Titley M, Steger B, Fernández-Vega-Cueto L, Meana A, Merayo-Lloves J, Diego P, Akhtar R, Levis HJ, Ferrari S, Kaye SB, Parekh M. Eye bank versus surgeon prepared DMEK tissues: influence on adhesion and re-bubbling rate. Br J Ophthalmol. 2022;106:177–83. https://doi.org/10.1136/bjophthalmol-2020-317608.

100. Romano V, Pagano L, Gadhvi KA, Coco G, Titley M, Fenech MT, Ferrari S, Levis HJ, Parekh M, Kaye S. Clinical outcomes of pre-loaded ultra-thin DSAEK and pre-loaded DMEK. BMJ Open Ophthalmol. 2020;5:e000546. https://doi.org/10.1136/bmjophth-2020-000546.

101. Jirsova K, Jones GLA. Amniotic membrane in ophthalmology: properties, preparation, storage and indications for grafting - a review. Cell Tissue Bank. 2017;18:193–204. https://doi.org/10.1007/s10561-017-9618-5.

102. Dua HS, Gomes JA, King AJ, Maharajan VS. The amniotic membrane in ophthalmology. Surv Ophthalmol. 2004;49:51–77.

103. Krysik K, Dobrowolski D, Wylegala E, Lyssek-Boron A. Amniotic membrane as a main component in treatments supporting healing and patch grafts in corneal melting and perforations. J Ophthalmol. 2020;2020:4238919. https://doi.org/10.1155/2020/4238919.

104. European Directorate for the Quality of Medicines & HealthCare (EDQM). Guide to the quality and safety of tissues and cells for human application, vol. 1. Strasbourg: Council of Europe; 2015. p. 349–55.

105. Burgos H, Sergeant RJ. Lyophilized human amniotic membranes used in reconstruction of the ear. J R Soc Med. 1983;76:433.

106. Hodge C, Sutton G, Devasahayam R, Georges P, Treloggen J, Cooper S, Petsoglou C. The use of donor scleral patch in ophthalmic surgery. Cell Tissue Bank. 2017;18:119–28. https://doi.org/10.1007/s10561-016-9603-4.

107. Mehta JS, Franks WA. The sclera, the prion, and the ophthalmologist. Br J Ophthalmol. 2002;86:587–92.

108. Eye Bank Association of America (EBAA). Medical standards. Washington, DC: EBAA; 2020. https://restoresight.org/wp-content/uploads/2020/07/Med-Standards-June-20-2020_7_23.pdf. Accessed 22 Feb 2022.

109. Barza M, Baum JL, Kane A. Comparing radioactive and trephine-disk bioassays of dicloxacillin and gentamicin in ocular tissues in vitro. Am J Ophthalmol. 1977;83:530–9.

110. Antonios SR, Cameron JA, Badr IA, Habash NR, Cotter JB. Contamination of donor corneas: postpenetrating keratoplasty endophthalmitis. Cornea. 1991;10:217–20.

111. Lau N, Hajjar Sesé A, Augustin VA, Kuit G, Wilkins MR, Tourtas T, Kruse FE, Højgaard-Olsen K, Manuel R, Armitage WJ, Larkin DF, Tuft SJ. Fungal infection after endothelial keratoplasty: association with hypothermic corneal storage. Br J Ophthalmol. 2019;103:1487–90. https://doi.org/10.1136/bjophthalmol-2018-312709.

112. Zanetti E, Bruni A, Mucignat G, Camposampiero D, Frigo AC, Ponzin D. Bacterial contamination of human organ-cultured corneas. Cornea. 2005;24:603–7.

113. Laun D, Suffo S, Kramp K, Bischoff M, Huber M, Langenbucher A, Seitz B. How implementing a quality management system at the LIONS Eye Bank Saar-Lor-Lux, Trier/Western Palatinate from 2006 to 2016 impacted the rate and reasons for discarding human organ-cultured corneas. Klin Monbl Augenheilkd. 2021;239:717–23.

114. Clover J. Slit-lamp biomicroscopy. Cornea. 2018;37(Suppl 1):5–6. https://doi.org/10.1097/ICO.0000000000001641.

115. Borderie VM, Scheer S, Touzeau O, Vedie F, Carvajal-Gonzalez S, Laroche L. Donor organ cultured corneal tissue selection before penetrating keratoplasty. Br J Ophthalmol. 1998;82:382–8. https://doi.org/10.1136/bjo.82.4.382.

116. Langenbucher A, Seitz B, Nguyen NX, Naumann GO. Corneal endothelial cell loss after nonmechanical penetrating keratoplasty depends on diagnosis: a regression analysis. Graefes Arch Clin Exp Ophthalmol. 2002;240:387–92. https://doi.org/10.1007/s00417-002-0470-2.

117. Bourne WM. Cellular changes in transplanted human corneas. Cornea. 2001;20:560–9. https://doi.org/10.1097/00003226-200108000-00002.

118. Schaub F, Enders P, Adler W, Bachmann BO, Cursiefen C, Heindl LM. Impact of donor graft quality on deep anterior lamellar keratoplasty (DALK). BMC Ophthalmol. 2017;17:204. https://doi.org/10.1186/s12886-017-0600-6.

119. Shaw EI, Rao GN, Arthur EJ, Aquavella VJ. The functional reserve of corneal endothelium. Trans Ophthalmol. 1978;85:640–9.

120. Sperling S. Evaluation of the endothelium of human donor corneas by induced dilation of intracellular spaces and trypan blue. Graefes Arch Clin Exp Ophthalmol. 1986;224:428–34.

121. Schroeter J, Rieck P. Endothelial evaluation in the Cornea Bank. In: Bredehorn-Mayr T, Duncker GIW, Armitage WJ, editors. Eye banking. Developments in ophthalmology, vol. 43. Basel: Karger; 2009. p. 47–62.

122. Fargione RA, Channa P. Cornea donors who have had prior refractive surgery; data from the Eye Bank Association of America. Curr Opin Ophthalmol. 2016;27:323–6. https://doi.org/10.1097/ICU.0000000000000278.

123. de Mello Farias RJ, Parolim A, de Sousa LB. [Corneal transplant utilizing a corneal graft that had undergone laser surgery - case report]. Arq Bras Oftalmol. 2005;68:266–9. https://doi.org/10.1590/s0004-27492005000200022.

124. Michaeli-Cohen A, Lambert AC, Coloma F, Rootman DS. Two cases of a penetrating keratoplasty with tissue from a donor who had undergone LASIK surgery. Cornea. 2002;21:111–3. https://doi.org/10.1097/00003226-200201000-00023.

125. Mifflin M, Kim M. Penetrating keratoplasty using tissue from a donor with previous LASIK surgery. Cornea. 2002;21:537–8. https://doi.org/10.1097/00003226-200207000-00024; author reply 538–9.

126. Kang SJ, Schmack I, Edelhauser HF, Grossniklaus HE. Donor corneas misidentified with prior laser in situ keratomileusis. Cornea. 2010;29:670–3. https://doi.org/10.1097/ICO.0b013e3181c325cc.

127. Mootha VV, Dawson D, Kumar A, Gleiser J, Qualls C, Albert DM. Slitlamp, specular, and light microscopic findings of human donor corneas after laser-assisted in situ keratomileusis. Arch Ophthalmol. 2004;122:686–92. https://doi.org/10.1001/archopht.122.5.686.

128. Vavra DE, Enzenauer RW. Predictive value of slit lamp examinations in screening donor corneas for prior refractive surgery. Arch Ophthalmol. 2005;123:707–8. https://doi.org/10.1001/archopht.123.5.707-c; author reply 708–709.

129. Ousley PJ, Terry MA. Objective screening methods for prior refractive surgery in donor tissue. Cornea. 2002;21:181–8. https://doi.org/10.1097/00003226-200203000-00011.

130. Ousley PJ, Terry MA. Use of a portable topography machine for screening donor tissue for prior refractive surgery. Cornea. 2002;21:745–50. https://doi.org/10.1097/00003226-200211000-00002.

131. Stoiber J, Ruckhofer J, Hitzl W, Grabner G. Evaluation of donor tissue with a new videokeratoscope: the Keratron Scout. Cornea. 2001;20:859–63. https://doi.org/10.1097/00003226-200111000-00016.

132. Terry MA, Ousley PJ. New screening methods for donor eye-bank eyes. Cornea. 1999;18(4):430–6. https://doi.org/10.1097/00003226-199907000-00007.

133. Lin RC, Li Y, Tang M, McLain M, Rollins AM, Izatt JA, Huang D. Screening for previous refractive surgery in eye bank corneas by using optical coherence tomography. Cornea. 2007;26:594–9. https://doi.org/10.1097/ICO.0b013e31803c5535.

134. Priglinger SG, Neubauer AS, May CA, Alge CS, Wolf AH, Mueller A, Ludwig K, Kampik A, Welge-Luessen U. Optical coherence tomography for the detection of laser in situ keratomileusis in donor corneas. Cornea. 2003;22:46–50. https://doi.org/10.1097/00003226-200301000-00011.

135. Damian A, Seitz B, Langenbucher A, Eppig T. Optical coherence tomography-based topography determination of corneal grafts in eye bank cultivation. J Biomed Opt. 2017;22:16001. https://doi.org/10.1117/1.JBO.22.1.016001.

136. Janunts E, Langenbucher A, Seitz B. In vitro corneal tomography of donor cornea using anterior segment OCT. Cornea. 2016;35:647–53. https://doi.org/10.1097/ICO.0000000000000761.

137. Mäurer S, Asi F, Rawer A, Damian A, Seitz B, Langenbucher A, Eppig T. [Concept for 3D measurement of corneal donor tissue using a clinical OCT]. Ophthalmologe. 2019;116:640–6. https://doi.org/10.1007/s00347-018-0801-2.

138. Tomey GmbH. CASIA2. 2022. https://assets.website-files.com/60c345b08518d0bd95024abf/60ddc04f9c8b48347261217a_CASIA2_brochure.pdf. Accessed 3 Feb 2022.

139. Eppig T, Mäurer S, Daas L, Seitz B, Langenbucher A. Imaging the cornea, anterior chamber and lens in

corneal and refractive surgery. In: Lanza M, editor. Clinical application of OCT in ophthalmology. London: IntechOpen; 2018. p. 133–52. https://doi. org/10.5772/intechopen.74129.

140. Quintin A, Hamon L, Mäurer S, Langenbucher A, Seitz B. OCT application for sterile corneal graft screening in the eye bank. Monbl Augenheilkd. 2021;238:688–92. https://doi. org/10.1055/a-1443-5451.

141. Seitz B, Asi F, Mäurer S, Hamon L, Quintin A, Langenbucher A. Anterior segment OCT: application to improve graft selection for corneal transplantation. In: Alió JL, Alió del Barrio JL, editors. Atlas of anterior segment optical coherence tomography. Cham: Springer; 2021. p. 223–36.

142. Mäurer S, Seitz B, Langenbucher A. "Harmonization" of donor and recipient tomography in corneal transplantation. Z Med Phys. 2021;31:73–7. https://doi. org/10.1016/j.zemedi.2020.05.006.

143. Seitz B, Langenbucher A, Naumann GOH. Astigmatismus bei Keratoplastik. In: Seiler T, editor. Refraktive Chirurgie der Hornhaut. Stuttgart: Enke; 2000. p. 197–252.

144. Quintin A, Hamon L, Mäurer S, Langenbucher A, Seitz B. [Comparison of sterile donor tomography in the eye bank and graft tomography after penetrating keratoplasty]. Ophthalmologe 2021;118:1038–44. https://doi.org/10.1007/s00347-020-01256-6.

145. Son H-S, Villarreal G, Meng H, Eberhart CG, Jun AS. On the origin of 'guttae'. Br J Ophthalmol. 2014;98:1308–10.

146. Vogt A. [Other results of slit lamp microscopy of the anterior segment of the bulb: (cornea, anterior chamber, iris, lens, anterior vitreous, conjunctiva, eyelid margins.) I. Section: cornea]. Graefes Arch Clin Exp Ophthalmol. 1921;106:63–103.

147. Waring GO III, Rodrigues MM, Laibson PR. Corneal dystrophies. II. Endothelial dystrophies. Surv Ophthalmol. 1978;23:147–68.

148. Adamis AP, Filatov V, Tripathi BJ, Tripathi RC. Fuchs' endo thelial dystrophy of the cornea. Surv Ophthalmol. 1993;38:149–68.

149. Weiss JS, Møller HU, Aldave AJ, Seitz B, Bredrup C, Kivelä T, Munier FL, Rapuano CJ, Nischal KK, Kim EK, Sutphin J, Busin M, Labbé A, Kenyon KR, Kinoshita S, Lisch W. IC3D classification of corneal dystrophies – edition 2. Cornea. 2015;34:117–59.

150. Borboli S, Colby K. Mechanisms of disease: Fuchs' endothelial dystrophy. Ophthalmol Clin North Am. 2002;15:17–25.

151. Wilson SE, Bourne WM. Fuchs' dystrophy. Cornea. 1988;7:2–18.

152. Yee RW, Matsuda M, Schultz RO, et al. Changes in the normal corneal endothelial cellular pattern as a function of age. Curr Eye Res. 1985;4:671–8.

153. Eghrari AO, Gottsch JD. Fuchs' corneal dystrophy. Expert Rev Ophthalmol. 2010;5:147–59.

154. Zoega GM, Fujisawa A, Sasaki H, Kubota A, Sasaki K, Kitagawa K, Jonasson F. Prevalence and risk factors for cornea guttata in the Reykjavik Eye Study. Ophthalmology. 2006;113:565–9. https://doi. org/10.1016/j.ophtha.2005.12.014.

155. Giasson CJ, Solomon LD, Polse KA. Morphometry of corneal endothelium in patients with corneal guttata. Ophthalmology. 2007;114:1469–75.

156. McCarey BE, Edelhauser HF, Lynn MJ. Review of corneal endothelial specular microscopy for FDA clinical trials of refractive procedures, surgical devices and new intraocular drugs and solutions. Cornea. 2008;27:1–16.

157. Schmitz LM, Safi T, Munteanu C, Seitz B, Daas L. Prevalence and severity of cornea guttata in the graft following Descemet Membrane Endothelial Keratoplasty (DMEK). Acta Ophthalmol. 2022;100(8):e1737–45. https://doi.org/10.1111/ aos.15195.

158. Schönit S, Maamri A, Zemova E, Munteanu C, Safi T, Daas L, Seitz B. Prevalence and impact of cornea guttata in the graft following penetrating keratoplasty in Germany. Cornea. 2022;41(12):1495–502. https://doi.org/10.1097/ICO.0000000000002971.

159. Nuzzi R, Boscia G, Marolo P, Ricardi F. The impact of artificial intelligence and deep learning in eye diseases: a review. Front Med. 2021;8:710329. https:// doi.org/10.3389/fmed.2021.710329.

160. Pels E, Rijneveld WJ. Organ culture preservation for corneal tissue. Technical and quality aspects. Dev Ophthalmol. 2009;43:31–46. https://doi. org/10.1159/000223837.

161. Kramp K, Suffo S, Laun D, Bischoff-Jung M, Huber M, Langenbucher A, Seitz B. Analysis of factors influencing the suitability of donor corneas in the LIONS Cornea Bank Saar-Lor-Lux, Trier/Westpfalz from 2006 to 2016. Klin Monbl Augenheilkd. 2020;237:1334–42.

162. Eye Bank Association of America (EBAA). 2019 eye bank statistical report. Washington, DC: EBAA; 2019. https://restoresight.org/wp-content/ uploads/2020/04/2019-EBAA-Stat-Report-FINAL. pdf. Accessed 24 Feb 2022.

163. Garcin T, Gauthier AS, Crouzet E, He Z, Herbepin P, Perrache C, Acquart S, Cognasse F, Forest F, Thuret G, Gain P. Innovative corneal active storage machine for long-term eye banking. Am J Transplant. 2019;19:1641–51. https://doi. org/10.1111/ajt.15238.

164. Garcin T, Gauthier AS, Crouzet E, He Z, Herbepin P, Perrache C, Acquart S, Cognasse F, Forest F, Gain P, Thuret G. Three-month storage of human corneas in an active storage machine. Transplantation. 2020;104:1159–65. https://doi.org/10.1097/ TP.0000000000003109.

165. Batista A, Breunig HG, König A, Schindele A, Hager T, Seitz B, Morgado AM, König K. Assessment of human corneas prior to transplantation using high-resolution two-photon imaging. Invest Ophthalmol Vis Sci. 2018;59:176–84. https://doi.org/10.1167/ iovs.17-22002.

Risk Classification and Management of Corneal Grafts, Human Leukocyte Antigen Matching, and Options for Immunosuppression Therapy

3

Paula W. Feng and Guillermo Amescua

Key Points
This chapter discusses:

- Risk factors affecting graft success in corneal transplantation
- The role of lymphangiogenesis in mediating graft rejection and associated mitigation strategies
- The role of Human leukocyte antigen (HLA) matching in donor selection and graft survival
- Topical and systemic strategies for prevention of corneal graft rejection
- Special considerations for immunosuppression limbal stem cell transplantation

Introduction

Corneal transplantation is the most common solid tissue transplant performed in humans. Over 180,000 transplants are performed annually worldwide [1, 2]. The cornea has traditionally been considered to have immune privilege, and although survival rates vary significantly depending on associated risk factors, low-risk transplants generally portend a high allograft survival rate. Proposed immune mechanisms responsible for this immune privilege include the cornea's relative absence of corneal lymph and blood vessels, relative lack of lymphatic drainage, diminished T-cell proliferation, and natural killer cell activation, allograft inducement of regulatory T-cells which inhibit the function and induction of alloimmune T-cells, protection from complement-mediated cytolysis, and induced apoptosis of neutrophils and T-cells at the graft-host interface [3, 4]. During implantation of corneal allografts, endothelial cells from allografts are theoretically sloughed off, enter the anterior chamber, and while there exposed to anti-inflammatory and immunosuppressive molecules. Antigen-specific suppression of delayed-type hypersensitivity responses, exclusion of complement-fixing antibodies, and preferential production of noncomplement-fixing antibody isotypes result from this exposure, promoting graft survival via a spectrum of immune responses known as anterior chamber autoimmune deviation (ACAID) [4].

However, immune privilege alone is insufficient to completely prevent corneal transplant rejection. Certain host risk factors increase the risk profile for corneal transplant rejection. For example, patients with ongoing ocular inflam-

Supplementary Information The online version contains supplementary material available at https://doi.org/10.1007/978-3-031-32408-6_3.

P. W. Feng · G. Amescua (✉)
Bascom Palmer Eye Institute, University of Miami, Miami, FL, USA
e-mail: gamescua@med.miami.edu

mation, preexisting corneal neovascularization, or a history of previous corneal graft rejection, among other risk factors, experience loss of immune privilege and have a high rate of immune rejection [4–6]. In the setting of ongoing inflammation, vascularization of the corneal bed alters multiple immune aspects, including lymphangiogenesis, antigen presentation, and anterior chamber-associated immune deviation. In solid organs, allospecific primed effector T-cells are recruited into the site of transplantation, a critical step in the rejection cascade. Early inflammation after surgery of vascularized organs causes more production of chemokines and late production of T-cell chemoattractants [7]. Among patients with such risk factors, the risk of acute rejection or graft failure can be similar to that seen in solid organ transplants. High-risk grafts have poor survival despite the use of systemic and topical immunosuppressive therapy [7, 8]. In the Collaborative Corneal Transplantation Study (CCTS), corneas with two or more quadrants of deep stromal vascularization or previous graft rejection were considered to be "high-risk" transplants [9]. In addition, we consider grafts in eyes with a history of HSV, VZV, uveitis, or atopy to be high-risk (see "Risk Factors" section below). Optimal management strategies for mitigating the risk of graft rejection must be taken into consideration in light of each patient's risk profile. In this chapter, we discuss the risk stratification of corneal transplants and consider strategies for immune suppression.

Risk Stratification

Risk Factors

Risk factors for an immune rejection or graft failure include primary diagnosis, increasing quadrants of host neovascularization, previous glaucoma, ocular inflammation or history of uveitis, herpetic infection, and previous graft failures, among others [10–12].

Table 3.1 Risk factors for corneal transplantation according to indication for transplantation and patient history

Minor	Major
Fuchs dystrophy	Infectious leukoma
Keratoconus, corneal ectasia	Chemical burn
Pseudophakic and aphakic corneal edema	Trauma
	HSV/VZV
	Previous transplantation
	Active inflammation
	Atopy
	Corneal neovascularization

Primary Diagnosis

One large retrospective study of 895 penetrating keratoplasties found that patients with keratoconus had the best 10-year survival outcome (95%), followed by endothelial and stromal dystrophies (55%), infectious leukomas (49%), trauma (33%), and chemical burns (14%) (Table 3.1) [13]. Given these widely varying results, it should be emphasized that graft survival varies widely based on the indication for transplantation. Other large cohorts of penetrating keratoplasties have found similar results, with the best survival for keratoconus and endothelial dystrophies and worse survival for patients with a history of anterior segment inflammation, herpetic infection, corneal neovascularization, and raised intraocular pressure [5, 10, 12, 14].

Previous Transplantation

This same large retrospective study demonstrated that the 10-year survival rate for primary penetrating keratoplasties was highest at 81%, followed by second grafts (33%), followed by third or more grafts (16%) [13]. The comparative immune privilege of the cornea and anterior chamber decrease with successive corneal grafts [4]. Pathogenic mechanisms include sensitization due to previous grafts and greater previous exposure of the recipient immune system to cornea-derived antigens, a heightened alloimmune response, and subsequent loss of immunological privilege, preceding recipient corneal neovascularization, and lymphangiogenesis, loss of avascularity, along with the higher likelihood of the presence of other risk factors predisposing to graft failure [15, 16]. See the sections below on active inflammation, the role of lymphangiogenesis, and anti-angiogenic and lymphangiogenic activity.

Glaucoma

The Cornea Donor Study was a multicenter prospective, double-masked, controlled clinical trial conducted at 80 clinical sites which followed 1090 moderate-risk corneal transplants, principally performed for pseudophakic or aphakic corneal edema or Fuchs dystrophy. History of glaucoma before penetrating keratoplasty was a significant risk factor for graft failure within 10 years. In one study, 58% of patients with previous glaucoma surgery and 22% without a history of glaucoma surgery or medication sustained graft failure within 10 years [6]. In the Australian Corneal Graft Registry (ACGR), a study of 1035 penetrating corneal grafts in Australia, elevated intraocular pressure was a common cause of graft failure [10]. In the Collaborative Corneal Transplantation Studies, glaucoma was also associated with an elevated chance of graft failure [17]. Glaucoma and ocular inflammation were both found to be independent risk factors for graft failure at 1 year in multivariate analysis by Tourkmani et al. as well [12].

Mechanisms for the association between glaucoma and graft failure are multifactorial. Elevated intraocular pressure after penetrating keratoplasty has been associated with accelerated chronic endothelial cell loss [18]. Direct endothelial compression due to elevated intraocular pressure has been proposed as a cause of endothelial cell loss [19–21]. In addition, in patients with acute or chronic angle closure

glaucoma, iridocorneal touch may cause endothelial trauma, disrupt the aqueous flow, induce hypoxia, and affect nutritional support to the endothelium [21–24]. It has additionally been hypothesized that toxicity from the chronic use of topical glaucoma medication and congenital alteration of the endothelium and trabecular meshwork may contribute to endothelial cell loss at baseline in glaucoma patients [21]. Additionally, glaucoma drainage implantation or filtration surgery is associated with significant loss of endothelial density. Studies have reported between 3 and 23% endothelial cell loss over 3 months to 3 years after glaucoma drainage implantations or filtration surgery [21]. The less the distance between a glaucoma shunt tube and the corneal endothelium, the greater the rate of endothelial cell attrition [25, 26]. Altered aqueous flow in the setting of glaucoma drainage implantation or trabeculectomy may theoretically also affect the nutritional support of the endothelium.

Active Inflammation

In patients who subsequently developed graft failure, histopathologic analysis of excised host corneas showed higher counts of leukocyte-common antigen, class II major histocompatibility complex antigens, myeloid-lineage markers, and peripheral T-cell markers. Higher leukocyte counts in recipient graft beds were correlated with subsequent graft failure [27]. In the Australian Corneal Graft Registry, patients with inflammation at the site of the graft or in the past at the graft site had a 9.6 relative risk of graft failure compared to those who had never been inflamed ($P < 0.001$) [10]. Lymphatic vessels are thought to regress earlier than blood vessels after acute inflammatory insults, suggesting that delaying transplantation after the resolution of inflammation may be of benefit [28]. In ideal circumstances, corneal transplantation should be avoided when the recipient eyes are actively inflamed [4].

Herpetic Infection

Past Herpes simplex eye and Herpes zoster disease are major risk factors for graft failure, and patients are at risk of disease reactivation after transplantation. In addition to having a higher rate of graft rejection, patients with a history of herpetic eye disease also demonstrate a higher rate of postkeratoplasty corneal neovascularization and corneal epithelial defects [29, 30]. In addition, immunosuppression with topical and oral steroids and steroid-sparing immunosuppressive therapy may lead to the reactivation of herpetic eye disease [31, 32]. Long-term maintenance high doses of oral antivirals for graft failure prophylaxis postkeratoplasty is recommended [29, 31, 33, 34]. In patients who do not receive antiviral prophylaxis, more than half of postpenetrating keratoplasty patients develop recurrence of herpetic stromal keratitis or graft rejection. Long-term antiviral therapy has been shown to reduce the rate of graft failure at 5 years by more than two-thirds compared to no prophylaxis [29, 35].

Neovascularization

Increasing quadrants of stromal neovascularization due to lymphangiogenesis and hemangiogenesis is associated with an increased likelihood of graft failure. In the ACGR, neovascularization of the graft was associated with a 6.8 relative risk of graft failure compared to no neovascularization ($P < 0.001$) [10]. This causes loss of the angiogenic privilege state of the host cornea. Blood vessels carry immune effector cells into the graft, and lymphatic vessels carry graft antigens that interact with host T-cells [16]. That removal of lymph nodes in mice enhances corneal graft survival suggests a role of lymphangiogenesis in mediating graft rejection [36]. See "Role of Lymphangiogenesis" and "Antiangiogenic and Lymphangiogenic Therapy" section.

Atopy

Patients with a history of atopy have a higher risk of rejection, perhaps due to the loss of immune privilege related to corneal inflammation at or before the time of transplantation unrelated to the allergy itself [4, 37–40]. Given the frequent co-occurrence of atopy with keratoconus, this is an especially important consideration in this group [41]. Patients with a history of atopic dermatitis have a higher rate of graft rejection, suggesting that systemic atopy may contribute to graft rejection [38]. In mouse models, exposure to airway allergens increases the likelihood of allograft rejection [42]. Mouse models have also demonstrated accelerated rejection of corneal transplants in mice with active allergic conjunctivitis at the time of transplantation [43]. Postkeratoplasty atopic sclerokeratitis can potentially have severe consequences, including loosening of running sutures and wound leakage, microbial suture abscess, persistent epithelial defects, and corneal perforation [44, 45]. Atopic rhinitis has been associated with spontaneous wound dehiscence after keratoplasty [46]. Although the reasons for this association are unclear, eye rubbing could be a potential contributor. Careful pre- and postoperative immunosuppression as well as control of atopic meibomian gland dysfunction and blepharitis with eyelid hygiene, warm compresses, and oral tetracyclines may lead to success in these cases [41, 47, 48]. Because of the risk of postkeroplasty atopic sclerokeratitis, patients should be closely monitored for control of atopy both before and after keratoplasty.

Aphakia

Data conflict on whether aphakia affects graft survival. The Australian Corneal Graft Registry found that aphakia before or after penetrating keratoplasty was associated with decreased survival [10]. However, no association between aphakia and graft survival was found in the

American Cornea Donor Study [6]. A retrospective study of penetrating keratoplasty found that aphakia was a significant risk factor for rejection and graft failure in univariate, but not multivariate analysis, after accounting for other risk factors [12].

Age

The Cornea Donor Study found an increased risk of graft failure in patient recipients over 70 compared to under 60 years of age, though the effect was moderate (29% vs. 19%, $P = 0.04$) [6]. The ACGR corroborated this trend; recipients over 50 years of age had a 3.0 relative risk of graft failure compared to those less than or equal to 50 years of age at transplantation ($P < 0.001$) [10].

Limbal Stem Cell Deficiency

In eyes with total limbal stem cell deficiency, secondary keratoplasty after keratolimbal allograft is associated with poor outcomes [16, 49–52]. A retrospective, noncomparative case series compared the long-term outcome of keratolimbal allograft and amniotic membrane transplantation with or without subsequent secondary penetrating keratoplasty. Keratolimbal allograft with amniotic membrane alone had significantly better visual outcomes than keratolimbal allograft with secondary penetrating keratoplasty; at 2 years, 86% versus 47% retained ambulatory vision in these groups, respectively [50, 53]. In the same study, central corneal graft survival was only 14% at 3 years in the secondary penetrating keratoplasty group. Given the poor prognosis and less-than-ideal visual outcomes, penetrating keratoplasty should be avoided in cases of total limbal stem cell deficiency even after a successful keratolimbal allograft. Although some studies have advocated waiting at least 9–12 months between keratolimbal allograft transplantation and secondary keratoplasty, similarly dismal

long-term success rates of penetrating keratoplasty have been reported [51, 52, 54]. In one such series, the majority of eyes developed glaucoma or ocular hypertension, and only half of the patients achieved any visual acuity gain after a mean follow-up time of 24 months [52]. Some suggest that lamellar keratoplasty after keratolimbal allograft transplantation may have more success than penetrating keratoplasty, but available data are limited to small case series [54]. In eyes with only partial limbal stem cell deficiency, keratoplasty may be carefully considered on a case-by-case basis.

Additional Factors

History of smoking was found to be associated with increased risk, as was African American background [6]. Most studies on graft failure are limited by short-term outcomes. One study examined at 500 consecutive PKs by a single surgeon. Over 20 years, the most common reason for graft failure over the long term was progressive endothelial cell loss and low endothelial cell count [5].

Mitigation Strategies for Corneal Graft Rejection

Role of Lymphangiogenesis

Lymphangiogenesis is a crucial role in the pathogenesis of graft rejection, as the outgrowth of new lymphatic vessels enables and hastens the exit of antigen-presenting cells, immunomodulatory cytokines, and memory T-cells from the graft to regional lymph nodes, leading to alloimmunization and subsequent rejection [55]. The significance of lymphangiogenesis is demonstrated by the fact that lymphadenectomy in mouse models of high-risk corneal transplantation results in increased survival of grafts. However, lymph node removal was ineffective in mice who had previous transplantation preoperatively, likely because they had already been allosensitized by the previous graft [36, 56]. However, such studies have not been replicated in humans, and this practice is uncommonly performed outside of experimental models. Molecular targets for inhibition of lymphangiogenesis, such as VEGF-receptor 3, are currently under investigation [55].

Anti-angiogenic and Lymphangiogenic Therapy

Topical and subconjunctival bevacizumab effectively reduces corneal neovascularization and causes regression of corneal vessels [57, 58].

In mouse models of corneal transplantation, the application of anti-vascular endothelial growth factor agents to corneal grafts preoperatively as well as postoperatively, or into recipient host beds, reduces hemangiognesis as well as lymphangiognesis, recruitment of mononuclear phagocytes into the graft, dendritic cell trafficking to draining lymph nodes, induction of delayed hypersensitivity reactions and improves graft survival [59–64].

In humans, one small retrospective case-control study of 37 eyes with preoperative corneal neovascularization covering at least one-quarter of the corneal surface compared patients who underwent 3 months of preoperative subconjunctival and/or intrastromal 5 mg/0.2 mL bevacizumab injections at the limbus before penetrating keratoplasty or deep anterior lamellar keratoplasty with patients who did not receive treatment. One-third of patients receiving bevacizumab treatment were able to completely avoid transplantation due to regression of the pathologic process. The remaining patients who received bevacizumab preoperatively and underwent transplantation had a higher graft survival rate (80%) compared to controls (64%). However, this improvement did not reach significance in this small sample ($P = 0.43$) [65]. Complicating the interpretation of the results of this study, 80% of the failures in the bevacizumab group had elevated intraocular pressure, which could have artificially elevated the potential rejection rate in the treatment group; confounding cannot be excluded.

A multicenter, prospective, randomized, placebo-controlled clinical trial examining the safety and efficacy of bevacizumab in high-risk corneal transplantation is currently underway. Preliminary data show that subconjunctival injection of 2.5 mg/0.1 mL bevacizumab at the time of surgery and topical 1% bevacizumab four times daily for 4 weeks postoperatively has a modest effect on reducing endothelial rejection and improving overall graft failure compared to placebo over 52 weeks of follow-up. However, the results did not reach significance in the small sample size ($n = 43$) presented [66].

Histocompatibility Matching

Human leukocyte antigen (HLA) matching has been shown to be effective in reducing the rejection rate and improving survival in solid organ transplants [67, 68]. Modern techniques for HLA typing are reliable, enabling HLA typing and matching among donors and recipients. However, there is no consensus on the cost efficacy and benefit of HLA matching in corneal graft survival, and the technique remains relatively underutilized.

The American Collaborative Corneal Transplantation Studies was a double-masked antigen masking study on the basis of HLA-A, -B, and -DR antigen matches conducted in the 1990s. The study did not demonstrate the benefit of HLA matching [9]. However, the success of this study may have been limited by the poorer reliability of more primitive typing techniques; in 55% of cases, serology-based tissue typing in this study differed from the results of molecular technique typing [15]. When recipients enrolled in this trial were later retyped as part of a quality assurance program, the agreement between the original and retyping laboratories was poor, especially for HLA-DR, which had structural similarities among DR3, DR5, and DR6 [69]. Subsequently, the Corneal Transplant Follow-up Study (CTFS) examined 2777 corneal grafts in the United Kingdom from 1987 to 1991 among

400 surgeons and yielded conflicting results. Poor HLA class I antigen matching was associated with an increased risk of rejection, but mismatched HLA-DR grafts had improved rejection rates over those with no mismatched HLA-DR grafts. The authors concluded that HLA-DR mismatching is associated with minimal harm at worst and should not be considered [70]. A later study suggested the utility of HLA-DR typing on 1681 transplants performed by a single surgeon based on a typing performed by a single experienced laboratory and suggested that the negative effect in the previous study was the result of laboratory technique and the accuracy of HLA typing. Simulations demonstrated that errors in as few as 5% of tissue types could sufficiently reduce the efficacy of HLA-DR matching [71]. Given the previous studies demonstrating poor reliability of typing techniques, some authors suggested retyping and verifying typing results at least once after initial testing [69].

Evidence suggests that HLA matching based on modern, reliable HLA typing techniques is likely to be of benefit, especially in high-risk grafts [71–73]. Additionally, efficacy has been demonstrated in HLA typing in limbal allogeneic stem cell transplantation. One prospective study of 12 eyes undergoing allogenic conjunctival transplantation found that eyes with incompatible HLA donor-recipient pairs were most likely to experience a rejection episode than those with matched HLA allotypes [74]. A retrospective, noncomparative case series of nine living-related donors, eight recipients (ten eyes) with the ocular surface disease found success with HLA-matched conjunctival limbal allografts, and the only two cases that experienced allograft rejection had two class I HLA mismatches [54]. The Cornea Transplant Follow-Up Study II (CTFS II) is a prospective, longitudinal clinical trial on the efficacy of HLA class II typing in improving the success of corneal transplantation which has completed enrollment and is currently underway [75].

In addition to the matching of major HLA antigens above, evidence has shown that matching of minor H-Y antigens is likely of benefit [76]. Indeed, a large retrospective study of over 17,000 endothelial, lamellar, and penetrating keratoplasties performed for moderate- and low-risk indications including Fuchs, keratoconus, infections, PBK, posttraumatic scars in inherited dystrophies, demonstrated that gender-matching between donors and recipients increased graft survival between 20 and 40% compared to nongender-matched donor-recipient pairs, likely on the basis of H-Y matching [77].

As another barrier to widespread adoption, the wait time for HLA-matched corneal grafts may be logistically prohibitive for at least some transplants, including high-risk transplants necessitating urgent intervention, which may most benefit from HLA matching [78]. A simulated model of wait times based on data from the Cornea Lions Bank in Germany suggested that waiting for zero mismatches would result in an estimated average wait time of 17 ± 14 months, whereas waiting for as many as two mismatches would result in a wait time of 1 ± 3 months [78]. With increasing numbers of corneal transplants performed each year, low donor availability and high wait times can be expected to increase [79]. An algorithm has been proposed that can help balance waiting times and histocompatibility for patients with rare HLA phenotypes [80]. Since it is thought that HLA typing improves long-term graft survival, HLA typing of major and minor histocompatibility antigens could conceivably become a highly cost-effective strategy by reducing the need for care of corneal graft rejections and repeat transplantation [81].

Strategies for Immunosuppression

Topical Therapy

Steroids

Topical steroids are a mainstay of immunosuppressive therapy after corneal transplantation. The overwhelming majority of practitioners use topical steroids for at least 6 months postoperatively, which likely explains the low rate of graft rejection during this period [82, 83]. In addition, a survey by United States-based Cornea Society revealed that 75% of cornea specialists who responded to the survey used intraoperative subconjunctival corticosteroids for avascular corneas receiving penetrating keratoplasty, and 68% said they did so for endothelial keratoplasty [83]. The overwhelming majority of cornea specialists surveyed preferred prednisolone, likely at least in part due to its ubiquitous availability in the United States, and a minority used fluoroethylene, loteprednol, or difluorinated. The latter was most commonly used in high-risk eyes, and loteprednol use increased after 6 months postoperatively, likely to reduce the effect of intraocular pressure [83]. In addition, long-term usage of topical steroids significantly decreases the risk of graft rejection and increases the cumulative survival rate of corneal grafts without any episode of endothelial allograft rejection [84, 85]. However, risks of long-term topical steroid use include the development of cataracts and glaucoma, the latter of which is a risk factor for graft failure [86]. Patients should be monitored long-term for the development of late graft rejection as well as treatment side effects from prolonged use of anti-inflammatory medication.

Cyclosporine

Cyclosporine binds cyclophilin, which inhibits IL-2 transcription, which suppresses T-cell activation and subsequent graft rejection [87]. Topical cyclosporine A 0.05% and 0.09% is commonly available for the treatment of dry eye, posterior blepharitis, ocular rosacea, atopic keratoconjunctivitis, graft-versus-host disease, and herpetic stromal keratitis, among other uses [88]. Higher dosages such as cyclosporine A 2% and 5% have been utilized for immunosuppression after corneal transplantation. A recent meta-analysis of four small randomized clinical trials and a retrospective cohort study examined supplemental topical cyclosporine treatment in addition to postoperative topical corticosteroids in penetrating keratoplasty. Supplemental cyclosporine led to an overall benefit in rejection-free graft survival at 12-months and 24-months postoperatively in both high-risk and normal populations of penetrating keratoplasties [87, 89–92]. Most studies in the meta-analysis utilized cyclosporine A 2%. In the two studies in this meta-analysis that used cyclosporine A 0.05% (Restasis, Allergan), there was no improvement on graft survival or rates of rejection [90, 91]. When cyclosporine 0.05% was substituted for prednisolone after 13-weeks posttransplant in low-risk transplants, there was a higher rate of rejection and rejection occurred earlier.

According to the Cornea Society survey, about 13–14% of respondents use cyclosporine routinely for penetrating and endothelial keratoplasty, respectively. This number increases to 48% and 40% in high-risk penetrating and endothelial keratoplasties, respectively [83]. Higher doses of topical cyclosporine A such as cyclosporine A 2% over 0.05% may be necessary to achieve the desired immunosuppressive effect for graft rejection prophylaxis. Based on current randomized clinical trials and meta-analyses, there is insufficient evidence to support the usage of topical cyclosporine A at any concentration in resolving or reversing acute rejection episodes [87, 89, 91].

Tacrolimus

Tacrolimus (FK506) is a macrolide antibiotic. Its mechanism of action is in suppression calcineurin, which, like cyclosporine A, then inhibits T-cell activation and subsequent T-cell signal transduction and IL-2 transcription, affecting the downstream release of cytokines such as interleukins, TNF-alpha, interferon-gamma [16, 93]. In addition, topical and systemic tacrolimus effectively cause regression of neovascularization and decreased VEGF expression in neovascularized murine corneas [94]. Topical tacrolimus effectively penetrates the cornea into the aqueous humor [93, 95]. Topical tacrolimus 0.03% is FDA-approved for atopic dermatitis and has been used off-label, and has been shown to be safe and effective in a variety of ophthalmic conditions such as atopic and vernal keratoconjunctivitis [96–98], necrotizing and nodular scleritis [99], Mooren ulcer [99], keratoconjunctivitis sicca due to Sjogren's syndrome [100, 101], ocular cicatricial pemphigoid [99], Stevens-Johnson syndrome [99], graft-versus-host disease [102], and superior limbic keratoconjunctivitis [93]. There have been no adverse effects reported with long-term use [103–105].

Topical 0.03% tacrolimus was effective in preventing corneal graft rejection in a retrospective cohort of 72 high-risk eyes which had undergone more than one penetrating keratoplasty in the same eye or had a severe chemical burn (Video 3.1). The patients receiving topical tacrolimus 0.03% twice daily had half the graft rejection rate compared to topical prednisolone alone [106].

Compared to cyclosporine, there is greater among of and stronger evidence for the usage of topical tacrolimus in preventing as well as reversing graft rejection in high-risk keratoplasty. However, the current evidence is of moderate quality and limited by small sample sizes and lack of blinding in randomized controlled trials. A randomized, prospective clinical trial of 49 eyes by Zhai and colleagues in high-risk penetrating keratoplasty compared the addition of tacrolimus 0.1% versus cyclosporine 1% to traditional therapy with tobramycin-dexamethasone for 3 weeks postoperatively. Patients were followed for an average of 23–24 months. In the tacrolimus group, the graft rejection rate was 16% and there were no irreversible graft rejections. In the cyclosporine group, the graft rejection rate was 45.8% ($P = 0.02$) [107]. Dhaliwal and colleagues presented a prospective case series of four eyes that underwent high-risk penetrating keratoplasty and had all developed steroid-induced glaucoma and had failed traditional immunosuppressant therapy. All four cases developed acute rejection which reversed with topical tacrolimus treatment at 0.03% twice daily. Patients were followed for 26–48 months, and none developed any repeat episodes of graft rejection [105].

In a prospective, randomized clinical trial of repeat penetrating keratoplasty comparing treatment with topical tacrolimus versus oral mycophenolate in addition to standard treatment with topical and oral corticosteroids, topical tacrolimus was equally effective as oral mycophenolate in preventing graft rejection at 1 year ($P = 0.74$) [108].

In a prospective case series of normal-risk penetrating keratoplasties, tacrolimus 0.06% was compared to traditional therapy with topical corticosteroids. The tacrolimus group had a 0% rejection rate at 12 months, compared to 16% in the control group, a small difference that did not reach significance in this small study ($P = 0.9$, $n = 40$). Larger series may be necessary to adequately assess the efficacy of topical tacrolimus in the immunosuppression of normal-risk grafts, given the high graft success rates in this population.

In the author's opinion, based on current evidence, topical tacrolimus is a relatively underutilized and likely effective immunosuppressive therapy for a variety of eye diseases as well as in immunosuppression of high-risk keratoplasty.

Systemic Therapy

Cyclosporine

Cyclosporine A is a protein derived from fungi. Systemic cyclosporine A increases graft survival in high-risk corneal transplantation. Risks of this medication are significant, and include hypertension, renal toxicity, neurotoxicity, hepatotoxicity, and posttransplant lymphoproliferative disorders [109–112].

A meta-analysis of 16 studies examining the utilization of systemic cyclosporine A in high-risk keratoplasty studied 518 patients using systemic cyclosporine for postkeratoplasty immunosuppression and 299 controls with a mean postoperative follow-up period of 26.5 ± 12.9 months. In the studies with 3 years or more of follow-up, 66% of rejection episodes were successfully reversed in patients on systemic cyclosporine A, compared to 27.8% in controls ($P = 0.02$) [113]. The study conducted a meta-analysis of ten studies that had 1-year or longer follow-up data and found that the odds ratio for clear graft survival in patients receiving cyclosporine versus controls was 2.43 (95% CI: 1.00–5.88, $I^2 = 37.9\%$) and 3.64 for rejection-free episodes (95% CI: 1.48–8.91, $I^2 = 64.8\%$) [113] Individual studies may be limited by low power, however, the meta-analysis provides strong evidence for the benefit of systemic cyclosporine administration.

A randomized control trial of 38 high-risk eyes trialed the usage of systemic cyclosporine and topical steroid in 20 patients, compared with 18 patients who only received topical steroid for postkeratoplasty immunosuppression. No difference was found in graft survival or rejection among both groups, but the rate of graft rejection was extremely low in the study, with only one rejection in the control group and none in the treatment group [114]. Another randomized control trial of 40 high-risk corneal transplants found no differences in the rates of graft clarity loss or endothelial rejection among patients receiving systemic cyclosporine in combination with systemic steroids, compared to a control group that received topical steroids alone [115].

Mycophenolate

Mycophenolate mofetil is an antimetabolite, the morpholinoethylester of mycophenolenic acid. It inhibits inosine monophosphate dehydrogenase and T- and B-lymphocyte proliferation. Common side effects include gastric discomfort, myelosuppression, and gingival hyperplasia. Thus, regular monitoring of complete blood counts is recommended [116–118]. A meta-analysis of four studies examining the usage of systemic mycophenolate mofetil in high-risk corneal transplantation found that mycophenolate mofetil increased the reversibility of rejection episodes to 91.7% compared to 52.05% in the control group ($P = 0.01$) [113].

A prospective, multicenter, randomized trial examined the efficacy of mycophenolate in high-risk penetrating keratoplasties. In the control group, 41 patients received fluocortolone 1 mg/kg/day tapered over 3 weeks, topical prednisolone acetate 5×/day tapered over 5 months. The mycophenolate group received all the same medications as controls in addition mycophenolate 1 g twice daily for 6 months. Mycophenolate mofetil improved rejection-free graft survival. Over a mean follow-up time of 34.9 ± 16.3 months, immune-reaction-free graft survival was 83% in the mycophenolate group and 64.5% in the control group ($P = 0.04$). The control group had five

reversible and seven irreversible graft rejections, compared to six reversible, and two irreversible graft rejections in the mycophenolate group. However, the rate of adverse events in the mycophenolate group was considerable; the majority (63%) in the mycophenolate group experienced mostly reversible adverse events including gastrointestinal disturbances, infections such as bronchitis, pneumonia, oral candidiasis, elevated liver enzymes, weight loss or gain, paresthesias, and others. Irreversible adverse events in this study included myocardial infarction and malignancies such as prostate gland and gladder carcinoma in a small minority of subjects [119].

A randomized trial of patients with recurrent herpetic keratitis who underwent penetrating keratoplasty studied the effect of prophylactic acyclovir 200 mg five times/day for 3 weeks postoperatively, for 1 year postoperatively and the addition of mycophenolate 1 g BID for 1 year in addition to acyclovir. Graft rejection was decreased with the addition of mycophenolate mofetil [120].

Another randomized multicenter trial studied 86 patients undergoing high-risk penetrating keratoplasty, of whom 38 controls received fluocortolone 1 mg/kg body weight/day, tapered within 3 weeks, and topical prednisolone 1% tapered within 5 months, and the treatment group additionally received mycophenolate daily 2 × 1 g for the first six postoperative months. The mycophenolate group had higher graft survival and fewer rejection episodes [116].

Mycophenolate vs. Cyclosporine

In two randomized clinical trials comparing mycophenolate versus cyclosporine, there was no difference in graft rejection among both groups [117, 121].

A meta-analysis assessed four studies which compared the efficacy of mycophenolate mofetil and cyclosporine A in graft survival after high-risk penetrating keratoplasty. In the meta-analysis, 278 patients received mycophenolate mofetil, and 304 patients received cyclosporine A for postoperative immunosuppression over a mean follow-up time of 24.3 ± 12.7 months. In the meta-analysis, mycophenolate appears to have had a slightly higher rejection-free and clear graft survival rate compared to cyclosporine (88.6% and 97.3%, respectively, compared to 88.8% and 88.6%, respectively), but no statistical analysis was provided.

Retrospective studies comparing systemic mycophenolate mofetil and cyclosporine A have shown similar results [119]. A retrospective study of 417 high-risk keratoplasties receiving systemic cyclosporine at blood trough levels of 120–150 ng/mL or mycophenolate at a daily dose of 1 g twice daily found that patients receiving mycophenolate were less likely to experience graft rejection (72% rejection-free graft survival) compared to cyclosporine (60%) at 3 years. Clear graft survival was 87% in the mycophenolate group and 77% in the cyclosporine group at 3 years. This was statistically significant [118].

Based on these data, there is no convincing evidence of the superiority of mycophenolate versus cyclosporine in high-risk penetrating keratoplasty.

Tacrolimus

There is little evidence on systemic tacrolimus in high-risk keratoplasty, and case series are limited by lack of controls. A noncomparative case series of 17 high-risk corneal and limbal grafts treated with oral tacrolimus found that no patient had irreversible graft rejection while receiving tacrolimus, while three patients had reversible graft rejection in the setting of low levels of tacrolimus [122]. Another case series explored the effect of systemic tacrolimus on ten high-risk penetrating keratoplasties which developed graft failure while on treatment with systemic cyclosporine. After treatment with tacrolimus, there were significantly fewer episodes of graft rejection ($P = 0.03$) and longer graft survival on Kaplan-Meier survival plots ($P = 0.04$) [122].

Selecting Immunosuppression According to Risk Stratification

Despite the large plethora of immunosuppressive therapies available, no standardized protocol has been proposed for corneal immunosuppression, likely because much of the above evidence is of moderate quality and limited by small study sizes. For ocular surface limbal stem cell transplantation, the Cincinnati protocol was highly effective in a retrospective study of 225 eyes [123]. Additionally, there is scant evidence for the role of immunosuppression in the highest-risk patients and those with severe graft rejection. Nevertheless, immunosuppression is widely utilized in such patients in order to provide the highest theoretical probability of graft survival.

Special Considerations for Limbal Stem Cell Transplantation

Traditionally, limbal stem cell transplantation has relied on allogeneic or, in the case of keratolimbal allograft, cadaveric limbal stem cell allografts, which require systemic immunosuppression due to highly vascularized and immunogenic donor tissue. The need for systemic immunosuppression limits recipients to those who can safely receive immunosuppression. Elderly patients and patients with comorbidities such as obesity, diabetes, cardiac, liver, or renal disease are not candidates [50, 123–126]. Due to the need for long-term systemic immunosuppression, allogeneic simple limbal epithelial transportation (SLET) should be performed with caution in children [127]. Preliminary studies suggest the success of allogeneic simple limbal epithelial transplantation with less intensive or minimal immunotherapy, but no long-term data are available [128, 129].

Living-related conjunctival limbal allografts rely on conjunctival and limbal tissue derived from an HLA-matched living relative and may have a lower rate of rejection by reducing the potential antigenic burden of the allograft [50, 130, 131].

Cultivated limbal epithelial transplantation is a modern advancement that requires shorter-term immunosuppression [132]. Because allogeneic donor DNA material is not present 9 months following transplantation [133], and the volume of tissue transplanted is smaller. Cultivated limbal epithelial transplantation only requires immunosuppression for a year.

Autologous limbal autografts do not carry the risk of immunoreactivity and thus bypass the need for immunosuppression [132, 134, 135].

Conclusion

Corneal transplantation is overall a highly successful procedure, with a low risk of graft rejection. Certain risk factors can alter immune privilege and increase the risk of rejection. Human leukocyte antigen matching has been shown to be useful in large series in which typing was performed by experienced laboratories, but larger-scale studies have failed to show benefit, potentially due to a high error rate in serological typing. In addition to traditional treatment with topical and systemic corticosteroids, topical tacrolimus and cyclosporine, and systemic cyclosporine, mycophenolate, and tacrolimus may be useful adjuncts in improving graft survival. Future work remains to be done in exploring the benefit of these promising therapies and antigen matching in improving graft survival.

Take Home Notes
- Fuchs dystrophy, keratoconus, corneal ectasias, pseudophakic, and aphakic corneal edema are primary transplant indications associated with high rates of corneal transplant survival. Risk factors for corneal transplant failure include a history of infectious leukoma, chemical burn, trauma, HSV/VZV, previous transplantation, glaucoma, active inflammation at the time of transplantation, atopy, and corneal neovascularization, among others.
- Lymphangiogenesis plays a crucial role in the pathogenesis of graft rejection. Anti-angiogenic and lymphangiogenic therapy have demonstrated promise in animal and human studies in reducing graft rejection rate.
- Human leukocyte antigen (HLA) matching has been shown to be effective in reducing the rejection rate and improving survival in solid organ transplants but may be costly and logistically prohibitive for many transplant centers.
- Topical therapy with steroids, cyclosporine, tacrolimus, and systemic therapy with cyclosporine, mycophenolate, and tacrolimus and their efficacy in corneal graft rejection prophylaxis are reviewed.
- Limbal stem cell transplantation and the recommended strategies for immunosuppression are discussed.

References

1. Williams KA, Brereton HM, Coster DJ. Prospects for genetic modulation of corneal graft survival. Eye (Lond). 2009;23(10):1904–9. https://doi.org/10.1038/eye.2008.378.
2. Gain P, Jullienne R, He Z, et al. Global survey of corneal transplantation and eye banking. JAMA Ophthalmol. 2016;134(2):167–73. https://doi.org/10.1001/jamaophthalmol.2015.4776.
3. van Essen TH, Roelen DL, Williams KA, Jager MJ. Matching for human leukocyte antigens (HLA) in corneal transplantation – to do or not to do. Prog Retin Eye Res. 2015;46:84–110. https://doi.org/10.1016/j.preteyeres.2015.01.001.
4. Niederkorn JY, Larkin DFP. Immune privilege of corneal allografts. Ocul Immunol Inflamm. 2010;18(3):162–71. https://doi.org/10.3109/09273948.2010.486100.
5. Patel SV, Diehl NN, Hodge DO, Bourne WM. Donor risk factors for graft failure in a 20-year study of penetrating keratoplasty. Arch Ophthalmol. 2010;128(4):418–25. https://doi.org/10.1001/archophthalmol.2010.27.
6. Writing Committee for the Cornea Donor Study Research Group, Sugar A, Gal RL, et al. Factors associated with corneal graft survival in the cornea donor study. JAMA Ophthalmol. 2015;133(3):246–54. https://doi.org/10.1001/jamaophthalmol.2014.3923.
7. Amescua G, Collings F, Sidani A, et al. Effect of CXCL-1/KC production in high risk vascularized corneal allografts on T cell recruitment and graft rejection. Transplantation. 2008;85(4):615–25. https://doi.org/10.1097/TP.0b013e3181636d9d.

8. Coster DJ, Williams KA. Management of high-risk corneal grafts. Eye (Lond). 2003;17(8):996–1002. https://doi.org/10.1038/sj.eye.6700634.

9. Collaborative Corneal Transplantation Studies Research Group. The Collaborative Corneal Transplantation Studies (CCTS): effectiveness of histocompatibility matching in high-risk corneal transplantation. Arch Ophthalmol. 1992;110(10):1392–403. https://doi.org/10.1001/archopht.1992.01080220054021.

10. Williams KA, Roder D, Esterman A, Muehlberg SM, Coster DJ. Factors predictive of corneal graft survival. Report from the Australian Corneal Graft Registry. Ophthalmology. 1992;99(3):403–14. https://doi.org/10.1016/s0161-6420(92)31960-8.

11. Thompson RW Jr, Price MO, Bowers PJ, Price FW. Long-term graft survival after penetrating keratoplasty. Ophthalmology. 2003;110(7):1396–402. https://doi.org/10.1016/S0161-6420(03)00463-9.

12. Tourkmani AK, Sánchez-Huerta V, De Wit G, et al. Weighing of risk factors for penetrating keratoplasty graft failure: application of Risk Score System. Int J Ophthalmol. 2017;10(3):372–7. https://doi.org/10.18240/ijo.2017.03.08.

13. Barraquer RI, Pareja-Aricò L, Gómez-Benlloch A, Michael R. Risk factors for graft failure after penetrating keratoplasty. Medicine. 2019;98(17):e15274. https://doi.org/10.1097/MD.0000000000015274.

14. Williams KA, Muehlberg SM, Lewis RF, Coster DJ. Long-term outcome in corneal allotransplantation. Transplant Proc. 1997;29(1–2):983. https://doi.org/10.1016/S0041-1345(96)00335-1.

15. Armitage WJ, Goodchild C, Griffin MD, et al. High-risk corneal transplantation: recent developments and future possibilities. Transplantation. 2019;103(12):2468–78. https://doi.org/10.1097/TP.0000000000002938.

16. Di Zazzo A, Kheirkhah A, Abud TB, Goyal S, Dana R. Management of high-risk corneal transplantation. Surv Ophthalmol. 2017;62(6):816–27. https://doi.org/10.1016/j.survophthal.2016.12.010.

17. Maguire MG, Stark WJ, Gottsch JD, et al. Risk factors for corneal graft failure and rejection in the collaborative corneal transplantation studies. Collaborative Corneal Transplantation Studies Research Group. Ophthalmology. 1994;101(9):1536–47. https://doi.org/10.1016/s0161-6420(94)31138-9.

18. Reinhard T, Böhringer D, Sundmacher R. Accelerated chronic endothelial cell loss after penetrating keratoplasty in glaucoma eyes. J Glaucoma. 2001;10(6):446–51. https://doi.org/10.1097/00061198-200112000-00002.

19. Cho SW, Kim JM, Choi CY, Park KH. Changes in corneal endothelial cell density in patients with normal-tension glaucoma. Jpn J Ophthalmol. 2009;53(6):569–73. https://doi.org/10.1007/s10384-009-0740-1.

20. Gagnon MM, Boisjoly HM, Brunette I, Charest M, Amyot M. Corneal endothelial cell density in glaucoma. Cornea. 1997;16(3):314–8.

21. Janson BJ, Alward WL, Kwon YH, et al. Glaucoma-associated corneal endothelial cell damage: a review. Surv Ophthalmol. 2018;63(4):500–6. https://doi.org/10.1016/j.survophthal.2017.11.002.

22. Ferreira TB, Ribeiro FJ, Silva D, Matos AC, Gaspar S, Almeida S. Comparison of refractive and visual outcomes of three presbyopia-correcting intraocular lenses. J Cataract Refract Surg. 2022;48(3):280–7. https://doi.org/10.1097/j.jcrs.0000000000000743.

23. Jonas JB, Aung T, Bourne RR, Bron AM, Ritch R, Panda-Jonas S. Glaucoma. Lancet. 2017;390(10108):2183–93. https://doi.org/10.1016/S0140-6736(17)31469-1.

24. Chen M-J, Liu CJ-L, Cheng C-Y, Lee S-M. Corneal status in primary angle-closure glaucoma with a history of acute attack. J Glaucoma. 2012;21(1):12–6. https://doi.org/10.1097/IJG.0b013e3181fc800a.

25. Tan AN, Webers CAB, Berendschot TTJM, et al. Corneal endothelial cell loss after Baerveldt glaucoma drainage device implantation in the anterior chamber. Acta Ophthalmol. 2017;95(1):91–6. https://doi.org/10.1111/aos.13161.

26. Koo EB, Hou J, Han Y, Keenan JD, Stamper RL, Jeng BH. Effect of glaucoma tube shunt parameters on cornea endothelial cells in patients with ahmed valve implants. Cornea. 2015;34(1):37. https://doi.org/10.1097/ICO.0000000000000301.

27. Williams KA, White MA, Ash JK, Coster DJ. Leukocytes in the graft bed associated with corneal graft failure. Analysis by immunohistology and actuarial graft survival. Ophthalmology. 1989;96(1):38–44. https://doi.org/10.1016/s0161-6420(89)32949-6.

28. Cursiefen C, Maruyama K, Jackson DG, Streilein JW, Kruse FE. Time course of angiogenesis and lymphangiogenesis after brief corneal inflammation. Cornea. 2006;25(4):443. https://doi.org/10.1097/01.ico.0000183485.85636.ff.

29. Goodfellow JFB, Nabili S, Jones MNA, et al. Antiviral treatment following penetrating keratoplasty for herpetic keratitis. Eye. 2011;25(4):470–4. https://doi.org/10.1038/eye.2010.237.

30. Halberstadt M, Machens M, Gahlenbek KA, Böhnke M, Garweg JG. The outcome of corneal grafting in patients with stromal keratitis of herpetic and non-herpetic origin. Br J Ophthalmol. 2002;86(6):646. https://doi.org/10.1136/bjo.86.6.646.

31. Gessa-Sorroche M, Kanclerz P, Alio J. Evidence in the prevention of the recurrence of herpes simplex and herpes zoster keratitis after eye surgery. Archivos De La Sociedad Española De Oftalmología Engl Ed. 2022;97(3):149–60. https://doi.org/10.1016/j.oftale.2022.02.003.

32. Lee JJ, Kim MK, Wee WR. Adverse effects of low-dose systemic cyclosporine therapy in high-risk penetrating keratoplasty. Graefes Arch Clin Exp Ophthalmol. 2015;253(7):1111–9. https://doi.org/10.1007/s00417-015-3008-0.

33. Abdelmassih Y, Dubrulle P, Sitbon C, et al. Therapeutic challenges and prognosis of Descemet's

membrane endothelial keratoplasty in herpes simplex eye disease. Cornea. 2019;38(5):553–8. https://doi.org/10.1097/ico.0000000000001891.

34. Tambasco FP, Cohen EJ, Nguyen LH, Rapuano CJ, Laibson PR. oral acyclovir after penetrating keratoplasty for herpes simplex keratitis. Arch Ophthalmol. 1999;117(4):445–9. https://doi.org/10.1001/archopht.117.4.445.

35. Sterk CC, Jager MJ, Swart M, Berg VD. Recurrent herpetic keratitis in penetrating keratoplasty. Doc Ophthalmol. 1995;90(1):29–33. https://doi.org/10.1007/bf01203291.

36. Plšková J, Holáň V, Filipec M, Forrester JV. Lymph node removal enhances corneal graft survival in mice at high risk of rejection. BMC Ophthalmol. 2004;4:3.

37. Küchle M, Cursiefen C, Nguyen NX, et al. Risk factors for corneal allograft rejection: intermediate results of a prospective normal-risk keratoplasty study. Graefes Arch Clin Exp Ophthalmol. 2002;240(7):580–4. https://doi.org/10.1007/s00417-002-0496-5.

38. Nguyen NX, Martus P, Seitz B, Cursiefen C. Atopic dermatitis as a risk factor for graft rejection following normal-risk keratoplasty. Graefes Arch Clin Exp Ophthalmol. 2009;247(4):573–4. https://doi.org/10.1007/s00417-008-0959-4.

39. Watson SL, Tuft SJ, Dart JKG. Patterns of rejection after deep lamellar keratoplasty. Ophthalmology. 2006;113(4):556–60. https://doi.org/10.1016/j.ophtha.2006.01.006.

40. Reinhard T, Möller M, Sundmacher R. Penetrating keratoplasty in patients with atopic dermatitis with and without systemic cyclosporin A. Cornea. 1999;18(6):645–51. https://doi.org/10.1097/00003226-199911000-00003.

41. Shimmura-Tomita M, Shimmura S, Satake Y, et al. Keratoplasty postoperative treatment update. Cornea. 2013;32:S60. https://doi.org/10.1097/ICO.0b013e3182a2c937.

42. Niederkorn JY, Chen PW, Mellon J, Stevens C, Mayhew E. Allergic airway hyperreactivity increases the risk for corneal allograft rejection. Am J Transplant. 2009;9(5):1017–26.

43. Flynn TH, Ohbayashi M, Ikeda Y, Ono SJ, Larkin DF. Effect of allergic conjunctival inflammation on the allogeneic response to donor cornea. Invest Ophthalmol Vis Sci. 2007;48(9):4044–9. https://doi.org/10.1167/iovs.06-0973.

44. Tomita M, Shimmura S, Tsubota K, Shimazaki J. Postkeratoplasty atopic sclerokeratitis in keratoconus patients. Ophthalmology. 2008;115(5):851–6. https://doi.org/10.1016/j.ophtha.2007.07.018.

45. Lyons CJ, Dart JKG, Aclimandos WA, Lightman S, Buckley RJ. Sclerokeratitis after keratoplasty in atopy. Ophthalmology. 1990;97(6):729–33. https://doi.org/10.1016/S0161-6420(90)32523-X.

46. Jayaram H, Falcon MG. Atopic rhinitis: a risk factor for spontaneous wound dehiscence following removal of a continuous penetrating keratoplasty suture. Graefes Arch Clin Exp Ophthalmol. 2005;243(9):958–9. https://doi.org/10.1007/s00417-005-1136-7.

47. Ghoraishi M, Akova YA, Tugal-Tutkun I, Foster CS. Penetrating keratoplasty in atopic keratoconjunctivitis. Cornea. 1995;14(6):610–3.

48. Geggel HS. Successful penetrating keratoplasty in a patient with severe atopic keratoconjunctivitis and elevated serum IgE level treated with long-term topical cyclosporin A. Cornea. 1994;13(6):543.

49. Solomon A, Ellies P, Anderson DF, et al. Long-term outcome of keratolimbal allograft with or without penetrating keratoplasty for total limbal stem cell deficiency. Ophthalmology. 2002;109(6):1159–66.

50. Atallah MR, Palioura S, Perez VL, Amescua G. Limbal stem cell transplantation: current perspectives. Clin Ophthalmol. 2016;10:593–602. https://doi.org/10.2147/OPTH.S83676.

51. Ozer MD, Altinkurt E, Alparslan N. The long-term surgical outcomes of conjunctival-limbal autograft procedure with or without penetrating keratoplasty in eyes with unilateral limbal stem cell deficiency. Taiwan J Ophthalmol. 2020;10(1):22–8. https://doi.org/10.4103/tjo.tjo_55_19.

52. Krysik K, Dobrowolski D, Tarnawska D, Wylegala E, Lyssek-Boroń A. Long-term outcomes of allogeneic ocular surface reconstruction: keratolimbal allograft (KLAL) followed by penetrating keratoplasty (PK). J Ophthalmol. 2020;2020:5189179. https://doi.org/10.1155/2020/5189179.

53. Solomon A, Pires RT, Tseng SC. Amniotic membrane transplantation after extensive removal of primary and recurrent pterygia. Ophthalmology. 2001;108(3):449–60. https://doi.org/10.1016/s0161-6420(00)00567-4.

54. Daya SM, Ilari FA. Living related conjunctival limbal allograft for the treatment of stem cell deficiency. Ophthalmology. 2001;108(1):126–33. https://doi.org/10.1016/s0161-6420(00)00475-9; discussion 133–4.

55. Cursiefen C, Chen L, Dana MR, Streilein JW. Corneal lymphangiogenesis: evidence, mechanisms, and implications for corneal transplant immunology. Cornea. 2003;22(3):273.

56. Yamagami S, Dana MR. The critical role of lymph nodes in corneal alloimmunization and graft rejection. Invest Ophthalmol Vis Sci. 2001;42(6):1293–8.

57. Bahar I, Kaiserman I, McAllum P, Rootman D, Slomovic A. Subconjunctival bevacizumab injection for corneal neovascularization in recurrent pterygium. Curr Eye Res. 2009. https://doi.org/10.1080/02713680701799101.

58. Kim SW, Ha BJ, Kim EK, Tchah H, Kim T-I. The effect of topical bevacizumab on corneal neovascularization. Ophthalmology. 2008;115(6):e33–8. https://doi.org/10.1016/j.ophtha.2008.02.013.

59. Bachmann BO, Bock F, Wiegand SJ, et al. Promotion of graft survival by vascular endothelial growth factor a neutralization after high-risk corneal transplan-

tation. Arch Ophthalmol. 2008;126(1):71–7. https://doi.org/10.1001/archopht.126.1.71.

60. Chen L, Hamrah P, Cursiefen C, et al. Vascular endothelial growth factor receptor-3 mediates induction of corneal alloimmunity. Nat Med. 2004;10(8):813–5. https://doi.org/10.1038/nm1078.

61. Zhang W, Schönberg A, Hamdorf M, Georgiev T, Cursiefen C, Bock F. Preincubation of donor tissue with a VEGF cytokine trap promotes subsequent high-risk corneal transplant survival. Br J Ophthalmol. 2022;106(11):1617–26. https://doi.org/10.1136/bjophthalmol-2021-319745.

62. Su W, Sun S, Tian B, et al. Efficacious, safe, and stable inhibition of corneal neovascularization by AAV-vectored anti-VEGF therapeutics. Mol Ther Methods Clin Dev. 2021;22:107–21. https://doi.org/10.1016/j.omtm.2021.06.007.

63. Salabarria A-C, Braun G, Heykants M, et al. Local VEGF-A blockade modulates the microenvironment of the corneal graft bed. Am J Transplant. 2019;19(9):2446–56. https://doi.org/10.1111/ajt.15331.

64. Dohlman TH, Omoto M, Hua J, et al. VEGF-trap aflibercept significantly improves long-term graft survival in high-risk corneal transplantation. Transplantation. 2015;99(4):678–86. https://doi.org/10.1097/TP.0000000000000512.

65. Fasciani R, Crincoli E, Mosca L, Guccione L, Caristia A, Rizzo S. Role of pre-transplant corneal injective anti VEGF treatment in high risk transplantation corneas. 2021. https://doi.org/10.21203/rs.3.rs-246503/v1.

66. Stodola E. Applications for bevacizumab in corneal surgery. EyeWorld. 2021.

67. Opelz G, Döhler B. Effect of human leukocyte antigen compatibility on kidney graft survival: comparative analysis of two decades. Transplantation. 2007;84(2):137–43. https://doi.org/10.1097/01.tp.0000269725.74189.b9.

68. Loupy A, Hill GS, Jordan SC. The impact of donor-specific anti-HLA antibodies on late kidney allograft failure. Nat Rev Nephrol. 2012;8(6):348–57. https://doi.org/10.1038/nrneph.2012.81.

69. Hopkins KA, Maguire MG, Fink NE, Bias WB. Reproducibility of HLA-A, B, and DR typing using peripheral blood samples: results of retyping in the collaborative corneal transplantation studies. Collaborative Corneal Transplantation Studies Group (corrected). Hum Immunol. 1992;33(2):122–8. https://doi.org/10.1016/0198-8859(92)90062-r.

70. Vail A, Gore SM, Bradley BA, Easty DL, Rogers CA, Armitage WJ. Conclusions of the corneal transplant follow up study. Collaborating Surgeons. Br J Ophthalmol. 1997;81(8):631–6. https://doi.org/10.1136/bjo.81.8.631.

71. Völker-Dieben HJ, Claas FH, Schreuder GM, et al. Beneficial effect of HLA-DR matching on the survival of corneal allografts. Transplantation. 2000;70(4):640–8. https://doi.org/10.1097/00007890-200008270-00018.

72. Sundmacher R, editor. Adequate HLA matching in keratoplasty. Dusseldorf: Karger Medical and Scientific Publishers; 2003.

73. Völker-Dieben HJ, Schreuder GMT, Claas FHJ, et al. Histocompatibility and corneal transplantation. Dev Ophthalmol. 2003;36:22–41. https://doi.org/10.1159/000067653.

74. Kwitko S, Marinho D, Barcaro S, et al. Allograft conjunctival transplantation for bilateral ocular surface disorders. Ophthalmology. 1995;102(7):1020–5. https://doi.org/10.1016/s0161-6420(95)30918-9.

75. Armitage WJ, Winton HL, Jones MNA, et al. Corneal transplant follow-up study II (CTFS II): a prospective clinical trial to determine the influence of HLA class II matching on corneal transplant rejection: baseline donor and recipient characteristics. Br J Ophthalmol. 2019;103(1):132–6. https://doi.org/10.1136/bjophthalmol-2017-311342.

76. Böhringer D, Spierings E, Enczmann J, et al. Matching of the minor histocompatibility antigen HLA-A1/H-Y may improve prognosis in corneal transplantation. Transplantation. 2006;82(8):1037–41. https://doi.org/10.1097/01.tp.0000235908.54766.44.

77. Hopkinson CL, Romano V, Kaye RA, et al. The influence of donor and recipient gender incompatibility on corneal transplant rejection and failure. Am J Transplant. 2017;17(1):210–7. https://doi.org/10.1111/ajt.13926.

78. Böhringer D, Reinhard T, Böhringer S, Enczmann J, Godehard E, Sundmacher R. Predicting time on the waiting list for HLA matched corneal grafts. Tissue Antigens. 2002;59(5):407–11. https://doi.org/10.1034/j.1399-0039.2002.590507.x.

79. Alió Del Barrio JL, et al. Corneal transplantation after failed grafts: options and outcomes. Surv Ophthalmol. 2021;66(1):20–40. https://doi.org/10.1016/j.survophthal.2020.10.003.

80. Duquesnoy RJ, Askar M. HLAMatchmaker: a molecularly based algorithm for histocompatibility determination. V. Eplet matching for HLA-DR, HLA-DQ, and HLA-DP. Hum Immunol. 2007;68(1):12–25. https://doi.org/10.1016/j.humimm.2006.10.003.

81. Böhringer D, Sundmacher R, Reinhard T. Histocompatilibility matching in penetrating keratoplasty. In: Reinhard T, Larkin F, Larkin DFP, editors. Cornea and external eye disease. Berlin: Springer; 2006. https://books.google.com/books/about/Cornea_and_External_Eye_Disease.html?id=uAfeQjUKTf4C.

82. Shimazaki J, Iseda A, Satake Y, Shimazaki-Den S. Efficacy and safety of long-term corticosteroid eye drops after penetrating keratoplasty: a prospective, randomized, clinical trial. Ophthalmology. 2012;119(4):668–73. https://doi.org/10.1016/j.ophtha.2011.10.016.

83. Kharod-Dholakia B, Randleman JB, Bromley JG, Stulting RD. Prevention and treatment of corneal graft rejection: current practice patterns of the Cornea Society (2011). Cornea. 2015;34(6):609. https://doi.org/10.1097/ICO.0000000000000403.

84. Nguyen NX, Seitz B, Martus P, Langenbucher A, Cursiefen C. Long-term topical steroid treatment improves graft survival following normal-risk penetrating keratoplasty. Am J Ophthalmol. 2007;144(2):318–9. https://doi.org/10.1016/j.ajo.2007.03.028.

85. Ross AH, Jones MNA, Nguyen DQ, et al. Long-term topical steroid treatment after penetrating keratoplasty in patients with pseudophakic bullous keratopathy. Ophthalmology. 2009;116(12):2369–72. https://doi.org/10.1016/j.ophtha.2009.06.006.

86. Butcher JM, Austin M, McGalliard J, Bourke RD. Bilateral cataracts and glaucoma induced by long term use of steroid eye drops. BMJ. 1994;309(6946):43. https://doi.org/10.1136/bmj.309.6946.43.

87. Marques RE, Leal I, Guerra PS, Barão RC, Quintas AM, Rodrigues W. Topical corticosteroids with topical cyclosporine A versus topical corticosteroids alone for immunological corneal graft rejection. Eur J Ophthalmol. 2022;32(3):1469–81. https://doi.org/10.1177/11206721211023320.

88. Donnenfeld E, Pflugfelder SC. Topical ophthalmic cyclosporine: pharmacology and clinical uses. Surv Ophthalmol. 2009;54(3):321–38. https://doi.org/10.1016/j.survophthal.2009.02.002.

89. Javadi MA, Feizi S, Karbasian A, Rastegarpour A. Efficacy of topical ciclosporin A for treatment and prevention of graft rejection in corneal grafts with previous rejection episodes. Br J Ophthalmol. 2010;94(11):1464–7. https://doi.org/10.1136/bjo.2009.172577.

90. Ünal M, Yücel I. Evaluation of topical ciclosporin 0.05% for prevention of rejection in high-risk corneal grafts. Br J Ophthalmol. 2008;92(10):1411–4. https://doi.org/10.1136/bjo.2008.143024.

91. Poon A, Constantinou M, Lamoureux E, Taylor HR. Topical cyclosporin A in the treatment of acute graft rejection: a randomized controlled trial. Clin Experiment Ophthalmol. 2008;36(5):415–21. https://doi.org/10.1111/j.1442-9071.2008.01808.x.

92. Sinha R, Jhanji V, Verma K, Sharma N, Biswas NR, Vajpayee RB. Efficacy of topical cyclosporine A 2% in prevention of graft rejection in high-risk keratoplasty: a randomized controlled trial. Graefes Arch Clin Exp Ophthalmol. 2010;248(8):1167–72. https://doi.org/10.1007/s00417-010-1388-8.

93. Shoughy SS. Topical tacrolimus in anterior segment inflammatory disorders. Eye Vis (Lond). 2017;4(1):1–7. https://doi.org/10.1186/s40662-017-0072-z.

94. Turgut B, Guler M, Akpolat N, Demır T, Celıker U. The impact of tacrolimus on vascular endothelial growth factor in experimental corneal neovascularization. Curr Eye Res. 2011;36(1):34–40. https://doi.org/10.3109/02713683.2010.516620.

95. Shoughy SS, Aljassar FM, Tabbara KF. Aqueous penetration of topical tacrolimus. Am J Ophthalmol Case Rep. 2020;17:100582. https://doi.org/10.1016/j.ajoc.2019.100582.

96. Taddio A, Cimaz R, Caputo R, et al. Childhood chronic anterior uveitis associated with vernal keratoconjunctivitis (VKC): successful treatment with topical tacrolimus. Case series. Pediatr Rheumatol Online J. 2011;9(1):34. https://doi.org/10.1186/1546-0096-9-34.

97. Kheirkhah A, Zavareh MK, Farzbod F, Mahbod M, Behrouz MJ. Topical 0.005% tacrolimus eye drop for refractory vernal keratoconjunctivitis. Eye (Lond). 2011;25(7):872–80. https://doi.org/10.1038/eye.2011.75.

98. Miyazaki D, Fukushima A, Ohashi Y, et al. Steroid-sparing effect of 0.1% tacrolimus eye drop for treatment of shield ulcer and corneal epitheliopathy in refractory allergic ocular diseases. Ophthalmology. 2017;124(3):287–94. https://doi.org/10.1016/j.ophtha.2016.11.002.

99. Lee YJ, Kim SW, Seo KY. Application for tacrolimus ointment in treating refractory inflammatory ocular surface diseases. Am J Ophthalmol. 2013;155(5):804–13. https://doi.org/10.1016/j.ajo.2012.12.009.

100. Moscovici BK, Holzchuh R, Chiacchio BB, Santo RM, Shimazaki J, Hida RY. Clinical treatment of dry eye using 0.03% tacrolimus eye drops. Cornea. 2012;31(8):945–9. https://doi.org/10.1097/ICO.0b013e31823f8c9b.

101. Moscovici BK, Holzchuh R, Sakassegawa-Naves FE, et al. Treatment of Sjögren's syndrome dry eye using 0.03% tacrolimus eye drop: prospective double-blind randomized study. Cont Lens Anterior Eye. 2015;38(5):373–8. https://doi.org/10.1016/j.clae.2015.04.004.

102. Abud TB, Di Zazzo A, Kheirkhah A, Dana R. Systemic immunomodulatory strategies in high-risk corneal transplantation. J Ophthalmic Vis Res. 2017;12(1):81–92. https://doi.org/10.4103/2008-322X.200156.

103. Durazzo TS, Frencher S, Gusberg R. Influence of race on the management of lower extremity ischemia: revascularization vs amputation. JAMA Surg. 2013;148(7):617–23. https://doi.org/10.1001/jamasurg.2013.1436.

104. Jung JW, Lee YJ, Yoon SC, Kim T-I, Kim EK, Seo KY. Long-term result of maintenance treatment with tacrolimus ointment in chronic ocular graft-versus-host disease. Am J Ophthalmol. 2015;159(3):519–27.e1. https://doi.org/10.1016/j.ajo.2014.11.035.

105. Dhaliwal JS, Mason BF, Kaufman SC. Long-term use of topical tacrolimus (FK506) in high-risk penetrating keratoplasty. Cornea. 2008;27(4):488. https://doi.org/10.1097/ICO.0b013e3181606086.

106. Magalhaes OA, Marinho DR, Kwitko S. Topical 0.03% tacrolimus preventing rejection in high-risk corneal transplantation: a cohort study. Br J Ophthalmol. 2013;97(11):1395–8. https://doi.org/10.1136/bjophthalmol-2013-303639.

107. Zhai L-Y, Zhang X-R, Liu H, Ma Y, Xu H-C. Observation of topical tacrolimus on high-risk penetrating keratoplasty patients: a randomized

clinical trial study. Eye (Lond). 2020;34(9):1600–7. https://doi.org/10.1038/s41433-019-0717-3.

108. Faramarzi A, Abbasi H, Feizi S, et al. Topical 0.03% tacrolimus versus systemic mycophenolate mofetil as adjuncts to systemic corticosteroids for preventing graft rejection after repeat keratoplasty: one-year results of a randomized clinical trial. Eye (Lond). 2021;35(10):2879–88. https://doi.org/10.1038/s41433-020-01375-z.

109. Hill JC. The use of cyclosporine in high-risk keratoplasty. Am J Ophthalmol. 1989;107(5):506–10. https://doi.org/10.1016/0002-9394(89)90494-7.

110. Hill JC. Systemic cyclosporine in high-risk keratoplasty: short- versus long-term therapy. Ophthalmology. 1994;101(1):128–33. https://doi.org/10.1016/S0161-6420(13)31253-6.

111. Algros M-P, Angonin R, Delbosc B, Cahn J-Y, Kantelip B. Danger of systemic cyclosporine for corneal graft. Cornea. 2002;21(6):613.

112. Abudou M, Wu T, Evans JR, Chen X. Immunosuppressants for the prophylaxis of corneal graft rejection after penetrating keratoplasty. Cochrane Database Syst Rev. 2015;(8):CD007603. https://doi.org/10.1002/14651858.CD007603.pub2.

113. Bali S, Filek R, Si F, Hodge W. Systemic immunosuppression in high-risk penetrating keratoplasty: a systematic review. J Clin Med Res. 2016;8(4):269–76. https://doi.org/10.14740/jocmr2326w.

114. Den S, Omoto M, Shimmura S, Tsubota K, Shimazaki J. Prospective, randomized study on efficacy of systemic cyclosporine a in high–risk corneal transplantation. Invest Ophthalmol Vis Sci. 2006;47(13):1286.

115. Shimazaki J, Den S, Omoto M, Satake Y, Shimmura S, Tsubota K. Prospective, randomized study of the efficacy of systemic cyclosporine in high-risk corneal transplantation. Am J Ophthalmol. 2011;152(1):33–39.e1. https://doi.org/10.1016/j.ajo.2011.01.019.

116. Reinhard T, Mayweg S, Sokolovska Y, et al. Systemic mycophenolate mofetil avoids immune reactions in penetrating high-risk keratoplasty: preliminary results of an ongoing prospectively randomized multicentre study. Transpl Int. 2005;18(6):703–8. https://doi.org/10.1111/j.1432-2277.2005.00126.x.

117. Reinhard T, Reis A, Böhringer D, et al. Systemic mycophenolate mofetil in comparison with systemic cyclosporin A in high-risk keratoplasty patients: 3 years' results of a randomized prospective clinical trial. Graefes Arch Clin Exp Ophthalmol. 2001;239(5):367–72. https://doi.org/10.1007/s004170100285.

118. Birnbaum F, Böhringer D, Sokolovska Y, Sundmacher R, Reinhard T. Immunosuppression with cyclosporine A and mycophenolate mofetil after penetrating high-risk keratoplasty: a retrospective study. Transplantation. 2005;79(8):964. https://doi.org/10.1097/01.TP.0000158022.62059.F2.

119. Birnbaum F, Mayweg S, Reis A, et al. Mycophenolate mofetil (MMF) following penetrating high-risk keratoplasty: long-term results of a prospec-

tive, randomised, multicentre study. Eye (Lond). 2009;23(11):2063–70. https://doi.org/10.1038/eye.2008.402.

120. Mayer K, Reinhard T, Reis A, Voiculescu A, Sundmacher R. Synergistic antiherpetic effect of acyclovir and mycophenolate mofetil following keratoplasty in patients with herpetic eye disease: first results of a randomised pilot study. Graefes Arch Clin Exp Ophthalmol. 2003;241(12):1051–4. https://doi.org/10.1007/s00417-003-0724-7.

121. Reis A, Reinhard T, Voiculescu A, et al. Mycophenolate mofetil versus cyclosporin A in high risk keratoplasty patients: a prospectively randomised clinical trial. Br J Ophthalmol. 1999;83(11):1268–71. https://doi.org/10.1136/bjo.83.11.1268.

122. Sloper CM, Powell RJ, Dua HS. Tacrolimus (FK506) in the management of high-risk corneal and limbal grafts. Ophthalmology. 2001;108(10):1838–44. https://doi.org/10.1016/s0161-6420(01)00759-x.

123. Holland EJ, Mogilishetty G, Skeens HM, et al. Systemic immunosuppression in ocular surface stem cell transplantation: results of a 10-year experience. Cornea. 2012;31(6):655. https://doi.org/10.1097/ICO.0b013e31823f8b0c.

124. Baradaran-Rafii A, Eslani M, Djalillian AR. Complications of keratolimbal allograft surgery. Cornea. 2013;32(5):561. https://doi.org/10.1097/ICO.0b013e31826215eb.

125. Holland EJ. Living related conjunctival limbal allograft for the treatment of stem cell deficiency - discussion. Ophthalmology. 2001;108(1):133–4.

126. Chan CC, Holland EJ. Keratolimbal allograft. In: Mannis MJ, Holland EJ, editors. Cornea. 5th ed. New York: Elsevier; 2022.

127. Shanbhag SS, Patel CN, Goyal R, Donthineni PR, Singh V, Basu S. Simple limbal epithelial transplantation (SLET): review of indications, surgical technique, mechanism, outcomes, limitations, and impact. Indian J Ophthalmol. 2019;67(8):1265–77. https://doi.org/10.4103/ijo.ijo_117_19.

128. Iyer G, Srinivasan B, Agarwal S, Tarigopula A. Outcome of allo simple limbal epithelial transplantation (alloSLET) in the early stage of ocular chemical injury. Br J Ophthalmol. 2017;101(6):828–33. https://doi.org/10.1136/bjophthalmol-2016-309045.

129. Kaur A, Jamil Z, Priyadarshini SR. Allogeneic simple limbal epithelial transplantation: an appropriate treatment for bilateral stem cell deficiency. BMJ Case Rep. 2021;14(2):e239998. https://doi.org/10.1136/bcr-2020-239998.

130. Férnandez-Buenaga R, Aiello F, Zaher SS, Grixti A, Ahmad S. Twenty years of limbal epithelial therapy: an update on managing limbal stem cell deficiency. BMJ Open Ophthalmol. 2018;3(1):e000164. https://doi.org/10.1136/bmjophth-2018-000164.

131. Serna-Ojeda JC, Basu S, Vazirani J, Garfias Y, Sangwan VS. Systemic immunosuppression for limbal allograft and allogenic limbal epithelial cell

transplantation. Med Hypothesis Discov Innov Ophthalmol J. 2019;9(1):23–32.

132. Graue-Hernandez EO. Simple limbal epithelial transplantation. In: Mannis MJ, Holland EJ, editors. Cornea. New York: Elsevier; 2022. p. 1634. e1–e1638.

133. Daya SM, Watson A, Sharpe JR, et al. Outcomes and DNA analysis of ex vivo expanded stem cell allograft for ocular surface reconstruction. Ophthalmology. 2005;112(3):470–7. https://doi.org/10.1016/j.ophtha.2004.09.023.

134. Eslani M, Cheung AY, Holland EJ. 3-s2.0-B9780323672405001645?indexOverride=GLOBAL. In: Mannis MJ, Holland EJ, editors. Cornea, 5th ed. New York: Elsevier; 2022. p. 1607.e1–14.e1.

135. Basu S, Sureka SP, Shanbhag SS, Kethiri AR, Singh V, Sangwan VS. Simple limbal epithelial transplantation: long-term clinical outcomes in 125 cases of unilateral chronic ocular surface burns. Ophthalmology. 2016;123(5):1000–10. https://doi.org/10.1016/j.ophtha.2015.12.042.

Management of the Vascularized Cornea Before Corneal Graft Surgery: Fine-Needle Diathermy and Inhibition of VEGF

4

Nadim S. Azar, Matias Soifer, and Victor L. Perez

Key Points

- Corneal neovascularization (CNV) is a pathological condition that appears as a result of chronic persistence of different infectious, immune-related and mechanical factors.
- Preoperative CNV is a key risk factor for graft rejection. It is necessary to treat corneal neovascularization prior to corneal transplant surgery to prevent rejection.
- Many surgical techniques exist for the management of corneal neovascularization prior to corneal transplantation, namely fine-needle diathermy and laser therapy.
- Medical therapies are also used for corneal neovascularization prior to corneal transplantation, notably anti-VEGF therapy via topical drops, subconjunctival injections and delivered through scleral lens.

Introduction and Epidemiology

Corneal neovascularization is a condition that affects around ten million people in the world. In the USA, it constitutes a feature of roughly 5% of all ophthalmic presentations, with an estimated incidence of 1.4 million new cases yearly [1]. The angiogenic drive emanates as a response to the presence of an irritating ocular surface pathogen over time, such as allergies, microbial keratitis, immune-mediated processes, persistent epithelial defects, limbal stem cell deficiency, chronic contact lens use and more. A chronic angiogenic response that persists as a response to the different etiologies can lead to a pathological CNV that may affect visual acuity. [2]

Corneal neovascularization represents a high-risk factor for rejection in patients that will undergo a corneal transplant. This was reported in a study by Cursiefen et al., where around 20% of human corneal buttons obtained by penetrating keratoplasty (PK) showed signs of neovascularization and angiogenesis [3, 4]. It is also

Supplementary Information The online version contains supplementary material available at https://doi.org/10.1007/978-3-031-32408-6_4.

N. S. Azar · M. Soifer
Foster Center for Ocular Immunology, Duke Eye Institute, Durham, NC, USA

Department of Ophthalmology, Duke University Medical Center, Durham, NC, USA
e-mail: nadim.azar@duke.edu;
matias.soifer@duke.edu

V. L. Perez (✉)
Foster Center for Ocular Immunology, Duke Eye Institute, Durham, NC, USA

Department of Ophthalmology, Duke University Medical Center, Durham, NC, USA

Foster Center for Ocular Immunology at Duke Eye Center, Duke University School of Medicine, Durham, NC, USA
e-mail: victor.perez.quinones@duke.edu

necessary to study corneal neovascularization prior to corneal transplant surgery, as CNV per se is a well-known risk predictor of graft rejection and subsequently failure [3, 5]. In fact, in this same study, histopathologic evaluation of neovascularized corneal buttons that underwent PK was done and showed that graft rejection was present in around 30% of the buttons [4]. CNV has shown to increase corneal edema, inflammation, scarring and lipid deposition and to worsen the prognosis of following PKs, thereby corroborating the necessity to treat it prior to PK [3]. In fact, the collaborative corneal transplantation studies (CCTS) evaluated the survival of corneal transplants in high-risk patients defined as having two or more quadrants of corneal stromal vascularization and/or a history of graft rejection previously, and observed that corneal rejection rate ranged between 16% and 41% regardless of human leukocyte antigen (HLA) or ABO-compatibility matching [6]. CNV prior to, but also following PK can adversely affect graft longevity [7]. Importantly, CNV presence can be recognized on slit lamp, and since it is a clinically visible objective biomarker, it can be noted, graded and treated adequately in order to prevent rejection, increase graft survival and inform the patient about the transplant prognosis. As such, management of the vascularized cornea before corneal graft surgery, and more specifically PK surgery, is vital and easy to detect and is a predictor of graft stability and decreased rejection.

Surgical and Medical Treatments for Corneal Neovascularization Prior to Corneal Transplantation

Many treatments are available for the management of corneal neovascularization prior to corneal transplants. These are commonly aimed at ablating the vessels (laser photocoagulation, cauterization or fine-needle diathermy) or regulating angiogenesis (anti-VEGF antibodies). The upcoming sections highlight modern management techniques for corneal neovascularization with their associated efficacy and pertinent side effects (Video 4.1).

Clinical Considerations for Treatment Administration and Management

There are important clinical considerations to be taken into account in treatment and management of CNV prior to PK. A comprehensive patient and slit lamp evaluation is essential toward identifying, staging, and managing the corneal neovascularization and its associated risk of rejection/failure of the patient's transplant. The principal risk factor for postoperative corneal graft rejection is the presence of host neovascularization prior to surgery. In fact, the risk is proportional to the area and depth of corneal vascularity [8]. Therefore, a thorough and complete clinical assessment of the corneal vessels is mandatory. Another important consideration is noting whether the vessels are epithelial (superficial) or stromal (deep) since the depth may offer clues to their etiology and establish a prognosis. In short, superficial neovascularization represent the "benign" spectrum of etiologies that occurs as a result of ocular surface disorders or contact lens wear. However, stromal vascularization points toward serious causes such as interstitial keratitis, which can be microbial or autoimmune. These warrant investigation since they may present a recurrent course and flare again, which results in poor graft survival. It has also been shown that deep corneal angiogenesis is more associated with risk of graft failure than superficial vascularization, which itself is more correlated with direct postoperative visual acuity [9].

Significantly, it is crucial to assess whether there is active inflammation on the hosts ocular surface and dampen as much of it as possible. Active inflammation conducts increased vessel formation and predisposes to rejection and overall failure. Every ophthalmic inflammatory disease should be in remission before doing elective corneal transplantation, at least for 6 months [10]. Although CNV is the biggest risk factor for graft rejection, an ocular surface evaluation is mandatory to correct potential additive features such as inflammatory dry eye syndrome [11] or lid abnormalities prone to increased inflammation and, consequently, a worse prognosis.

Treating inflammatory conditions that can be associated with corneal neovascularization such as the ones described previously in the risk factors is necessary for the reduction of neovascularization. Finally, the patient should be counseled regarding the high-risk category of their transplant [12]. A strict anti-inflammatory and antimicrobial protocol has to be explained with its rationale to help the patient understand the need for frequent postoperative topical drops, the possibility of a graft rejection, and its management given their prognosis.

Surgical and Laser Treatments for Management of Corneal Neovascularization

Fine-Needle Diathermy

Fine-needle diathermy (FND) is a mainstay and an important method of targeting corneal neovascularization (Table 4.1). It consists of applying thermal energy to the corneal layers up to the deep stroma in order to obliterate corneal neovascularization. It involves using a stainless-steel cutting needle attached to a nylon suture. The needle is usually inserted around the limbus in a parallel fashion to the blood vessels targeted. It can also be inserted directly into the blood vessel lumen in case the vessel is large. A diathermy unit set at a low current setting (around 0.5–1 mA) is put in contact with the needle for around 1 s, which blanches the selected blood vessels [1]. This technique was studied and described by Pillai et al. [13].

Although there is limited literature assessing the efficacy and safety of the technique, it has been used for the management of CNV. Our group, among other surgical teams, has adopted the use of FND during corneal transplant surgery. We target the diathermy treatment toward bleeding stromal vessels in the host bed. This usually happens after removing the recipient tissue but before performing the transplant. This technique's efficacy relies on its ability to be used during surgery while taking advantage of clear visualization of blood vessels and neovascularization, but also direct access to them.

Fine-needle diathermy, however, can potentially damage the corneal endothelium beneath the treated area, but also corneoscleral limbus [14]. It has also been noted that FND releases proangiogenic factors, which would lead to the stimulation of vascularization, which goes against its intended effect and limits its use [15]. Some of the downsides include the necessity for retreatments for optimal results, but also serious side effects such as corneal perforations, notably in thin corneas, as it involves the use of a needle [1, 16]. Other side effects might include striae creation, corneal scarring and intracorneal bleeding that usually resolves in weeks [17]. To counteract intrastromal bleeding, FND guided by angiography can be used to selectively treat afferent feeder vessels [18, 19]. In some instances, whitening of the stromal cornea occurs near the needle pricks, but it is usually resolvable over a day or 2 [16, 17]. Overall, it appears as a reasonable treatment modality due to the fact that is affordable, simple and effective. It is usually

Table 4.1 Surgical therapies for managing corneal neovascularization prior to corneal transplant: clinical benefits, drawbacks and complications

Surgical therapies	Clinical benefits	Drawbacks	Complications
Fine-needle diathermy	Relatively cheap, simple and effective, it can penetrate into different depths of neovascularization invasion	Afferent both afferent and efferent corneal vessels, retreatment necessary, can release proangiogenic factors	Corneal perforations and scarring, striae formation, intracorneal and intrastromal bleeding, corneal opacification
Laser	Simple procedure, patient tolerability, very targeted: only corneal efferent vessels are affected	Afferent corneal vessel re-budding does not show significant effects when neovascularization is sizeable or when corneas are very inflamed, costly and several sessions needed	Damage to corneal endothelium and lens, corneal thinning and bleeding, iris deposits and atrophy, pupil peaking

done under topical anesthesia and, unlike laser treatment, it destroys both afferent and efferent corneal vessels. FND has recently been altered by using an electrolysis needle that is thinner and more flexible than the previously described [20]. It involves direct thermal energy to cauterize the vessels instead of electrical currents, as originally described in diathermy. It was reported in three cases of lipid keratopathy on whom no postoperative complications were observed [20], but the sample size was small, and more extensive research should be done to assess this procedure.

Laser Treatment

Another effective strategy for targeting corneal vascularization is through the use of laser therapy (Table 4.1). In general, laser photocoagulation works by destruction of corneal efferent vessels, specifically as these are wide and have a slow blood flow relatively, in comparison to the afferent vessels that are deeper and thinner and have a much faster blood flow [16]. Targeting of afferent vessels would thus lead to their reappearance and the necessity to resort to different modalities of treatments. Frequency-doubled Nd:YAG (532 nm), an important type of laser photocoagulation, is an effective treatment that can decrease the area of corneal vascularization without causing any significant side effects, as stromal hemorrhage was a rare noted complication by Parsa et al., in a patient where an attempt to reduce

CNV prior to PK was done [21]. Although practical in an outpatient setting and tolerable by patients, laser treatment is not as effective in cases in cases of sizeable corneal neovascularization [22]. Overall general side effects of laser therapy might include damage to corneal endothelium or even the lens, but also corneal thinning and bleeding, iris deposits and atrophy, and pupil peaking [16, 23].

Medical Antiangiogenic Treatments for Management of Corneal Neovascularization

Anti-VEGF/VEGF receptor agents have appeared as notable players in the anti-angiogenesis therapy prior to PK. Many antiangiogenic therapeutic techniques interfere with the VEGF system, the most important ones consisting of VEGF neutralizing direct antibodies, VEGF receptor antibodies and receptor tyrosine kinase inhibitors that act downstream in the VEGF pathway. VEGF is a member of a family of proteins consisting of several subtypes (VEGF-A, VEGF-B, VEGF-C and VEGF-D), with the VEGF-A isoforms being the most studied and notable inducer of pathologic CNV. The main categories we will discuss in the chapter are VEGF neutralizing antibodies and also use of scleral devices incorporating anti-VEGF on the ocular surface (Table 4.2).

Table 4.2 Antiangiogenic medical therapies for corneal neovascularization prior to corneal transplant: clinical benefits, drawbacks and side effects

Medical therapies	Clinical benefits	Drawbacks	Side effects
Anti-VEGF agents	Work on newly formed vessels, extensive data regarding use, different modes of administration, safer and more effective than anti-inflammatory drugs, directed mechanism of action	Costly, reduced antiangiogenic effects on mature already existing vessels, resistance to treatment, nonresponsiveness to treatment, short half-lives	Subconjunctival injection: risk of vasospasm and vascular effects, local side effects from injection
			Topical injections: adhesions between corneal epithelium and basement membrane, stromal thinning, delayed wound healing, epithelial defects
Scleral lens devices with anti-VEGF	Constantly bathes ocular surface and increases the bioavailability of drugs, mechanical protective effects on cornea, custom-fitted	Costly, scarcity of data regarding scleral lens devices prior to PK, similar drawbacks to anti-VEGF treatments that are administered under the device	Adhesions, stromal thinning, delayed wound healing in some cases

VEGF vascular endothelial growth factor, *PK* penetrating keratoplasty

Anti-VEGF Local Therapy

VEGF is as a corneal angiogenic factor that stems from inflammation and is described as an essential component of neovascularization in rat corneas [24]. VEGF is proven to be involved in a causal relationship in corneal neovascularization through extensive research and evidence [25–30]. VEGF-A, a subtype from the VEGF family of proteins, augments the replication of endothelial cells through mitosis and facilitates their migration but is also involved in the creation of blood vessels [25].

Anti-VEGF antibodies, which are currently used as intravitreal injections for retinal proliferative vascular disorders, offer promising applications for the management of corneal neovascularization [31]. These can be administrated via topical drops, subconjunctival injection, and with the use of scleral lenses. Anti-VEGF antibodies help in corneal graft survival, as initial mouse models report improvement in murine graft survival [32, 33].

Bevacizumab is the most studied anti-VEGF therapy: it consists of a humanized murine monoclonal IgG1 antibody that reduces corneal neovascularization [34]. Many clinical studies, mainly prospective case series and case reports, were effectuated using bevacizumab therapy for corneal neovascularization. These studies involve different etiologies from which the corneal neovascularization emanates, such as preceding a PK [35, 36], after a PK [37], and on rejected/rejecting PK [38–41]. Experimental bevacizumab studies have demonstrated statistically significant effects in decreasing neovascularization, by using different parameters such as length, density and area of CNV [27, 32, 39, 42–46]. It has shown particularly good results on newly formed vessels rather than already existing ones [35, 38, 39, 47, 48]. This discrepancy is theorized to occur as pre-existing vessels become less dependent on VEGF for growth and survival [49] and are covered by pericytes [47, 50]. Moreover, bevacizumab effects were also greater when vessels were smaller and less numerous and early in the CNV course [38, 48, 51].

In terms of route of administration, topical, subconjunctival and intraocular formulations of bevacizumab have been shown to decrease neovascularization to some extent, thereby improving corneal clarity [52, 53]. A direct comparison between subconjunctival and topical administrations has shown that both are equally as effective in reducing corneal angiogenesis [54]. Subconjunctival injection has three main drawbacks: it has a limited duration of action in the cornea [55], may result in the quicker entry of the drug into the systemic circulation, thus exposing the patient to the risk of vasospasm and vascular effects and finally, local side effects from the injection. However, topical drop administration is estimated to affect adhesion between epithelium and basement membrane in comparison to subconjunctival injection, resulting in stromal thinning and delayed wound healing [40, 56–59]. This effect is duration and dose-dependent [58] and has been shown to reverse after treatment [60].

In short, anti-VEGF therapy studies are still small and cannot provide extremely conclusive evidence. Anti-VEGF agents may be safer and more effective than anti-inflammatory drugs as they generally present with less side effects and have a more directed mechanism of action rationale. As a whole, they appear to be especially useful for the treatment of newly created vessels which signify ongoing disease, while they are less effective in treating mature previously present vessels in chronic neovascularization. As such, they might be used in conjunction with steroids and other anti-inflammatory drugs to target both immature and mature vessels [1]. Major challenges to anti-VEGF antibody use mainly pertain to high costs of the modality, resistance to treatment, short half-life and partial to nonresponsiveness to the treatment [61–63].

Scleral Lens Devices with the Use of Anti-VEGF Therapy

The use of scleral lens devices such as the prosthetic replacement of the ocular surface (PROSE) provide a reservoir for the antiangiogenic molecules so that it these are constantly bathing the ocular surface, thus increasing the bioavailability of the drug. The PROSE lens is a large, rigid, gas-permeable, custom-designed lens that vaults over the corneal surface. Despite its advantages, there is still scarcity of data observing outcomes on scleral lens or PROSE with Bevacizumab prior to corneal transplants. On an interventional case series of 13 patients with corneal neovascularization, one drop of 1% bevacizumab was instilled each morning in the fluid reservoir of the PROSE device. This was repeated after 6 h with a second drop of bevacizumab for a median of 6 months. The response was highly positive as 12/13 cases presented regression of the neovascularization and 10/13 improved their visual acuity [64]. Another case series of five patients with a similar protocol had similar results and followed patients for up to 2 years without noting epithelial side effects [65]. Although neither of these studies tackled corneal transplantation outcomes in these populations, their results suggest that the use of bevacizumab with scleral lens devices may improve the success of grafts if surgery is undertaken.

Conclusion

Corneal neovascularization can appear as a pathologic response to different factors affecting the ocular surface, such as infectious, immune-mediated and mechanical effects. It is important to treat CNV prior to corneal transplants, especially on penetrating keratoplasties, as it has been shown to increase graft longevity and prevent rejection. Prevention of CNV is very challenging, but many different modalities have been used to treat it prior to PK. Many surgical and medical therapies have offered significant therapeutic benefits for the management of CNV prior to PK, mainly the use of fine-needle diathermy, lasers and medical management with antiangiogenic treatments such as anti-VEGF antibodies and coupling it with scleral lens devices. It is necessary to address the clinical benefits of each therapy prior to initiating it, but also to target the specific side effects discussed in this chapter that are associated with the different modalities in question, in order to optimize patient response and promote corneal graft survival. Overall, research done on corneal neovascularization is mainly focused on basic science in animal models. It is vital to expand our knowledge regarding corneal neovascularization in order to target more specific molecular angiogenic pathways and reduce the burden of a worldwide health problem.

Take Home Notes

- Corneal neovascularization is a pathologic phenomenon that can happen as a result of different infectious or immune-related insults to the ocular surface.
- Corneal neovascularization treatment prior to corneal transplantation has been shown to increase the longevity of the graft and prevent rejection.
- Fine-needle diathermy is a cheap and effective method that uses thermal energy to cauterize vessels.
- Laser therapy is a simple and tolerable procedure but is less effective on sizeable neovascularization.
- Anti-VEGF local therapy, albeit costly, is a very effective method to treat corneal neovascularization and offers several modes of administration.
- Novel scleral lens devices bathe the corneal surface with anti-VEGF therapy and increase the bioavailability of the therapy, but they are expensive.

References

1. Gupta D, Illingworth C. Treatments for corneal neovascularization: a review. Cornea. 2011;30(8):927–38.
2. Lee P, Wang CC, Adamis AP. Ocular neovascularization: an epidemiologic review. Surv Ophthalmol. 1998;43(3):245–69.
3. Chang JH, Gabison EE, Kato T, Azar DT. Corneal neovascularization. Curr Opin Ophthalmol. 2001;12(4):242–9.
4. Cursiefen C, Küchle M, Naumann GO. Angiogenesis in corneal diseases: histopathologic evaluation of 254 human corneal buttons with neovascularization. Cornea. 1998;17(6):611–3.
5. Mayer DJ, Casey TA. Reducing the risk of corneal graft rejection. A comparison of different methods. Cornea. 1987;6(4):261–8.

6. The collaborative corneal transplantation studies (CCTS). Effectiveness of histocompatibility matching in high-risk corneal transplantation. The Collaborative Corneal Transplantation Studies Research Group. Arch Ophthalmol. 1992;110(10):1392–403.

7. Dana MR, Schaumberg DA, Kowal VO, Goren MB, Rapuano CJ, Laibson PR, et al. Corneal neovascularization after penetrating keratoplasty. Cornea. 1995;14(6):604–9.

8. Maguire MG, Stark WJ, Gottsch JD, Stulting RD, Sugar A, Fink NE, et al. Risk factors for corneal graft failure and rejection in the collaborative corneal transplantation studies. Collaborative Corneal Transplantation Studies Research Group. Ophthalmology. 1994;101(9):1536–47.

9. Vail A, Gore SM, Bradley BA, Easty DL, Rogers CA. Corneal graft survival and visual outcome. A multicenter study. Corneal Transplant Follow-up Study Collaborators. Ophthalmology. 1994;101(1):120–7.

10. Jabbehdari S, Rafii AB, Yazdanpanah G, Hamrah P, Holland EJ, Djalilian AR. Update on the management of high-risk penetrating keratoplasty. Curr Ophthalmol Rep. 2017;5(1):38–48.

11. Soifer M, Mousa HM, Stinnett SS, Galor A, Perez VL. Matrix metalloproteinase 9 positivity predicts long term decreased tear production. Ocul Surf. 2021;19:270–4.

12. Soifer M, Mousa HM, Levy RB, Perez VL. Understanding immune responses to surgical transplant procedures in Stevens Johnsons Syndrome Patients. Front Med. 2021;8:656998. https://www.frontiersin.org/article/10.3389/fmed.2021.656998.

13. Pillai CT, Dua HS, Hossain P. Fine needle diathermy occlusion of corneal vessels. Invest Ophthalmol Vis Sci. 2000;41(8):2148–53.

14. Kirwan RP, Zheng Y, Tey A, Anijeet D, Sueke H, Kaye SB. Quantifying changes in corneal neovascularization using fluorescein and indocyanine green angiography. Am J Ophthalmol. 2012;154(5):850–858.e2.

15. Junghans BM, Collin HB. The limbal vascular response to corneal injury. An autoradiographic study. Cornea. 1989;8(2):141–9.

16. Feizi S, Azari AA, Safapour S. Therapeutic approaches for corneal neovascularization. Eye Vis Lond Engl. 2017;4:28.

17. Faraj LA, Elalfy MS, Said DG, Dua HS. Fine needle diathermy occlusion of corneal vessels. Br J Ophthalmol. 2014;98(9):1287–90.

18. Romano V, Steger B, Kaye SB. Fine-needle diathermy guided by angiography. Cornea. 2015;34(9):e29–30.

19. Spiteri N, Romano V, Zheng Y, Yadav S, Dwivedi R, Chen J, et al. Corneal angiography for guiding and evaluating fine-needle diathermy treatment of corneal neovascularization. Ophthalmology. 2015;122(6):1079–84.

20. Wertheim MS, Cook SD, Knox-Cartwright NE, Van DL, Tole DM. Electrolysis-needle cauterization of corneal vessels in patients with lipid keratopathy. Cornea. 2007;26(2):230–1.

21. Parsa CF, Temprano J, Wilson D, Green WR. Hemorrhage complicating YAG laser feeder vessel coagulation of cornea vascularization. Cornea. 1994;13(3):264–8.

22. Baer JC, Foster CS. Corneal laser photocoagulation for treatment of neovascularization. Efficacy of 577 nm yellow dye laser. Ophthalmology. 1992;99(2):173–9.

23. Marsh RJ. Argon laser treatment of lipid keratopathy. Br J Ophthalmol. 1988;72(12):900–4.

24. Amano S, Rohan R, Kuroki M, Tolentino M, Adamis AP. Requirement for vascular endothelial growth factor in wound- and inflammation-related corneal neovascularization. Invest Ophthalmol Vis Sci. 1998;39(1):18–22.

25. Andreoli CM, Miller JW. Anti-vascular endothelial growth factor therapy for ocular neovascular disease. Curr Opin Ophthalmol. 2007;18(6):502–8.

26. Cursiefen C, Rummelt C, Küchle M. Immunohistochemical localization of vascular endothelial growth factor, transforming growth factor alpha, and transforming growth factor beta1 in human corneas with neovascularization. Cornea. 2000;19(4):526–33.

27. Gan L, Fagerholm P, Palmblad J. Vascular endothelial growth factor (VEGF) and its receptor VEGFR-2 in the regulation of corneal neovascularization and wound healing. Acta Ophthalmol Scand. 2004;82(5):557–63.

28. Hosseini H, Nejabat M, Mehryar M, Yazdchi T, Sedaghat A, Noori F. Bevacizumab inhibits corneal neovascularization in an alkali burn induced model of corneal angiogenesis. Clin Exp Ophthalmol. 2007;35(8):745–8.

29. Kim B, Tang Q, Biswas PS, Xu J, Schiffelers RM, Xie FY, et al. Inhibition of ocular angiogenesis by siRNA targeting vascular endothelial growth factor pathway genes: therapeutic strategy for herpetic stromal keratitis. Am J Pathol. 2004;165(6):2177–85.

30. Philipp W, Speicher L, Humpel C. Expression of vascular endothelial growth factor and its receptors in inflamed and vascularized human corneas. Invest Ophthalmol Vis Sci. 2000;41(9):2514–22.

31. Heier JS, Antoszyk AN, Pavan PR, Leff SR, Rosenfeld PJ, Ciulla TA, et al. Ranibizumab for treatment of neovascular age-related macular degeneration: a phase I/II multicenter, controlled, multidose study. Ophthalmology. 2006;113(4):633.e1–4.

32. Cursiefen C, Cao J, Chen L, Liu Y, Maruyama K, Jackson D, et al. Inhibition of hemangiogenesis and lymphangiogenesis after normal-risk corneal transplantation by neutralizing VEGF promotes graft survival. Invest Ophthalmol Vis Sci. 2004;45(8):2666–73.

33. Yatoh S, Kawakami Y, Imai M, Kozawa T, Segawa T, Suzuki H, et al. Effect of a topically applied neutralizing antibody against vascular endothelial growth factor on corneal allograft rejection of rat. Transplantation. 1998;66(11):1519–24.

34. Rodrigues EB, Farah ME, Maia M, Penha FM, Regatieri C, Melo GB, et al. Therapeutic monoclonal antibodies in ophthalmology. Prog Retin Eye Res. 2009;28(2):117–44.

35. Mackenzie SE, Tucker WR, Poole TRG. Bevacizumab (avastin) for corneal neovascularization--corneal light shield soaked application. Cornea. 2009;28(2):246–7.
36. Gerten G. Bevacizumab (avastin) and argon laser to treat neovascularization in corneal transplant surgery. Cornea. 2008;27(10):1195–9.
37. DeStafeno JJ, Kim T. Topical bevacizumab therapy for corneal neovascularization. Arch Ophthalmol. 2007;125(6):834–6.
38. Awadein A. Subconjunctival bevacizumab for vascularized rejected corneal grafts. J Cataract Refract Surg. 2007;33(11):1991–3.
39. Bock F, König Y, Kruse F, Baier M, Cursiefen C. Bevacizumab (Avastin) eye drops inhibit corneal neovascularization. Graefes Arch Clin Exp Ophthalmol. 2008;246(2):281–4.
40. Dastjerdi MH, Al-Arfaj KM, Nallasamy N, Hamrah P, Jurkunas UV, Pineda R, et al. Topical bevacizumab in the treatment of corneal neovascularization: results of a prospective, open-label, noncomparative study. Arch Ophthalmol. 2009;127(4):381–9.
41. Doctor PP, Bhat PV, Foster CS. Subconjunctival bevacizumab for corneal neovascularization. Cornea. 2008;27(9):992–5.
42. Manzano RPA, Peyman GA, Khan P, Carvounis PE, Kivilcim M, Ren M, et al. Inhibition of experimental corneal neovascularisation by bevacizumab (Avastin). Br J Ophthalmol. 2007;91(6):804–7.
43. Bachmann BO, Bock F, Wiegand SJ, Maruyama K, Dana MR, Kruse FE, et al. Promotion of graft survival by vascular endothelial growth factor a neutralization after high-risk corneal transplantation. Arch Ophthalmol. 2008;126(1):71–7.
44. Habot-Wilner Z, Barequet IS, Ivanir Y, Moisseiev J, Rosner M. The inhibitory effect of different concentrations of topical bevacizumab on corneal neovascularization. Acta Ophthalmol. 2010;88(8): 862–7.
45. Han YS, Lee JE, Jung JW, Lee JS. Inhibitory effects of bevacizumab on angiogenesis and corneal neovascularization. Graefes Arch Clin Exp Ophthalmol. 2009;247(4):541–8.
46. Kim TI, Kim SW, Kim S, Kim T, Kim EK. Inhibition of experimental corneal neovascularization by using subconjunctival injection of bevacizumab (Avastin). Cornea. 2008;27(3):349–52.
47. Cursiefen C, Hofmann-Rummelt C, Küchle M, Schlötzer-Schrehardt U. Pericyte recruitment in human corneal angiogenesis: an ultrastructural study with clinicopathological correlation. Br J Ophthalmol. 2003;87(1):101–6.
48. You IC, Kang IS, Lee SH, Yoon KC. Therapeutic effect of subconjunctival injection of bevacizumab in the treatment of corneal neovascularization. Acta Ophthalmol. 2009;87(6):653–8.
49. Jo N, Mailhos C, Ju M, Cheung E, Bradley J, Nishijima K, et al. Inhibition of platelet-derived growth factor B signaling enhances the efficacy of anti-vascular endothelial growth factor therapy in multiple models of ocular neovascularization. Am J Pathol. 2006;168(6):2036–53.
50. Ferrari G, Dastjerdi MH, Okanobo A, Cheng SF, Amparo F, Nallasamy N, et al. Topical ranibizumab as a treatment of corneal neovascularization. Cornea. 2013;32(7):992–7.
51. Lin CT, Hu FR, Kuo KT, Chen YM, Chu HS, Lin YH, et al. The different effects of early and late bevacizumab (Avastin) injection on inhibiting corneal neovascularization and conjunctivalization in rabbit limbal insufficiency. Invest Ophthalmol Vis Sci. 2010;51(12):6277–85.
52. Avisar I, Weinberger D, Kremer I. Effect of subconjunctival and intraocular bevacizumab injections on corneal neovascularization in a mouse model. Curr Eye Res. 2010;35(2):108–15.
53. Lee SH, Leem HS, Jeong SM, Lee K. Bevacizumab accelerates corneal wound healing by inhibiting TGF-beta2 expression in alkali-burned mouse cornea. BMB Rep. 2009;42(12):800–5.
54. Ozdemir O, Altintas O, Altintas L, Ozkan B, Akdag C, Yüksel N. Comparison of the effects of subconjunctival and topical anti-VEGF therapy (bevacizumab) on experimental corneal neovascularization. Arq Bras Oftalmol. 2014;77(4):209–13.
55. Mohammadpour M. Deep intrastromal injection of bevacizumab for the management of corneal neovascularization. Cornea. 2013;32(1): 109–10.
56. Kim T-i, Chung JL, Hong JP, Min K, Seo KY, Kim EK. Bevacizumab application delays epithelial healing in rabbit cornea. Invest Ophthalmol Vis Sci. 2009;50(10):4653–9.
57. Koenig Y, Bock F, Horn F, Kruse F, Straub K, Cursiefen C. Short- and long-term safety profile and efficacy of topical bevacizumab (Avastin) eye drops against corneal neovascularization. Graefes Arch Clin Exp Ophthalmol. 2009;247(10):1375–82.
58. Kim SW, Ha BJ, Kim EK, Tchah H, Kim T-i. The effect of topical bevacizumab on corneal neovascularization. Ophthalmology. 2008;115(6): e33–8.
59. Murata M, Takanami T, Shimizu S, Kubota Y, Horiuchi S, Habano W, et al. Inhibition of ocular angiogenesis by diced small interfering RNAs (siRNAs) specific to vascular endothelial growth factor (VEGF). Curr Eye Res. 2006;31(2):171–80.
60. Carrasco MA. Subconjunctival bevacizumab for corneal neovascularization in herpetic stromal keratitis. Cornea. 2008;27(6):743–5.
61. Chames P, Van Regenmortel M, Weiss E, Baty D. Therapeutic antibodies: successes, limitations and hopes for the future. Br J Pharmacol. 2009;157(2):220–33.
62. Bergers G, Hanahan D. Modes of resistance to anti-angiogenic therapy. Nat Rev Cancer. 2008;8(8):592–603.
63. Tranos P, Vacalis A, Asteriadis S, Koukoula S, Vachtsevanos A, Perganta G, et al. Resistance to antivascular endothelial growth factor treatment in

age-related macular degeneration. Drug Des Dev Ther. 2013;7:485–90.

64. Yin J, Jacobs DS. Long-term outcome of using Prosthetic Replacement of Ocular Surface Ecosystem (PROSE) as a drug delivery system for bevacizumab in the treatment of corneal neovascularization. Ocul Surf. 2019;17(1):134–41.

65. Lim M, Jacobs DS, Rosenthal P, Carrasquillo KG. The Boston Ocular Surface Prosthesis as a novel drug delivery system for bevacizumab. Semin Ophthalmol. 2009;24(3):149–55.

Suggested Reading

Perez VL. Corneal vessel cauterization. Durham: Duke Eye Center; 2022.

Part II

Penetrating Keratoplasty

Main Issues to Overcome in Modern Penetrating Keratoplasty

Farideh Doroodgar, Sana Niazi, Hassan Hashemi, and Mohammad Ali Javadi

Key Points

- Immunologic rejection and endothelial decompensation are two important causes of graft failure.
- Special attention should be paid to the condition of the Ocular Surface when deciding on Penetrating keratoplasty as it may negatively influence its outcomes significantly.
- The large enough second graft with no remnants of the first transplant, systemic steroid, and immunosuppressive medications before surgery and continue for a long time afterward, avoiding raising eye pressure and hastening infectious crystalline keratopathy (ICK) development, removing any loose or vascularized sutures as soon as possible are measures that can be taken to increase the chances of survival in regraft.
- In this chapter, we discuss the pitfalls of modern penetrating keratoplasty (PK) along with other issues and techniques in order to achieve the best possible results by taking adequate action on the variables that negatively influence the outcomes of PKP, avoiding or controlling the associated risks.

Supplementary Information The online version contains supplementary material available at https://doi.org/10.1007/978-3-031-32408-6_5.

F. Doroodgar (✉) · S. Niazi
Translational Ophthalmology Research Center, Tehran University Medical Science, Tehran, Iran

Negah Aref Ophthalmic Research Center, Shahid Beheshti University of Medical Science, Tehran, Iran
e-mail: f-doroodgar@farabi.tums.ac.ir;
sananiazi@sbmu.ac.ir

H. Hashemi
Noor Ophthalmology Research Center, Noor Eye Hospital, Tehran, Iran

Eye Research Center, Farabi Eye Hospital, Tehran University of Medical Sciences, Tehran, Iran
e-mail: hhashemi@noorvision.com

M. A. Javadi
Department of Ophthalmology, Labbafinezhad Hospital, Shahid Beheshti University of Medical Sciences, Tehran, Iran

Introduction

Corneal blindness is a significant cause of reversible blindness, making corneal transplantation the most prevalent type of human organ transplantation. Corneal transplantation, performed for therapeutic, tectonic, and optical purposes, is thus a procedure that successfully restores vision in thousands of patients each year. Different surgical techniques have been suggested for corneal transplantation; penetrating keratoplasty (PK) ranks among the oldest and most common surgical techniques, which offers good long-term visual rehabilitation, most suitable in the presence of endothelial dysfunction or severe deep corneal scarring, affecting the visual axis up to the Descemet membrane (DM) level. Other surgical techniques have also been proposed for reducing complications in special indications [1]. In this chapter, we focus on the pitfalls of modern PK and technical issues of the trephination, suturing technique, and immunological aspects in a review of randomized controlled trials of penetrating keratoplasty techniques [2]. There was no indication that any one technique was superior in increased quality of life or cost-effectiveness.

In modern keratoplasty, selectivity is the main principle, i.e., whether to replace only the affected corneal layer through layer-by-layer or interlayer transplantation. One of the important modern advances that aim to improve clinical outcomes is replacing manual surgical incision of the cornea with new techniques, like a laser. Production of surgical graft profiles such as "top-hat," "mushroom," and "zig-zag" shapes (which increases the wound surface area, decreases surgically associated astigmatism and nonastigmatic aberrations, and thus improves wound healing and biomechanical stability), higher precision, the inherent automatability and repeatability (which eases the learning curve and decreases complications), earlier suture removal, and improved visual outcomes (short- and long-term) are the main advantages of using an infrared femtosecond laser (FSL) [3, 4]. The use of other lasers, such as nonmechanical excimer-assisted lasers and pulsed ultraviolet light from excimer lasers, has also been announced with improved outcomes in PK and other surgical procedures [5]. However, like any other surgery, this type of surgery has complications, including minor (astigmatism, slow rehabilitation, and prolonged use of topical steroids) and major complications (graft failure). Considering the diversity of operative incisions in different keratoplasty modifications, clarification is required to evaluate their postoperative complications; therefore, in the present chapter, we discuss the pitfalls of modern PK alongside other issues and techniques.

First, we discuss the reasons for early and late graft rejection after penetrating keratoplasty, which can help a better comprehension of the mechanisms of this complication. Regarding the direct association of visual acuity after PK with patients' quality of life [6], we pay attention to the short-term and long-term visual outcomes of PK in section "The Short-Term and Long-Term Functional and Refractive Outcomes of Penetrating Keratoplasty". In section "Clinical Aspects of Graft Failure After Penetrating Keratoplasty", we focus on graft rejection and failure, which is considered the measure of surgical success, and explain the risk factors of graft failure after PK. Knowing about the risk factors can provide a better understanding of the indications of PK and the implementation of effective prevention and treatments in high-risk patients [7]. sections "Management of Postpenetrating Keratoplasty Astigmatism" and "Postoperative Care" include postoperative care and management.

The Reasons for Early and Late Graft Rejection After Penetrating Keratoplasty

Graft rejection is the most common cause of corneal graft failure, defined as the irreversible loss of refractive quality. Immunologic rejection (allograft) is the leading cause of graft failure. More than half the cases of graft decompensation are caused by allograft rejection [8]. Another important cause of graft failure is endothelial decompensation.

Immunological Rejection

Allograft rejection after PK is the main cause of graft failure. Despite immunosuppressive agents prescribed to high-risk patients, immunologic rejection occurs by destroying the donor tissue by the host's immune system. This causes reversible or irreversible damage to the grafted cornea [9]. A corneal graft failure is result of an activated sequence of complex immune responses. The host immune system has an efferent immune response against these foreign antigens. This response culminates in rejection and graft decompensation, resulting in irreversible damage to the cornea [9]. The details of the cellular mechanisms of immunologic rejection are described elsewhere [9, 10]. Preoperative major histocompability complex (MHC) and non-MHC antigens matching, and new treatment modalities are still controversial and under investigation.

Endothelial Cell Failure

The most common form of graft rejection is endothelial rejection, while epithelial and subepithelial rejections are infrequent. Epithelial rejection occurs in roughly 2% of graft rejections, beginning days to weeks earlier as a line (which consists of lymphocytes, plasma cells, and neutrophils) located near engorged limbal vessels. The commonest consists of a line of Keratic Precipitates (KP) beginning inferiorly at the graft-host junction and marching superiorly [11, 12]. Molecular evidence shows a steadily decreasing trend of endothelial cell density (ECD) after PK, predictive of graft failure due to endothelial decompensation [13, 14].

Other reasons have also been described for corneal graft failure, which serves as risk factors rather than causes; factors such as glaucoma, nonviral infections, endothelial cell failure, viral herpetic infections [15], intraocular pressure (IOP) elevation/glaucoma, diseases of the ocular surface, recurrence of the primary disease, wound dehiscence/hypotonia and trauma [16], uncorrectable refractive error, and primary donor failure [17]. Risk factors for corneal allograft rejection are the presence of stromal blood vessels in one or more quadrants of the recipient cornea (high risk), preoperative glaucoma, young age, prior anterior segment surgery, active ocular inflammation, ocular surface disease, herpes simplex keratitis, neurotrophic keratopathy, large and eccentric grafts, and anterior synechiae. Of note, all studies report a high rate for other or undetected causes, which shows that the cause of graft failure is still not well-established [10]. Others have reported the main risk factors of immunologic rejection as new vascularization of the recipient cornea over two or more quadrants, corneal opacity due to an infectious origin, posttraumatic corneal opacity or congenital glaucoma, graft diameter >8 mm, and a therapeutic indication of PK [17]. In another study, the risk factors of allograft rejection after PK included corneal vascularization, long operation time, and younger donor age [18]. The presented risk factors for graft failure and allograft rejection should be considered by surgeons when contemplating PK.

Graft survival should be interpreted with caution when comparing different studies to assess the success of corneal transplantation. There is no consensus on graft failure; some define it as the loss of optical clarity, whereas others have a variable effect on vision. Late endothelial failure's gradual loss of clarity could give an uncertain endpoint.

Measures that can be taken to increase the chances of survival of corneal transplantation in those who have a second operation are:

If the immunological system is to blame for the first operation's success:

1. The second operation should be performed as soon as feasible after the first, and no evidence of inflammation should be seen throughout the procedure.

2. The second graft should be large enough to incorporate all of the previously grafted tissue, with no remnants of the first transplant unless the previous transplantation was, particularly huge and off-center.

3. Systemic steroid and immunosuppressive medications should be started 2–7 days before surgery and continued for a long time afterward.

4. After surgery, immunosuppressive drops such as tacrolimus, in addition to topical steroids, should be given indefinitely as supplementary therapy. At the same time, caution should be exercised to avoid raising eye pressure and hastening ICK development.
5. After surgery, any loose or vascularized sutures should be removed as soon as possible, and the patient should have unrestricted access to the treating physician.

Topical administration of Adhesion Molecules AB enhanced graft survival in animal experiments, but this has yet to be investigated in humans. Several adhesion molecules are implicated in corneal transplant rejection, two of which are VLA-4 (Very Late Antigen) and LFA-1 (Leukocyte Function Adhesion) [19].

Ocular Surface Problems and Dry Eye Disease

One crucial reason for graft rejection is ocular surface problems and dry eye disease (DED), affecting millions globally. Immunopathological graft failure is one of the most prevalent ocular surface problems. Hyperosmolarity is also crucial in dry eye disease's inflammatory cycle [20].

Maintaining a healthy and moist ocular surface depends on healthy epithelia, tear film, and eyelid, increasing corneal graft survival. Several previous studies revealed that dry eye disease, as a form of the ocular surface disorder (OSD), can lead to graft rejection and has two known causes, lipid or aqueous tear deficiency [21, 22]. Mild inflammatory processes can progress to serious chronic diseases (i.e., cicatrizing conjunctivitis) that are contraindications for whole penetrating keratoplasty.

The goal of managing dry eye or OSD is to manage the tear film's hyperosmolarity state to decrease the immune system's expression of a response to any foreign substances and inflammatory antigens. Although the cornea has immunological privilege because of its avascular and lymph node-free nature, effective immune rejection avoidance is preferable to immune suppression with immune modifying agents [23].

Following transplantation, treatments such as gene therapy may be used. Because of its inexpensive cost, minor histocompatibility complex tissue matching can be performed. ABO antigen testing, on the other hand, is not as specific as significant histocompatibility tests. The cornea remains the only organ with the unique immune privilege to assess major histocompatibility complex tissue matching [15].

Specifically, most major histocompatibility testing only works for class II and has not been demonstrated successful for class I. Unfortunately, because significant human histocompatibility complex genes are highly polymorphic, any random allocation of human leukocyte antigens (HLA) will take a very long time to obtain the required matching level, which is highly unethical for our patients [15]. Suppose a highly specific, low-cost, and time-efficient HLA matching is developed in the future. In that case, HLA testing may be used as a routine evaluation to increase the number of grafts that survive in transplant recipients.

As noted in the literature, high-risk situations such as corneal vascularization, DED, and prolonged use of antiglaucoma medicine can lower the corneal graft survival rate [24]. In light of this, the injection of anti–vascular endothelial growth factor therapy (anti-VEGF) [25] into the subconjunctival, the use of Lifitegrast [26], an antagonist of LFA-1 and an inhibitor of T cell formation, in dry eye management as well as subconjunctival, an adjunct nonpreservative topical lubricant in glaucoma treatment [27], will likely be beneficial and produce a promising result related to a higher graft survival rate in the future.

The aforementioned items conclude that a prospective clinical trial examining the impact of preexisting DED on corneal transplant survival is warranted. An immunological understanding of HLA's function in corneal graft rejection and a thorough understanding of the need for HLA tissue matching will open up new avenues for preventing graft rejection. Due to continuing research into potential pharmacotherapies with novel targets, several viable therapy options for DED are envisaged.

The Short-Term and Long-Term Functional and Refractive Outcomes of Penetrating Keratoplasty

While anatomic success is relatively frequent, functional failure is relatively common. A systematic review of 13 studies (530 eyes) on visual outcomes of PK reported mean best-corrected visual acuity (BCVA) in the logarithm of the minimum angle of resolution (Log-MAR) within the range of 0.05–0.40 Log-MAR; notably, studies with longer follow-ups (>2 years) have reported a mean BCVA of 0.05 or 0.1 Log-MAR [28]. Fukuoka reported mean BCVA of 1.54 ± 0.68, 0.06 ± 0.22, 0.03 ± 0.17, and 0.14 ± 0.42 Log-MAR after 10 years, 20 years, and 25 years, respectively [21, 29]. A mean follow-up of 14 years also revealed 73.2% of patients having a BSCVA of 20/40 or better and an open-angle glaucoma rate of 5.4% [30, 31]. The application of new microkeratome-assisted with transplantation of a two-piece mushroom-shaped graft showed favorable visual outcomes comparable to conventional PK; BCVA of 20/40 and 20/20 were observed in 100% and >50% of eyes, respectively [32]. Studies comparing the quality of vision after PK with other surgical techniques, such as deep anterior lamellar keratoplasty (DALK), have also reported better BCVA after PK in the long run [28, 33]. The difference in techniques used during modern PK can also impact the visual outcome.

At least 1 year is usually required for the PK wound to heal sufficiently. Up to 30% of eyes still have astigmatism, uncorrectable with spectacles, and considered an important cause of poor visual outcomes of keratoplasty [34, 35]. The incidence of astigmatism can be reduced by better separation of the corneal button from the cornea of donor and recipient, termed trephination. Trephination systems include handheld, motor trephine, excimer laser, or FSL-based (Fig. 5.1; Video 5.1). The modifications of the different recommended protocols have been discussed in a section on postoperative management of penetrating keratoplasty [36–38].

The new FSL technique, which cuts both recipient and donor within a liquid interface, could solve this problem. Excimer-assisted trephination has shown better alignment in all sutures-out keratoplasty patients. It leaves the cornea's curvature undisturbed, reducing shear and compression artifacts in the tissue [5, 36, 39].

FS technology has enabled perfect limbal-oriented centration through optical coherence tomography. This solves the problem of centration with trephination in the recipient's eye. FSL can use side-cut profiles that improve the fitting between donor disc and recipient bed. They combine the optical benefits of PK and increased visual rehabilitation [4, 40]. Different side-cut profiles can be chosen in FSL PK; mushroom-shaped incisions can be performed manually with an FSL or a microkeratome, but a zig-zag incision can only be performed with FSL (Fig. 5.2).

The mushroom PK aims to minimize the replacement of the recipient healthy endothelium (typically keratoconus eyes) and maintain a large diameter of the superficial, refractive part of the graft for optimizing the postoperative refractive results. The top-hat design was intended to also address the advantage of supplying a larger amount of donor cells to eyes with decompensated endothelial cells [41–44]. The potential advantages of these profiles include improved graft adaptation, better and more stable wound healing leading to earlier suture removal, and eventually prolonged graft survival; however, none of these potential advantages have been approved by reliable studies until now, except for more favorable visual outcomes [45].

Apart from the visual acuity of the patients after PK, most of which can be corrected by spectacles, an important outcome after PK is graft failure/rejection, the clinical aspects of which are explained in the following.

F. Doroodgar et al.

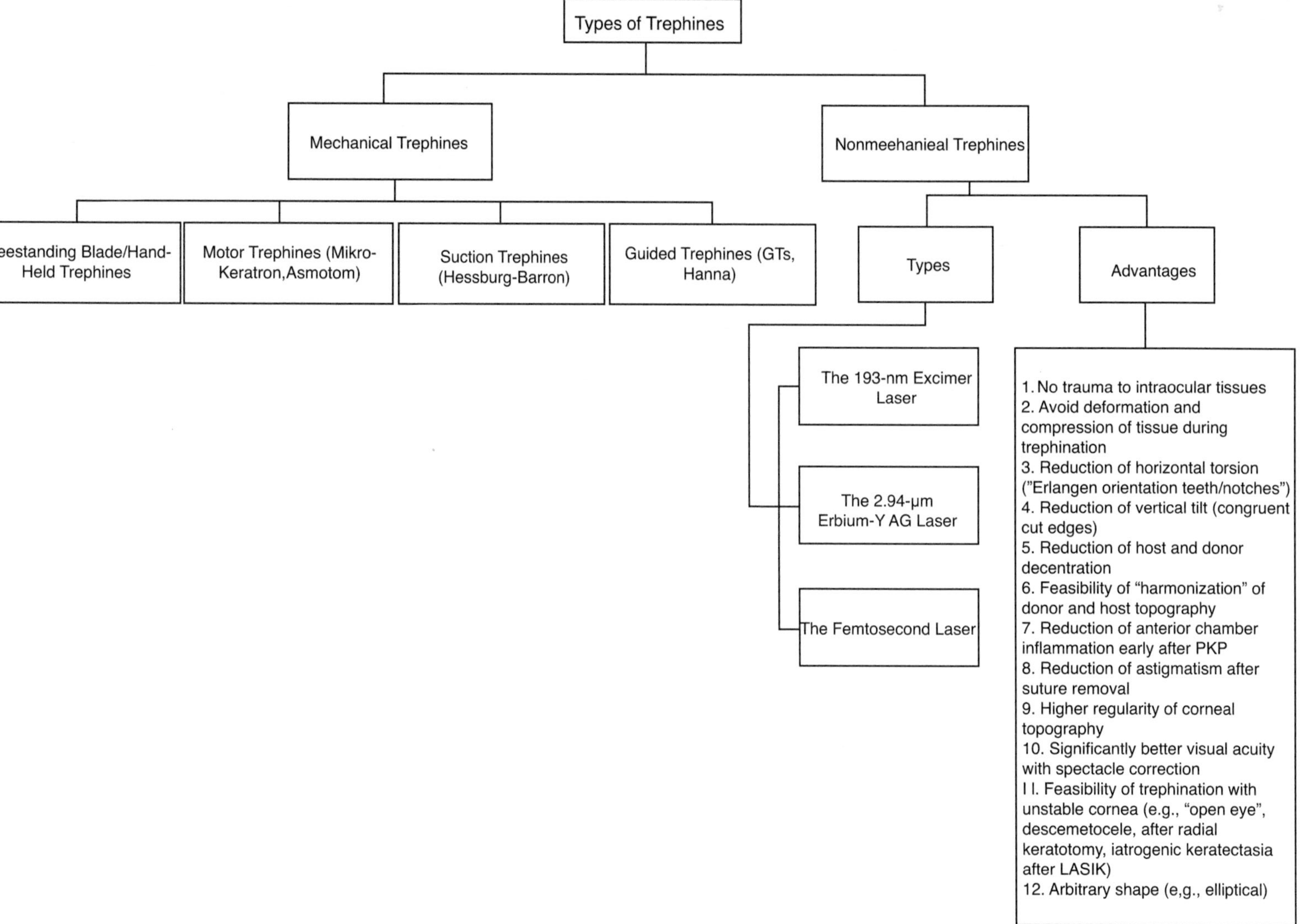

Fig. 5.1 Different types of trephines

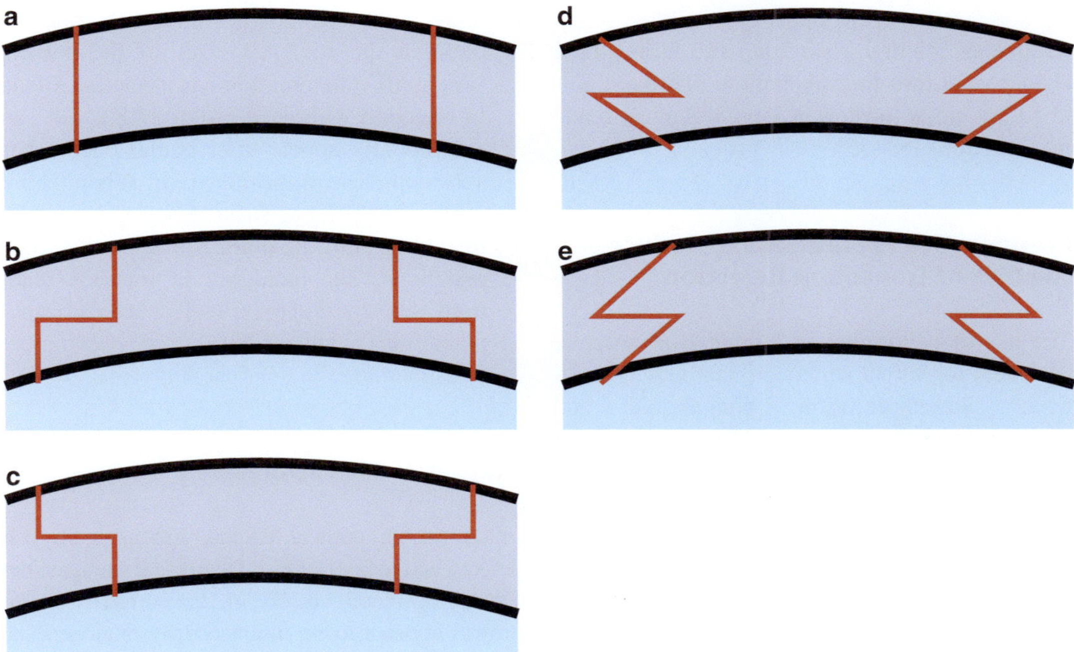

Fig. 5.2 The shapes of sidecuts used in laser-assisted keratoplasty. Standard cut (**a**), top hat (**b**), mushroom (**c**), zig-zag (**d**), and Christmas tree (**e**)

Clinical Aspects of Graft Failure After Penetrating Keratoplasty

In PK, all five layers of the cornea are removed and replaced with donor tissue. The rejection rates reported for PK range from 5.8% to 41%, depending on the duration of follow-up. Rejection can occur a few weeks after a cornea transplant, but it is more common after several months [46, 47], while others have reported favorable short-term (91% survival at 1 year) [48] and long-term outcomes (25-year graft survival rate of 85.4% [31] and 98.8%, 97.0%, and 93.2% at 10 years, 20 years, and 25 years after surgery, respectively) [29]. One of the main causes of graft failure after PK is the progressive donor endothelial cell loss (ECL) after PK, migration from areas with high to low-density ECD. The higher probability of ECL after PK for bullous keratopathy than after PK for keratoconus suggested the positive role of a healthy recipient endothelium (with high ECD) on the long-term survival of donor tissue [49, 50].

Graft survival of PK has been compared with other keratoplasty procedures, such as DALK, and some have claimed worse graft survival of cornea after PK compared with DALK. The use of new microkeratome-assisted transplantation of a two-piece mushroom-shaped graft showed a graft immunologic rejection rate of <5% and graft survival >95% for 5 years. Any independent postoperative risk factors, including infection, rejection, disease recurrence, eyelid or glaucoma surgery, or a repeat graft, decreased graft survival to 34% at 10 years [32, 48, 51, 52].

Clinical Aspects for Prevention and Treatment of Corneal Transplant Rejection

No standard or uniform guideline for preventing transplant rejection in high-risk cases of corneal transplantation exists. A history of HSK, a history of rejection, and transplantation in actively infected eyes are all factors to consider before surgery. Despite advances in anti-inflammatory drug regimens, glaucoma surgery, and other treatments, the high-risk group still faces a 60% chance of cornea transplantation. The main goal of follow-up is to prevent immunological rejection reactions [53–55].

Preoperative Precautions to Reduce the Risk of Transplant Rejection

The use of tacrolimus as a topical or systemic treatment for vernal keratoconjunctivitis is beneficial. Stevens-Johnson, pemphigoid and Mooren's ulcer should be postponed for at least 1 year after the inflammation have been controlled. Blepharitis, eyelid inflammation, infection, and eyelid disorders like ectropion and entropion can all be treated. A stem cell transplant should be performed at least 3 months before corneal transplant surgery if the patient has a large corneal stem cell defect (due to factors such as chemical burns or atopic keratoconjunctivitis) [54].

The Ways of Diagnosing Corneal Transplant Rejection

1. Look into the patient's complaints, such as eye pain or photosensitivity, as well as slit lamp findings, like the presence of KP or cells in the anterior chamber. The disadvantage of this method is that it does not allow for early detection of rejection before clinical rejection occurs.
2. The number of KPs, which can only show an increase in the thickness of the laryngeal and endothelial layers and cannot detect inflammatory cells, is also being tracked [56–58].
3. In-Vivo Confocal Microscopy is able to show microstructural changes in corneal cells and shows an increase in ICs (Immune Cells, Activated Keratocytes) in the early stages of transplant rejection. They can be found in all layers of the cornea, particularly in the subbasal region and endothelium [56–59]. There is a relationship between clinical symptoms and IC (AK) density. The patient experiences more severe pain when there are more of them in the subbasal layer of the cornea. Low-graft inflammation can sometimes lead to rejection without the start of KP. KP can occasionally appear after ocular edema has subsided. The appearance of subepithelial infiltrates (SEIs) or stromal edema should be treated as fully as other full-thickness graft rejections. The incidence of immune reactions was reported to be 10% in layered transplantation and 23% in complete transplantation in a 3-year study.

Angiogenesis Suppression

Inflammation, corneal edema, limbus stem cell defects, and hypoxia are all factors that stimulate the growth of blood vessels in the cornea. Corneal growth appears to be influenced by angiogenesis. There is growth from both bone marrow precursors and lymphatic vessels when it comes to lymphatic vessel growth. Although VEGF is the most important molecule in vascular endothelial cell proliferation, other factors such as nitric oxide and proinflammatory cytokines are also involved. Although VEGF is the most important molecule in vascular endothelial cell proliferation, other factors such as nitric oxide, matrix metalloproteinases, proinflammatory cytokines, and some growth factors (platelet-derived growth factor (PDGF) and fibroblast growth factor b (bFGF)) are also involved [60].

Inatomi et al. introduced a clinical classification for corneal vascular growth that includes four levels.

The first level is vascular growth in the corneal environment, then vascular growth in the mid-periphery. In the third level, moderate vascular growth is seen throughout the cornea, and at the end, severe vascular growth throughout the cornea [60].

The location, depth, length, and diameter of vessels, their branched appearance, and the state of blood flow in the arteries should all be considered when assessing corneal arteries. Long-term contact lens use after deep anterior lamellar keratoplasty (DALK) is an example of lipid keratopathy [60, 61].

Treatment of Corneal Angiogenesis

The removal of the angiogenic stimulus is the primary treatment for corneal angiogenesis. Despite the risk of side effects, topical corticosteroids are still the first line of defense. Immunosuppressive drugs such as 0.05% cyclosporine A and tacrolimus are other anti-inflammatory drugs [60].

Cyclosporine A systemically inhibits endothelial cell migration and inhibits angiogenesis. There are conflicting studies on the effect of topical cyclosporine A [60].

Tacrolimus inhibits the production of cytokines by T lymphocytes. It also reduces the production of immunoglobulins [60].

Anti-VEGF monoclonal antibodies, such as bevacizumab and ranibizumab, are another class of drugs used to treat corneal arteries. These drugs work by slowing the growth of young, active vessels while having no effect on mature or older vessels. Bevacizumab drops (5 mg/mL five times daily) have been shown in animal studies to be effective in reducing corneal vessels that do not respond to anti-inflammatory therapies [62].

Various studies have shown that subconjunctival injections of pegaptanib and aflibercept have antiangiogenic effects [63, 64].

FD006 is a new monoclonal antibody with potent antiangiogenic properties that have recently been introduced [65].

The safety of using topical monoclonal antibodies on the eye's surface has been questioned. Although there have been reports of delays in epithelial defect repair and increased expression of matrix metalloproteinases after topical application, there do not appear to be any serious side effects [60, 66].

Drugs in the tetracycline family, such as minocycline and doxycycline, have antiangiogenic properties in addition to anti-collagenase properties. Recently, a gel and solution containing 2% doxycycline were developed, and antiangiogenic effects were observed in animal and human studies [60, 67].

Fasudil is a Rho Kinase Inhibitor (ROCK Inhibitor) drug that has been shown to have anti-angiogenic properties in laboratory studies [68].

Various studies have suggested several methods for blocking blood vessels in addition to pharmacological treatments, including cryotherapy, laser thermal cauterization, fine needle diathermy (FND), and photodynamic therapy (PDT). Although these methods are most effective in treating adult arteries, they can also be used to treat young and immature arteries when combined with monoclonal antibodies.

Clinical studies have used vascular cauterization with argon lasers and Nd:YAG lasers.

Fine needle diathermy is effective in the treatment of corneal arteries in 80% of cases and is an effective, easy, safe, and inexpensive method. In a study using the Nd: YAG laser, 53% of the arteries were completely blocked after 3 months, while 37% reopened. Because fine needle diathermy can increase VEGF production, it is best combined with the topical application of anti-VEGF monoclonal antibodies to reduce the risk of corneal recurrence [60, 69].

Verteporfin photodynamic therapy is a method of selectively blocking corneal arteries. However, this method is costly, and there is a risk of laser-related side effects as well as the generation of oxygen-free radicals [70].

Amniotic membrane transplantation (AMT) is a surgical technique used to repair corneal epithelial defects and reduce inflammation and angiogenesis. Less invasive surgical procedures, such as sequential sector conjunctival epitheliectomy (SSCE), have been used in cases of damage to part of the corneal stem cells. Corneal vascular growth was associated with this damage. Amniotic Membrane Transplantation has anti-inflammatory and antiangiogenic properties [71].

A **conjunctival and limbus autograft (CLAU)** is removed from one eye when only one eye is affected, and the other eye is perfectly healthy. It is the most effective treatment of corneal stem cells associated with damage to more than two-thirds of limbus stem cells. Another option is cultured limbal epithelial transplants, which are used for complete defects in the stem cells of one or both eyes. Living-related conjunctival **limbal allograft (lr-CLAL)**, as well as keratolimbal allograft (KLAL), are recommended in cases where there is a significant corneal stem cell defect [60]. Other surgical procedures recommended for stem cell defects include **simple limbal epithelial transplant (SLET) and cultivated oral mucosal epithelial transplantation (COMET)**. The advantage of autograft methods over allogeneic methods is that there is no risk of allogeneic transplant rejection, and there is no need for suppressive drugs in the postoperative treatment regimen [72].

The blood vessels in the cornea should be investigated to determine the source of their presence. Anti-herpes medication is required in addition to transplant rejection treatment. Obviously, the blood vessels will regress as well, but if the blood vessels remain active despite immunological treatment, cautery or a topical injection of 2.5 mg bevacizumab 0.1% should be employed as an additional therapy. If the cause is a specific underlying condition (e.g., HSK), anti-herpes medication is required in addition to transplant rejection treatment.

The Risk Factors of Graft Failure

The risk factors of graft failure after PK include the following.

Graft Characteristics: Donor's Age and Sex, Graft Size, and Eye Banking Practices

Donor's Age

The effect of donor's sex and age on the graft survival rate is controversial. Gal and colleagues suggested no effect on donor's age. In a study by Barraquer and colleagues, grafts from donors aged 80 were at a slightly higher risk of failure than patients under 80 years [73–75]. The Corneal Donor Study (CDS) has reported no or weak association between donor age and failure up to 97 years of age, with follow-up ranging from <1 year to 22 years. A comparison of grafts that survived for 5 years postoperatively also showed a higher ECL in the donors aged between 70 and 76 years [46, 76–79]. This difference in the results of studies can be related to the different methodologies used for the statistical analysis,

such as age ranges compared or considering age as a continuous variable; also, the results can differ based on the preoperative estimation of the likelihood of graft survival [73, 77].

There was no significant difference in results between PK and DALK in pediatric keratoconus. Low-quality donor tissues increased the incidence of graft epithelium abnormalities. With adequate therapy, graft clarity and visual results may be good. In chronic or delayed-onset mustard gas keratitis, PKP should be considered a high-risk transplant[1] [80, 81] (Fig. 5.3).

Donor's Sex

The higher risk of failure in female patients (hazard ratio = 1.42) has also been reported as the spurious result of analysis with multiple comparisons [74, 75]. Female grafts from male donors may be subject to alloimmune reactivity in female recipients, as Y gene antigens are only not expressed in females. Lass and colleagues have also observed that the higher ECD in females at baseline did not influence the failure of PK at 5 years [79, 82, 83].

Graft Size

A study by Barraquer and colleagues shows graft diameters of 7.0–7.4 and 8.0 mm had the best 10-year survival estimate (70% and 69%) in PKs larger than 8.75 mm. The mechanism of graft failure and rejection is supposed to be the proximity of lumbar vasculature to conjunctival vessels and, thus, antigenic materials, which makes immunologic rejection more probable. In the first half of the twentieth century, a diameter of 8.00–8.25 mm was suggested as optimal for full-thickness grafts. In PKs for bullous keratopathy or Fuchs' dystrophy (with insufficient recipient ECD), an inverse association was observed between ECL and trephine diameter [50, 75, 82–88].

In keratoconus, the cone is frequently inferiorly displaced and should be completely removed to prevent residual or recurrent disease. In advanced scarred conus, corneal topography is unreliable and should not be used for surgical

---

[1] If there are no risk factors, transplant rejection reduces as the recipient becomes older.

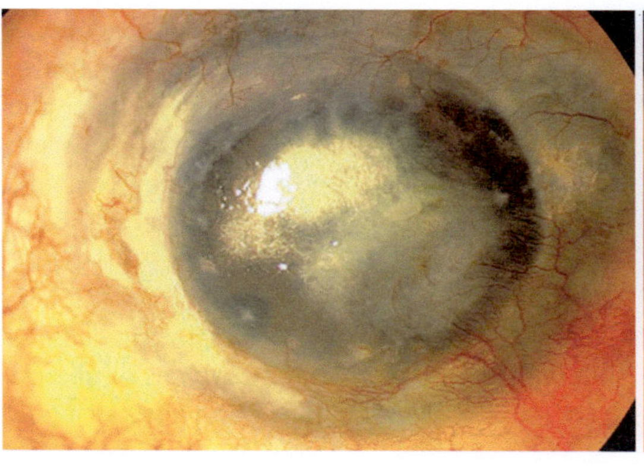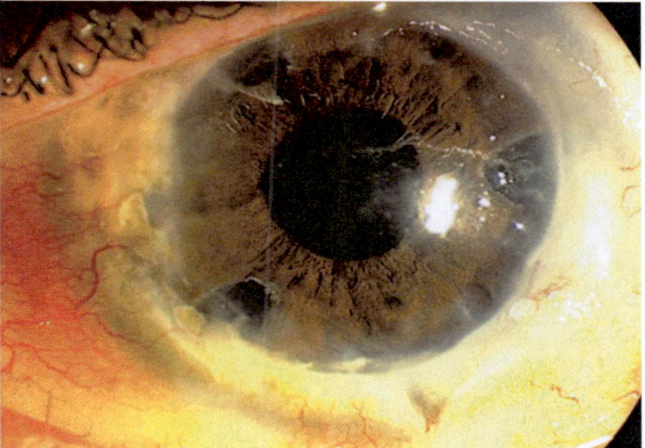

Fig. 5.3 PKP in chronic or delayed-onset mustard gas keratitis should be considered as a high-risk graft; however, with appropriate management, graft clarity and visual outcomes may be favorable

planning. Donor size will be adjusted in relation to the host limbal white-to-white measurement and conus extension, so grafts larger than 8.5 mm may be required [1].

In a phakic eye undergoing penetrating keratoplasty, a larger donor button is used to ensure the greatest fit. The donor cornea is predicted to be 0.26 mm smaller than the donor corneas cut from the endothelial side. Penetrating grafts used to treat keratoconus had a superior visual outcome and graft survival rate[2] [89] (Video 5.2).

- A corneal transplant size of about 7.5 mm is associated with a higher rate of rejection, researchers have found. Because of the graft's small size, a portion of the cone may remain, causing significant astigmatism and, in some cases, graft failure.
- In cases of keratoconus, the graft should be large enough to cover the entire cone in order to avoid damaging eye orbits.
- However, no clinical investigation has been conducted to prove that a smaller transplant size is related to a lower rejective reaction than a corneal transplant rejection [90]. Some factors that increase the chances of corneal transplant rejection include closeness to most receptor and receptor Langer cells and proximity to more blood vessels in the limbus area [91, 92].

____

[2]Considering size to prevent rejection.

Eye Banking Practices

DALK has shown that poor-quality corneas are not associated with an increased risk of graft failure in penetrating keratoplasty, following transplantation. Other conditions of the graft, such as preservation status and time between donor's death and transplant (enucleation within 12 h), have not been identified as significant risk factors. By reducing the requirement for a perfectly healthy endothelium and a high ECD, DALK increases the number of donor cornea available for transplantation—but more follow-up is required immediately after DALK [75, 76, 93–97].

Recipient-Related Factors: Primary Diagnosis, Number of Surgeries, Neovascularization, and Comorbidities

Primary Diagnosis

The Asian Cohort (Singapore) and Cornea donor study (CDS) showed a higher failure rate in pseudophakic bullous keratopathy than Fuch's dystrophy grafts. The presence of trauma and chemical burns at the time of PK also deserves special mention, considering the worst prognosis among all diagnoses. It has been postulated that the lower ECL in these patients may be the main cause of lower graft survival rates. Based on the results of 895 PK from 778 patients, patients with keratoconus (the most frequent diagnosis) showed the best 10-year survival estimate (95%), followed by endothelial and stromal dystrophies (both 55%), infectious leukomas (corneal ulcers with different infectious etiologies; 49%), trauma (33%), and chemical burns (14%); other diagnoses resulted in a 10-year survival rate of 37%, which showed a 4.6-fold higher odds (hazard ratio) of failure in patients with stromal dystrophies, sixfold for endothelial dystrophies, 7.4-fold for infectious leukomas, tenfold for trauma, and 11.9-fold for the chemical burn; 9.5 for other diagnoses, compared with keratoconus[3] [48, 75, 98].

Primary or Repeat PK

Another recipient-related factor impacting the outcome is the primary or repeat PK performance. The prognosis of repeat surgeries has been suggested by several studies. This is probably due to deteriorated condition of the corneal bed, increased IOP during the previous keratoplasty, and violation of anterior chamber immunological privilege. In an earlier study by Thompson and colleagues, similar results were obtained, considering the better survival of primary grafts and keratoconus. The patient's age had less impact on the second or more grafts when compared to first grafts[4] [9, 75, 93, 100–104] (Video 5.3).

Corneal Neovascularization

The loss of corneal angiogenic privilege after PK increases the risk of graft failure. Barraquer and colleagues also showed that primary PK grafts with avascular recipient corneas had the best

---

[3]The benefits of steroid treatment should be weighed against the risks of long-term steroid therapy, especially in those with an underlying condition that causes damage to the eyes.

[4]Systemic sensitization to donor antigens is more likely than local alterations caused by the main graft to hasten the rejective reaction. This rejection is unrelated to MHC congruence and could be caused by MHC components shared by both the first and second donors. The survival of the second link will not be improved by matching the donor-recipient HLA17. Therefore, the chance of rejection increases after the second corneal transplant operation [99]. No increases in the chances of transplant rejection have been observed in the other eye of someone whose first eye has had a rejection corneal transplant in any of the authors' clinical studies.

10-year survival estimate. Corneal vascularization quadrants are another characteristic associated with graft failure and rejection after keratoplasty. Preoperative administration of anti-angiogenic pharmacologic agents may be able to improve survival [75, 105–112].

Infections

Corneal infectious disease is a major cause of blindness worldwide. Different types of keratitis may influence the long-term prognosis of grafts. Active microbial infection at the time of PK increases the graft failure rate (hazard ratio = 5.10). The use of oral antivirals and immunosuppression with cyclosporin A or Mycophenolate Mofetil has reduced the recurrence rate of herpes simplex [54, 113–116].

In summary, keratitis induced by herpes simplex has a lower likelihood of successful corneal transplantation if:

- During surgery, there has been inflammation.
- In the cornea, blood vessels have formed.
- Due to decreased tear production and decreased corneal sensitivity, there is a higher risk of persistent epithelial defects (PED) after surgery. Suture loosening, corneal invasion, and graft failure are all symptoms of PED [91, 92, 117].

A prophylactic dose of antiviral drug should be started 1–2 weeks before corneal transplantation and continue for at least 6 months after. In endothelial insufficiency caused by herpes simplex that is treated with DSEAK/DMEK antiviral drugs can last for up to a year [118].

Glaucoma

This effect has not been approved in subgroup analysis, separated based on the indication of PK. More studies are needed to establish the exact mechanism of this effect. CDS also showed that cases with a history of glaucoma (before PK and those who used IOP-lowering medications at PK) had a higher graft failure rate than those with no history of glaucoma (58% vs. 22%, respectively; hazard ratio = 7.2). Considering the higher rate of endothelial decompensation in patients with glaucoma, the higher failure is related to ECL decline. Stewart and colleagues showed a 3-year transplant survival rate of 86% in eyes without glaucoma, 72% in eyes with glaucoma (73% in eyes with medically managed glaucoma and 63% in surgically managed glaucoma) [98, 119–121].

Antiglaucoma drugs increase the risk of corneal transplant rejection for three reasons as follows:

- Graft rejection is higher as a result of increased intraocular inflammation.
- Epithelial cell surface abnormalities cause persistent inflammation.
- Decomposition of endothelial cells without immunological responses [122].
- There have been reports of pilocarpine drops when a rejection occurs, which subside after the medicine is stopped and topical steroids are started [123].
- Dorzolamide is a reversible carbonic anhydrase II inhibitor that does not build up inside the cornea with repeated use. It acts as a selective inhibitor of type II and has a minor effect on type I. All of the patients in the study had complicated ocular histories, which included several surgeries and compromised corneas [124].

Ocular Surface Diseases

The ocular surface is formed by three-component tissues: the cornea, conjunctiva, and limbus. Corneal infection in any form of bacterial, fungal (Video 5.4), or viral infection can increase the possibility of corneal graft failure. Any disease that endangers the healthy and moist surface accelerates corneal transplant rejection [22].

Inflammation

Anterior synechiae on the iris can impair ocular immune privilege and increase the risk of graft rejection. Auto-immune diseases include uveitis, ocular mucous membrane pemphigoid, eye-involved collagen vascular disorders, Steven-Johnson syndrome, and atopic keratoconjunctivitis. Both glaucoma and traction,

induced by synechyma on the corneal endothelium, may lead to graft failure[5] [54].

Systemic Chronic Diseases

Children with Peters' anomaly and those with associated cataracts and glaucoma are at risk for graft failure. Smoking and poor outcomes in the first decade of life may also play a role. African-Americans and nonwhite race have also been noted as risk factors but not confirmed as independent risk factors [48, 98, 116, 122, 127–130].

During endothelial transplantation, roughly 10% of immune reactions and transplant rejection are delicate and dispersed KPs on the endothelium's surface, less as Khodadoust lines, and respond well to topical steroids. The reasons for this response are:

1. The limbus area's distance from the endothelium layer.
2. A less amount of stroma is transferred with the tissue.
3. In connective tissue, there is no corneal epithelium.
4. Receptor dendritic cells are unable to access the grafted layer. Thereby, selective endothelial keratoplasty should be considered in cases where only the endothelium is affected.

Surgery-Related Factors

The exact effect of the surgical details on the outcome has been only evaluated scantly. Some factors related to surgery, such as loose sutures and iris synechiae to the graft margin, have been demonstrated as risk factors for graft failure. The possibility of combined surgeries as a risk factor has also been raised. Still, combined surgery lost its effect in multivariate analysis [12, 75]. Others have also shown that combined surgeries did not significantly affect graft survival [95, 131]. This

---

[5]Immune reactions can occur after any inflammation in the eyes that have had corneal transplantation, and YAG laser capsulotomy is no exception. To decrease these immunological reactions, steroid drops should be used following capsulotomy [125, 126].

is while Fasolo et al. showed a 2.8-fold greater risk of graft failure after PK with pars plana vitrectomy [93]. The low number of combined surgeries in study populations is the main limitation in the available literature [132].

Other surgical interventions at the time of surgery, including cataract extraction, removal, and insertion of IOL, did not alter the odds of rejection. The study also found that none of the surgical procedures combined with PK, including posterior-lens implantation or pars plana vitrectomy, influenced graft survival [130, 131, 133]. Others have also confirmed higher graft failure rates in children who received PK combined with other intraocular surgeries than those without. Others have also claimed that concurrent vitrectomy results in a higher rate of immunologic rejection. As stated in the literature, the surgical procedures, considered as "combined," are variable. Cox regression analysis of 37 variables showed concurrent cataract extraction or IOL removal without lens implantation and intraocular silicone oil after the PK as significant predictors of graft failure after PK; two-thirds of these patients experienced graft failure eventually [116, 134–136].

The main focus of this section was on the risk factors of graft rejection/failure after PK; however, the rates reported among different studies are different for several reasons. First, various predictive treatments have been suggested for reducing the graft rejection rate after PK, especially in high-risk patients, such as immunosuppressive agents [15], and variation in their use for the study population of different studies can be a source of different rates reported. Another issue that must be considered is that the surgical details of PK are continually evolving, and several modifications have been introduced since its introduction (1950) [137]. Therefore, the difference in the surgical techniques used during each procedure can be an important source of diverse results of studies. A review of seven comparative studies showed that FSL PK was not superior to conventional PK in postoperative topographic astigma-

tism, spherical equivalent, graft rejection, graft failure, and complications. However, it resulted in higher ECD and better BCVA [40].

Further studies are required to compare the surgical outcome of modern vs. conventional PK. The large studies considered a strict inclusion criterion that comprises only a specific group of patients (with moderate risk) and is performed on specific races. It has to be noted that the frequency of these risk factors varied among studies, based on the study population.

Penetrating Keratoplasty in Keratoconus

An elective PK is now reserved in extreme cases when the DM and endothelium appear to be separated due to previous corneal hydrops. In such cases, a lamellar approach can still be used, especially if the scars do not disrupt the visual axis. The procedure will need to be modified to a PK intraoperatively if a large tear is discovered (longer than 2–3 clock hours). Although the PK strategy for keratoconus is not dissimilar to that used for other etiologies, there are a few things to keep in mind:

Decentered Grafts
Decentered grafts can also create significant irregular astigmatism in the visual axis, requiring the patient to wear stiff glasses for visual rehabilitation and, in certain situations, a second-centered graft. Keratoconus patients may benefit from employing same-diameter trephines for both donor and host tissues, which shrinks the donor button and lowers postoperative myopia. Reducing donor size when the anterior lens-to-retina length is less than 20.19 mm could result in significant postoperative hyperopia [138–142].

Suturing Technique
The surgeon can use one of the following suture techniques after placing the four cardinal 10-0

nylon sutures: single continuous suture (SCS), double continuous suture (DCS), combination of continuous and interrupted suture (CCIS), or interrupted suture (IS). IS should always be the closure method in cases where partial or complete suture removal is required. These include pediatric keratoplasty (sutures becoming loose too quickly), vascularization in the host cornea, multiple previous rejections, or inflammatory concomitant conditions [143].

Furthermore, research comparing astigmatism in keratoconus patients treated with a single continuous suture against a DCS found that astigmatism was identical in both groups after removing the sutures (DCS 4.6 D, SCS 5.2 D) [144]. As a result, it is apparent that any suture closure technique can work. The final choice is made by the surgeon. The needle is placed 90% deep into the donor cornea and then through the host cornea to provide a rudimentary idea of normal graft suturing. The ideal bite is as close to DM as possible, and a similar amount of tissue should be acquired in both the donor and host corneas to approximate Bowman's layer.

They hypothesized that the time between transplanting and recurrence with DALK would be shorter than with PK, albeit this has yet to be confirmed or supported by other investigations [145]. More research on long-term results is needed to assess the influence of DALK on keratoconus [1].

Penetrating keratoplasty is a safe and successful treatment for patients with keratoconus who are contact lens intolerant or have poor corrected visual acuity. The severity of the problem and the trephination and suturing techniques performed does not affect the ultimate visual results [30].

DALK is the first surgical option for patients with keratoconus and possibly other corneal stromal pathologies with normal endothelium. Because of its benefits, such as better globe integrity preservation, reduced intraoperative complications, and elimination of endothelial graft rejection, DALK can be considered an alternative to PK for this condition [146] (Fig. 5.4).

Management of Postpenetrating Keratoplasty Astigmatism

When astigmatism is too severe to be treated with the excimer laser alone, it can be reduced to a level where PRK or LASIK can be performed with or without relaxing incisions. Similarly, emmetropia-like refractive outcomes could be achieved by combining relaxing incisions with IOL implantation or IOL implantation with an excimer laser [147].

Postoperative Care

Intraocular Pressure Measurement after Penetrating Keratoplasty

The Goldmann applanation tonometry (GAT) remains the gold standard of IOP assessment, despite changes in corneal anatomy that occur after PK. The iCare, Tono-Pen XL, ocular response analyzer, and PDCT contour tonometry are gaining attention. All save the iCare tend to overstate IOP when compared to GAT. Future developments may improve the method's dependability even more. Although Goldmann tonometry is still the most appropriate modality for IOP measurement in post-PK eyes, its limitations in these situations underscore the need for new approaches that are more accessible and convenient to employ other tonometers have yielded inconsistent results, with some promising and others discouraging [148].

Management of Patients after Surgery to Reduce the Risk of Corneal Transplant Rejection

After a high-risk corneal transplant, the main goals are prevention, early diagnosis, and appropriate treatment. The patient should be educated on the symptoms of transplantation and suture loosening in order to make an early diagnosis. Topical steroids and antibiotics should be prescribed to prevent transplant rejection and infection after suturing. Regular follow-up can

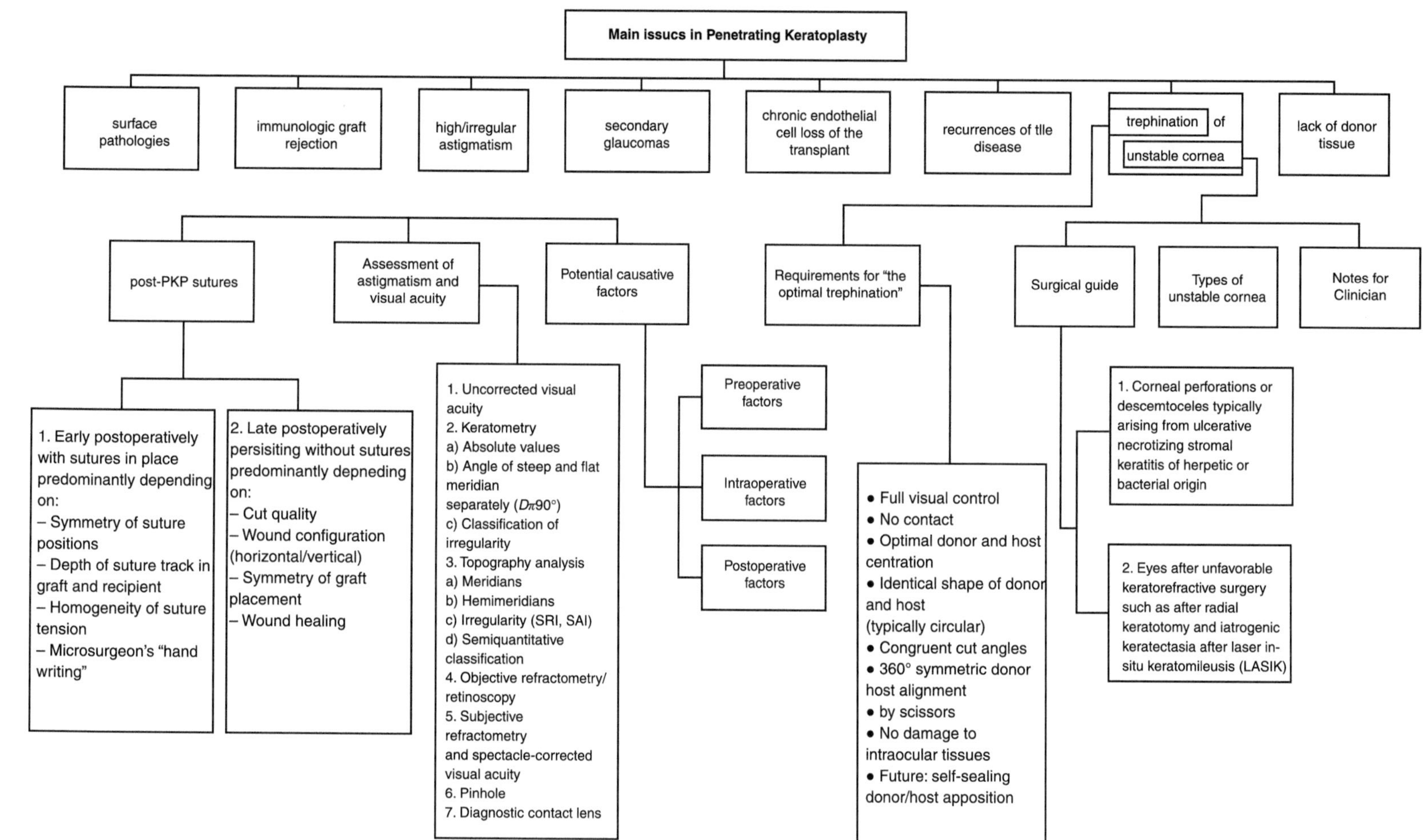

Fig. 5.4 Comprehensive schematic illustration of key penetrating keratoplasty considerations

Table 5.1 Comparison of different topical corticosteroids in terms of available types, potency, penetration, and side effects

Increasing intraocular pressure	Penetrating eyes	Anti-inflammatory effect	Dosages	Available types	Topical corticosteroid
Low	Low	Medium	0.10%	Drops	Fluorometholone (acetate)
			0.10%	Ointment	
Low	Low	High	0.2–0.5%	Drops	Loteprednol (etabonate)
High	Medium	High	0.10%	Drops	Dexamethasone (sodium phosphate)
			Complex	Ointment	
High	High	High	0.125–1%	Drops	Prednisolone (acetate, phosphate)
Very high	High	Very high	0.05%	Drops	Difluprednate
High	High	Very high	0.10%	Drops	Betamethasone (acetate and sodium phosphate)
			0.10%	Ointment	
Low	Low	High	0.5–1%	Drops	Hydrocortisone
			1–3%	Ointment	
Low	Low	Medium	1%	Drops	Medrysone
Low	Low	High	1%	Drops	Rimexolone

also aid in the early detection of cornea transplant rejection.

Corticosteroids

Corticosteroids are still the most commonly prescribed drugs for corneal transplant prevention and treatment [53, 54, 72]. In cases of high-risk corneal transplant rejection, specific immunosuppressive drugs are used.

The most commonly prescribed drugs to prevent and treat rejection in all types of corneal transplants are topical corticosteroids (betamethasone and prednisolone acetate 1%). How these drugs are administered in postcorneal transplant regimens varies greatly [53]. Table 5.1 Introduce widely used steroids in ophthalmology [149, 150].

How Important Topical Steroids Work and What Are They Used For

The ideal steroid will pass through the stromal fluid layer, depending on how much-unchanged drug enters the systemic circulation. The penetration of acetate derivatives is lower in the case of an epithelial defect, but regardless of that, acetate and alcohol derivatives are more effective than phosphate derivatives in inhibiting corneal inflammation [149].

Prednisolone acetate 1% (the preferred and most commonly prescribed topical corticosteroid for preventing corneal transplant rejection according to a 2011 survey [53]) reaches a high level in the aqueous humor in 120 min and persists for a day [151].

Topical corticosteroid drops (**betamethasone 0.1%** or prednisolone acetate 1%) in two doses, four times a day for 3 months, are used to prevent transplant rejection in penetrating keratoplasty transplants with no risk factors and a low risk of rejection (ACAID time), and at a daily dose of 4–6 months and gradually reducing the dose over 6–12 months, they are used in penetrating keratoplasty transplants with a high risk of corneal transplant rejection. Patients with herpes simplex keratopathy complications should be treated with an oral prophylactic dose of acyclovir or valaciclovir for a long time. Although anterior layer grafting eliminate graft rejection, graft rejection in the stromal layer and epithelium remains a possibility. Prednisolone acetate drops 6–4 times a day are recommended for these patients in the first days after surgery, with the dose gradually decreasing over 6–12 months because the majority of transplant rejection after endothelium transplantation has been observed when topical corticosteroid drops are completely stopped[6] [152, 153].

---

[6]Topical steroid after Low-Risk surgery should be used for at least 2 months until ACAID is created, with eye

If the pseudo facial and intraocular pressures are normal, topical corticosteroid drops can be safely continued for longer, but the dose must be limited or less potent drugs such as loteprednol etabonate or fluorometholone be used to prevent cataracts in patients with clear crystalline lenses.

Shimazaki discovered that long-term use of **fluorometholone 0.1%** was effective in preventing corneal transplant rejection in low-risk penetrating keratoplasty (PKP) patients with no significant side effects, but considering the condition of the lens in terms of the onset of posterior subcapsular cataracts (PSC), eye pressure control is required at each visit [151]. It is recommended that the daily dose of **topical corticosteroids be continued for a long time** until the surgeon sees significant side effects. For 1 year after transplantation, some surgeons use Fluorometholone drops or Prednisolone lotion drops on a daily basis. If the transplant is not in the high-risk group, the immune privilege (IP) mode will be restored after some time, making the patient no different from other patients [154, 155].

Difluprednate 0.05% is *not currently available* in Iran and many other countries.

Injecting 20–40 mg of **Triamcinolone** subconjunctival capsule during surgery is helpful in patients who are unlikely to cooperate postoperatively or have a high risk of corneal transplant rejection. Some surgeons perform a conjunctival injection of 40 mg methylprednisolone acetate 1 mL or 0.1% dexamethasone disodium phosphate. In terms of improved transplant rejection and relapse, there was no statistically significant difference between the two groups at the end of the study [156].

Corticosteroid injections into the conjunctiva have not been shown to prolong epithelial defect repair. There is no evidence that using oral corticosteroids to prevent corneal transplant rejection is beneficial. The probability of rejective reactions is very low when dynamic mechanisms are

activated and cause ACAID, but the probability of graft rejection is very high until the ACAID phenomenon occurs in 6–8 weeks after surgery [155].

The first corneal transplant rejection can occur after 3–4 weeks and a week in a low-risk or high-risk operation, respectively. Start a topical steroid and, depending on the response, taper and discontinue within 3–4 weeks. If KP occurs during follow-up, we will continue with the rejection treatment as planned. If the patient's corneal transplantation was due to keratoconus or corneal dystrophies, start topical steroids immediately, and if the patient's corneal transplantation was due to herpes, start an oral antiviral drug or prophylactic dose.

Long-Term Topical Steroid Use

In high-risk cases, such as a history of glaucoma [157] or vitreous and retinal surgery, multiple cases of rejection attacks, as well as pseudophakic patients who have one eye [158], recommend taking topical steroids for a long time.

There is no general rule for all patients, and the risk of developing Infectious Crystalline Keratopathy is the worst part. In a patient with a history of corneal transplantation, during a routine examination, start topical steroids every 2–4 h and reduce them within 2–3 months.

Immunosuppressive Therapies

Immunosuppressive therapies, either topical or systemic, are frequently required to prevent graft rejection. According to Holland et al.'s research, the use of corticosteroid-sparing diets is recommended in high-risk transplants to prevent corneal transplant rejection due to the many side effects of oral corticosteroids [159]. Calcineurin Inhibitors, Anti-proliferative drugs, and blocking the activation and action of T cells are all included in these diets. Calcineurin inhibitors include Cyclosporine A and Tacrolimus. In low-risk transplants, systemic immunosuppressive therapy usually has no place [160]. However, in high-risk patients, the use of these drugs is recommended (Fig. 5.5).

Cyclosporine is a cyclic undecapeptide, while tacrolimus is a macrocyclic lactone; However,

---

pressure and lens position monitored regularly. In patients with a low risk of rejection, steroid treatment should be started at 2- to 3-h intervals and continued until the KP has entirely disappeared. Even daily use of a steroid drop can cause eye strain, cataracts in phakic patients, and corneal infectious crystalline keratopathy (ICK).

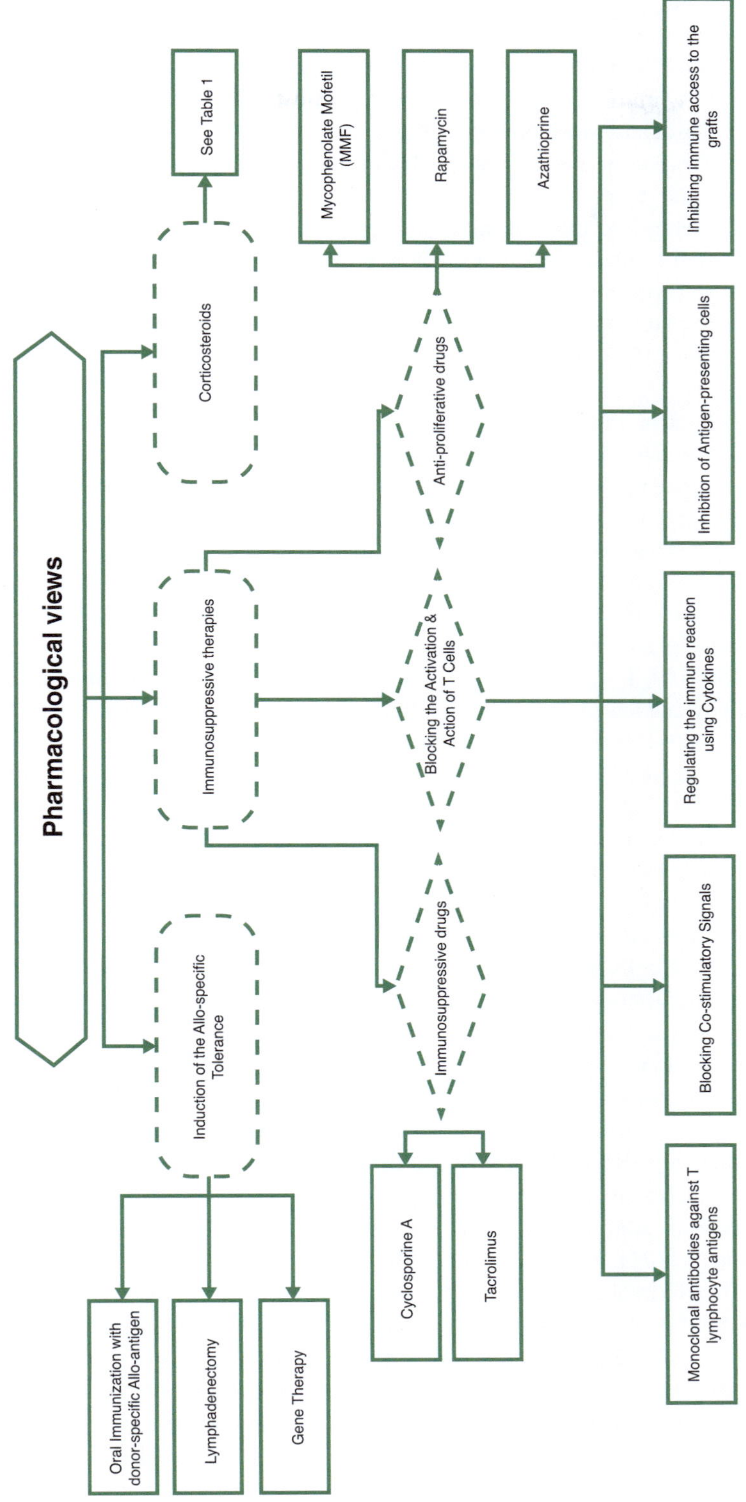

Fig. 5.5 Management of patients after surgery to reduce the risk of corneal transplant rejection

both inhibit calcineurin and are classified as immunosuppressive drugs [161]. Tacrolimus blocks calcineurin to limit T lymphocyte IL-2 production. Cyclosporine A inhibits T lymphocyte migration, and vascular development increases lymphocyte infiltration in the conjunctiva and lacrimal gland and tears production. Despite differences in potency, tacrolimus, and cyclosporine both have high graft survival rates [162, 163]. However, cyclosporine A has low efficiency in avoiding transplant rejection and is not frequently used nowadays [53, 54, 150, 159, 164, 165].

The use of anti-proliferative drugs (such as mycophenolate mofetil, rapamycin, and azathioprine) along with the mentioned immunosuppressive drugs can be more effective in preventing transplant rejection. Mycophenolate mofetil (MMF-known as CellCept) inhibits T and B lymphocyte proliferation. It had fewer side effects and a more significant effect in preventing graft rejection than cyclosporin A [53, 54, 150, 159, 164]. Rapamycin inhibits B and T cell activity and lowers Ig production, with an effect that is 80–100 times stronger than cyclosporine A. It is a good substitute for mycophenolate mofetil [53, 54, 150, 159, 164, 166]. In complicated patients, azathioprine is currently used as a supplement to oral cyclosporine A or oral tacrolimus [53, 54, 150, 159, 164].

Some experimental approaches to blocking the activation and action of T cells are monoclonal antibodies against T lymphocyte antigens, blocking co-stimulatory signals, regulating the immune response with cytokines and peptides, inhibiting antigen-presenting cells, and inhibiting immune access to grafts [53, 54, 167–170].

Monoclonal antibodies against CD3, CD4, CD8, IL-12, and αβ T-cell receptors have beneficial effects after parenteral administration in experimental animal models [171]. Xanax (daclizumab) and Simulect (basiliximab) bind to the alpha subunit (Tac/CD25) of interleukin 2 to prevent T lymphocyte activation [54, 168, 170]. Alemtuzumab (CD52 receptor antibody), in a small number of studies, has been shown to improve transplant survival [169].

Abatacept (cytotoxic T-lymphocyte-associated protein 4) is a high affinity-bonded recombinant fusion protein to B7 molecules. The CD28 receptor T lymphocyte is responsible for CLTA4-Ig's. Both topical CLTA2g drops and monoclonal antibodies against CD28 have improved connective tissue survival in various studies [169, 172–174]. Belatacept (more fusion to B7) has not yet been used to prevent corneal transplantation rejection [169, 173]. Also, a study showed that Tocilizumab may promote corneal allograft survival, possibly by modulating the Treg-Th17 balance in rat [175].

Regulating the immune reaction using cytokines also could be a beneficial approach to management transplantation. Transfection of interleukin-4 (IL-4) and interleukin-10 (IL-10) genes into transplanted corneal epithelium via viral carriers increases its survival in animal studies [169, 170]. In rat eyes, topical administration of α-melanocytic stimulating hormone [176], α-Tumor necrosis factor, or α-TNF, in a mouse study, less transplant rejection [177].

Despite the effect of inhibition of antigen-presenting cells to reduce inflammation, it did not affect reducing the rate of corneal transplant rejection [54, 169, 178].

Inhibiting immune access to the grafts has significant effects in preventing graft rejection via obstructing the movement of immune cells and corneal vascularization attenuation. Among the methods of obstructing the movement of immune cells, we can mention: Leukocyte function antigen 1 or LFA-on T lymphocytes attach to intracellular adhesion molecule 1 (ICAM-1). As a result, cytokine production increases [54, 167, 169, 178]. Antigen function of white blood cells and very late antigens 1 and 4 are among these antibodies (VLA-1 and VLA-4). Liftegrast 5% (Xiidra) is one of the topical treatments for dry eye that has been shown to help transplanted corneas survive longer. Its structure is similar to that of ICAM-1 [178–180].

Several genes are involved in increasing transplant survival. Induction of the allospecific Tolerance could be effective in combination with anti-inflammatory and other immune-regulating properties to prevent transplant rejection. For example, in a study, oral immunization with donor-specific alloantigen tolerance was induced in animals [181]. Also, lymphadenectomy, another offered treatment, prevents antigen-presenting by blocking the function of VEGF-3 [182, 183]. The transfer of the interleukin-10 gene in animal studies and programmed cell death ligand (PDL-1) gene transfer (decreasing CD8 lymphocytes, natural killer proinflammatory cytokines) [54, 184–186] showed that gene therapy could be a different and impressive treatment method in the future.

The Stages and Approach to the Corneal Transplant Rejection

1. When a corneal transplant that is already clear and free of problems develops edema without any inflammatory or clinical signs, it is considered "possible."
2. When corneal edema is accompanied by inflammation, but there is no endothelial rejection line, it is considered "probable."
3. When corneal edema is accompanied by an endothelial rejection line, this is referred to as "definite rejection."

Corneal transplant rejection usually starts with photophobia, then mild to moderate AC reaction, then the emergence of subtle pigmented KPs, then the pigmentation of KPs, and finally the formation of Khodadoust line and corneal edema.

Basically, hyperacute rejection does not occur during corneal transplant rejection. The term "hyperacute rejection" has been used in some articles to rule out corneal transplantation, but this is a phenomenon unique to organ transplantation. The rejection of the graft in the stromal layer is mentioned immediately after the endothelial layer is expelled in the articles that have used this term, which starts with the sign of corneal opacity and involves the center of the cornea for a short time [9].

Up to one-third of transplant rejection cases result in transplant failure. Two to 3 months before the onset of clinical symptoms, a confocal microscopic examination of the stroma reveals the presence of activated keratocytes (AK). It is a way to diagnose corneal transplant rejection before the clinical signs begin. The density of immune cells in different layers of the cornea was studied in a study of 38 patients who underwent corneal transplantation (15 with rejection and 23 without rejection) using in vivo confocal microscopy (IVCM). The authors concluded that the density of these cells increases in patients with corneal transplant rejection, particularly in the subbasal and endothelial layers, and that this increase is linked to pain and light sensitivity in these patients [56]. In a separate study, 45 patients who had corneal transplants were followed up prospectively, with AK cells counted with IVCM on the first and seventh days after surgery, as well as monthly. In this study, patients who had rejective transplant reactions 2 months ago had an increase in AK cells. The number of cells in the other group remained constant for 4 months after transplantation [187].

Rapid diagnosis and initiation of treatment with high and frequent doses of the drug according to the stage, KPs, and clinical findings is the second most effective strategy in the management of corneal transplant rejection.

Better Management of Transplantation Considering KPs, Vascularization, and Iris Adhesions

A subconjunctival injection of betamethasone 2–4 mg is helpful if the rejection is more severe. Oral steroids and intravenous injections may be added to the regimen in addition to the above. Steroid drops are started at 1-h intervals, and betamethasone ointment can be used at night while sleeping.

KP is not pigmented at first and disappears with proper treatment, but due to the severity of the reaction, large, and pigmented KP can occur, which may disappear or remain for a long time (old KPs) after treatment except for inflammation. No special treatment is required in such cases where the number, size, and color of KPs have not changed over time.

When severe corneal edema prevents KP from being seen, the edema can be treated and reduced to allow KP to be seen. KP may be gone, but edema persists in the final stages of complete transplant rejection, which cannot be improved. If there are predisposing factors for rejective reactions, they should be removed at the same time as starting treatment because stromal edema may prevent KPs from being seen after KP edema has resolved. The presence of active blood vessels, especially the cornea, is one of the active factors in the rejection of corneal transplantation, which should be eliminated by subconjunctival injection of anti-VEGF or fine needle courtesy.

As a supplement, it has been suggested that iris adhesions to the cornea be isolated. It is emphasized that treatment for corneal transplant rejections should be continued until the KPs have vanished completely. During this time, the eye pressure should be recorded at each visit, and the clarity or onset of opacity in keratoconus patients should be observed more than in other people [55].

Pharmaceuticals and Clinical Aspects of Different Drugs in Keratoplasty

The clinical factors that should be taken into account when using various corticosteroids as the cornerstone of treatment, immunosuppressants, and antibodies are summarized in Tables 5.2, 5.3, and 5.4, respectively [156, 169, 177, 188–196]. Figure 5.6 also includes a summary of safeguards that should be taken before undergoing corneal transplantation.

In conclusion, the most effective strategy for treating corneal transplantation is prevention and

Table 5.2 Clinical points in using corticosteroid drugs

Drugs	Using
Betamethasone 0.1%, Prednisolone Acetate 1%, or Dexamethasone 0.1%	As previously stated, the most commonly used drug for corneal transplantation is prednisolone acetate drops 1%.
	Corticosteroids are usually prescribed at a dose of one drop every 3 h at the start of treatment, with the dose gradually decreasing depending on the severity of the transplant rejection and the clinical response to treatment. Corticosteroid drops should be used until the KPs (keratic precipitate) deposits on the cornea are completely gone.
	In a patient with corneal transplant rejection, we usually stop treatment 2–3 weeks after no KPs or cells are seen in the anterior chamber, and the KPs resolve after starting the steroid after 4–5 weeks, but a re-examination is needed a few weeks later to ensure there is no recurrence of KPs.
	Patients with a history of recurrent corneal transplant rejection should continue to use low-dose corticosteroid drops on a long-term basis (once daily or every other day).
Betamethasone eye ointment	Betamethasone eye ointment can also be used once a night before bed as a complementary treatment in patients with a history of recurrence. However, keep in mind that the ointment's bioavailability is lower than that of frequent drops.
	Patients should be followed up on a regular basis. In patients with a history of high blood pressure or herpes simplex keratopathy, corticosteroids should be used with caution.
Injection of 20 mg of Triamcinolone acetonide or 2 mg of Dexamethasone	In case of severe rejection or patients who cannot use the drug frequently, an injection of 20 mg of triamcinolone acetonide or 2 mg of dexamethasone can be used.
	Increased intraocular pressure is the most serious side effect of triamcinolone acetonide injection or dexamethasone submucosal injection, and patients should be closely monitored for it.
Oral corticosteroids (Prednisolone)	There is no agreement on the use of oral corticosteroids (prednisolone) at a daily dose of 1 mg/kg body weight in the treatment of corneal transplant rejection, and a small clinical study has been done.

(continued)

Table 5.2 (continued)

Drugs	Using
Intravenous corticosteroids (single-dose methylprednisolone, 125–500 mg)	Several studies have been performed on the use of intravenous corticosteroids (single-dose methyl prednisolone, 125–500 mg) in the acute phase of corneal transplant rejection. Patients with acute endothelial layer transplant rejection were randomly divided into two groups in one clinical study: Topical corticosteroids were combined with a single pulse of methylprednisolone (500 mg) in one group, while topical corticosteroids were used alone in the other. In both groups, topical corticosteroid treatment consisted of a single subconjunctival injection of 2 mg of betamethasone followed by treatment with 0.01% dexamethasone drops for the first 24 h. In terms of transplant rejection, relapse, recurrence, and posttransplant rejection failure, there was no statistically significant difference between the two groups at the end of the study.
Oral Prednisolone	The use of oral prednisolone in the treatment of corneal transplant rejection seems to be useful only in cases where 6 months or less have elapsed since corneal transplant surgery, and on examination, in addition to the rejection symptoms, there is corneal edema.
Subconjunctival injection of 20 mg Triamcinolone	Another study also showed that endothelial transplant rejection after penetrating keratoplasty (PKP) with subconjunctival injection of 20 mg triamcinolone acetonide with 1% prednisolone acetate compared with the intravenous pulse of 500 mg methylprednisolone with prednisolone acetate 1% was preferred.
Intracameral injection of Triamcinolone and Dexamethasone	In several studies, the effect of intracameral injection of triamcinolone and dexamethasone in endothelial layer transplantation and penetrating keratoplasty (PKP) was investigated. Because of the risk of infection and cataracts from injecting into the anterior chamber, this method is not recommended.

Table 5.3 Clinical points in using immunosuppressive drugs

Drugs	Using
Topical and systemic tacrolimus	Some studies have recommended the use of immunoregulator drugs such as topical and systemic tacrolimus as well as CellCept. The patient's condition, whether he or she has only one eye or the other eye is healthy, and whether or not there is a systemic disease such as diabetes or kidney failure, will determine how to begin and how long to use them. The anterior segment specialist is consequently compelled to choose. Topical steroids and tacrolimus drops are used for a long time, and in some cases forever, after the inflammation has been controlled.
Cyclosporine 0.05% drops	Other clinical studies have shown that cyclosporine 0.05% drops have no effect in the treatment of acute corneal transplant rejection.
Tacrolimus drops 0.05%	In another study, the therapeutic effect of tacrolimus drops 0.05% on endothelial layer transplantation after PKP was evaluated, and patients were randomly divided into two groups: Both groups received corticosteroid therapy, with tacrolimus drops 0.05% added as an adjunct drug in one group. A single subconjunctival injection of 1 mg betamethasone, 1% prednisolone acetate drops, and 1 mg oral prednisolone tablets per weight (1 mg/kg) was given to both groups as corticosteroid treatment. Treatment with 0.05% tacrolimus drops was found to be ineffective in treating the acute phase of corneal endothelial rejection at the conclusion of the study, though during recurrences, it might reduce rejection.

Table 5.4 Clinical points in using antibodies

Drugs	Using
CD3 receptor antibody (muromonab or OKT3)	The first monoclonal antibody approved by the US Food and Drug Administration (FDA) to prevent kidney transplant rejection is the CD3 receptor antibody (muromonab or OKT3).
	CD3 is one of the receptors on T lymphocytes, and its systemic consumption causes a significant reduction in the number of T lymphocytes and immune system suppression. Diets containing this monoclonal antibody have been used to prevent and treat acute renal, liver, and heart transplants. Acute corneal transplant rejection has also been treated with this antibody. The use of this antibody systemically has a number of negative consequences, including an increased risk of infection and cytokine release syndrome.
Muromonab	In one case, muromonab was injected into the anterior chamber to treat acute corneal transplant rejection, which resulted in a severe inflammatory intraocular response.
α-Tumor necrosis factor or α-TNF	α-Tumor necrosis factor or α-TNF is associated with apoptosis, and therefore its inhibition can greatly inhibit immune function.
	In a study in mice, after corneal allograft transplantation for one of the groups, α-TNF factor receptor drops were started and decreased corneal transplant rejection in that group.
	Antibodies have no place in the treatment of corneal transplant rejection.

quickly diagnose to start treatment with high, frequent doses of corticosteroids.

Take Home Notes
- In high-risk cases, the main goals of corneal follow-up are transplantation rejection prevention, rapid diagnosis, and appropriate treatment.
- The following steps are currently recommended as a treatment regimen for preventing transplant rejection:
  - Use high-dose topical corticosteroids that are gradually reduced and kept at a low dose for a long time.
  - Topical tacrolimus or topical cyclosporine 2% in combination with topical corticosteroids for a long time.
  - Preoperative oral corticosteroids and systemic mycophenolate mofetil prescriptions, rapamycin, and azithromycin may be used as substitutes.
  - Combination of oral tacrolimus or oral cyclosporine and oral Mycophenolate Mofetil.
  - With more research being done on monoclonal antibodies, these drugs will play a bigger role in transplant rejection prevention regimens in the future.
- The most effective treatment for acute corneal transplant rejection is still corticosteroid drops. Because of its high penetration of healthy corneal epithelium and strong immunosuppressive effect, 1% prednisolone acetate is the most widely used corticosteroid drop in the treatment of acute corneal transplantation, but in Iran, betamethasone 0.1% drops are the drug of choice.

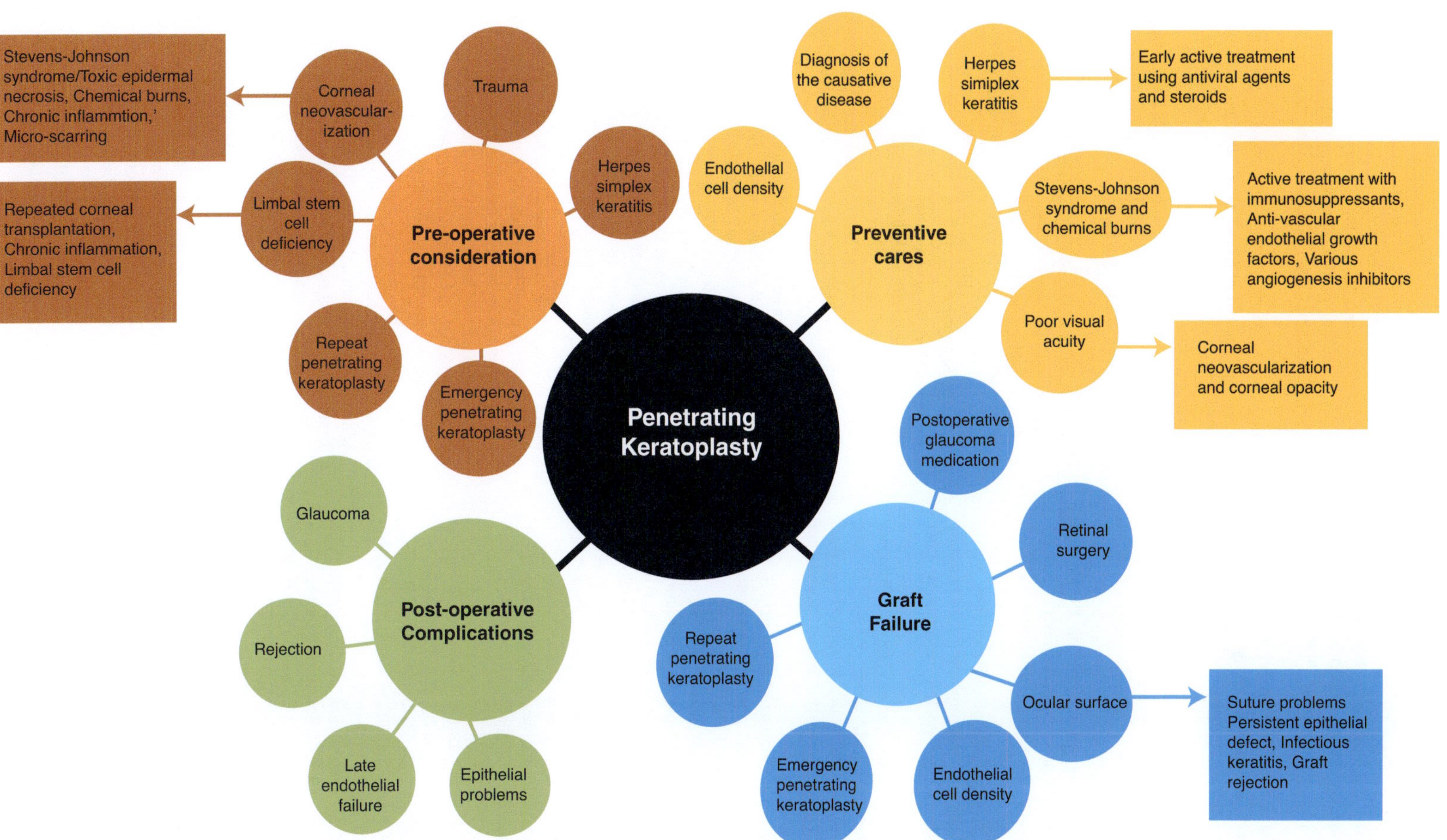

Fig. 5.6   An overview of preventative, preoperative, and postoperative measures

References

1. Arnalich-Montiel F, Alió del Barrio JL, Alió JL. Corneal surgery in keratoconus: which type, which technique, which outcomes? Eye Vis. 2016;3:2.
2. Frost NA, Wu J, Lai TF, Coster DJ. A review of randomized controlled trials of penetrating keratoplasty techniques. Ophthalmology. 2006;113:942–9.
3. Trufanov SV, Budnikova EA, Rozinova VN [Modern modifications of penetrating keratoplasty with complex operative incision]. Vestn oftalmol. 2019;135:260–6.
4. Adeyoju J, Konstantopoulos A, Mehta JS, Hossain P. Femtolaser-assisted keratoplasty: surgical outcomes and benefits. J EuCornea. 2020;8: 1–13.
5. Tóth G, et al. Comparison of excimer laser versus femtosecond laser assisted trephination in penetrating keratoplasty: a retrospective study. Adv Ther. 2019;36:3471–82.
6. Castellanos-González JA, Orozco-Vega R, González Ojeda A, Martínez Ruiz AM, Fuentes-Orozco C. Evaluation of the quality of life related to vision after penetrating keratoplasty. Archiv Soc Espan Oftalmol. 2021;96:69–73.
7. Selver OB, Karaca I, Palamar M, Egrilmez S, Yagci A. Graft failure and repeat penetrating keratoplasty. Exp Clin Transplant. 2021;19:72–6.
8. Chotikavanich S, Prabhasawat P, Satjapakasit O. Ten-year survival of optical penetrating keratoplasty and risk factors for graft failure in Thai patients. J Med Assoc Thail. 2020;103:883–90.
9. Panda A, Vanathi M, Kumar A, Dash Y, Priya S. Corneal graft rejection. Surv Ophthalmol. 2007;52:375–96.
10. Qazi Y, Hamrah P. Corneal allograft rejection: immunopathogenesis to therapeutics. J Clin Cell Immunol. 2013;2013:006.
11. Guilbert E, et al. Long-term rejection incidence and reversibility after penetrating and lamellar keratoplasty. Am J Ophthalmol. 2013;155:560–569.e562.
12. Anderson E, Chang V. Corneal allograft rejection and failure. Am Acad Ophthalmol. 2015;
13. Benetz BA, et al. Endothelial morphometric measures to predict endothelial graft failure after penetrating keratoplasty. JAMA Ophthalmol. 2013;131:601–8.
14. Lass JH, et al. Endothelial cell density to predict endothelial graft failure after penetrating keratoplasty. Arch Ophthalmol. 2010;128:63–9.
15. Di Zazzo A, Kheirkhah A, Abud TB, Goyal S, Dana R. Management of high-risk corneal transplantation. Surv Ophthalmol. 2017;62:816–27.
16. Gómez-Benlloch A, et al. Causes of corneal transplant failure: a multicentric study. Acta Ophthalmol. 2021;99:e922–8.
17. Sellami D, et al. Epidemiology and risk factors for corneal graft rejection. Transplant Proc. 2007;39:2609–11. (Elsevier).
18. Inoue K, Amano S, Oshika T, Tsuru T. Risk factors for corneal graft failure and rejection in penetrating keratoplasty. Acta Ophthalmol Scand. 2001;79:251–5.
19. Hori J, Isobe M, Yamagami S, Tsuru T. Acceptance of second corneal allograft by combination of anti-VLA-4 and anti-LFA-1 monoclonal antibodies in mice. Transplant Proc. 1998;1:200–1.
20. Baratta RO, Schlumpf E, Buono BJD, DeLorey S, Calkins DJ. Corneal collagen as a potential therapeutic target in dry eye disease. Surv Ophthalmol. 2022;67:60–7.
21. Alio JL, et al. Corneal graft failure: an update. Br J Ophthalmol. 2021;105:1049.
22. Siregar S. How ocular surface disorder affected corneal graft survival. In: Dry eye syndrome-modern diagnostic techniques and advanced treatments. Rijeka: IntechOpen; 2021.
23. Beining MW, et al. In-office thermal systems for the treatment of dry eye disease. Surv Ophthalmol. 2022;67:1405–18.
24. Alió del Barrio JL, et al. Corneal transplantation after failed grafts: options and outcomes. Surv Ophthalmol. 2021;66:20–40.
25. Ji YW, et al. Corneal lymph angiogenesis facilitates ocular surface inflammation and cell trafficking in dry eye disease. Ocul Surf. 2018;16:306–13.
26. Perez VL, Pflugfelder SC, Zhang S, Shojaei A, Haque R. Lifitegrast, a novel integrin antagonist for treatment of dry eye disease. Ocul Surf. 2016;14:207–15.
27. Zhang X, Vadoothker S, Munir WM, Saeedi O. Ocular surface disease and glaucoma medications: a clinical approach. Eye Contact Lens. 2019;45:11–8.
28. Song Y, Zhang J, Pan Z. Systematic review and meta-analysis of clinical outcomes of penetrating keratoplasty versus deep anterior lamellar keratoplasty for keratoconus. Exp Clin Transplant. 2019;18:417–28.
29. Fukuoka S, et al. Extended long-term results of penetrating keratoplasty for keratoconus. Cornea. 2010;29:528–30.
30. Javadi MA, et al. Outcomes of penetrating keratoplasty in keratoconus. Cornea. 2005;24:941–6.
31. Pramanik S, Musch DC, Sutphin JE, Farjo AA. Extended long-term outcomes of penetrating keratoplasty for keratoconus. Ophthalmology. 2006;113:1633–8.
32. Busin M, Madi S, Scorcia V, Santorum P, Nahum Y. A two-piece microkeratome-assisted mushroom keratoplasty improves the outcomes and survival of grafts performed in eyes with diseased stroma and healthy endothelium (An American Ophthalmological Society Thesis). Trans Am Ophthalmol Soc. 2015;113:T1.
33. Garrido C, Cardona G, Güell JL, Pujol J. Visual outcome of penetrating keratoplasty, deep anterior

lamellar keratoplasty and Descemet membrane endothelial keratoplasty. J Opt. 2018;11:174–81.

34. Lam F, Rahman M, Ramaesh K. Traumatic wound dehiscence after penetrating keratoplasty—a cause for concern. Eye. 2007;21:1146–50.

35. Tzelikis PF, et al. Traumatic wound dehiscence after corneal keratoplasty. Arq Bras Oftalmol. 2015;78:310–2.

36. Latz C, Asshauer T, Rathjen C, Mirshahi A. Femtosecond-laser assisted surgery of the eye: overview and impact of the low-energy concept. Micromachines. 2021;12:122.

37. Seitz B, Hager T, Langenbucher A, Naumann GO. Reconsidering sequential double running suture removal after penetrating keratoplasty: a prospective randomized study comparing excimer laser and motor trephination. Cornea. 2018;37:301–6.

38. Seitz B, et al. Penetrating keratoplasty for keratoconus – excimer versus femtosecond laser trephination. Open Ophthalmol J. 2017;11:225–40.

39. Boden KT, et al. Novel liquid interface for femtosecond laser-assisted penetrating keratoplasty. Curr Eye Res. 2020;45:1051–7.

40. Liu Y, Li X, Li W, Jiu X, Tian M. Systematic review and meta-analysis of femtosecond laser–enabled keratoplasty versus conventional penetrating keratoplasty. Eur J Ophthalmol. 2021;31:976–87.

41. Maier P, Böhringer D, Birnbaum F, Reinhard T. Improved wound stability of top-hat profiled femtosecond laser-assisted penetrating keratoplasty in vitro. Cornea. 2012;31:963–6.

42. Seitz B, et al. Inverse mushroom-shaped nonmechanical penetrating keratoplasty using a femtosecond laser. Am J Ophthalmol. 2005;139:941–4.

43. Saelens IE, Bartels MC, Van Rij G. Manual trephination of mushroom keratoplasty in advanced keratoconus. Cornea. 2008;27:650–5.

44. McAllum P, Kaiserman I, Bahar I, Rootman D. Femtosecond laser top hat penetrating keratoplasty: wound burst pressures of incomplete cuts. Arch Ophthalmol. 2008;126:822–5.

45. Maier P, Birnbaum F, Reinhard T. Therapeutic applications of the femtosecond laser in corneal surgery. Klinische Monatsblatter fur Augenheilkunde. 2010;227:453–9.

46. Williams KA, et al. How effective is penetrating corneal transplantation? Factors influencing long-term outcome in multivariate analysis. Transplantation. 2006;81:896–901.

47. Borderie VM, et al. Predicted long-term outcome of corneal transplantation. Ophthalmology. 2009;116:2354–60.

48. Anshu A, et al. Long-term review of penetrating keratoplasty: a 20-year review in Asian eyes. Am J Ophthalmol. 2021;224:254–66.

49. Reinhard T, Böhringer D, Hüschen D, Sundmacher R. Chronic endothelial cell loss of the graft after penetrating keratoplasty: influence of endothelial cell migration from graft to host. Klinische Monatsblatter fur Augenheilkunde. 2002;219:410–6.

50. Chung S-H, Kim HK, Kim MS. Corneal endothelial cell loss after penetrating keratoplasty in relation to preoperative recipient endothelial cell density. Ophthalmologica. 2010;224:194–8.

51. Arundhati A, et al. Comparative study of long-term graft survival between penetrating keratoplasty and deep anterior lamellar keratoplasty. Am J Ophthalmol. 2021;224:207–16.

52. Borderie VM, Guilbert E, Touzeau O, Laroche L. Graft rejection and graft failure after anterior lamellar versus penetrating keratoplasty. Am J Ophthalmol. 2011;151:1024–1029.e1021.

53. Azevedo Magalhaes O, Shalaby Bardan A, Zarei-Ghanavati M, Liu C. Literature review and suggested protocol for prevention and treatment of corneal graft rejection. Eye. 2020;34:442–50.

54. Jabbehdari S, et al. Update on the management of high-risk penetrating keratoplasty. Curr Ophthalmol Rep. 2017;5:38–48.

55. Javadi M. Corneal graft rejection: mechanism, clinical manifestations, diagnosis, and treatment. Bina J Ophthalmol. 2004;10:90–105.

56. Chirapapaisan C, et al. In vivo confocal microscopy demonstrates increased immune cell densities in corneal graft rejection correlating with signs and symptoms. Am J Ophthalmol. 2019;203:26–36.

57. Abou Shousha M, et al. In vivo characteristics of corneal endothelium/descemet membrane complex for the diagnosis of corneal graft rejection. Am J Ophthalmol. 2017;178:27–37.

58. Van Den Berg R, et al. Descemet's membrane thickening as a sign for the diagnosis of corneal graft rejection: an ex vivo study. Cornea. 2017;36:1535.

59. Eleiwa TK, et al. Diagnostic performance of three-dimensional endothelium/descemet membrane complex thickness maps in active corneal graft rejection. Am J Ophthalmol. 2020;210:48–58.

60. Roshandel D, et al. Current and emerging therapies for corneal neovascularization. Ocul Surf. 2018;16:398–414.

61. Javadi MA, Feizi S. Mustard gas eye injuries in chemical warfare victims; 2015. (Farhang Farda).

62. Koenig Y, et al. Short-and long-term safety profile and efficacy of topical bevacizumab (Avastin®) eye drops against corneal neovascularization. Graefes Arch Clin Exp Ophthalmol. 2009;247:1375–82.

63. Dastjerdi MH, Sadrai Z, Saban DR, Zhang Q, Dana R. Corneal penetration of topical and subconjunctival bevacizumab. Invest Ophthalmol Vis Sci. 2011;52:8718–23.

64. Oliveira HB, et al. VEGF TrapR1R2 suppresses experimental corneal angiogenesis. Eur J Ophthalmol. 2010;20:48–54.

65. Wang Q, et al. Pharmacological characteristics and efficacy of a novel anti-angiogenic antibody FD006 in corneal neovascularization. BMC Biotechnol. 2014;14:1–9.

66. Dekaris I, Gabrić N, Drača N, Pauk-Gulić M, Miličić N. Three-year corneal graft survival rate in high-

risk cases treated with subconjunctival and topical bevacizumab. Graefes Arch Clin Exp Ophthalmol. 2015;253:287–94.

67. Jovanovic V, Nikolic L. The effect of topical doxycycline on corneal neovascularization. Curr Eye Res. 2014;39:142–8.

68. Hata Y, et al. Antiangiogenic properties of fasudil, a potent Rho-Kinase inhibitor. Jpn J Ophthalmol. 2008;52:16–23.

69. Faraj LA, Elalfy MS, Said DG, Dua HS. Fine needle diathermy occlusion of corneal vessels. Br J Ophthalmol. 2014;98:1287–90.

70. Al-Torbak AA. Photodynamic therapy with verteporfin for corneal neovascularization. Mid E Afr J Ophthalmol. 2012;19:185.

71. Lee HS, Lee JH, Kim CE, Yang JW. Anti-neovascular effect of chondrocyte-derived extracellular matrix on corneal alkaline burns in rabbits. Graefes Arch Clin Exp Ophthalmol. 2014;252:951–61.

72. Ferrari G, et al. Topical ranibizumab as a treatment of corneal neovascularization. Cornea. 2013;32:992.

73. Group, C.D.S.I. The effect of donor age on corneal transplantation outcome: results of the cornea donor study. Ophthalmology. 2008;115:620–626.e626.

74. Stulting RD, et al. Effect of donor and recipient factors on corneal graft rejection. Cornea. 2012;31:1141.

75. Barraquer RI, Pareja-Aricò L, Alba Gómez-Benlloch RM. Risk factors for graft failure after penetrating keratoplasty. Medicine. 2019;98:e15274.

76. Williams KA, Lowe M, Bartlett C, Kelly T-L, Coster DJ. Risk factors for human corneal graft failure within the Australian corneal graft registry. Transplantation. 2008;86:1720–4.

77. Mannis MJ, et al. The effect of donor age on penetrating keratoplasty for endothelial disease: graft survival after 10 years in the Cornea Donor Study. Ophthalmology. 2013;120:2419–27.

78. Group, C.D.S.I. Donor age and corneal endothelial cell loss 5 years after successful corneal transplantation: specular microscopy ancillary study results. Ophthalmology. 2008;115:627–632.e628.

79. Lass JH, et al. Baseline factors related to endothelial cell loss following penetrating keratoplasty. Arch Ophthalmol. 2011;129:1149–54.

80. Feizi S, et al. Penetrating keratoplasty versus deep anterior lamellar keratoplasty in children and adolescents with keratoconus. Am J Ophthalmol. 2021;226:13–21.

81. Velásquez-Monzón K, Navarro-Peña MC, Klunder-Klunder M, Tsatsos M, Ramírez-Ortiz MA. Pediatric penetrating keratoplasty and graft rejection: experience at the Hospital Infantil de México Federico Gómez. Boletín médico del Hospital Infantil de México. 2020;77:23–7.

82. Anshu A, Lim LS, Htoon HM, Tan DT. Postoperative risk factors influencing corneal graft survival in the Singapore Corneal Transplant Study. Am J Ophthalmol. 2011;151:442–448.e441.

83. Böhringer D, et al. Matching of the minor histocompatibility antigen HLA-A1/HY may improve prognosis in corneal transplantation. Transplantation. 2006;82:1037–41.

84. Skeens HM, Holland EJ. Large-diameter penetrating keratoplasty: indications and outcomes. Cornea. 2010;29:296–301.

85. Lass JH, et al. Donor age and factors related to endothelial cell loss 10 years after penetrating keratoplasty: specular Microscopy Ancillary Study. Ophthalmology. 2013;120:2428–35.

86. Epstein AJ, de Castro TN, Laibson PR, Cohen EJ, Rapuano CJ. Risk factors for the first episode of corneal graft rejection in keratoconus. Cornea. 2006;25:1005–11.

87. Williams KA, Roder D, Esterman A, Muehlberg SM, Coster DJ. Factors predictive of corneal graft survival: report from the Australian Corneal Graft Registry. Ophthalmology. 1992;99:403–14.

88. Bidaut-Garnier M, et al. Evolution of corneal graft survival over a 30-year period and comparison of surgical techniques: a cohort study. Am J Ophthalmol. 2016;163:59–69.

89. Goble RR, Lea SJH, Falcon MG. The use of the same size host and donor trephine in penetrating keratoplasty for keratoconus. Eye. 1994;8:311–4.

90. Li C, et al. Effect of corneal graft diameter on therapeutic penetrating keratoplasty for fungal keratitis. Int J Ophthalmol. 2012;5:698.

91. Beekhuis WH. Current clinician's opinions on risk factors in corneal grafting. Results of a survey among surgeons in the eurotransplant area. Cornea. 1995;14:39–42.

92. Wilson SE. Graft failure after penetrating keratoplasty. Surv Ophthalmol. 1990;34:325–56.

93. Fasolo A, et al. Risk factors for graft failure after penetrating keratoplasty: 5-year follow-up from the corneal transplant epidemiological study. Cornea. 2011;30:1328–35.

94. Patel SV. Graft survival after penetrating keratoplasty. Am J Ophthalmol. 2011;151:397–8.

95. Sugar J, et al. Donor risk factors for graft failure in the cornea donor study. Cornea. 2009;28:981.

96. Dunn SP, et al. The effect of ABO blood incompatibility on corneal transplant failure in conditions with low-risk of graft rejection. Am J Ophthalmol. 2009;147:432–438.e433.

97. Feizi S, Javadi MA, Kanavi MR, Javadi F. Effect of donor graft quality on clinical outcomes after deep anterior lamellar keratoplasty. Cornea. 2014;33:795–800.

98. The Writing Committee for the Cornea Donor Study Research Group, et al. Factors predictive of corneal graft survival in the cornea donor study. JAMA Ophthalmol. 2015;133:246.

99. Banerjee S, Dick AD, Nicholls SM. Factors affecting rejection of second corneal transplants in rats1. Transplantation. 2004;77:492–6.

100. Kitazawa K, et al. Moderately long-term safety and efficacy of repeat penetrating keratoplasty. Cornea. 2018;37:1255–9.
101. Al-Mezaine H, Wagoner M. Repeat penetrating keratoplasty: indications, graft survival, and visual outcome. Br J Ophthalmol. 2006;90:324–7.
102. Khairallah AS. Outcome of repeat penetrating keratoplasty in eyes with failed penetrating keratoplasty. Saudi Med J. 2016;37:1029–32.
103. Yalniz-Akkaya Z, et al. Repeat penetrating keratoplasty: indications and prognosis, 1995–2005. Eur J Ophthalmol. 2009;19:362–8.
104. Thompson RW Jr, Price MO, Bowers PJ, Price FW Jr. Long-term graft survival after penetrating keratoplasty. Ophthalmology. 2003;110:1396–402.
105. Bachmann B, Taylor RS, Cursiefen C. Corneal neovascularization as a risk factor for graft failure and rejection after keratoplasty: an evidence-based meta-analysis. Ophthalmology. 2010;117:1300–1305. e1307.
106. Merz PR, Röckel N, Ballikaya S, Auffarth GU, Schmack I. Effects of ranibizumab (Lucentis®) and bevacizumab (Avastin®) on human corneal endothelial cells. BMC Ophthalmol. 2018;18:1–8.
107. Al-Debasi T, Al-Bekairy A, Al-Katheri A, Al Harbi S, Mansour M. Topical versus subconjunctival anti-vascular endothelial growth factor therapy (Bevacizumab, Ranibizumab and Aflibercept) for treatment of corneal neovascularization. Saudi J Ophthalmol. 2017;31:99–105.
108. Fasciani R, Mosca L, Giannico MI, Ambrogio SA, Balestrazzi E. Subconjunctival and/or intrastromal bevacizumab injections as preconditioning therapy to promote corneal graft survival. Int Ophthalmol. 2015;35:221–7.
109. Hos D, et al. Risk of corneal graft rejection after high-risk keratoplasty following fine-needle vessel coagulation of corneal neovascularization combined with bevacizumab: a pilot study. Transplant Dir. 2019;5:e452.
110. Koenig Y, Bock F, Kruse FE, Stock K, Cursiefen C. Angioregressive pretreatment of mature corneal blood vessels before keratoplasty: fine-needle vessel coagulation combined with anti-VEGFs. Cornea. 2012;31:887–92.
111. Cursiefen C, et al. Antisense oligonucleotide eye drops against IRS-1 inhibit corneal neovascularization: interim results of a randomized phase II clinical trial. Invest Ophthalmol Vis Sci. 2009;50:4953.
112. Cursiefen C, et al. Aganirsen antisense oligonucleotide eye drops inhibit keratitis-induced corneal neovascularization and reduce need for transplantation: the I-CAN study. Ophthalmology. 2014;121:1683–92.
113. Altenburger AE, Bachmann B, Seitz B, Cursiefen C. Morphometric analysis of postoperative corneal neovascularization after high-risk keratoplasty: herpetic versus non-herpetic disease. Graefes Arch Clin Exp Ophthalmol. 2012;250:1663–71.
114. Serna-Ojeda JC, et al. Long-term outcomes of pediatric penetrating keratoplasty for herpes simplex virus keratitis. Am J Ophthalmol. 2017;173:139–44.
115. Kuffova L, et al. High-risk corneal graft rejection in the setting of previous corneal herpes simplex virus (HSV)-1 infection. Invest Ophthalmol Vis Sci. 2016;57:1578–87.
116. Shiuey EJ, et al. Development of a nomogram to predict graft survival after penetrating keratoplasty. Am J Ophthalmol. 2021;226:32–41.
117. Whitcup SM, Nussenblatt RB, Price FW Jr, Chan C-C. Expression of cell adhesion molecules in corneal graft failure. Cornea. 1993;12:475–80.
118. Tan DT, et al. Penetrating keratoplasty in Asian eyes: the Singapore corneal transplant study. Ophthalmology. 2008;115:975–982.e971.
119. Banitt M, Lee R. Management of patients with combined glaucoma and corneal transplant surgery. Eye. 2009;23:1972–9.
120. Hollander DA, et al. Graft failure after penetrating keratoplasty in eyes with Ahmed valves. Am J Ophthalmol. 2010;150:169–78.
121. Stewart RM, et al. Effect of glaucoma on corneal graft survival according to indication for penetrating keratoplasty. Am J Ophthalmol. 2011;151:257–262. e251.
122. Price MO, Thompson RW, Price FW. Risk factors for various causes of failure in initial corneal grafts. Arch Ophthalmol. 2003;121:1087–92.
123. Massry GG, Assil KK. Pilocarpine-associated allograft rejection in postkeratoplasty patients. Cornea. 1995;14:202–5.
124. Konowal A, et al. Irreversible corneal decompensation in patients treated with topical dorzolamide. Am J Ophthalmol. 1999;127:403–6.
125. Cahane M, Ashkenazi I, Urinowski E, Avni I. Corneal graft rejection after neodymium-yttrium-aluminum-garnet laser posterior capsulotomy. Cornea. 1992;11:534–7.
126. DeBacker CM, El-Naggar S, Sugar J, Lai WW. Effect of neodymium: YAG laser posterior capsulotomy on corneal grafts. Cornea. 1996;15:15–7.
127. Lass JH, et al. The effect of donor diabetes history on graft failure and endothelial cell density 10 years after penetrating keratoplasty. Ophthalmology. 2015;122:448–56.
128. Zhang X, et al. Association of smoking and other risk factors with Fuchs' endothelial corneal dystrophy severity and corneal thickness. Invest Ophthalmol Vis Sci. 2013;54:5829–35.
129. Jurkunas UV, Bitar MS, Funaki T, Azizi B. Evidence of oxidative stress in the pathogenesis of fuchs endothelial corneal dystrophy. Am J Pathol. 2010;177:2278–89.
130. Karadag R, et al. Survival of primary penetrating keratoplasty in children. Am J Ophthalmol. 2016;171:95–100.
131. Alice LY, et al. Perioperative and postoperative risk factors for corneal graft failure. Clin Ophthalmol. 2014;8:1641.

132. Hayashi T, et al. Pars plana vitrectomy combined with penetrating keratoplasty and transscleral-sutured intraocular lens implantation in complex eyes: a case series. BMC Ophthalmol. 2020;20:369.

133. Rahman I, Carley F, Hillarby C, Brahma A, Tullo A. Penetrating keratoplasty: indications, outcomes, and complications. Eye. 2009;23:1288–94.

134. Zhang Y, et al. Indications and outcomes of penetrating keratoplasty in infants and children of Beijing, China. Cornea. 2018;37:1243–8.

135. Majander A, Kivelä TT, Krootila K. Indications and outcomes of keratoplasties in children during a 40-year period. Acta Ophthalmol. 2016;94:618–24.

136. Sugar A, et al. Factors associated with corneal graft survival in the cornea donor study. JAMA Ophthalmol. 2015;133:246–54.

137. Young AL, Kam K, Jhanji V, Cheng LL, Rao SK. A new era in corneal transplantation: paradigm shift and evolution of techniques. Hong Kong Med J. 2012;18:509–16.

138. Olson RJ. Variation in corneal graft size related to trephine technique. Arch Ophthalmol. 1979;97:1323–5.

139. Wilson SE, Bourne WM. Effect of recipient-donor trephine size disparity on refractive error in keratoconus. Ophthalmology. 1989;96:299–305.

140. Javadi MA, Mohammadi MJ, Mirdehghan SA, Sajjadi SH. A comparison between donor-recipient corneal size and its effect on the ultimate refractive error induced in keratoconus. Cornea. 1993;12:401–5.

141. Kuryan J, Channa P. Refractive surgery after corneal transplant. Curr Opin Ophthalmol. 2010;21:259–64.

142. Lanier JD, Bullington RH, Prager TC. Axial length in keratoconus. Cornea. 1992;11:250–4.

143. Javadi MA, et al. Comparison of the effect of three suturing techniques on postkeratoplasty astigmatism in keratoconus. Cornea. 2006;25:1029–33.

144. Solano JM, Hodge DO, Bourne WM. Keratometric astigmatism after suture removal in penetrating keratoplasty: double running versus single running suture techniques. Cornea. 2003;22:716–20.

145. Romano V, Iovieno A, Parente G, Soldani AM, Fontana L. Long-term clinical outcomes of deep anterior lamellar keratoplasty in patients with keratoconus. Am J Ophthalmol. 2015;159:505–11.

146. Javadi MA, Feizi S, Yazdani S, Mirbabaee F. Deep anterior lamellar keratoplasty versus penetrating keratoplasty for keratoconus: a clinical trial. Cornea. 2010;29:365–71.

147. Feizi S, Zare M. Current approaches for management of postpenetrating keratoplasty astigmatism. J Ophthalmol. 2011;2011:708736.

148. Dumitrescu O-M, Istrate S, Macovei M-L, Gheorghe AG. Intraocular pressure measurement after penetrating keratoplasty. Diagnostics. 2022;12:234.

149. McGhee C. Pharmacokinetics of ophthalmic corticosteroids. Br J Ophthalmol. 1992;76:681.

150. Abud TB, Di Zazzo A, Kheirkhah A, Dana R. Systemic immunomodulatory strategies in high-risk corneal transplantation. J Ophthal Vis Res. 2017;12:81.

151. Shimazaki J, Iseda A, Satake Y, Shimazaki-Den S. Efficacy and safety of long-term corticosteroid eye drops after penetrating keratoplasty: a prospective, randomized, clinical trial. Ophthalmology. 2012;119:668–73.

152. Ang M, Soh Y, Htoon HM, Mehta JS, Tan D. Five-year graft survival comparing Descemet stripping automated endothelial keratoplasty and penetrating keratoplasty. Ophthalmology. 2016;123:1646–52.

153. Jordan CS, Price MO, Trespalacios R, Price FW. Graft rejection episodes after Descemet stripping with endothelial keratoplasty: part one: clinical signs and symptoms. Br J Ophthalmol. 2009;93:387–90.

154. Niederkorn JY. High risk corneal allografts and why they lose their immune privilege. Curr Opin Allergy Clin Immunol. 2010;10:493.

155. Niederkorn JY. Corneal transplantation and immune privilege. Int Rev Immunol. 2013;32:57–67.

156. Hudde T, Minassian D, Larkin D. Randomised controlled trial of corticosteroid regimens in endothelial corneal allograft rejection. Br J Ophthalmol. 1999;83:1348–52.

157. Dunn SP, et al. Corneal graft rejection ten years after penetrating keratoplasty in the cornea donor study. Cornea. 2014;33:1003.

158. Armitage WJ, et al. High-risk corneal transplantation: recent developments and future possibilities. Transplantation. 2019;103:2468.

159. Holland EJ, et al. Systemic immunosuppression in ocular surface stem cell transplantation: results of a 10-year experience. Cornea. 2012;31:655–61.

160. Streilein JW. Immunobiology and immunopathology of corneal transplantation. Chem Immunol. 1999;73:186–206.

161. Barbarino JM, Staatz CE, Venkataramanan R, Klein TE, Altman RB. PharmGKB summary: cyclosporine and tacrolimus pathways. Pharmacogenet Genomics. 2013;23:563–85.

162. Fahr A. Cyclosporin clinical pharmacokinetics. Clin Pharmacokinet. 1993;24:472–95.

163. Thomson A, Bonham C, Zeevi A. Mode of action of tacrolimus (FK506): molecular and cellular mechanisms. Ther Drug Monit. 1995;17:584–91.

164. Kharod-Dholakia B, Randleman JB, Bromley JG, Stulting RD. Prevention and treatment of corneal graft rejection: current practice patterns of the Cornea Society (2011). Cornea. 2015;34:609–14.

165. Xie L, Shi W, Wang Z, Bei J, Wang S. Prolongation of corneal allograft survival using cyclosporine in a polylactide-co-glycolide polymer. Cornea. 2001;20:748–52.

166. Thompson P, Xu D, Brunette I, Chen H. Combined effect of rapamycin and cyclosporine in the prevention of rat corneal allograft rejection. Transplant Proc. 1998;4:1033–5.

167. Fu H, Larkin DF, George AJ. Immune modulation in corneal transplantation. Transplant Rev. 2008;22:105–15.
168. Williams KA, Coster DJ. Use of monoclonal antibodies in corneal transplantation. Clin Immunotherapeut. 1994;2:32–41.
169. Thiel M, Kaufmann C, Coster D, Williams K. Antibody-based immunosuppressive agents for corneal transplantation. Eye. 2009;23:1962–5.
170. Singh S, et al. Monoclonal antibodies: a review. Curr Clin Pharmacol. 2018;13:85–99.
171. Thiel MA, Coster DJ, Williams KA. The potential of antibody-based immunosuppressive agents for corneal transplantation. Immunol Cell Biol. 2003;81:93–105.
172. Merediz S, Zhang E-P, Wittig B, Hoffmann F. Ballistic transfer of minimalistic immunologically defined expression constructs for IL4 and CTLA4 into the corneal epithelium in mice after orthotopic corneal allograft transplantation. Graefes Arch Clin Exp Ophthalmol. 2000;238:701–7.
173. Bluestone JA, St Clair EW, Turka LA. CTLA4Ig: bridging the basic immunology with clinical application. Immunity. 2006;24:233–8.
174. Thiel MA, et al. Local or short-term systemic costimulatory molecule blockade prolongs rat corneal allograft survival. Clin Exp Ophthalmol. 2005;33:176–80.
175. Wu X-S, et al. Tocilizumab promotes corneal allograft survival in rats by modulating Treg-Th17 balance. Int J Ophthalmol. 2019;12:1823.
176. Hamrah P, et al. Local treatment with alpha-melanocyte stimulating hormone reduces corneal allorejection. Transplantation. 2009; 88:180.
177. Qian Y, Dekaris I, Yamagami S, Dana MR. Topical soluble tumor necrosis factor receptor type I suppresses ocular chemokine gene expression and rejection of allogeneic corneal transplants. Arch Ophthalmol. 2000;118:1666–71.
178. Amouzegar A, Chauhan SK. Effector and regulatory T cell trafficking in corneal allograft rejection. Mediat Inflamm. 2017;2017:8670280.
179. Donnenfeld ED, et al. Safety of lifitegrast ophthalmic solution 5.0% in patients with dry eye disease: a 1-year, multicenter, randomized, placebo-controlled study. Cornea. 2016;35:741.
180. Semba CP, Gadek TR. Development of lifitegrast: a novel T-cell inhibitor for the treatment of dry eye disease. Clin Ophthalmol. 2016;10:1083.
181. Ma D, Mellon J, Niederkorn JY. Oral immunisation as a strategy for enhancing corneal allograft survival. Br J Ophthalmol. 1997;81:778–84.
182. Plšková J, Holáň V, Filipec M, Forrester JV. Lymph node removal enhances corneal graft survival in mice at high risk of rejection. BMC Ophthalmol. 2004;4:1–7.
183. Chen L, et al. Vascular endothelial growth factor receptor-3 mediates induction of corneal alloimmunity. Nat Med. 2004;10:813–5.
184. Gong N, Pleyer U, Volk H, Ritter T. Effects of local and systemic viral interleukin-10 gene transfer on corneal allograft survival. Gene Ther. 2007;14:484–90.
185. Nosov M, et al. Role of lentivirus-mediated overexpression of programmed death-ligand 1 on corneal allograft survival. Am J Transplant. 2012;12:1313–22.
186. Pleyer U, et al. Survival of corneal allografts following adenovirus-mediated gene transfer of interleukin-4. Graefes Arch Clin Exp Ophthalmol. 2000;238:531–6.
187. Kocaba V, Colica C, Rabilloud M, Burillon C. Predicting corneal graft rejection by confocal microscopy. Cornea. 2015;34:S61–4.
188. Webster AC, Pankhurst T, Rinaldi F, Chapman JR, Craig JC. Monoclonal and polyclonal antibody therapy for treating acute rejection in kidney transplant recipients: a systematic review of randomized trial data. Transplantation. 2006;81:953–65.
189. Hashemian MN, et al. Topical tacrolimus as adjuvant therapy to corticosteroids in acute endothelial graft rejection after penetrating keratoplasty: a randomized controlled trial. Cornea. 2018;37: 307–12.
190. Reinhard T, Sundmacher R. Adjunctive intracameral application of corticosteroids in patients with endothelial immune reactions after penetrating keratoplasty: a pilot study. Transpl Int. 2002;15:81–8.
191. Maris PJGJ, Correnti AJ, Donnenfeld ED. Intracameral triamcinolone acetonide as treatment for endothelial allograft rejection after penetrating keratoplasty. Cornea. 2008;27:847–50.
192. Kim BZ, et al. New Zealand trends in corneal transplantation over the 25 years 1991-2015. Br J Ophthalmol. 2017;101:834–8.
193. Alldredge OC, Krachmer JH. Clinical types of corneal transplant rejection: their manifestations, frequency, preoperative correlates, and treatment. Arch Ophthalmol. 1981;99:599–604.
194. Hill JC, Maske R, Watson P. Corticosteroids in corneal graft rejection: oral versus single pulse therapy. Ophthalmology. 1991;98:329–33.
195. Randleman JB, Stulting RD. Prevention and treatment of corneal graft rejection: current practice patterns (2004). Cornea. 2006;25:286–90.
196. Poon A, Constantinou M, Lamoureux E, Taylor HR. Topical Cyclosporin A in the treatment of acute graft rejection: a randomized controlled trial. Clin Exp Ophthalmol. 2008;36:415–21.

Improvements in Surgical Techniques and Suturing in Penetrating Keratoplasty

Abdo Karim Tourkmani and Colm McAlinden

Key Points

- Full-thickness corneal transplantation has stood the test of time and is still a boon to corneal surgeons in the twenty-first century. From the first description by Reisinger in 1824 and the landmark case report by Zirm in 1905, many modifications ensued including the switching of square grafts to round grafts by Castroviejo. The development of the surgical microscope, suture materials, and topical steroids has had a profound impact on the success of penetrating keratoplasty (PKP). The femtosecond laser is one of the latest developments which adds precision to depth and diameter of tissue penetration as well as the ability to create various edge profiles for grafts, such as mushroom, top hat and zigzag configurations.
- The most important aspect of pre-operative planning is an assessment of the contribution to visual impairment by corneal disease. One needs to consider how likely the patient will benefit from corneal transplantation, what impact surgery may have on other conditions, and what impact other conditions may have on graft success and survival.
- PKP is indicated for corneal diseases affecting all layers of the cornea, except the epithelium, including Combined endothelial and stromal diseases (e.g. Fuchs endothelial dystrophy with keratoconus), endothelial disease (e.g. Fuchs endothelial dystrophy) with significant secondary stromal scarring and keratoconus with previous hydrops.

Supplementary Information The online version contains supplementary material available at https://doi.org/10.1007/978-3-031-32408-6_6.

A. K. Tourkmani (✉)
Department of Ophthalmology, Royal Gwent Hospital, Newport, UK

C. McAlinden
Corneo Plastic Unit & Eye Bank, Queen Victoria Hospital, East Grinstead, UK

History of Penetrating Keratoplasty (PKP)

In 1905, Austrian Ophthalmologist Eduard Zirm was the first surgeon to successfully perform a full-thickness corneal transplant which remained clear [1]. Interestingly, the indication was for a bilateral chemical injury, which even today would be deemed a poor candidate for transplantation. There were many attempts prior to the report from Zirm, dating back to the early 1800s, which all failed, with graft transparency not lasting more than 2–3 weeks [2]. Franz Reisinger first introduced the term keratoplasty in 1824 [3], and Michael Marcus described the first set of basic steps of full-thickness keratoplasty in 1840 [4]. Towards the end of the 1800s, there was great interest and work on lamellar corneal grafting;

however, with the turn of the century, following the landmark case report by Zirm, there was a resurgence in interest in full-thickness keratoplasty.

In the 50 years following the publication by Zirm, many advances in keratoplasty ensued. One of the most notable was the work of Ramon Castroviejo, progressing from square-shaped grafts to circular grafts as well as progressing from overlay sutures to appositional sutures [5]. Richard Townley Paton developed the first eye bank in 1944 in New York, USA, which paved the way for greater access to corneal tissue [6]. Other advances such as the development of the surgical microscope, suture materials, and topical steroids have had a profound impact on the success of penetrating keratoplasty (PKP). In more recent times, the femtosecond laser has added to the evolution of PKP [7]. The laser adds precision to depth and diameter of tissue penetration as well as the ability to create various edge profiles for grafts, such as mushroom, top hat and zigzag configurations [8].

Pre-operative Considerations

In the past two decades, lamellar corneal grafting has superseded PKP, with the selective replacement of only the diseased layers of the cornea. However, PKP still has a very important role. Perhaps, the most important aspect of pre-operative planning is an assessment of the contribution to visual impairment by corneal disease. Ocular co-morbidities need to be carefully considered. One needs to consider how likely the patient will benefit from corneal transplantation, what impact surgery may have on other conditions, and what impact other conditions may have on graft success and survival.

The following co-morbidities require specific consideration:

- Ocular surface disease (OSD):
  - This is the leading cause of graft failure, and hence it is imperative that pre-operative OSD is aggressively treated. These measures need to be maintained in the post-operative period also. Those with limbal

stem cell deficiency may require stem cell transplantation prior to PKP [9].
- Inflammation/infection:
  - Active inflammation/infection is a risk factor for graft failure. Inflammation should be well controlled prior to surgery. In eyes with infections such as fungal, acanthamoeba and herpetic keratitis, they should be quiescent for many months prior to PKP. The exception to this would be tectonically grafting in co-existing perforation [10].
- Lid abnormalities:
  - Lid conditions such as ectropion and entropion should be surgically corrected prior to PKP to reduce the risk of failure post-operatively.
- Glaucoma:
  - Glaucoma is an independent risk factor for graft failure. Further, poorly controlled intraocular pressure (IOP) is associated with endothelial cell loss [11]. Hence good IOP control is essential pre-operatively. Glaucoma drainage devices (GDD) are highly associated with graft failure occurring in approximately 45% of eyes at 3 years [12]. The optimal glaucoma procedure and timing in PKP eyes remain to be established [13].

Patients need to understand the lengthy postoperative period of visual rehabilitation as well as post-operative topical therapy as well as the life-long risk of rejection and graft failure. A full ophthalmic and systemic history is vital as well as anaesthetic considerations. With advancing patient age, there are lower rejection rates [14]; however, advanced age is a risk factor for suprachoroidal haemorrhage.

Generally, PKP is indicated for corneal diseases affecting all layers of the cornea except the epithelium. These include:

- Combined endothelial and stromal diseases (e.g. Fuchs endothelial dystrophy with keratoconus)
- Endothelial disease (e.g. Fuchs endothelial dystrophy) with significant secondary stromal scarring
- Keratoconus with previous hydrops

Relative contraindications to PKP include:

- Epithelial disease (e.g. limbal stem cell failure and severe dry eye)
- Significant stromal vascularisation
- Multiple previous failed grafts

However, even in cases of full-thickness scars or perforations, some surgeons may consider deep anterior lamellar keratoplasty (DALK) or Descemet Stripping Endothelial Keratoplasty (DSEK) [15], particularly in higher-risk eyes, to avoid the risk of endophthalmitis or expulsive haemorrhage with open-sky PKP. It can be surprising how well some patients see despite small residual scars.

Surgical Techniques

A clear surgical plan is a prerequisite to safe surgery, with efficient use of time to maintain as short as possible operating time (Video 6.1). Modifications need to be planned such as if cataract surgery is planned with PKP.

Povidone iodine pre-operatively is important in reducing post-operative endophthalmitis. This can be administered as 5% eye drops many minutes prior to draping and further with 10% painted to the lashes and peri-ocular region. In patients undergoing combined PKP with cataract surgery, the pupil is dilated pre-operatively, whereas, in those who are phakic, 2% pilocarpine drops are administered.

Suprachoroidal haemorrhage is a dreaded complication with the main risk factors being age, glaucoma (and in particular, high pre-operative IOP), previous surgery, hypertension, anticoagulant therapy, tachycardia, arteriosclerosis and previous suprachoroidal haemorrhage [16]. Steps should be taken to reduce these factors pre-operatively, e.g. ensure good blood pressure control and safely stop anticoagulants pre-operatively. Ingraham and colleagues reported, in a group of 714 patients undergoing PKP under general anaesthesia, 4 patients (0.56%) developed suprachoroidal haemorrhages, and in 116 patients under local anaesthesia, 5 patients (4.3%) developed suprachoroidal haemorrhages [17]. Sudden drops in intraocular pressure intraoperatively should be avoided; when entering the anterior chamber, this should be performed slowly, followed by an injection of viscoelastic. The duration of the eye left open should be kept to a minimum.

There are many variations to the surgical technique of PKP; however, the main goals are to safely perform surgery without complications and achieve good wound apposition with minimal astigmatism induction. The main general steps of the procedure are summarised below:

- Scleral fixation ring: the purpose of this ring is to provide scleral structural support when the eye is open to reduce the risk of suprachoroidal haemorrhage. The ring is sized just within the interpalpebral opening and sutured to the sclera, typically with 7-0 silk sutures.
- The diameter of the host cornea is measured, and the centre is marked with a marking pen. Sizing depends on numerous factors including pathology, the extent of pathology, host corneal diameter and risk of rejection. A trephine to make a circular cut on both the donor and recipient cornea. These can be hand-held, motor (e.g. Asmotom), suction (e.g. Hessburg-Barron) or guided (e.g. Hanna). However, the most modern method of performing the cuts is with the use of a femtosecond laser. A 7.5–8 mm trephination to the host cornea is a typical size. The trephination is ideally centred on the corneal marking; however, it may need to be decentred to account for the pathology, e.g., peripheral thinning. It is a trade-off with increasing astigmatism induction with larger decentrations.
- Donor cornea trephination: the punch trephination is performed with the corneal endothelial side up and is sized 0.25 mm larger than the planned host cornea trephination. Alternatively, the femtosecond laser may be used (Fig. 6.1).
- Host cornea trephination: the size of the host corneal trephination is 0.25–0.5 mm less than the donor cornea. The trephine is placed on the host cornea, and most commonly, suction

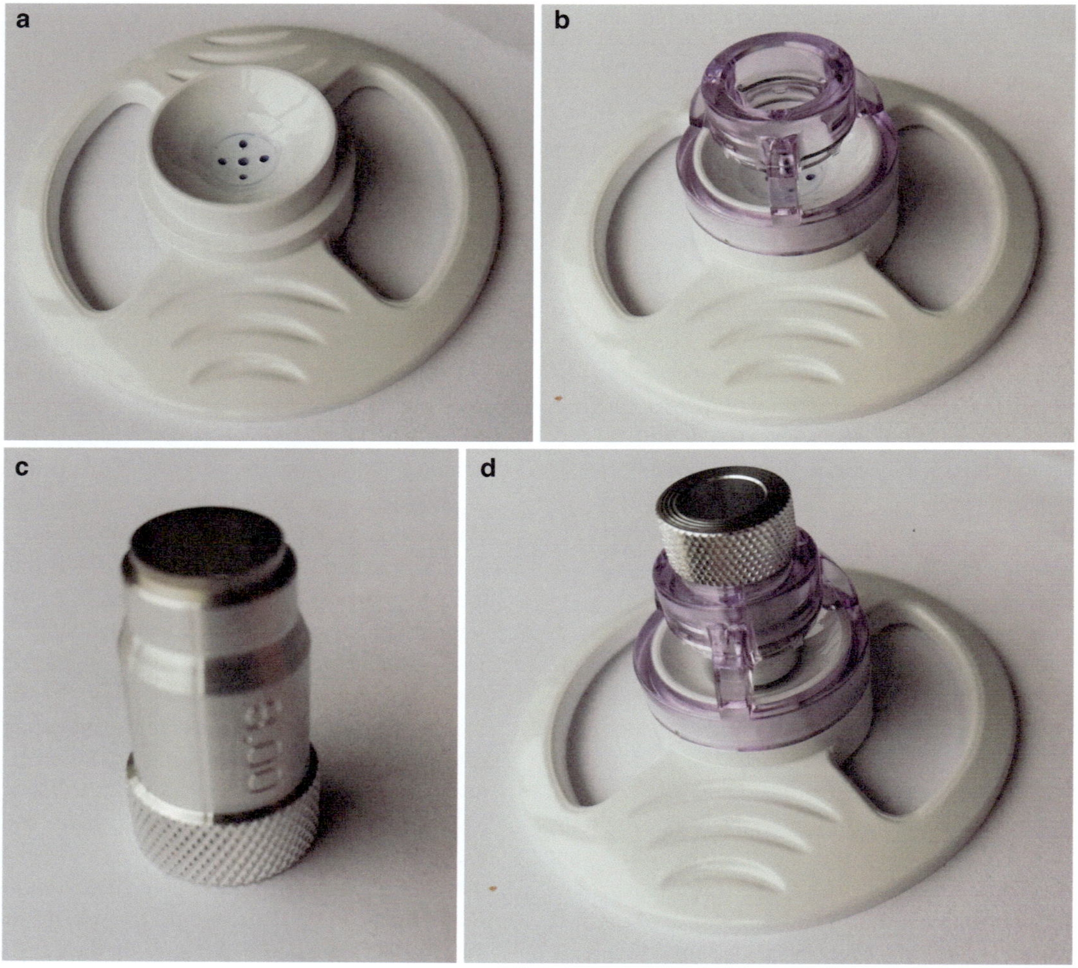

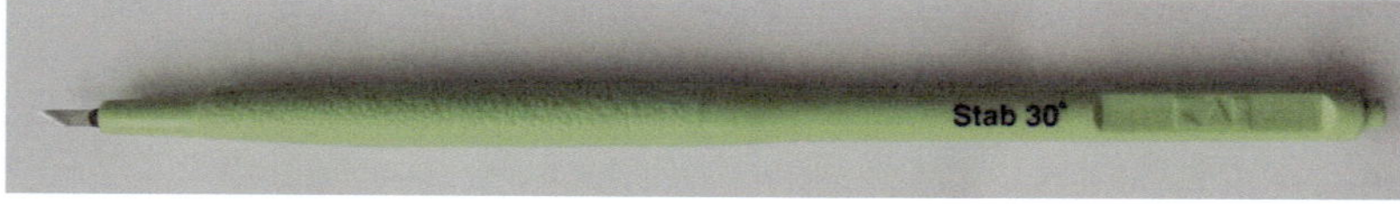

Fig. 6.1 The CORONET® donor corneal trephine punch. (**a**) Base to place donor cornea epithelium side down (i.e. endothelium side up), (**b**) trephine guide added, (**c**) independent trephine, (**d**) trephine added to the system

Fig. 6.2 30° blade used to penetrate the anterior chamber after almost full-thickness trephination

is applied. Alternatively, a free-hand trephine without suction may be used. The cutting blade is lowered by rotating the dial. The trephine can be made to almost full-thickness or full-thickness, whereby a small aqueous leak is usually observed. In almost full-thickness trephinations, a blade (e.g. MVR or 30° blade, Fig. 6.2) can be used to gently penetrate the anterior chamber in a controlled manner. Viscoelastic can then be injected into the anterior chamber.

- Right and left-bevelled corneal scissors are used to excise the host cornea in a perpendicular fashion; however, slight inward angling creates a posterior wound ledge that may assist with a watertight wound.

- With a Paton spatula, the donor cornea is carefully positioned and sutured into the host, and suturing may begin. This starts with four cardinal 10-0 nylon interrupted sutures, typically starting at the 12 o'clock position, followed by 6 o'clock, then 3 and 9 o'clock. The second suture is the most important in terms of astigmatism and graft alignment. Fine double-toothed forceps are used to grasp the donor cornea and the suture passed, aiming for 90% depth. The suture is tied in a 3-1-1 fashion or a slipknot. A further 8–12 interrupted sutures are placed (16 in total is typical) (Fig. 6.3). Alternatively, a running suture may be placed after eight interrupted sutures. Suture knots should be buried in the donor graft as this will be further from the limbus. One should avoid the temptation to over-tighten sutures, as this can lead to cheese wiring, flatter corneas, high astigmatism, hyperopia and surface healing issues. A Bowman-to-Bowman layer alignment and apposition should be the aim. Further details on suturing techniques and types will be discussed later in this chapter. A typical PKP instrument set is shown in Fig. 6.4.
- Suture modifications can be made to optimise astigmatism, aided with the use of an intraoperative keratoscope or aberrometry.
- Surgery is completed with an injection of subconjunctival steroids and antibiotics.

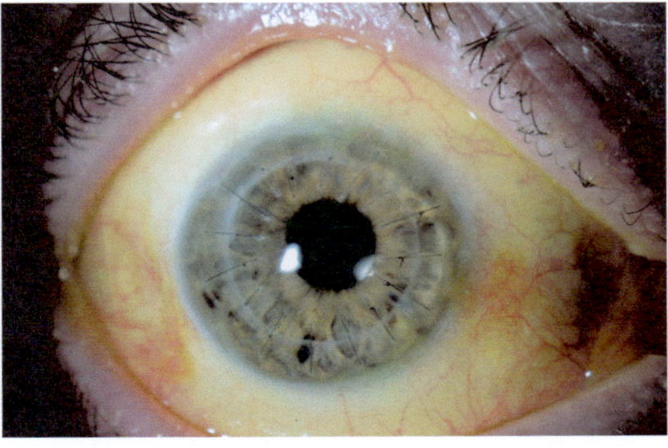

Fig. 6.3 16 interrupted 10-0 nylon corneal sutures

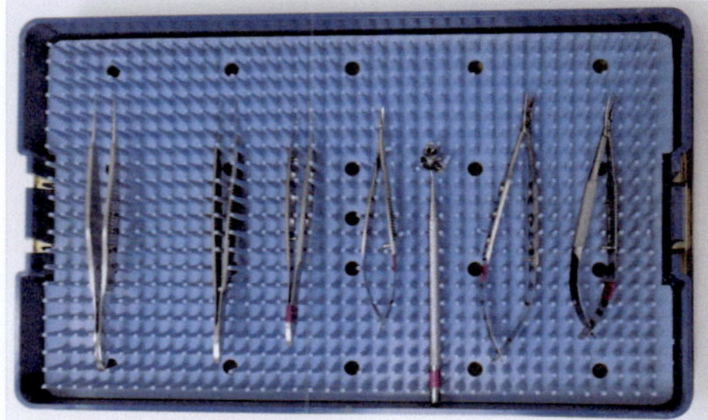

Fig. 6.4 Instrument set with commonly used PKP instruments (not exhaustive). From left to right: straight tying forceps, toothed forceps, rhexis forceps (for cataract extraction), Vannas scissors, keratoplasty suture marker, spring scissors and needle holder

Suture Materials and Sizes

Suture material can be classified into non-absorbable or absorbable, and structurally, mono-filament or multi-filament. It can also be classified as natural or synthetic. Absorbable sutures are used for temporary wound closure and undergo enzymatic degradation or hydrolysis with time. Non-absorbable sutures are used for longer-term wound closure, and although they are non-absorbable, they may degrade with time and, in the process, loose tensile strength. Monofilament sutures contain a single strand of the material, which is more resistant to harbouring microorganisms. Multi-filament sutures have multiple strands that are braided together, permitting good handling properties but may attract microorganisms.

Absorbable

- Synthetic
  - Polygalactin 910 (Vicryl)
  - Polydioxanone (PDS)
- Natural:
  - Fast/plain/chromic gut

Non-absorbable

- Synthetic
  - Nylon (e.g. Ethilon)
  - Polypropylene (e.g. Prolene)
  - Polyester (e.g. Dacron, Ethibond, Mersilene)
- Natural:
  - Silk

Nylon is the most effective suture material in keratoplasty surgery. Its relatively elastic, biocompatible and strength properties are superior to other materials for this purpose. Prolene or Mersilene can cause stromal fibrosis. Also, the lack of elasticity can cause issues when post-operative corneal oedema resolves. Silk is commonly used to suture the scleral fixation ring intraoperatively. It is very easy to handle and knot but is associated with significant tissue reaction; hence its use is limited to intraoperative in PKP surgery.

Suture sizes are based on the United States Pharmacopeia (USP) system. The initial sizes introduced were #1 to #6, with higher numbers indicating larger suture diameter. Later, size 0 was introduced as a thinner suture. Further thinner suture diameters were introduced, and the system was modified to 1-0 to 12-0, with 1-0 being the thickest and 12-0 being the thinnest. The diameter of 10-0 is approximately 20 μm.

Suturing in Penetrating Keratoplasty

Correct suturing is of paramount importance for an appropriate wound apposition, ensuring the chances of wound leaks, loose stitches or any other graft-host junction problems are reduced to the minimum possible [18]. Several suturing techniques have been described in penetrating keratoplasty (PKP). These include interrupted suturing, continuous single suturing and continuous double suturing. For continuous suturing, whether single or double, they can be classified as torque or anti-torque suturing [19].

We will describe each one of these types in greater detail later in this text, however, it is important to emphasise some principles that are common to whichever type of suturing is chosen.

- The material chosen for suturing would be a nylon suture. Only in the case of a double continuous suture, the surgeon may choose a 10-0 nylon for both sutures, or 10-0 for one and 11-0 for the second suture [20].
- The depth of the needle passage in both graft and host should be around 90%. This reduces the chance of having steps at the level of the graft-host junction [21].
- The length of the bite should be tailored to each individual case, however, the longer the bite, the greater the compression area (hence less chance of post-operative leaks).
- Whether using interrupted sutures or continuous sutures, there is a need for implanting first the initial four cardinal sutures. The surgeon usually starts with the suture at the 12 o'clock position, then the one opposite to it (6 o'clock), aiming for an equal distribution of the graft over the trephination area. Then, two sutures would be placed along the 3–9 o'clock meridian, choosing first the clock hour in which the gap between graft and host is larger.
- The knot has to be locked, so that it does not loosen; then buried into the cornea, so that it is not exposed (to avoid the risk of suture-related infection and corneal neovascularisation, amongst others) [22].

We will now proceed with a more detailed explanation of each one of the suturing techniques referenced above.

Interrupted Suturing

This is the technique usually employed at the beginning of the learning curve for a PKP surgeon [23]. It is usually easier than the others, and the surgeon does not rely on the same suture for the whole process. It is more forgiving with a needle becoming bent or blunt from numerous (both successful and unsuccessful) passes, or a suture breaking halfway through the surgery (common events for any surgeon irrespective of the experience, but far more common in the early learning curve).

The surgeon would start the suturing by placing the four cardinal sutures, as explained earlier in the text. Then, the surgeon would continue by placing interrupted sutures halfway between the sutures that have been already placed (45–225° meridian and 135–315° meridian). The principles to follow would be:

- Start in the quadrant where the gap between graft and host is greatest.
- Continue with suturing along the same axis but in the opposite quadrant.
- Repeat the action on the meridian 90° from of the meridian that has just been sutured.

At this stage, the donor button has been fixed to the recipient's eye with eight interrupted sutures in the 90–270° meridian, 0–180° meridian, 45–225° meridian and 135–315° meridian. Ideally, each one of the sutures should be equidistant from one another.

The surgeon then should continue by placing the next interrupted suture in the area where the gap between the graft and host is greatest, equidistantly from the sutures to either side; then continue with the suture along the same meridian but in the opposite quadrant; then repeat the action in the meridian 90° away.

As a rule of thumb, the above steps should be repeated until 16 interrupted 10-0 nylon sutures have been placed. However, for non-standard PKPs (very large or very small, irregular trephinations, etc.), more or less sutures may be required (Figs. 6.5 and 6.6).

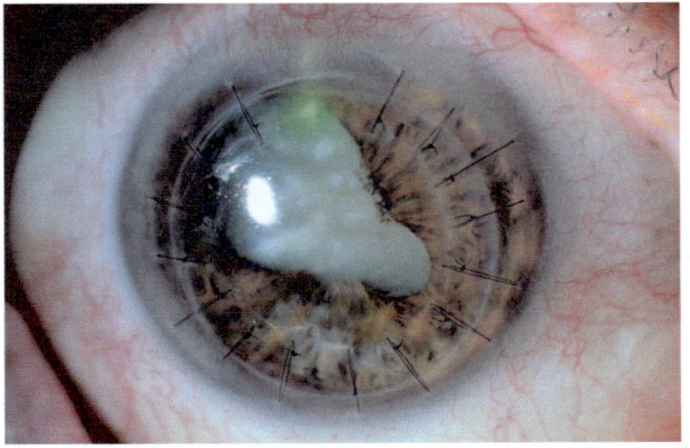

Fig. 6.5 PKP for herpetic corneal perforation with 15 interrupted 10-0 nylon corneal sutures. The superior cardinal suture became loose and had been removed. Note this patient later developed a white dense cataract with posterior synechiae

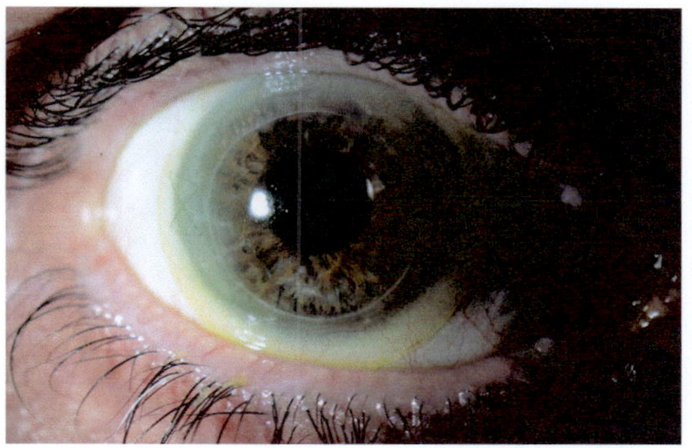

Fig. 6.6 This image is of the same patient as in Fig. 6.5, following cataract surgery and removal of all interrupted graft sutures. Note, a suture to the main corneal wound is shown in this image

Continuous Suturing (Single)

The operating surgeon may choose to use a single continuous suture. The basic principles would still apply. Preferably, a 10-0 nylon suture would be used [23]. The first four interrupted cardinal sutures still need to be placed for an appropriate fixation of the donor button to the host recipient eye, which would then allow for an appropriate continuous suture to be placed.

The running suture would start in the outer lip of the graft-host junction (i.e. within the "host" lip), so that, at the completion of the suture, it would exit from the inner lip (i.e. within the "donor" lip), allowing for the knot to be buried in the graft-host junction. Approximately three equidistant bites would be placed per quadrant, plus a bite overriding the cardinal interrupted sutures. Thus, usually, 16 bites are applied. The four cardinal interrupted sutures can be removed, the running suture is tightened and adjusted, and the knot is tied and buried.

The suture can be torque (the bites through the cornea are radial; the thread joining consecutive bites is oblique over the cornea) or anti-torque (the bites through the cornea are oblique; the thread joining consecutive bites are radial over the cornea). Typically, if a single continuous suture is chosen, a torque orientation is utilised (Fig. 6.7).

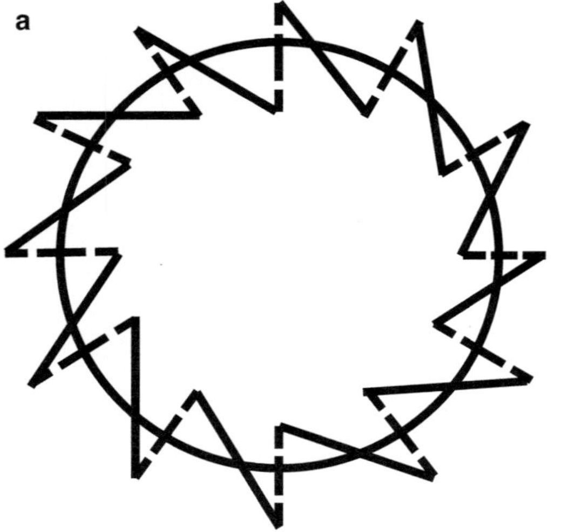

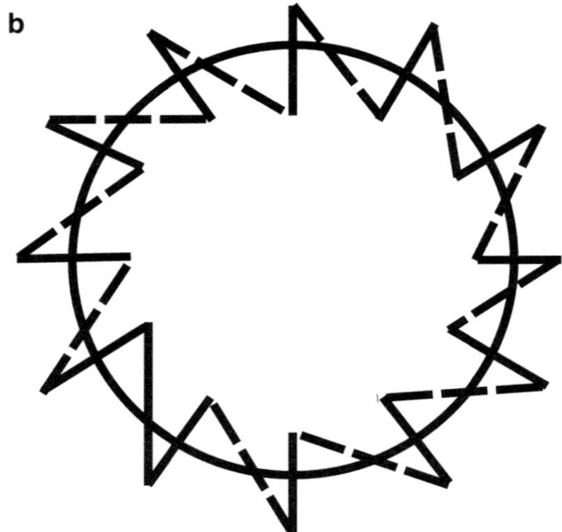

Fig. 6.7 Schematic diagram showing (**a**) Torque (the bites through the cornea are radial; the thread joining consecutive bites is oblique over the cornea) and (**b**) anti-torque (the bites through the cornea are oblique; the thread joining consecutive bites are radial over the cornea) running suture. The dashed lines depict the suture deep to the corneal surface. The solid lines depict the suture superficial to the corneal surface

Continuous Suturing (Double)

Double Torque

This would consist of a double torque type suture, in which the bites of the second suture would run in between the bites of the first suture [19]. The first suture would usually be 10-0 nylon, with the second suture being either again 10-0 nylon or 11-0 nylon.

Double Torque–Anti-torque

In this technique, the first suture would be a 10-0 nylon torque suture, with the second one being either a 10-0 or 11-0 anti-torque nylon suture. When placed correctly, these sutures create the appearance of equilateral triangles with geometrical perfection. Also, the theoretical advantage of using an anti-torque suture in combination with a torque suture would be "locking" the donor graft button in the current "post-torque suture" position, rather than inducing further rotation (hence increased cylinder) within the corneal donor button with a further second torque suture (Fig. 6.8).

Spadea et al. compared the outcomes of a single-running suture to a double torque–anti-torque suture in PKP [24]. The first group of 35 eyes received a 16 bite 10-0 nylon running suture, and the second group of 33 eyes received an 8 + 8 bite 10-0 nylon double running suture, with one running clockwise and one running anti-clockwise (i.e. double torque–anti-torque). In the single-running suture group, five patients had a suture adjustment in the post-operative period, and no adjustment was made in any patients with the double-running suture. Sutures were removed between 12 and 20 months post-operatively. Corneal topography was performed in all patients after all sutures were removed. The topographic astigmatism ranged from 1.07 to 8.09 D (mean 3.51 ± 1.93 SD) in the single-running suture group and from 1.13 to 9.36 D (3.42 ± 1.94) in the double-running torque–anti-torque group. The refractive cylinder ranged from 1.00 to 4.50 D (2.62 ± 1.20) in the single-running suture group and from 1.00 to 4.50 D (2.73 ±1.17) in the double-running torque–anti-torque group. The mean topographic keratometric values ranged from 37.45 to 52.24 D (45.47 ± 3.82) in the single-running suture group and from 40.90 to 51.84 D (46.25 ± 2.99) in the double-running

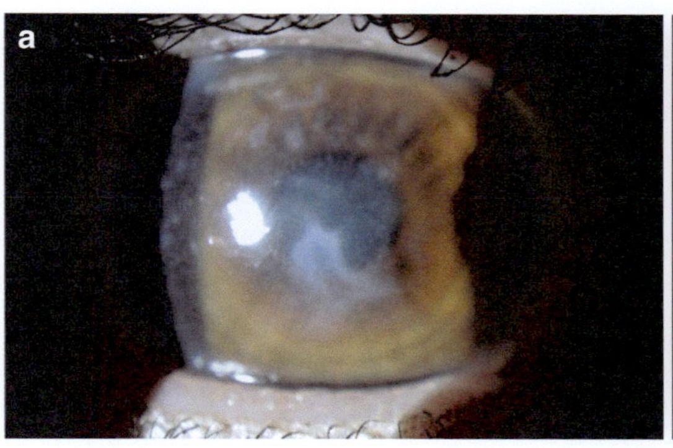
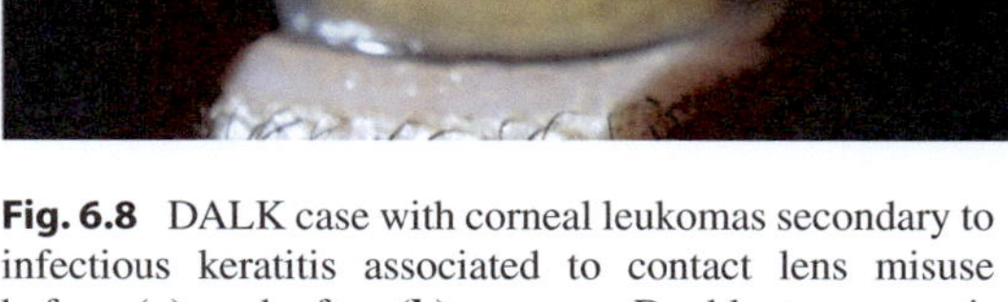
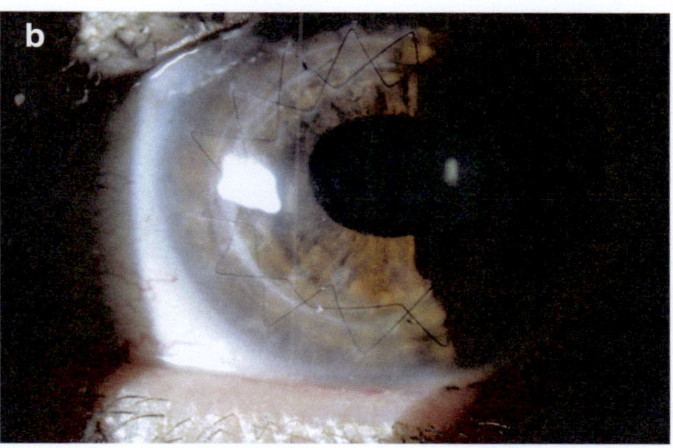

Fig. 6.8 DALK case with corneal leukomas secondary to infectious keratitis associated to contact lens misuse before (**a**) and after (**b**) surgery. Double torque–anti-torque suture is used in this case with an excellent astigmatic refractive outcome. (*Courtesy of Jorge L. Alio*)

torque–anti-torque group. No significant change in mean central corneal power and astigmatism occurred in either group before and after the suture removal. Comparing final astigmatism, the two groups' corneal curvature and refractive cylinder showed no statistically significant differences ($P > 0.05$). No patient developed post-operative glaucoma, wound dehiscence and suture-related complications during the 36 months of the follow-up period [24].

Vajpayee et al. compared three continuous running suture techniques, namely, torque, anti-torque and no torque in PKP [25]. Fifty-three patients were randomly assigned to one of the three suture types. In total, 17 eyes had torque, 18 eyes had anti-torque and 18 eyes had no torque. All patients with astigmatism of more than 3 D at 4 weeks underwent suture adjustment at the slit lamp. Astigmatism at 4 weeks (before any suture adjustment) was higher in the torque group on keratometry, refraction and topography, but this was not statistically significant. Thirty eyes had more than 3 D of astigmatism and underwent suture adjustment (12 torque group, 11 anti-torque group, 7 no-torque group). Four of these 30 eyes required a second suture adjustment (2 torque group, 2 no-torque group). One eye in the torque group required a third suture adjustment. There were no significant differences in astigmatism following suture adjustments between the three groups, and this remained the case at 3 and 6 months follow-up [25].

In a group of 40 patients, Sharma et al. studied the post-operative topographic patterns following torque, anti-torque and no torque continuous suturing in PKP [26]. Patients were randomly assigned to a group, and 10-0 nylon was used in all cases. Patients with 3 D or more astigmatism 1 month post-operatively underwent suture adjustment at the slit lamp. With a jeweller and tying forceps, the suture was pulled from the flatter meridians to the steeper meridians. The anti-torque group showed a significantly higher number of prolate pattern maps post-operatively compared with the other suture groups, and further, a significantly higher proportion of patients in the prolate group required suture adjustment. Following suture adjustment, the frequency of prolate patterns decreased, but most reverted to the prolate pattern at 3 months. Among the eyes with a prolate corneal pattern, the torque group had the highest astigmatism (11.21 ± 6.21 D), whereas the astigmatism in the anti-torque group was 6.1 ± 2.52 D, and in the no-torque group, it was 8.85 ± 2.6 D [26].

Nuzzi et al. recently compared five suturing techniques in a group of 100 eyes from 100 patients undergoing PKP [27]. Each patient was randomly assigned a suture technique group, which consisted of: interrupted (10-0 nylon, 16 bites), single running (10-0 nylon, 16–24 bites), double running (two 10-0 sutures, 12–16 bites), double running anti-torque (two 10-0 sutures with cross-stitch sutures in the opposite direction), and double running with 10-0 and 11-0 sutures. In the three double-running suture groups, the first suture was placed at 90% depth and the second at 50–90% depth. Patients with greater than 3 D of astigmatism post-operatively had suture adjustment. In the interrupted suture group, selective suture removal was performed along the corresponding meridian at 2–3 months post-operatively. In the single-running group, the suture was adjusted immediately post-operatively or at later follow-up visits. In the three double running groups, complete removal of a single 10-0 nylon suture was performed at 2–3 months post-operatively. At 12 months post-operatively, the mean keratometric astigmatism was 5.86 ± 1.87 D in the interrupted suture group, 5.34 ± 1.99 D in the single running suture group, 3.00 ± 1.38 D in the double 10-0 running suture group, 2.89 ± 1.11 D in the double 10-0 running anti-torque suture group and 3.06 ± 1.22 D in the double running 10-0 and 11-0 sutures. In terms of statistical significance of these differences, there was no difference between the interrupted suture group and single-running suture group; however, the difference between each of these two groups and the three double-running suture groups was statistically significant. There were no statistically significant differences between the three double-running suture groups. In terms of complications, no endophthalmitis or graft ulceration occurred in any group, however in terms of wound leak, this occurred in 10% in the interrupted suture group, 5.3% in the single-running suture group and 0% in all double-running suture groups [27].

Tying, Locking and Burying the Knot

Whichever technique is chosen by the surgeon, the suture knot would need to be locked (to avoid loosening of tension) then buried within the corneal tissue (ideally avoiding burying the knot in the graft-host junction). Once again, different techniques can be chosen for this purpose.

The two most commonly used techniques would be either a 3-1-1 knot or a 2-1-1-1 knot. Eventually, a 2-1-1 can be used. Some surgeons may choose a 1-1-1 technique. The author of this chapter favours using a 3-1-1 technique.

The 10-0 nylon suture would be passed through the donor cornea, then through the host corneal rim, leaving a short end of around 1–1.5 corneal diameters over the donor button, and a longer end peripherally. Holding the long end with a needle holder (or any other adequate holding instrument of the surgeon's preference), the longer end would be looped around a tying forceps three times; then the short end would be picked up with the tip of the tying forceps, and the knot tightened to an adequate tension—enough to appose the graft and host, but not too tight to induce high astigmatism or loosen up neighbouring sutures. When the desired tension is achieved, the long end can be pulled centripetally and held flat on the donor cornea. Then, the shorter end is pulled towards the long end (centripetally as well), locking the knot in position. Then, a one loop knot is performed, with care not to loosen up the initial knot, aiming for this second knot to be in line with the first one. The process is repeated with an extra loop. The 1-1 knots need to be tied with "opposite" orientation (clockwise/counterclockwise), otherwise if all the 3-1-1 knots are tied with the same orientation of the loop, it will end up being a sliding knot (i.e. loosening up with time).

The technique is largely similar for a 2-1-1 or a 2-1-1-1 technique. However it is different for a 1-1-1 technique. With this technique, a 1 loop knot is not possible to lock after the first knot, but rather after the second knot. Care needs to be taken that the second knot is aligned with the first knot, so as it is tightened, it is not locked before reaching the desired tension. This is usually less controlled than any of the other techniques and the only theoretical advantage is easier burial of the knot, which, if the technique is good, is easy to do with any of the other methods as well.

Wound Apposition

Appropriate wound apposition is of paramount importance to avoid early postoperative leaks, loose sutures, or steps between graft and host junction that may lead to delayed graft-host wound dehiscence (sometimes even at the time of removal of graft sutures, which would require re-suturing and a delayed healing process) [28].

A suture passage at approx. 90% depth in both graft and host would usually ensure that no steps occur on the corneal surface. This however may be more difficult to achieve when uneven thicknesses between graft and host are present (such as that typically seen in patients with keratoconus or corneal melting/thinning) [21]. As a rule of thumb, in a standard case, a 90% suture depth passage and a relatively longer bite would be recommended, to ensure a greater compression area, and reduce the chances of gaps in the interface at any level.

The knot would be tightened to appose both wound lips and not to have a loose stitch. Excessive tightening is to be avoided as very tight sutures induce high astigmatism, and in some cases, induce suture-related cheese wiring.

Intraoperative Suture Adjustment

Intraoperative suture adjustment differs depending on the suturing technique used (interrupted sutures vs. running sutures). For interrupted sutures, it has already been highlighted how these should be placed (four cardinal sutures, then four oblique sutures etc.). As the initial four sutures are placed, one should see a symmetrical distribution of the donor graft over the trephination area. One should also see tension lines between consecutive bites, conforming a "diamond" square configuration. As we continue with the next four sutures, then a rather homogenous "octagon" configuration should be seen. At this point, a keratoscope can be used every so often to check for the roundness of the corneal keratoscopic mires, and adjust the sutures accordingly—even repeat those that may be too tight or too loose.

For running sutures, intraoperative adjustment should be performed before the knot is tied, with the help of an intraoperative keratoscope. When the keratoscopic mires look round and regular, the knot can then be tied and buried.

Postoperative Suture Adjustment

For interrupted suturing, this can be rather simple, as the only way to do an adjustment would be via selective or complete suture removal [29]. A corneal suture can eventually stay in place for an unlimited period of time, as long as the suture is not loose or broken (which would represent a risk of infection and/or corneal neovascularisation). Sutures that become loose or broken in the early postoperative period may (or likely) need to be replaced. Sutures that break or become loose after several months can simply be removed.

From a refractive perspective, selective suture removal can be performed after 6–12 months. Time varies with the age of the patient and the indication for graft. As an example, younger keratoconic patients would have a quicker recovery time compared to elder patients with neurotrophic corneas. As such, a young keratoconic patient could be considered for suture removal 6 months after surgery, whereas an elderly patient with neurotrophic cornea may need the sutures in place for 18 months or longer. The interrupted suture can be removed corresponding to the steep axis as measured by corneal topography. Hence, by removing sutures along the steep axis, this would become flatter and by a coupling effect, the flatter meridian would become steeper.

In a running suture, the options are either removal or adjustment. In an adjustment, the suture tension can be locally modified, ideally under keratoscopic control, until the surgeon obtains a rounder keratoscopic reflex [30]. With suture removal, whether under the microscope or at the slit lamp, the recommendation would be to cut the suture at many different points after the application of topical anaesthesia and topical povidone-iodine. This way, the passes of the suture running intrastromally at the time of removal would be significantly less than pulling a full suture from the same point, hence reducing the chances of promoting a corneal abscess.

Take Home Notes

- Ocular surface disease (OSD) is the leading cause of graft failure and hence it is imperative that pre-operative OSD is aggressively treated. However, this needs to be maintained post-operatively.

- There are many variations to the surgical technique of penetrating keratoplasty; however, the main goals are to safely perform surgery without complications and achieve good wound apposition with minimal astigmatism induction.
- For a DALK procedure, the same principles would apply, bearing in mind that the suture should go full-thickness through the DALK donor button, and not 90% depth as for a PKP.
- Nylon is the most effective suture material in keratoplasty surgery. Its relatively elastic, biocompatible and strength properties are superior to other materials for this purpose. The 10-0 size is commonly used which has a diameter of approximately 20 μm.
- Correct suturing is of paramount importance for an appropriate wound apposition, ensuring the chances of wound leaks, loose stitches or any other graft-host junction problems are reduced to the minimum possible.
- The suture knot would need to be locked (to avoid loosening of tension) and then buried within the corneal tissue (ideally avoiding burying the knot in the graft-host junction). The two most commonly used techniques would be either a 3-1-1 knot or a 2-1-1-1 knot.

References

1. Zirm E. Eine erfolgreiche totale Keratoplastik. Graefes Arch Ophthalmol. 1906;64:580–93.
2. Armitage WJ, Tullo AB, Larkin DF. The first successful full-thickness corneal transplant: a commentary on Eduard Zirm's landmark paper of 1906. Br J Ophthalmol. 2006;90:1222–3.
3. Reisinger F. Die Keratoplastik, ein Versuch zur Erweiterung der Augenheilkunst. Bayerische Annalen. 1824;1:207–15.
4. Marcus M. Angabe eines Operationsverfahren zur Ausführung der Transplantatio Corneae. In: Schmidt CC, editor. Jahrbücher der in-und ausländischen gesamten Medicin. Leipzig: Otto Weigand; 1841. p. 89.
5. Keratoplasty CR. Comments on the technique of corneal transplantation. Source and preservation of donor's material. Report of new instruments. Am J Ophthalmol. 1941;24:1–20.
6. Farge EJ. Eye banking: 1944 to the present. Surv Ophthalmol. 1989;33:260–3.
7. Seitz B, Brunner H, Viestenz A, et al. Inverse mushroom-shaped nonmechanical penetrating keratoplasty using a femtosecond laser. Am J Ophthalmol. 2005;139:941–4.
8. Daniel MC, Bohringer D, Maier P, et al. Comparison of long-term outcomes of femtosecond laser-assisted keratoplasty with conventional keratoplasty. Cornea. 2016;35:293–8.
9. Tsubota K, Satake Y, Kaido M, et al. Treatment of severe ocular-surface disorders with corneal epithelial stem-cell transplantation. N Engl J Med. 1999;340:1697–703.
10. Hossain P, Tourkmani AK, Kazakos D, et al. Emergency corneal grafting in the UK: a 6-year analysis of the UK Transplant Registry. Br J Ophthalmol. 2018;102:26–30.
11. Reinhard T, Bohringer D, Sundmacher R. Accelerated chronic endothelial cell loss after penetrating keratoplasty in glaucoma eyes. J Glaucoma. 2001;10:446–51.
12. Kwon YH, Taylor JM, Hong S, et al. Long-term results of eyes with penetrating keratoplasty and glaucoma drainage tube implant. Ophthalmology. 2001;108:272–8.
13. Tourkmani AK, Sanchez-Huerta V, De Wit G, et al. Weighing of risk factors for penetrating keratoplasty graft failure: application of Risk Score System. Int J Ophthalmol. 2017;10:372–7.
14. Bradley BA. Rejection and recipient age. Transpl Immunol. 2002;10:125–32.
15. Tourkmani AK, Ansari AS, Hossain PN, et al. Tectonic Descemet stripping endothelial keratoplasty for the management of corneal perforation: a case series. Cornea. 2020;39:1571–5.
16. Bandivadekar P, Gupta S, Sharma N. Intraoperative suprachoroidal hemorrhage after penetrating keratoplasty: case series and review of literature. Eye Contact Lens. 2016;42:206–10.
17. Ingraham HJ, Donnenfeld ED, Perry HD. Massive suprachoroidal hemorrhage in penetrating keratoplasty. Am J Ophthalmol. 1989;108:670–5.
18. Melles GR, Binder PS. A comparison of wound healing in sutured and unsutured corneal wounds. Arch Ophthalmol. 1990;108:1460–9.
19. McNeill JI, Wessels IF. Adjustment of single continuous suture to control astigmatism after penetrating keratoplasty. Refract Corneal Surg. 1989;5:216–23.
20. Holland E. A comparison of suture types in the stimulation of corneal inflammation. Invest Ophthalmol Vis Sci Suppl. 1990;31(4):270.
21. Busin M, Arffa RC. Deep suturing technique for penetrating keratoplasty. Cornea. 2002;21:680–4.
22. Shahinian L Jr, Brown SI. Postoperative complications with protruding monofilament nylon sutures. Am J Ophthalmol. 1977;83:546–8.

23. Javadi MA, Naderi M, Zare M, et al. Comparison of the effect of three suturing techniques on post-keratoplasty astigmatism in keratoconus. Cornea. 2006;25:1029–33.
24. Spadea L, Cifariello F, Bianco G, et al. Long-term results of penetrating keratoplasty using a single or double running suture technique. Graefes Arch Clin Exp Ophthalmol. 2002;240:415–9.
25. Vajpayee RB, Sharma V, Sharma N, et al. Evaluation of techniques of single continuous suturing in penetrating keratoplasty. Br J Ophthalmol. 2001;85:134–8.
26. Sharma V, Sharma N, Vajpayee RB, et al. Study of corneal topographic patterns with single continuous suturing techniques in penetrating keratoplasty. Cornea. 2003;22:5–9.
27. Nuzzi R, Burato C, Tridico F, et al. Advantages of double running sutures in astigmatism after penetrating keratoplasty. Clin Ophthalmol. 2022;16:797–802.
28. Abou-Jaoude ES, Brooks M, Katz DG, et al. Spontaneous wound dehiscence after removal of single continuous penetrating keratoplasty suture. Ophthalmology. 2002;109:1291–6; discussion 1297.
29. Van Meter WS, Gussler JR, Soloman KD, et al. Postkeratoplasty astigmatism control. Single continuous suture adjustment versus selective interrupted suture removal. Ophthalmology. 1991;98:177–83.
30. Solano JM, Hodge DO, Bourne WM. Keratometric astigmatism after suture removal in penetrating keratoplasty: double running versus single running suture techniques. Cornea. 2003;22:716–20.

Closing the Wound: Can Sutures Be Avoided?

7

Luca Menabuoni, Alessandra Balestrazzi,
Luca Buzzonetti, Romina Fasciani,
Claudio Macaluso, Luigi Mosca, Roberto Pini,
Giada Magni, Paolo Matteini, Fulvio Ratto,
Michele Rossi, and Francesca Rossi

Key Points

- Description of the laser welding approach and its recent history
- Photothermal effects in laser welding of corneal tissue
- Mechanical load resistance of laser welded corneas in PK
- Laser welding in Deep Anterior Lamellar Keratoplasty (DALK): a clinical case
- The development of biocompatible patches to be welded as adhesives in ocular surgery

Supplementary Information The online version contains supplementary material available at https://doi.org/10.1007/978-3-031-32408-6_7.

L. Menabuoni
Casa di Cura Villa Donatello, Florence, Italy

A. Balestrazzi
Cornea and Ocular Surface Unit, ASL ROMA 2, Rome, Italy

L. Buzzonetti
Ophthalmology Department, Bambino Gesù IRCCS Children's Hospital, Rome, Italy
e-mail: luca.buzzonetti@opbg.net

R. Fasciani · L. Mosca
Cornea and Refractive Surgery Unit, Department of Opthalmology, Agostino Gemelli University Polyclinic Foundation-IRCCS, Rome, Italy
e-mail: romina.fasciani@policlinicogemelli.it;
luigi.mosca@policlinicogemelli.it

C. Macaluso
University of Parma, Parma, Italy

R. Pini · G. Magni · P. Matteini · F. Ratto · M. Rossi
F. Rossi (✉)
Institute of Applied Physics, Italian National Research Council, Florence, Italy
e-mail: r.pini@ifac.cnr.it; g.magni@ifac.cnr.it;
p.matteini@ifac.cnr.it; f.ratto@ifac.cnr.it;
f.rossi@ifac.cnr.it

Introduction

Suturing is a critical step in the surgical practice: it allows closuring an open wound and supports the recovery of the injured tissue. Nowadays, a variety of suturing techniques are available, while the fundamental goals remain the same: an excellent adhesion of the wound walls, providing a strong mechanical response of the treated tissue, prevention of inflammation and bacterial contamination, and a satisfactory functional and cosmetic outcome.

In ocular surgery, suturing is usually performed in corneal transplantation. It can be performed using interrupted sutures, continuous running single suture, double sutures or a combination of interrupted and continuous sutures [1, 2].

Needles and stitches are also used in cataract surgery and more in general in corneal wounds management.

However, the suturing procedure is time-consuming, and the post-treatment results can be affected by several side effects that might impair the surgery outcome. The use of needle and of the suturing thread induces a mechanical trauma in the tissue. The presence of the foreign body at the wound site can exacerbate or prolong the inflammatory phase. The emergence of infection, suture erosion, and granuloma are associated with further problems [3–5]. The poor apposition of the donor and recipient flaps due to sutures can result in post-operative astigmatism [1].

These possible adverse effects related to corneal transplantation may adversely affect the quality of the patient's post-operative course. In addition, in susceptible subjects, clinical conditions could worsen to the point of requiring medical care, representing an additional cost to the national health service.

On this basis, for about 20 years we have been working on corneal laser welding, implementing this consolidated technique with the use of new materials characterised by biocompatibility and low production costs. Laser welding is a technique that exploits the selective interaction between a specific wavelength and an absorber, resulting in a photothermal effect. This controlled and localised temperature increase determines the welding of the edges of biological tissue, especially if it consists of thermosensitive molecules such as collagen.

Different solutions were proposed to overcome all these problems: the use of the femtosecond laser for corneal tissue cutting can support the introduction of self-closuring wounds or the reduction of suturing need (e.g. in cataract surgery or intrastromal corneal surgery) [2]. The use of biocompatible adhesives or patches can support the realisation of a suture-less transplantation or the conjunctiva treatment [6].

In this chapter, we describe the proposed technique for a full laser-assisted corneal surgery and the biocompatible patches that can be used for the closuring or the local medication of ocular tissues.

Laser Closuring of Corneal Wounds

Laser welding of biological tissues is a technique used to join tissues by inducing a photothermal effect between the two edges of the wound. It has been proposed in several surgical specialities over the last 30 years: neurosurgery, eye surgery, dermatology, aesthetic medicine, dentistry, etc., are just some of the fields where laser welding is applied [7]. Laser welding hold the promise to provide instantaneous, watertight seals without the introduction of foreign materials. For this reason, laser welding has progressively gained relevance in the clinical setting, making surgery less invasive, faster and less risky, and appearing as a valid alternative to traditional surgical methods.

In the laser welding approach, optimised by our research team for corneal tissue, we proposed the application of the photo-enhancing dye Indocyanine Green (ICG) in the tissue and the use of a diode laser emitting at 810 nm. Most of biological tissues, and corneal tissue in particular, are transparent to the light in the near-infrared region, while the stained tissue presents the optical absorbance peak at this specific wavelength. In other words: only the presence of the biological tissue stained with the ICG absorbs the radiation emitted by the laser. This interaction triggers a confined photothermal effect resulting in the selective fusion of wound walls at low irradiation power per target area, thus reducing the risk of thermal damage to surrounding tissues. The welding effect may be modulated in the depth of the transparent tissue, thus resulting in a more effective closure of the wound.

Laser closuring of ocular tissues can be performed following different original approach, that has been studied and well-described over the past 20 years [7–23].

In the literature, the main absorption is due to the water content of the cornea: this means that the photothermal effect is not spatially confined and mainly located in the external corneal surface, immediately impacting the laser light. Moreover, to the best of our knowledge, only one of the designed protocols reached the test phase in animal models in vivo [19], and our original approach has been tested in the clinical practice in selected patients [12, 15, 18]: both are based on the combined use of the exogenous dye (typically ICG) and the 810 nm laser.

Photothermal Laser Welding in Keratoplasty

During the last 20 years of research activity, at the Institute of Applied Physics, we developed an original photothermal approach to the laser welding of corneal tissue, thus supporting the closuring of surgical wounds in corneal transplantation [7, 8, 12, 13, 15, 16, 24, 25].

It is based on the use of a near-infrared diode laser emitting at 810 nm and the topical application of the chromophore ICG, which shows high optical absorption at the laser wavelength emission. The protocol is as follows: (1) ICG is prepared in the form of a saturated aqueous solution of commercially available Indocyanine Green for biomedical applications (e.g. IC-GREEN Akorn, Buffalo Grove, IL or ICG-Pulsion Medical Systems AG, Germany). (2) The solution is accurately positioned within the surgical wound walls, staining the stromal tissue in depth. (3) The wound edges are approximated, and laser welding (8 W/cm^2 power density) is performed under a surgical microscope [18].

The laser used in pre-clinical tests and in clinical applications is typically an AlGaAs diode laser (e.g. Mod. WELD 800 by El.En. SpA, Italy) emitting at 810 nm and equipped with a fiberoptic delivery system.

This approach is of particular interest when combined with femtosecond laser approach in a fully laser-based transplantation: laser cutting enables to realise a clear-cut plane, with the same geometrical and morphological profile both in the donor and in the recipient tissues. By doing this, a perfect matching of the wound walls is obtained, thus reducing the occurrence of post-operative astigmatism or of reduced visual acuity [2]. The use of the laser welding approach supports the reduction of stitches, thus further improving the post-operative results and lowering the occurrence of astigmatism.

Another important aspect that the combination of the femtosecond laser with laser welding improves, is the possibility to design patient-tailored profiles, with enhanced mechanical resistance [26, 27]. Several donor/host-profiled configurations have been described in the literature, such as zigzag, Christmas tree, mushroom, top hat [28, 29] or anvil ones [17, 18]. Each profile choice is due to patient's anatomy and pathology and to the surgeon's experience. During clinical practice, it has been shown that the anvil cut shape leads to improved sealing: it has a larger surface of the donor/recipient wound edge, and an observed mechanical stability [30].

Theoretical studies [30, 31] and clinical observations [18, 24] pointed out that the femtosecond laser cut profiles support a stronger mechanical load resistance to IOP. The qualitatively theoretical studies showed that the overlap in the zigzag, Christmas tree, top hat, mushroom and anvil patterns led to higher pressure resistance as compared with non-profiled femtosecond laser-assisted trephination. The laser profiled flaps are stronger to mechanical stress and strain due to increasing internal pressure in respect to the traditional straight cut. Moreover, the femtosecond laser-assisted anvil wound configuration was found to be the most stable graft configuration. Thanks to the peripheral lamellar ring, in the anvil profiled PK, the donor cornea easily fit into the recipient bed: the angled edge created a key-hole effect between the donor and the host tissues and increased the surface area of junction, as the clinical practice evidenced (Fig. 7.1).

Thanks to the laser welding procedure, the donor flap presents very good mechanical stability not only in the immediate post-surgery times but even 1 year after the treatment [14]. Good mechanical stability after the treatment was clinically observed during a re-surgery after corneal rejection. It is well known that the photothermal effect underlying the laser welding of the wound walls is based on the controlled thermal denaturation of interfibrillar links [32–38]. During irra-

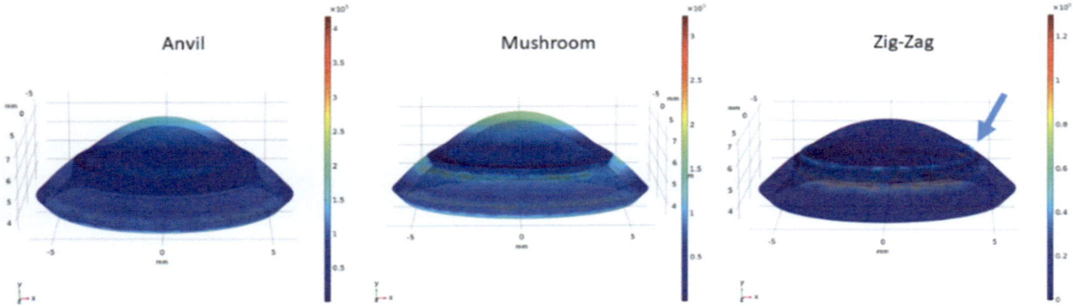

Fig. 7.1 Deformation (in mm) and stress evaluation (von Mises values in N/m², in false colours) in the transplanted cornea in anvil (left) mushroom (centre) zigzag profile (right). At high internal pressure load, the anvil profile maintains intact the connection at the donor/host interface, while at the same IOP values, the zigzag profile is losing contact (see arrow)

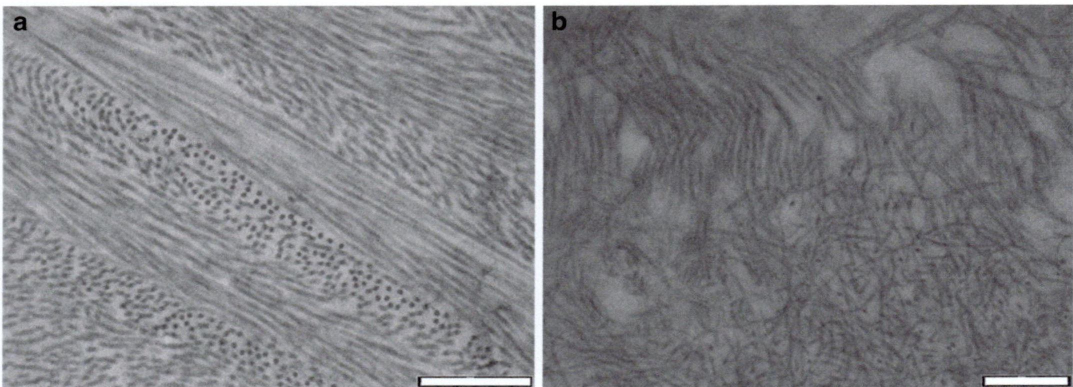

Fig. 7.2 TEM micrograph of a stromal region 50 μm far from the weld site (**a**). The appearance of a stromal region close to the welded area (**b**). Scale bar 500 nm

diation, the temperature in the stained tissue is at around 55 °C, thus preserving the morphology of the single collagen fibre. Its regular spatial distribution however is lost, as the interfibrillar bridges are denaturised at these temperatures. New bridges are realised immediately after irradiation, during the cooling phase. The result is an immediate closure of the wound walls, where the collagen from the two sides of the walls is interwoven, and thus, the wound is sealed.

The clinical observation in re-surgery was a clear resistance of the transplanted flap at the weld site (Fig. 7.2), very close to the mechanical resistance of a natural and closed cornea, while re-cutting a transplanted flap is usually an easy-to-perform procedure in sutured donor flaps (Fig. 7.3).

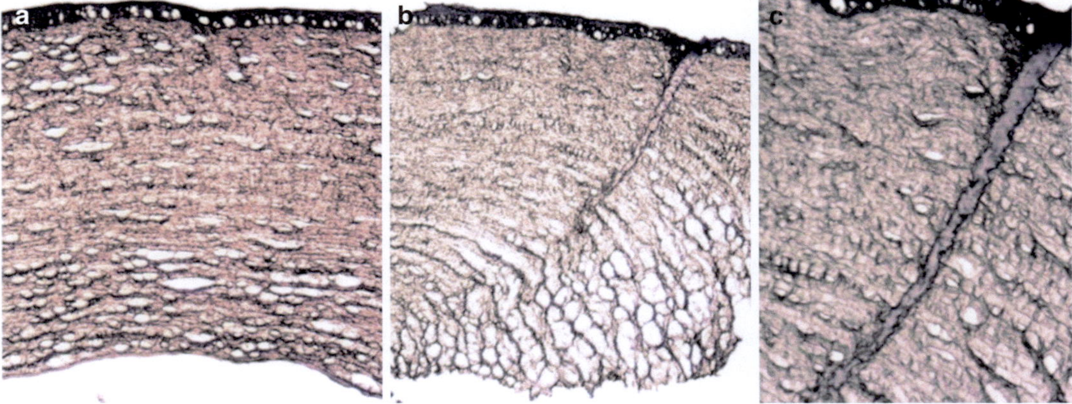

Fig. 7.3 Porcine cornea in laser welding tests, modelling the sealing of a surgical wound. Sections (10 μm thickness) coloured with standard histological staining (haematoxylin and eosin) of intact cornea (**a**), 10× image of the laser welded cut (**b**); 40× image of the surgical cut (**c**)

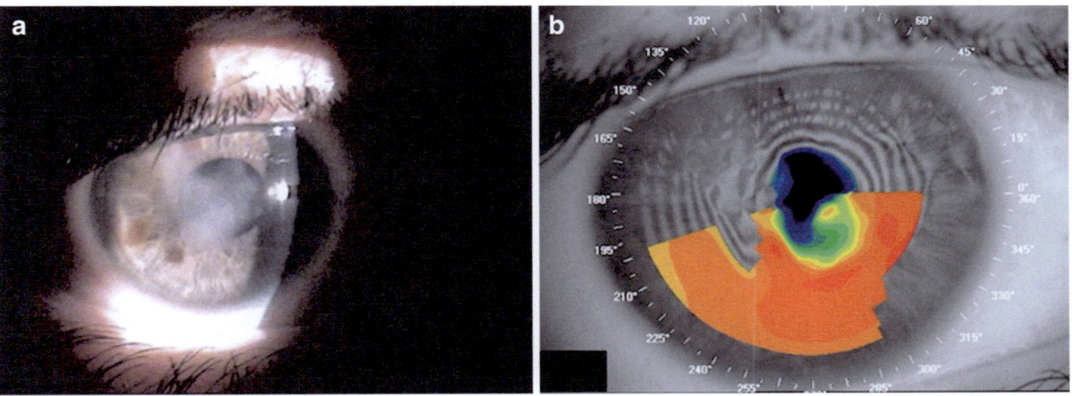

Fig. 7.4 Pre-operative slit-lamp image (**a**) and corneal map (**b**) of a patient's cornea (right eye) selected for a sutureless, laser-welded, DALK. The cornea presents a post-herpetic stromal scar in the central part

All-Laser Transplantation

The combined use of femtosecond laser and photothermal laser welding of the surgical wound supports the all-laser corneal transplantation, such as Deep Anterior Lamellar Keratoplasty (DALK) [25, 39].

In this particular approach, the first attempt to perform an all-laser DALK procedure with the support of laser welding was performed in Tuscany in 2006 [36]. In brief, this suture-less surgery has been performed on a 55 years-old patient with a dense scar in the central area of the cornea. The pre-operative BCVA was 1/20, and the intraocular pressure was 14 mmHg (Fig. 7.4). The pachymetry revealed a thinnest point of 430 μm. Donor and recipient corneal flaps were trephined with a femtosecond laser. After laser trephination, the donor lamella was applied in the recipient bed: no sutures were used to stabilise the donor cornea, while the laser welding procedure was selected and performed, as described in "Photothermal Laser Welding in Keratoplasty" section (see Video 7.1). No adverse events or complications occurred during surgery or in the post-operative period. A satisfactory intraoperative wound apposition was observed under the operating microscope at 360° before and after laser welding (Fig. 7.5). The central corneal was clear with a slight interface, and the wound was well-apposed on the 360° in each examination (Fig. 7.6).

In this laser welding procedure, it was possible to observe that, thanks to controlled heating of the graft–host junction, the structure of the collagen proteins denature and create a quick stabilisation and healing of the wound at the graft–host junction. The good apposition was maintained for all the follow-up, with an increasing CDVA during the 6 months period. This laser welding technique can support the more common suturing approach in DALK and PK or eventually totally substitute it, at least in the DALK procedure.

Monitoring the Thermal Effects of Laser Welding

The laser welding protocol is based on the induction of a controlled photothermal effect within the corneal tissue. A specific thermal range has to be reached: below 50 °C, the procedure is ineffective, while over 70 °C undesired thermal damages can occur [40]. The induced temperature values are related to the energy density, i.e. the fluence, delivered to the tissue, and this is related to the distance of the fibre tip from the target. The welding effect is thus due to the surgeon ability to maintain the correct distance during the irradiation. When the correct temperature is induced, the main clinical evidence is a whitening of the cornea at the welded site [9, 41]. It is thus obvious the whole procedure, and its efficacy is strongly surgeon-depended.

Over the last 10 years, the research activities were thus devoted to design a new approach to control and monitor the temperature effects during the welding procedure. Several attempts can be found in the literature [20, 23], almost based on the NIR monitoring of the temperature at the irradiation site. In our research group, we developed a robotic platform enabling to control and standardise the irradiation conditions: the movement of the fibre tip and its distance from the target is controlled by a robotic arm [42–46]. This solution enables to overcome the problems related to the manual procedure. The proposed platform is based on the teleoperation of a robot controlled with visual feedback, where machine vision and image processing are part of the control system. A collaborative robot arm was cho-

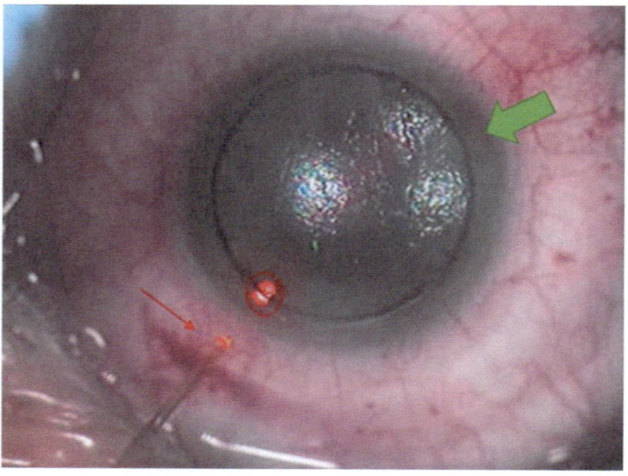

Fig. 7.5 Laser welding procedure in DALK. In the image, it is possible to see the stained wound walls (green arrow), the NIR laser tip (red arrow) and the red pointer (inside the green circle), indicating the welding area

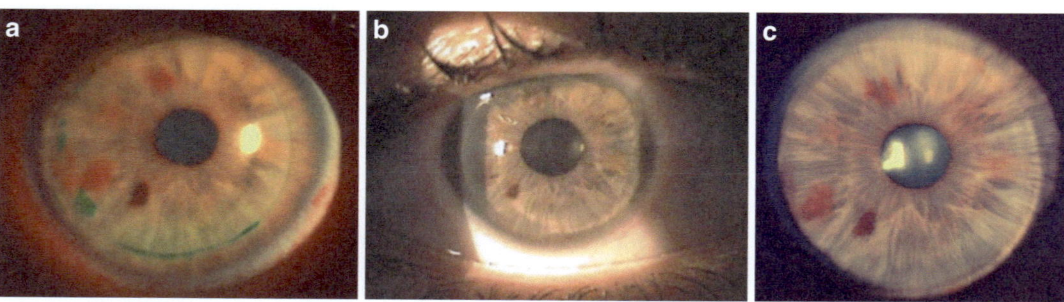

Fig. 7.6 Post-operative slit-lamp images of a laser welded DALK at 1 (**a**), 7 (**b**) and 30 (**c**) p.o. days

sen, with a control system that autonomously decides to stop the procedure in case of adverse events: two cameras, one dedicated to the general vision and the other one devoted to the control of the temperature, together with the general control system based on a visual servoing continuously adjust the trajectory. The system was tested on porcine corneas, with good welding results.

Laser Closuring with Biocompatible Materials

Recent research activities are focused on the design and optimisation of biocompatible patches. These new materials can be used for the closuring of wounds [47, 48] and for local medication by the controlled delivery of drugs in situ.

The first successful ex vivo tests were performed in our lab for the closuring of capsular tissue [49, 50]. The approach is similar to the photothermal welding described in the previous paragraphs. However, here the fibre tip is positioned onto the flap to be secured, which is previously stained with ICG (Fig. 7.7).

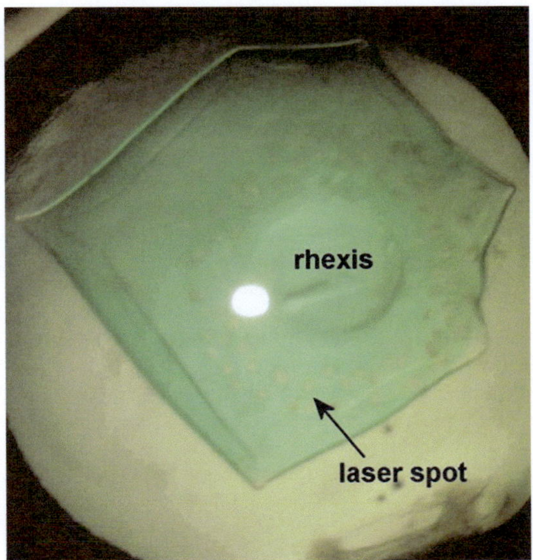

Fig. 7.7 ICG-stained capsular patch laser welded by diode laser radiation, to close a capsulorhexis. Laser spots are clearly evident at the periphery of the patch. Tests are performed ex vivo in porcine eyes

In the past, few attempts to close scleral wounds were performed [51], by the use of chitosan patches [52–54]. This was the starting point to push the research activities towards the design and optimisation of new biocompatible materials to support the healing of ocular tissues [55, 56].

The working principle is as follows: the biomaterial is casted or electro-spinned with the staining dye, typically ICG or cyanines. The biomaterials are designed in order to be biocompatible, biodegradable, to present a good handling, good chemical stability and good mechanical load resistance when necessary.

The 810 nm diode laser is used to seal the patch onto the tissue: as said, the tissue is transparent to this wavelength, while the stained patch directly absorbs the light. As a result, a photothermal effect is induced: as the realised patches are thin (thickness around 20–40 μm), the thermal effect is transferred towards the ocular tissue. In the area of the spot, we thus observe a confined denaturation of the biological tissue together with the denaturation of the patch, thus leading to the immediate sealing of the tissue and the patch.

The controlled photothermal effect can also be used to enable the release of drugs encapsulated within the patch [57].

Conclusions

The research activities offered a large variety of different solutions to the problems that can occur in the suturing procedure, in particular when ocular tissues are involved. The use of a NIR diode laser, in combination with an absorbing dye used to stain the biological tissue, is proposed to realise a suture-less surgery, while providing an immediate sealing of the surgical wounds and improving the healing process. The combined use of biocompatible materials is proposed for the local treatment of ocular tissues or to close extremely thin tissues.

Moreover, the laser welding procedure was tested in combination with the laser cutting approach in corneal transplantation, demonstrating to be a flexible tool for performing patient-tailored surgery.

Take Home Notes

- Suturing is a challenging procedure in PK: it can induce several side effects in the post-operative period, such as foreign body reaction, partial closuring of the wound walls, uneven healing in the corneal perimeter leading to astigmatism.
- Laser welding of the surgical wound walls can be performed with a NIR diode laser (810 nm) and the preliminary staining of the tissues.
- A spatially confined and controlled thermal effect is induced, thus resulting in an immediate sealing and in a stable flap over the healing time.
- New materials can be used as adhesives: once stained, they can be welded to the ocular tissues, thus improving local treatment of wounds and pathological tissues.

References

1. Krootila K, Wetterstrand O, Holopainen J. Post-keratoplasty astigmatism. In: Hjortdal J, editor. Corneal transplantation. Cham: Springer; 2016. https://doi.org/10.1007/978-3-319-24052-7_12.
2. Williams GP, Mehta JS. Technology: femtosecond laser in keratoplasty. In: Hjortdal J, editor. Corneal transplantation. Cham: Springer; 2016. https://doi.org/10.1007/978-3-319-24052-7_15.
3. Christo CG, van Rooij J, Geerards AJ, et al. Suture-related complications following keratoplasty: a 5-year retrospective study. Cornea. 2001;20(8):816–9. https://doi.org/10.1097/00003226-200111000-00008.
4. Bar-Sela SM, Spierer O, Spierer A. Suture-related complications after congenital cataract surgery: Vicryl versus Mersilene sutures. J Cataract Refract Surg. 2007;33(2):301–4. https://doi.org/10.1016/j.jcrs.2006.10.039.
5. Jeganathan SV, Ghosh S, Jhanji V, et al. Resuturing following penetrating keratoplasty: a retrospective analysis. Br J Ophthalmol. 2008;92(7):893–5. https://doi.org/10.1136/bjo.2007.133421.
6. Liu J, Huang Y, Yang W, Sun X, Yingni X, Peng Y, Song W, Yuan J, Li R. Sutureless transplantation using a semi-interpenetrating polymer network bioadhesive for ocular surface reconstruction. Acta Biomater. 2022;153:273–86. https://doi.org/10.1016/j.actbio.2022.09.049.
7. Pini R, Rossi F, Matteini P, et al. Laser tissue welding in minimally invasive surgery and microsurgery. In: Pavesi L, Fauchet PM, editors. Biophotonics. Berlin: Springer; 2008. p. 275–99.
8. Pini R, Rossi F, Menabuoni L, et al. Diode laser welding for cornea suturing: an experimental study of the repair process. In: Manns F, Soderberg PG, Ho A, editors. Ophthalmic technologies XIV; 2004. p. 245–52.
9. Rossi F, Pini R, Menabuoni L, et al. Experimental study on the healing process following laser welding of the cornea. J Biomed Opt. 2005;10(2). https://doi.org/10.1117/1.1900703.
10. Pini R, Rossi F, Menabuoni L, et al. Preliminary study on the closure of the lens capsule by laser welding - art. no. 61381C. In: Manns F, Soderberg PG, Ho A, editors. Ophthalmic technologies XVI; 2006. p. C1381.
11. Pini R, Rossi F, Menabuoni L. Laser welding of biological tissue: experimental studies in ophthalmology - art. no. 619103. In: Grzymala R, Haeberle O, editors. Biophotonics and new therapy frontiers; 2006. p. 19103.
12. Menabuoni L, Pini R, Rossi F, et al. Laser-assisted corneal welding in cataract surgery: retrospective study. J Cataract Refract Surg. 2007;33(9):1608–12. https://doi.org/10.1016/j.jcrs.2007.04.013.
13. Rossi F, Matteini P, Ratto F, et al. Laser tissue welding in ophthalmic surgery. J Biophotonics. 2008;1(4):331–42. https://doi.org/10.1002/jbio.200810028.
14. Rossi F, Matteini P, Pini R, et al. Long term observation of low power diode laser welding after penetrating keratoplasty in human patients. In: Manns F, Soderberg PG, Arthur HO, editors. Ophthalmic technologies XX; 2010.
15. Buzzonetti L, Capozzi P, Petrocelli G, et al. Laser welding in penetrating keratoplasty and cataract surgery in pediatric patients: early results. J Cataract Refract Surg. 2013;39(12):1829–34. https://doi.org/10.1016/j.jcrs.2013.05.046.
16. Rossi F, Menabuoni L, Malandrini A, et al. "All-Laser" endothelial corneal transplant in human patients. In: Manns F, Soderberg PG, Ho A, editors. Ophthalmic technologies XXII; 2012.
17. Menabuoni L, Canovetti A, Rossi F, et al. The 'anvil' profile in femtosecond laser-assisted penetrating keratoplasty. Acta Ophthalmol. 2013;91(6):e494–5. https://doi.org/10.1111/aos.12144.
18. Canovetti A, Malandrini A, Lenzetti I, et al. Laser-assisted penetrating keratoplasty: 1-year results in patients using a laser-welded anvil-profiled graft. Am J Ophthalmol. 2014;158(4):664–70. https://doi.org/10.1016/j.ajo.2014.07.010.
19. Rodriguez Galarza RM, McMullen RJ Jr. Descemet's membrane detachments, ruptures, and separations in ten adult horses: clinical signs, diagnostics, treatment options, and preliminary results. Vet Ophthalmol. 2020;23(4):611–23. https://doi.org/10.1111/vop.12793.
20. Strassmann E, Livny E, Loya N, et al. CO_2 laser welding of corneal cuts with albumin solder using radiometric temperature control. Ophthalmic Res. 2013;50(3):174–9.
21. Rasier R, Ozeren M, Artunay O, et al. Corneal tissue welding with infrared laser irradiation after clear cor-

neal incision. Cornea. 2010;29(9):985–90. https://doi.org/10.1097/ICO.0b013e3181cc7a3e.

22. Savage HE, Halder RK, Kartazayeu U, et al. NIR laser tissue welding of in vitro porcine cornea and sclera tissue. Lasers Surg Med. 2004;35(4):293–303. https://doi.org/10.1002/lsm.20094.

23. Barak A, Eyal O, Rosner M, et al. Temperature-controlled CO2 laser tissue welding of ocular tissues. Surv Ophthalmol. 1997;42 Suppl 1:S77–81. https://doi.org/10.1016/s0039-6257(97)80029-x.

24. Menabuoni L, Malandrini A, Canovetti A, Lenzetti I, Pini R, Rossi F. The use of femtosecond laser and corneal welding in the surgery of keratoconus. In: Alió J, editor. Keratoconus. Essentials in ophthalmology. Cham: Springer; 2017. https://doi.org/10.1007/978-3-319-43881-8_24.

25. Rossi F, Canovetti A, Malandrini A, et al. An "all-laser" endothelial transplant. J Vis Exp. 2015;(101):e52939. https://doi.org/10.3791/52939.

26. Nuzzo V, Aptel F, Savoldelli M, et al. Histologic and ultrastructural characterization of corneal femtosecond laser trephination. Cornea. 2009;28(8):908–13. https://doi.org/10.1097/ICO.0b013e318197ebeb.

27. Chamberlain WD, Rush SW, Mathers WD, et al. Comparison of femtosecond laser-assisted keratoplasty versus conventional penetrating keratoplasty. Ophthalmology. 2011;118(3):486–91. https://doi.org/10.1016/j.ophtha.2010.08.002.

28. Busin M, Robert CA. Microkeratome-assisted mushroom keratoplasty with minimal endothelial replacement. Am J Ophthalmol. 2005;140(1):138–40.

29. Farid M, Kim M, Steinert RF. Results of penetrating keratoplasty performed with a femtosecond laser zigzag incision initial report. Ophthalmology. 2007;114(12):2208–12. https://doi.org/10.1016/j.ophtha.2007.08.048.

30. Canovetti A, Rossi F, Rossi M, et al. Anvil-profiled penetrating keratoplasty: load resistance evaluation. Biomech Model Mechanobiol. 2019;18(2):319–25. https://doi.org/10.1007/s10237-018-1083-y.

31. Lee HP, Zhuang H. Biomechanical study on the edge shapes for penetrating keratoplasty. Comput Methods Biomech Biomed Engin. 2012;15(10):1071–9. https://doi.org/10.1080/10255842.2011.571677.

32. Matteini P, Rossi F, Menabuoni L, et al. Microscopic characterization of collagen modifications induced by low-temperature diode-laser welding of corneal tissue. Lasers Surg Med. 2007;39(7):597–604. https://doi.org/10.1002/lsm.20532.

33. Matteini P, Ratto F, Rossi F, et al. Photothermally-induced disordered patterns of corneal collagen revealed by SHG imaging. Opt Exp. 2009;17(6):4868–78.

34. Matteini P, Ratto F, Rossi F, et al. Investigation on fibrous collagen modifications during corneal laser welding by second harmonic generation microscopy. In: Manns F, Soderberg PG, Ho A, editors. Ophthalmic technologies XIX; 2009.

35. Matteini P, Rossi F, Ratto F, et al. Quantitative analysis of thermally-induced alterations of corneal stroma by second-harmonic generation imaging. In: Manns F, Soderberg PG, Arthur HO, editors. Ophthalmic technologies XX; 2010.

36. Matteini P, Cicchi R, Ratto F, et al. Thermal transitions of fibrillar collagen unveiled by second-harmonic generation microscopy of corneal stroma. Biophys J. 2012;103(6):1179–87. https://doi.org/10.1016/j.bpj.2012.07.055.

37. Rossi F, Pini R, Menabuoni L. Experimental and model analysis on the temperature dynamics during diode laser welding of the cornea. J Biomed Opt. 2007;12(1):014031. https://doi.org/10.1117/1.2437156.

38. Rossi F, Matteini P, Pini R, et al. Temperature control during diode laser welding in a human cornea - art. no. 663215. In: Vogel A, editor. Therapeutic laser applications and laser-tissue interaction III. Spie-Int Soc Optical Engineering: Bellingham; 2007. p. 63215.

39. Menabuoni L, Pini R, Fantozzi M, et al. "All–laser" sutureless lamellar keratoplasty (ALSL–LK): a first case report. Invest Ophthalmol Vis Sci. 2006;47(13):2356.

40. Niemz MH. Laser-tissue interactions. Berlin: Springer; 2007.

41. Rossi F, Pini R. Modeling the temperature rise during diode laser welding of the cornea. In: Ophthalmic technologies XV, vol. 5688; 2005. p. 185–193. https://doi.org/10.1117/12.610814.

42. Rossi F, Pini R, Menabuoni L, et al. Robotic consolle for ocular surgery: a preliminary study. In: Ophthalmic technologies XXIV; 2014.

43. Menabuoni L, Malandrini A, Canovetti A, et al. Laser assisted robotic surgery in keratoplasty. Investig Ophthalmol Vis Sci. 2017;58(8):3.

44. Rossi F, Micheletti F, Magni G, et al. A robotic platform for laser welding of corneal tissue. In: Novel biophotonics techniques and applications IV; 2017.

45. Rossi F, Micheletti F, Magni G, et al. Laser assisted robotic surgery in cornea transplantation. In: Design and quality for biomedical technologies X; 2017.

46. Russo S, Petroni G, Quaglia C, et al. ESPRESSO: a novel device for laser-assisted surgery of the anterior eye segment. Minim Invasive Ther Allied Technol. 2016;25(2):70–8. https://doi.org/10.3109/13645706.2015.1092450. PMID: 26429150.

47. Bal-Ozturk A, Cecen B, Avci-Adali M, et al. Tissue adhesives: from research to clinical translation. Nano Today. 2021;36:101049. https://doi.org/10.1016/j.nantod.2020.101049.

48. Smeets R, Tauer N, Vollkommer T, et al. Tissue adhesives in reconstructive and aesthetic surgery-application of silk fibroin-based biomaterials. Int J Mol Sci. 2022;23(14):7687. https://doi.org/10.3390/ijms23147687.

49. Pini R, Menabuoni L, Lenzetti I, et al.

50. Pini R, Rossi F, Menabuoni L, et al. A new technique for the closure of the lens capsule by laser welding. Ophthalmic Surg Lasers Imaging. 2008;39(3):260–1. https://doi.org/10.3928/15428877-20080501-12.

51. Rossi F, Matteini P, Menabuoni L, et al. Sutureless closure of scleral wounds in animal models by the use of laser welded biocompatible patches. In: Manns F, Soderberg PG, Ho A, editors. Ophthalmic technologies XXI; 2011.
52. Rossi F, Matteini P, Esposito G, et al. In vivo experimental study on laser welded ICG-loaded chitosan patches for vessel repair. In: Kollias N, Choi B, Zeng H, editors. Photonic therapeutics and diagnostics VII; 2011.
53. Rossi F, Matteini P, Esposito G, et al. In vivo laser assisted end-to-end anastomosis with ICG-infused chitosan patches. In: Sroka R, Lilge LD, editors. Medical laser applications and laser-tissue interactions V; 2011.
54. Rossi F, Matteini P, Ratto F, et al. Laser bonding with ICG-infused chitosan patches: preliminary experiences in suine dura mater and vocal folds. In: Biophotonics: photonic solutions for better health care IV, vol. 9129; 2014. https://doi.org/10.1117/12.2051487.
55. Milanesi A, Magni G, Centi S, et al. Optically activated and interrogated plasmonic hydrogels for applications in wound healing. J Biophotonics. 2020;13(9):e202000135. https://doi.org/10.1002/jbio.202000135.
56. Ratto F, Magni G, Aluigi A, et al. Cyanine-doped nanofiber mats for laser tissue bonding. Nanomaterials (Basel). 2022;12(9):1613. https://doi.org/10.3390/nano12091613.
57. Matteini P, Ratto F, Rossi F, et al. Chitosan films doped with gold nanorods as laser-activatable hybrid bioadhesives. Adv Mater. 2010;22(38):4313–6. https://doi.org/10.1002/adma.201002228.

Femtosecond-Assisted Penetrating Keratoplasty and Deep Anterior Lamellar Keratoplasty

Alfredo Vega-Estrada and Jorge L. Alió

Key Points

- Femtosecond laser-assisted keratoplasty provides highly reproducible corneal incisions.
- Incisions performed using the femtosecond laser heal faster and stronger. This may have the advantage of earlier suture removal.
- A significant investment, together with a learning curve period, is necessary when adopting femtosecond laser technology for assisting keratoplasty procedures.
- Femtosecond laser-assisted keratoplasty procedure induces healing patterns in the peripheral cornea that can be grade according to the degree of induced scaring.
- The potential of femtosecond-assisted surgery to improve wound healing and vision recovery has been observed in numerous animal and clinical studies.

Supplementary Information The online version contains supplementary material available at https://doi.org/10.1007/978-3-031-32408-6_8.

A. Vega-Estrada
Vissum, Grupo Miranza, Alicante, Spain

Universidad Miguel Hernández de Elche, Alicante, Spain

Hospital Virgen de los Lirios de Alcoy, Alicante, Spain
e-mail: alfredovega@vissum.com

J. L. Alió (✉)
Vissum Miranza, Miguel Hernández University, Alicante, Spain
e-mail: jlalio@vissum.com

Femtosecond Laser Action on Corneal Tissue

Femtosecond laser dissection is based on the creation of extremely precise incisions in the corneal tissue by separating lamellar fibers within the stroma. This effect is explained under the principles of optical breakdown and laser photodisruption. Achieving optical breakdown will produce two different effects that have in common tissue ablation. The first one, called plasma-induced ablation, determines a physics process, and the second one is called photodisruption and describes the mechanical behavior of matter.

Laser-induced optical breakdown (LIOB) plays a significant role in the mechanism of plasma-mediated photodisruption, the most important interaction between femtosecond pulses and tissues. LIOB requires a small focal spot size to achieve the threshold Fluence (energy/area) for plasma formation [1].

This spatial resolution is determined by the width of the free-electron distribution, which is the function of focalized size and peak intensity which at the same time is determined in the femtosecond laser systems by the numerical aperture (NA). NA is defined as the sine of the angle of the marginal ray coming from the focal point, multiplied by the refractive index of the medium from which the input beam comes (Fig. 8.1).

In femtosecond laser systems, NA represents one of the most important factors that determine laser precision. To achieve the larger NA possi-

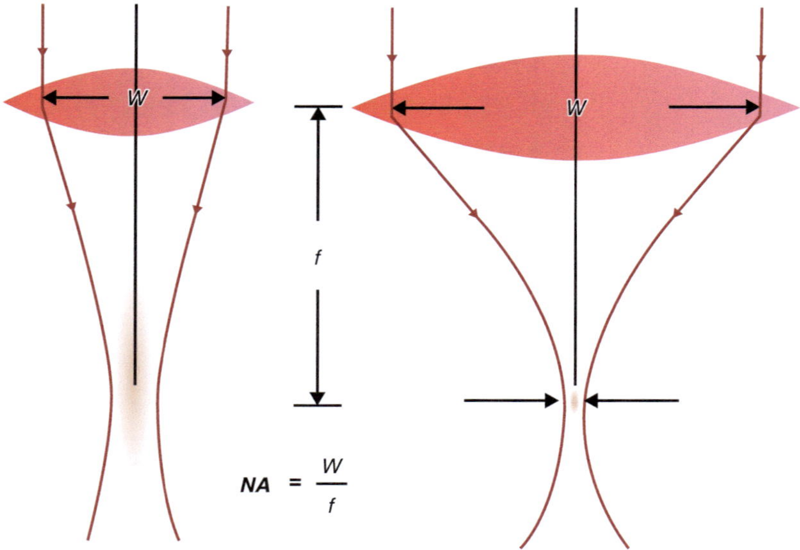

Fig. 8.1 Numerical aperture (NA). (Courtesy of Jaypee Brothers published in Femtosecond Laser Assisted Corneal Graft Surgery. Editor. Jorge L. Alio)

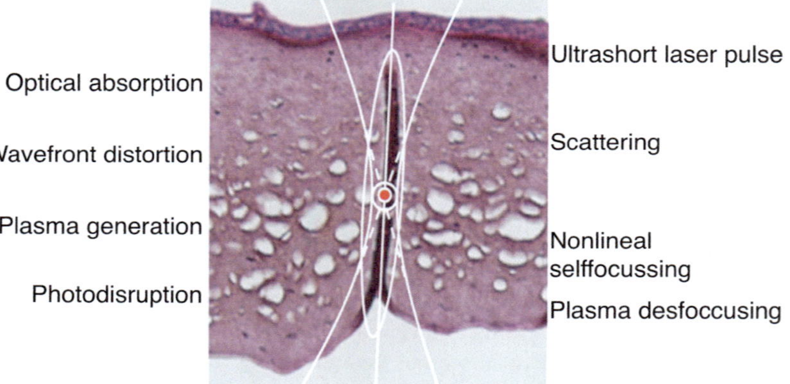

Fig. 8.2 Laser interaction with the corneal tissue. (Courtesy of Jaypee Brothers published in Femtosecond Laser Assisted Corneal Graft Surgery. Editor. Jorge L. Alio)

ble, the energy delivered will condense in a decreased spot size [2].

There are two ways that the systems use in order to increase the NA: one is to increase the lens diameter, and the other, is to decrease the focal distance (Figs. 8.1 and 8.2).

Thus, the optical breakdown process consists in focusing the photon energy beam at a specific depth into the corneal stroma, concentrating enough energy over the threshold level, which frees the chemical bonds, thus transforming the solid area of tissue covered by the photon beam into a vapor state, creating a cavitation gas bubble (Fig. 8.3).

Cavitation bubble size can vary depending on laser energy and occupies a greater space volume than previous solid material, which induces a lamellar tissue separation. The femtosecond laser can then be programmed to align several millions of cavitation bubbles to create larger tissue separation aiming to compose several patterns of corneal tissue dissection. Femtosecond laser incisions are composed of a great number of overlapped bubbles with a specific per-pulse energy. This bubble overlap will create micronsized tissue separation that, when placed all together, will be responsible for the tissue dissection.

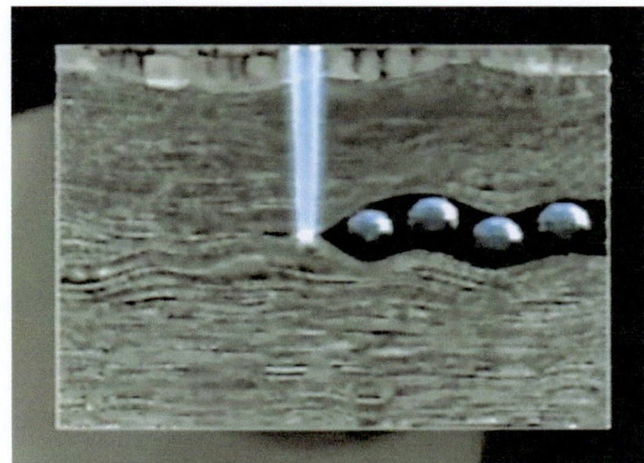

Fig. 8.3 Schematic view of cavitation bubble creation within the corneal stroma. (Courtesy of Jaypee Brothers published in Femtosecond Laser Assisted Corneal Graft Surgery. Editor. Jorge L. Alio)

This way, tissue dissection will depend on corneal tissue transparency, laser per-pulse energy, and spot separation. Selecting the appropriate balance when programming the femtosecond laser to obtain high-quality incisions is important. To optimize incision quality, femtosecond energy pulses must be precisely positioned within the corneal tissue to permit bubbles to interact [3]. That is why femtosecond lasers use a certain type of contact patient interface along with a suction ring that holds the eye in a fixed position during the entire treatment.

In summary, femtosecond laser dissection is based on a complex physical process, including the creation of millions of cavitation bubbles that, when placed together, can separate the tissue and therefore create a highly precise tissue dissection.

Femtosecond-Assisted Keratoplasty: Profiles, Outcomes, Advantages, and Disadvantages

Nowadays, there are many femtosecond laser platforms for dissecting corneal tissue. Each of these platforms uses independent algorithms and software to create its own incision architecture and dissection patterns in order to be used for performing keratoplasty procedures.

In the next section, we will describe the incision module used in the Intralase femtosecond laser platform, which is the one in which the authors have more experience.

Incision Design Software

IntraLase-enabled keratoplasty (IEK) module is the incision design software in the Intralase femtosecond laser system [4]. Corneal graft surgery includes several techniques, such as penetrating keratoplasty (PK), deep anterior lamellar keratoplasty (DALK), descemet's stripping automated keratopalsty (DSAEK), and others that can be used depending on the surgical technique. Tissue dissection design within the IEK module is based on the combination of different cutting elements that, when overlapping each other, creates complex graft incision in order to give more precise dissection when performing keraoplasty procedures (Fig. 8.4).

In the next section, we describe those cutting elements that are used by the IEK module:

Posterior Side Cut

Posterior side cut is a vertical cylindrical-shaped incision with a certain diameter that starts from the base of the cornea at its posterior depth and extends up to meet the lamellar incision at the anterior depth point.

This posterior cylinder can be warped into a conic section by adjusting the side cut angle parameter, as shown in the figure typically used in zigzag profiles.

Lamellar Cut

Lamellar cut is a planar incision parallel to the surface of the cornea that extends from the outer diameter to the inner diameter, where it is expected to meet the anterior side cut.

This forms a ring incision whenever the inner diameter is present and becomes a full lamellar incision with an inner diameter equal to zero.

Anterior Side Cut

Anterior side cut is the analog section to the posterior side cut, a cylindrical-shaped incision that

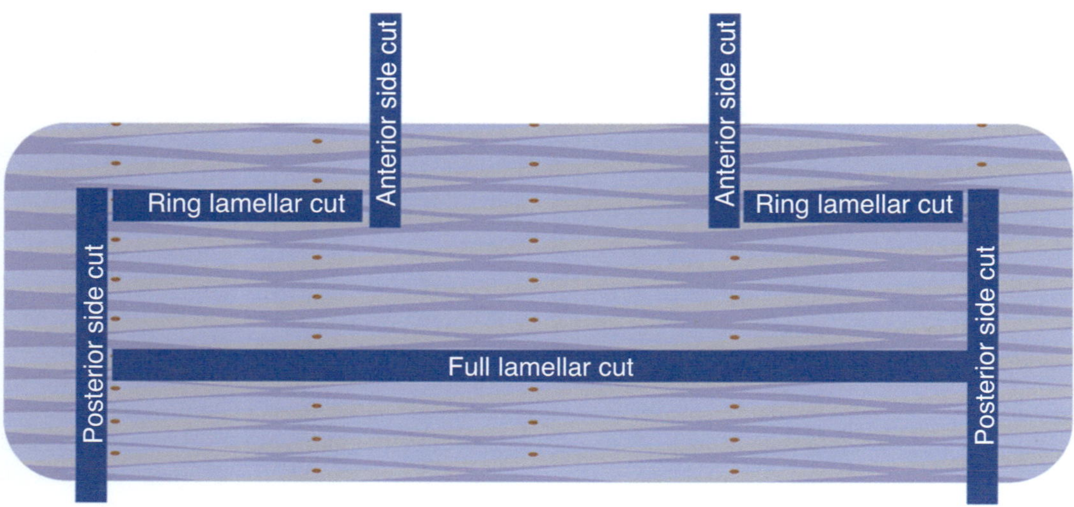

Fig. 8.4 Different incision uses in the Intralase-enabled keratoplasty module. (Courtesy of Jaypee Brothers published in Femtosecond Laser Assisted Corneal Graft Surgery. Editor. Jorge L. Alio)

extends from the posterior depth to the surface of the cornea. Anterior side cut is also used for astigmatic keratotomy to correct residual astigmatism following corneal graft surgery.

Keratoplasty Incision Profiles

Combining these previously described incisions produces a huge tool when designing the corneal graft, allowing the surgeon to perform tailored solutions to optimize clinical results in each case. Posterior side cut, anterior side cut, and lamellar cut can be combined in a limitless number of complex edge profile graft combinations [5] with a very high level of precision in dimensions and centration, which is not possible with other techniques [6].

Several profiles have been extensively tested, and it is up to the surgeon needs to adapt them to the specific case scenario in the field of corneal graft surgery.

In the following lines we will describe the tissue dissection profiles that the authors usually uses when performing corneal graft surgery.

Tophat-Based Profile

The most instructional and well-known shape might be the tophat profile, which is composed of three single steps imitating that typical hat morphology: (1) a wider posterior side cut; (2) ring lamellar cut;

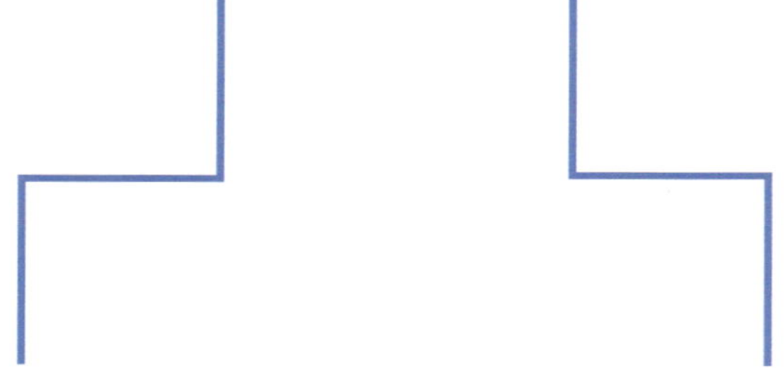

Fig. 8.5 Tophat profile

and (3) a narrower anterior side cut. This type of architecture maximizes the posterior tissue to the transplanted and may be better suited for posterior corneal disease such as endothelial defect, Fuchs dystrophy, or bullous keratopathy (Fig. 8.5).

Stepped incisions such as tophat were recognized long time ago to provide better wound healing responses [7, 8]. Thus, self-healing profile grafts such as tophat provide a superior tissue apposition, prevent wound leakage, and can potentially accelerate wound healing.

Original tophat incision uses 90° angulation as standard settings, and can evolve into different shapes by reducing the posterior side cut angle such as square-zag which reduces the deepest diameter which the objective of facilitating deep stromal dissection and direct visualization during deep lamellar surgery [9].

Mushroom-Based Profile

The inverted version of a tophat is known as a mushroom and is often used for anterior surface surgery, being composed of a narrower posterior side cut and a wider anterior side cut, both intersected by the ring lamellar cut (Fig. 8.6).

The broader anterior section maximizes the superficial stromal area of the transplanted, which makes it more suitable for anterior lamellar corneal graft surgeries such as those caused by corneal burns or scarring, keratoconus or marginal pellucid degeneration [10].

Zigzag-Based Profile

One of the more complex edge profile incisions is the zigzag graft, which compared to the squared angled profiles (tophat, mushroom), presents superior biomechanical, sealing, and coaptation properties [5]. Zigzag can be challenging in terms of graft configuration, which is the reason why it is considered a second step in the starting user learning curve. Zigzag profile is composed of a slanted anterior and posterior side cuts connected by the ring lamellar cut. It can be adapted to maximize either anterior or posterior surface, which makes it suitable to a wide variety of situations (Fig. 8.7).

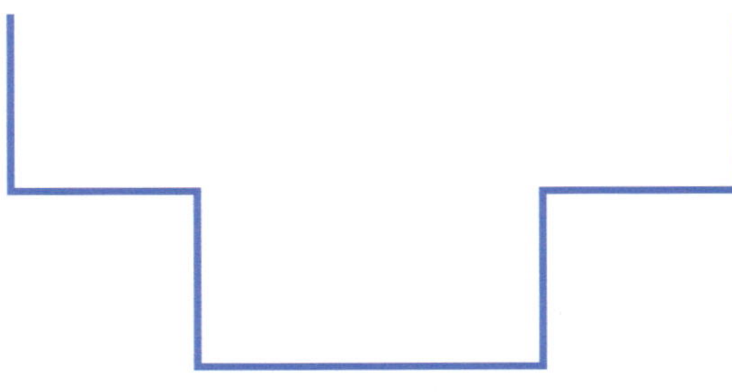

Fig. 8.6 Mushroom profile

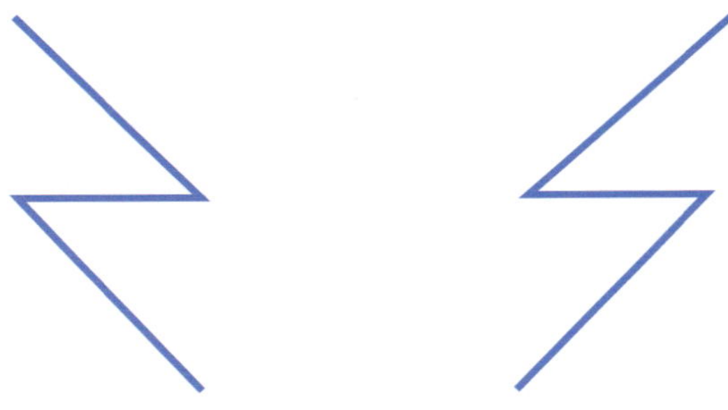

Fig. 8.7 Zigzag profile

Zigzag slanted incisions increase the wound apposition area, avoiding vertical cuts and offering superior biomechanical properties, as well as stronger wound healing and earlier postoperative period [5].

Femtosecond-Assisted Penetrating Keratoplasty Outcomes

For the conventional penetrating keratoplasty procedure (PKP) indications like advanced Fuchs' dystrophy, severe pseudophakic bullous keratopathy, extensive trauma, corneal amyloidosis, and severe keratoconus, the femtosecond laser-assisted PKP (FSPKP) has been done with high efficacy and safety outcomes [11–13]. There are some authors that have proposed that FSPKP could be superior to PKP in case of repeated PKP and global trauma with corneal laceration [14, 15]. Over the past decade, several researchers have demonstrated that FSPKP is highly safe and enables faster suture removal with better refractive and visual outcomes than conventional PKP [13, 16]. Farid et al. published a study comparing results between FSPKP (zigzag pattern) and PKP in relation with refractive and visual outcomes [17]. Significant differences in the average postoperative astigmatism between both groups after the first month ($P = 0.013$) and the third one ($P = 0.018$) were reported. By the third month, the average astigmatism was 3D in the zigzag FSPKP group and 4.46 D in the conventional PKP group. Additionally, significant differences in best spectacle-corrected visual acuity (BSCVA) were achieved after the first ($P = 0.0003$) and the third month ($P = 0.006$), with 81% of the FSPKP zigzag group versus 45% of the conventional group achieving BSCVA of more than or equal to 20/40 by the third month ($P = 0.03$). In the same line, Chamberlain et al. [13] and Gaster et al. [18] report similar results in terms of postoperative topographic astigmatism.

On the other hand, many authors have published the higher stability of the FS tophat dissection pattern with higher wound leakage pressure [12, 16, 18–21] together with other dissection patterns that could provide less risk of endothelial rejection and, therefore, less complications [22, 23].

Optical coherence tomography analysis reveals no wound dehiscence and excellent appearance of graft host tissue apposition and confirms that FSLAPKP offers benefits of rapid wound healing and predictable wound geometry [24].

Contrast sensitivity function, quality of vision, and higher orders aberration analysis were reported with favorable results using FSPKP [25, 26]. In terms of the ultrastructure and microbiological studies, it has been reported that femtosecond laser preserves the ultrastructure of the disrupted corneal collagen fibers [27], prompts an initial increase in keratocyte activation and dendritic cells that decrease over time [28], favors corneal reinnervation as early as 1 month postoperatively [28]. All these advantages support the safety and efficacy of femtosecond laser when performing penetrating keratoplasty procedures.

Additionally, from the standpoint of mechanical strength, femtosecond laser wound configurations are biomechanically more stable and create more surface area for healing than the conventional corneal trephination penetrating keratoplasty [29]. Additionally in theory less suture tension is required to achieve a water-tight wound in FSPK than in conventional PKP. In FSPK, laser cutting is precisely controlled, and the edge profile is predictable and controllable. Further, in FSPK, laser-produced radial alignment markers guarantee the accurate placement of cardinal sutures. With regard to manual trephination, tilting trephination and subsequent cuts with scissors could have an uneven or irregular edge profile [29].

Some authors believed that the application of the femtosecond laser might stimulate the proliferation of keratocytes, thereby enhancing the graft–bed connection and wound stability and enabling earlier suture removal [29].

In despite of the aforementioned results, in a recent review article that analyzed the published data since 2007 until 2019 comparing the outcomes of both FSPKP and conventional PKP, authors did not find significant results between both techniques [29]. Specifically, the authors reported that 12 months after the procedure, there was no significant difference in terms of visual acuity and rejection rate [29].

The few limitations of the femtosecond laser in PKP include difficulty to cut in peripheral corneal opacity and difficulty to achieve the desired planar cuts in eyes with significant anterior and posterior surface irregularities like descemetocele [30], which can be overcome by optimization and innovations of the femtosecond technology. Additionally, in order to perform FS laser dissection, you need to use the laser platform in both the patient and tissue donor that also needs to be dissected on an artificial anterior chamber which, in the end, increases the overall surgical time. Finally, femtosecond laser platforms are expensive to purchase and maintain, representing a high cost and not suitable for all ophthalmological departments.

Femtosecond-Assisted Deep Anterior Lamellar Keratoplasty Outcomes

There are several factors that make it difficult to carry out a proper analysis of the outcomes obtained after the deep anterior lamellar keratoplasty (DALK) procedure. The different methods of baring the Descemet membrane (DM), the technologies used to perform the dissection of the recipient and the donor tissue, and the different suturing techniques, among others, must be considered as factors that will impact the results obtained by different authors. Video 8.1 describes the different steps in both the donor's and the recipient's cornea during a FSDALK procedure.

Nevertheless, we can get an insight into the outcomes after the DALK procedure by analyzing the different scientific data that have been published over the last few years.

One of the main complications of keratoplasty procedures reported by several investigators is the significant amount of refractive error mainly related to the induction of irregular astigmatism [31]. A theoretical advantage of FSDALK in terms of postoperative corneal astigmatism is that the same configuration of the incisions should lead to a more regular corneal surface in, therefore, less astigmatism. Nevertheless, a recent review of femtosecond DALK (FSDALK) found that different authors report no significant difference in postoperative astigmatism when comparing FSDALK with conventional manual trephination procedure [32]. In the same line, our group report a few years ago showed no statistically significant difference in the corneal cylinder when comparing FSDALK with the conventional technique [33].

In terms of visual acuity, some authors that have analyzed the effect of the residual stromal bed after the DALK procedure have found that there is a correlation between the tissue remaining after baring the DM and the vision that the patient can achieve after the surgery [31]. Those authors have shown that the less the stromal residual tissue remains over the DM, the better the outcomes in terms of visual acuity after the procedure. Li et al. published, in 2016, a comparative study analyzing the outcomes of FSDALK and vacuum trephine and reported that FSDALK performed better in terms of visual acuity at 6 and 12 months postoperative [32]. It must be remarked that the FSDALK procedure did not involve Descemet membrane stromal baring in the abovementioned series [32]. On the other hand, other authors have not found significant differences when comparing FSDALK and conventional DALK in terms of visual outcomes. That is the case of Shehadeh–Mashor and col. that found better vision in the early postoperative in the FSDLAK group but not at 6 and 12 months after the surgery [32]. In the same way, Bleriot et al. did not observe significant differences in terms of vision when comparing FSDALK and manual technique [32]. Moreover, similar findings were reported by our research group when comparing the visual acuity of patients that underwent FSDALK and manual DALK [32].

Other advantages that FSDALK will theoretically have in terms of refraction, specifically in terms of managing postoperative astigmatism, is that the anterior aspect of the side cut from multiplanar incisions might be open in those areas where topographical astigmatism is higher and in this way reduce the corneal cylinder [32].

Regarding wound integrity, there are some reports which claim that FSDALK will perform better in terms of stronger incisions. Laboratory research demonstrates that FSDALK incision will support as high as 800 mmHg pressure which is significantly above physiological pressure [32]. The possibility of removing sutures early in the postoperative period is another factor that supports the fact that wound integrity will perform better than conventional PK [32].

In terms of graft rejection and endothelial cell loss, endothelial-mediated rejection is unlikely to occur in DALK procedures as this tissue is not being replaced during the surgery. In this line, a study comparing FSDALK and the manual technique found that FSDALK has a lower rejection rate when compared with the manual trepanation technique [32]. Another issue of interest is that the energy released by the FS laser when passing close to the Descemet membrane may reduce the endothelial cell population. Nevertheless, the few reports published in the scientific literature addressing this matter demonstrate no significant differences in the endothelial cell count when comparing the FSDALK with the conventional manual trepanation [32].

The few limitations of the femtosecond laser in DALK procedures include difficulty cutting in peripheral corneal opacity and achieving the desired planar cuts in eyes with significant anterior and posterior surface irregularities [11]. Additionally, in order to perform FS laser dissection, you need to use the laser platform in both the patient and tissue donor that also needs to be dissected on an artificial anterior chamber which, in the end, increases the overall surgical time. Finally, femtosecond laser platforms are expensive to purchase and maintain, representing a high cost and not suitable for all ophthalmological departments.

Healing Patterns in Femtosecond Laser-Assisted Keratoplasty

The cutting process in high pulse energy femto-laser is driven by mechanical forces applied by the expanding bubbles, which disrupt the tissue at a larger radius than the plasma created at the laser focus. While in low pulse energy femto-laser, spot separations smaller than the spot sizes are used for overlapping plasmas, which directly evaporate the tissue inside the plasma volume, effectively separating tissue without a need for secondary mechanical tearing [34].

Shtein et al. conducted in vivo confocal microscopic evaluation of corneal wound healing after femtosecond laser-assisted keratoplasty [28]. Their findings confirmed that keratocyte activation increased significantly following surgery in both the central ($p < 0.001$) and peripheral ($p = 0.002$) cornea. The level of activation then decreases over time, but it is unknown whether activated keratocytes can completely return to their original state or remain permanently biochemically altered. They also observed an increase in dendritic cells postoperatively which decreases after 6 months as wound healing progresses, and they found a significant association between the degree of keratocyte activation and dendritic cells.

They also observed accelerated nerve regeneration which may be an indicator of improved corneal healing after FLAK, as femtosecond laser allow shaped trephination with better wound apposition and less collateral damage when compared to potential crush injury from the mechanical trephine [28].

Early laboratory studies demonstrated that femtosecond laser-enabled keratoplasty using the tophat configuration provided better wound integrity compared with manual PKP [12, 20]. Laboratory experiments have shown an increased burst pressure indicating increased wound stability. This is difficult to test in human patients.

Earlier suture removal seems to support increased wound integrity [35].

The wound configurations in femtosecond-assisted DALK may combine the mechanical and wound healing advantages found for stepped corneal wounds in PKP with the advantages of lamellar surgery [35].

It also offers the advantages of better donor-recipient fit with increased surface area contact, which may accelerate wound healing and earlier suture removal [36].

Our group established a grading for the side cut corneal healing as observed and registered photographically by slit lamp photography with illumination at 45° light angle of incidence concerning the slit lamp observation optics placed orthogonal to the corneal vertex as observed by the first Purkinje reflex [33]. The grading of the scar was performed as follows: Grade 0 = transparent scar, Grade 1 = faint healing opacity, Grade 2 = evident healing opacity, Grade 3 = significant opacity with some cosmetic imbalance, and Grade 4 = highly significant opacity with very significant cosmetic imbalance (Table 8.1).

In a study made by our research group [33] for femtosecond laser-assisted mushroom configuration DALK, 52% of cases show healing pattern grade 3 or 4.

The reasons for the femtosecond-assisted DALK to show a more active wound healing leading to leucomatous wound could be either due to the larger area of contact between the donor and recipient tissues and/or to femtosecond laser-related biological activation of the corneal tissues, which should be related to the level of energy used for the creation of the side cut.

Another study compared Femtosecond-assisted DALK to mechanical DALK in 20 pediatric patients and concluded that femtosecond cuts could improve the success rate of big-bubble technique. By improving donor/recipient fit through femtosecond-created side cuts, the postoperative spherical equivalent is reduced, and healing is accelerated [10].

Table 8.1 Analysis of side cut corneal wound healing pattern

Grade 0 Transparent scar	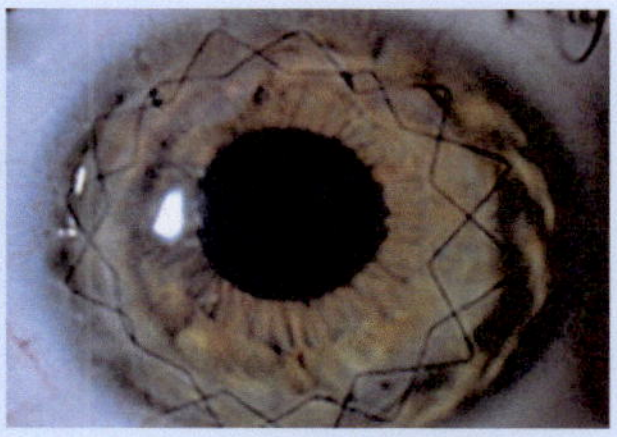
Grade 1 Faint healing opacity	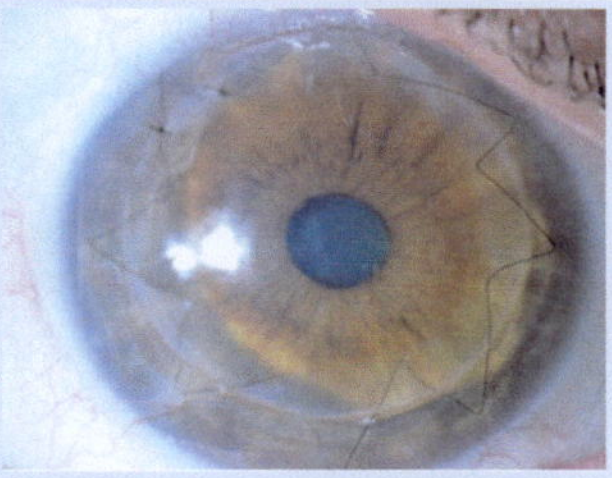
Grade 2 Evident healing opacity	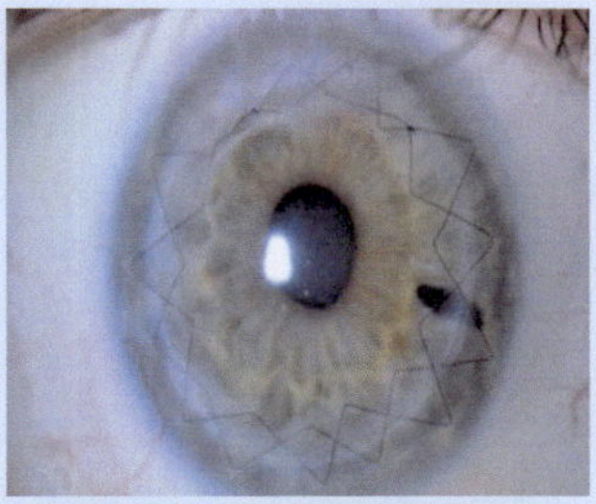
Grade 3 Significant opacity with some cosmetic imbalance	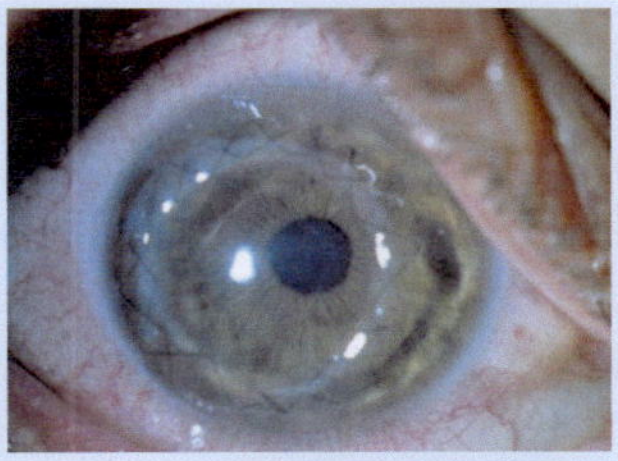
Grade 4 Highly significant opacity with very significant cosmetic imbalance	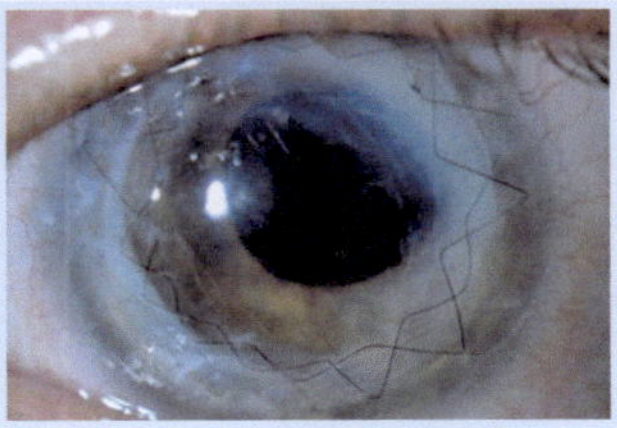

Future Perspective and Conclusions

In summary, we can say that femtosecond laser-assisted keratoplasty offers the surgeon the ability to create dissection patterns in the corneal tissue that are otherwise not possible with manual trephination. Many of the scientific work that has been published in the scientific literature demonstrates that femtosecond laser-assisted keratoplasty can provide multiplanar self-healing profiles, which provides better tissue coaptation and biomechanical stability helping to optimize clinical results, reduce the number of sutures and earlier suture removal compared to the mechanical procedure. Nevertheless, some of the review articles that have been recently published comparing FSPK and conventional PKP do not report a clear advantage of laser-assisted techniques. However, we must keep in mind that most of these studies have a limited methodology, so it would be necessary to carry out well-designed trials with a higher quality of scientific evidence in order to reach conclusive results.

The potential of femtosecond-assisted surgery to improve wound healing and vision recovery has been observed in numerous animal and clinical studies. As a result, more trials are underway to develop more desirable cutting shapes to enhance wound alignment and attachment for performing suture-less keratoplasty in the future. In addition, in the way that our understanding of the physical and mechanical forces involved in the process improves, we will be able to create custom shape dissections and increase biomechanical wound stability that, in the future, will allow us to perform early suture removal and decrease the amount of astigmatism related to keratoplasty procedures.

Take Home Notes

- Femtosecond laser keratoplasty procedure is highly accepted among corneal surgeons because it is highly reproducible and intuitive technology that provides and guarantees an excellent wound apposition. Today it is mostly used for PKP and DALK procedures, while the technique has limitations for its use in posterior lamellar techniques.
- Using femtosecond laser during keratoplasty procedures might have the potential advantages of earlier suture removal.

- Excellent wound apposition between the corneal donor and receptor can be achieved, providing more biomechanical and safer dissection patterns.
- Nowadays, there are no clear advantages in terms of outcomes of final corneal astigmatism or BCVA when comparing femtosecond-assisted keratoplasty and conventional keratoplasty procedures.
- Nowadays, several ongoing trials are on the way to develop more desirable cutting shapes in order to enhance wound alignment and attachment for performing suture-less keratoplasty in the future and to use femtosecond technology also for DSAEK.

References

1. Roach WP, Thompson ET. Selected papers on ultrashort laser pulse bioeffects. SPIE milestone series, vol. 174; 2002.
2. Slade S. Laser refractive cataract surgery, science, medicine and industry. Wayne: Bryn Mawr Communications LLC; 2012.
3. Binder PS, Sarayba M, Ignacio T, et al. Characterization of submicrojoule femtosecond laser corneal tissue dissection. J Cataract Refract Surg. 2008;34:146–52.
4. Ortiz JG, Alió JL. Femtosecond laser corneal graft applications with IntraLase technology. In: Alió JL, editor. Femtosecond laser assisted keratoplasty, vol. 3. p. 18; 30.
5. Farid M, Kim M, Steinert RF. Results of penetrating keratoplasty performed with a femtosecond laser zigzag incision initial report. Ophthalmology. 2007;114:2208–12.
6. Sarayba MA, Maguen E, Salz J, et al. Femtosecond laser keratome creation of partial thickness donor corneal buttons for lamellar keratoplasty. J Refract Surg. 2007;23:58–65.
7. Barraquer JI. Technique of penetrating keratoplasty. Am J Ophtalmol. 1950;33:6–17.
8. Busin M. A new lamellar wound configuration for penetrating keratoplasty surgery. Arch Ophthalmol. 2003;121:260–5.
9. Neuhann TF, Lege BB, Joergensen JS, et al. Femtosecond laser profiled penetrating Keratoplasty with the IntraLase FS60 IEK. Chicago: ASCRS; 2008.
10. Price FW, Price MO. Femtosecond laser shaped penetrating keratoplasty: one-year results utilizing a top-hat configuration. Am J Ophthalmol. 2008;145:210–4.
11. Alió JL, Soria F, Vega A, Abdou A. Femtosecond laser-assisted penetrating keratoplasty with IntraLase technology (use of the different technologies, surgical practical

pearls, outcomes). In: Alió JL, editor. Femtosecond laser assisted keratoplasty, vol. 8. p. 58; 74.

12. Steinert RF, Ignacio TS, Sarayba MA. "Top-hat"-shaped penetrating keratoplasty using the femtosecond laser. Am J Ophthalmol. 2007;143(4):689–91.

13. Chamberlain WD, Rush SW, Mathers WD, et al. Comparison of femtosecond laser-assisted keratoplasty versus conventional penetrating keratoplasty. Ophthalmology. 2011;118(3):486–91.

14. Rush SW, Fraunfelder FW, Mathers WD, et al. Femtosecond laser-assisted keratoplasty in failed penetrating keratoplasty and globe trauma. Cornea. 2011;30(12):1358–62.

15. Graef S, Maier P, Boehringer D, et al. Femtosecond laserassisted repeat keratoplasty: a case series. Cornea. 2011;30(6):687–91.

16. Bahar I, Kaiserman I, McAllum P, et al. Femtosecond laserassisted penetrating keratoplasty: stability evaluation of different wound configurations. Cornea. 2008;27(2):209–11.

17. Farid M, Steinert RF, Gaster RN, et al. Comparison of penetrating keratoplasty performed with a femtosecond laser zig-zag incision versus conventional blade trephination. Ophthalmology. 2009;116(9):1638–43.

18. Gaster RN, Dumitrascu O, Rabinowitz YS. Penetrating keratoplasty using femtosecond laser-enabled keratoplasty with zig-zag incisions versus a mechanical trephine in patients with keratoconus. Br J Ophthalmol. 2012;96(9):1195–9.

19. Ignacio TS, Nguyen TB, Chuck RS, et al. Top hat wound configuration for penetrating keratoplasty using the femtosecond laser: a laboratory model. Cornea. 2006;25(3):336–40.

20. Maier P, Böhringer D, Birnbaum F, et al. Improved wound stability of top-hat profiled femtosecond laser-assisted penetrating keratoplasty in vitro. Cornea. 2012;31(8):963–6.

21. Birnbaum F, Wiggermann A, Maier PC, et al. Clinical results of 123 femtosecond laser-assisted penetrating keratoplasties. Graefes Arch Clin Exp Ophthalmol. 2013;251(1):95–103.

22. Fung SS, Iovieno A, Shanmuganathan VA, et al. Femtosecond laser-assisted lock-and-key shaped penetrating keratoplasty. Br J Ophthalmol. 2012;96(1):136–7.

23. Gilmer W, McLeod SD, Jeng BH. Laboratory model of bursting pressures of femtosecond laser-assisted penetrating keratoplasty wounds using novel pattern designs. Br J Ophthalmol. 2012;96(9):1273–4.

24. Heur M, Tang M, Yiu S, et al. Investigation of femtosecond laser-enabled keratoplasty wound geometry using optical coherence tomography. Cornea. 2011;30(8):889–94.

25. Cheng YY, van den Berg TJ, Schouten JS, Pels E, Wijdh RJ, van Cleynenbreugel H, et al. Quality of vision after femtosecond laser-assisted descemet stripping endothelial keratoplasty and penetrating keratoplasty: a randomized, multicenter clinical trial. Am J Ophthalmol. 2011;152(4):556–66.

26. Chamberlain W, Omid N, Lin A, et al. Comparison of corneal surface higher-order aberrations after endothelial keratoplasty, femtosecond laser-assisted keratoplasty, and conventional penetrating keratoplasty. Cornea. 2012;31(1):6–13.

27. Nuzzo V, Aptel F, Savoldelli M, et al. Histologic and ultrastructural characterization of corneal femtosecond laser trephination. Cornea. 2009;28(8):908–13.

28. Shtein RM, Kelley KH, Musch DC, et al. In vivo confocal microscopic evaluation of corneal wound healing after femtosecond laser-assisted keratoplasty. Ophthalmic Surg Lasers Imaging. 2012;43(3):205–13.

29. Wen-yan P, Zhi-ming T, Xiu-fen L, Shi-you Z. Comparing the efficacy and safety of femtosecond laser-assisted vs conventional penetrating keratoplasty: a metaanalysis of comparative studies. Int Ophthalmol. 2021;41:2913–23.

30. Yoo SH, Hurmeric V. Femtosecond laser-assisted keratoplasty. Am J Ophthalmol. 2011;151(2):189–91.

31. Alió JL, Vega A, Soria F, Abdou A. Femtosecond laser-assisted anterior lamellar keratoplasty with IntraLase technology (use of the different technologies, surgical practical pearls, outcomes). In: Alió JL, editor. Femtosecond laser assisted keratoplasty, vol. 9. p. 78; 86.

32. Chamberlain WD. Femtosecond laser-assisted deep anterior lamellar keratoplasty. Curr Opin Ophthalmol. 2019;30:256–63.

33. Alio JL, Abdelghany AA, Barraquer R, et al. Femtosecond laser assisted deep anterior lamellar keratoplasty outcomes and healing patterns compared to manual technique. Biomed Res Int. 2015;2015:397891.

34. Latz C, Asshauer T, Rathjen C, Mirshahi A. Femtosecond-laser assisted surgery of the eye: overview and impact of the low-energy concept. Micromachines (Basel). 2021;12(2):122. https://doi.org/10.3390/mi12020122. PMID: 33498878; PMCID: PMC7912418.

35. Price FW Jr, Price MO, Grandin JC, Kwon R. Deep anterior lamellar keratoplasty with femtosecond-laser zigzag incisions. J Cataract Refract Surg. 2009;35(5):804–8. https://doi.org/10.1016/j.jcrs.2009.01.011. Erratum in: J Cataract Refract Surg. 2009 Jul;35(7):1325. PMID: 19393877.

36. Jonas JB, Vossmerbaeumer U. Femtosecond laser penetrating keratoplasty with conical incisions and positional spikes. J Refract Surg. 2004;20(4):397. https://doi.org/10.3928/1081-597X-20040701-15. PMID: 15307404.

Femtosecond Laser-Assisted Tuck-In Penetrating Keratoplasty

9

Jorge L. Alió del Barrio, Olena Al-Shymali, and Jorge L. Alió

Key Points

- Tuck-in lamellar keratoplasty provides structural support to those extremely weakened corneas with diffuse and severe thinning up to the periphery, such as keratoglobus.
- However, in patients where hydrops or endothelial damage is present, such tuck-in lamellar keratoplasty technique is not possible.
- Femtosecond laser-assisted tuck-in PKP is a 1-step technique that allows us to approach cases where extreme peripheral thinning and corneal endothelial damage are present.

Supplementary Information The online version contains supplementary material available at https://doi.org/10.1007/978-3-031-32408-6_9.

J. L. A. del Barrio · J. L. Alió (✉)
Vissum Miranza, Miguel Hernández University, Alicante, Spain
e-mail: jlalio@vissum.com

O. Al-Shymali
Cornea, Cataract and Refractive Surgery Unit, Vissum (Miranza Group), Alicante, Spain

Introduction

Keratoglobus (KTG) is a rare noninflammatory corneoscleral ectasia [1]. It is a bilateral disorder characterized by generalized corneal thinning especially peripherally [2], that results in the globular protrusion of the cornea. Previously, it was thought-out equivalent to congenital glaucoma and megalocornea until it was described by Verrey as an individual clinical entity in 1947 [3]. Afterward, this was backed by Cavara in 1950 [4].

Although the exact etiology of KTG remains unknown, it has been described in both acquired and congenital forms [1]. The former has been associated with vernal keratoconjunctivitis and chronic marginal blepharitis due to frequent eye rubbing, dysthyroid eye disease, and idiopathic orbital inflammation [5, 6]. Congenital KTG has been linked to Leber's congenital amaurosis, blue sclera syndrome, osteogenesis imperfecta, and connective tissue disorders like Ehlers–Danlons syndrome, type IV in particular, Marfan syndrome and Rubinstein–Tayabi syndrome [1, 7–9].

The extreme corneal thinning and protrusion in patients with KTG lead to visual deterioration due to extreme myopia, irregular astigmatism, and scaring [10]. The condition can be complicated by acute hydrops causing pain [11] or by corneal perforations occurring spontaneously or following minimal trauma [1, 12].

Since KTG is a rare ectasia, diverse algorithms were proposed. Still, no agreement on a standard method was reached. Using conservative methods such as spectacles or contact lenses to correct myopia, and astigmatism is not always possible, especially in children, and sometimes are ineffective with a corneal perforation risk owing to trauma. The surgical approach consists of various lamellar keratoplasty and epikeratoplasty techniques that provide structural support to these extremely weakened corneas. However, in patients where hydrops or endothelial damage are present, a two-step procedure with a second central corneal penetrating graft will be necessary, which means two corneoscleral buttons per eye are required [2, 10]. Although conventional penetrating keratoplasty (PKP) is the gold-standard procedure for many corneal diseases, it is impracticable in KTG because of peripheral thinning. Therefore, large limbus to limbus grafts is used, which may cause limbal stem cells and angle structure disruptions as well as increase the risk of neovascularization and graft rejection [1, 13].

Recently our team proposed a 1-step technique for KTG cases with endothelial damage, femtosecond laser-assisted tuck-in PKP, where both extreme peripheral thinning and corneal endothelial damage exists [14]. On account of the thinning disorders in KTG, the aim of our technique is to insure tectonic support and optimal thickness to the extremely subtle peripheral cornea, in addition to replacing the damaged central part of the cornea.

Indications

Femtosecond laser-assisted tuck-in PKP is indicated in patients with KTG that have both peripheral corneal thinning and endothelial damage due to hydrops or Descemet membrane tears. In this way, we enhance the thickness of the peripheral recipient stroma and simultaneously exchange the central damaged part of the KG cornea by a full-thickness penetrating corneal graft.

Surgical Technique

Preoperative Considerations

An explicit examination of the cornea in a KTG patient should be done under the slit lamp. Moreover, a detailed pachymetric map must be made, especially of the corneal periphery. For this technique, we advise a minimum thickness of 300 microns peripherally in order to have a higher chance of succeeding during this technically demanding surgery. If no Descemet membrane tears and endothelial damage are present, the surgeon may opt for conventional lamellar keratoplasty or a tuck-in lamellar keratoplasy technique [2, 15, 16]. However, when in addition to the peripheral thinning, we have a damaged Descemet membrane or endothelium, we have two options: the 2-step procedure [10] of a lamellar epikeratoplasty followed by a central corneal penetrating graft which takes a longer time and needs two corneoscleral buttons per eye, or we go for our described femtosecond laser-assisted tuck-in PKP [14], a 1-step surgery that requires only one corneoscleral button per eye.

Technique

Donor Cornea Preparation

In an artificial anterior chamber and assisted by the iFS femtosecond laser (AMO Inc, Irvine, CA), an anterior side cut of 8.5 mm in diameter and 310 microns deep is performed, continued by a 300 µm deep ring lamellar cut up to 9.5 mm of diameter (8.4–9.5 mm). Then, following the ring lamellar dissection plane through the anterior side cut, a crescent blade is used to complete the lamellar dissection until the limbal area. Once this maneuver is finished, a final full-thickness trephination with an 11 mm trephine from the endothelial side is done. Eventually, a donor button that is 11 mm in total diameter with an 8.5 mm central full-thickness area and a 1.25 mm partial-thickness circumferential peripheral edge is obtained (Fig. 9.1a).

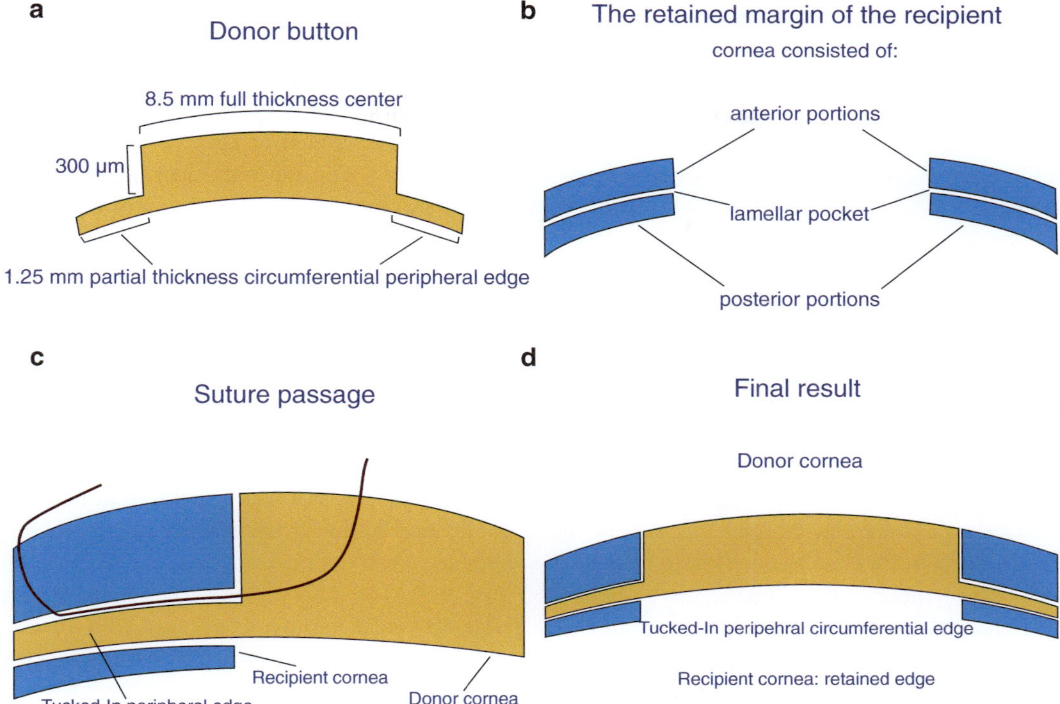

Fig. 9.1 Femtosecond laser-assisted Tuck-in PKP surgical diagram: (**a**) final appearance of the donor cornea; (**b**) final appearance of the peripheral recipient stromal pocket; (**c**) the thread passes through the central 8.5 mm portion of the donor cornea with partial-thickness bite and the anterior portion of the recipient's stromal pocket; (**d**) the peripheral circumferential donor rim remains tucked into the recipient's stromal pocket, enhancing the peripheral corneal thickness

Recipient Cornea Preparation

Once the preparation of the donor cornea is finished, the recipient cornea is prepared using the same pattern as the femtosecond laser, performing an anterior side cut of 8.5 mm in diameter at 160 microns depth and a ring lamellar cut depth of 150 μm with 9.5 mm in diameter (recipient side cut depth should be estimated as half of the mean preoperative peripheral recipient corneal thickness). Similarly to the donor cornea, a crescent blade is used to complete the peripheral lamellar dissection following the previously dissected ring lamellar plane, creating a lamellar pocket. The dissection is aimed at the most corneal periphery by reaching the limbus. After the injection of viscoelastic into the anterior chamber (AC) through a paracentesis, the AC is entered using a 15-degree sharp blade following the contour of the 8.5 mm diameter anterior side cut. Further, the central recipient cornea is excised with the assistance of Vannas scissors. Subsequently, a recipient peripheral stromal pocket made of an anterior and posterior portion is obtained (Fig. 9.1b).

Donor-Recipient Apposition

The donor cornea is then sutured using 10/0 nylon interrupted sutures. The thread is passed through the donor 8.5 mm full-thickness button in a partial-thickness manner (up to the level where the peripheral rim starts) and the anterior portion of the recipient stromal pocket as close as it could be to the limbus (Fig. 9.1c). Similarly, all 16 sutures are placed on the whole cornea. Then, in order to make sure that the peripheral donor edge remains within the peripheral recipient stromal pocket, this peripheral donor edge is unfolded and tucked in the stromal recipient pocket with the assistance of a blunt spatula (Fig. 9.1d) (Video 9.1).

Postoperative Management

Postoperative care does not differ from the one used for a standard PKP surgery: topical antibiotic four times a day for 1 week and topical steroids every 2 h for 1 week and four times a day thereafter.

Complications

The experience with this technique is still limited, and the only postoperative complications that we have observed were an Urrets-Zavalia syndrome due to retained viscoelastic and suture-related infectious keratitis. However, intra and postoperative potential complications with this Femto Tuck-In PKP technique should be equivalent to those described for standard PKP. Especially important for this technique is the fact of performing an adequate preoperative plan for the femtosecond laser dissection planes (diameters and depths) in relation to the peripheral preoperative pachymetry in order to avoid too superficial or too deep surgical planes with subsequent risk of anterior or posterior perfora-tion. Probably, the most challenging step is the manual expansion of the lamellar plane with the crescent blade on the recipient cornea, along with the creation of the lamellar recipient pocket. In this step, it is critical to keep the correct depth, but as we work inside a thin peripheral cornea, inadvertent tears of the anterior lip of the cornea may occur, requiring extra suturing to reconstruct the tear and ensure the correct positioning of the donor cornea.

Outcomes

As already discussed, published evidence with this technique is still short, and it is limited to a publication of our group describing the outcome obtained from both eyes of the same KG patient (Fig. 9.2) [14]. This patient experienced a great bilateral visual improvement (corrected distance vision of 20/50 in both eyes), with a residual refractive cylinder of five diopters. Corneal topography showed high but regular astigmatism, and the anterior segment optical coherence tomography (OCT) adequately restored the peripheral corneal thickness (Fig. 9.3).

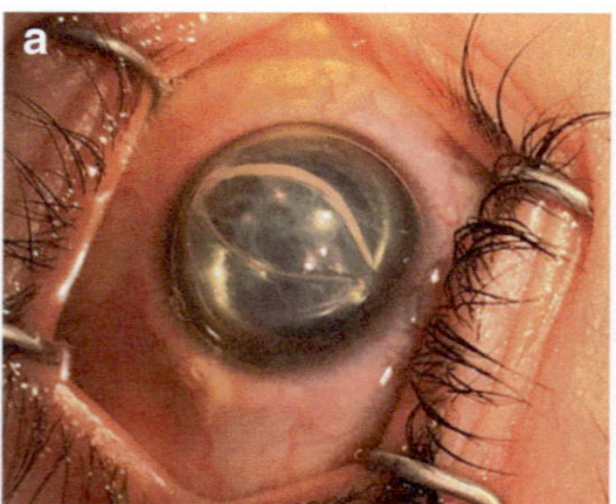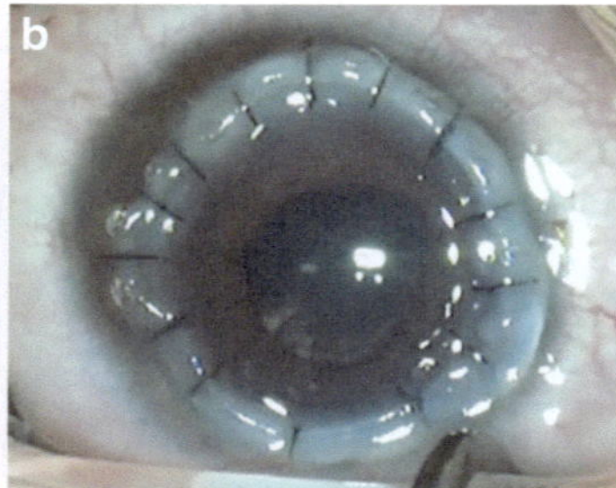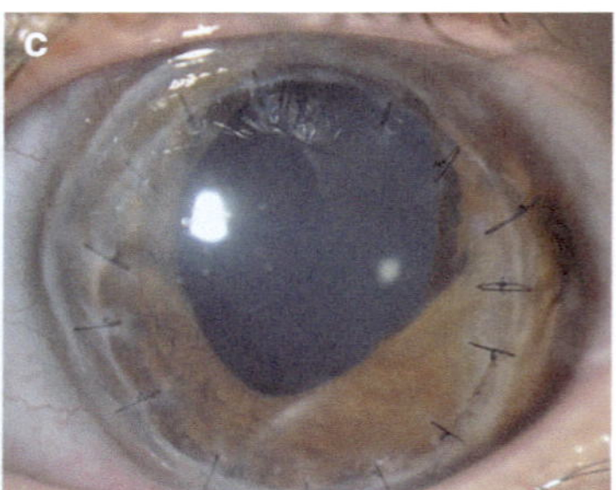

Fig. 9.2 Preoperative external anterior segment photograph after intracameral air injection of a patient with keratoglobus and chronic hydrops in relation to a severe tear of the corneal endothelium (**a**); Intraoperative photograph immediately after completing the Tuck-in PKP (**b**); Slit lamp postoperative anterior segment picture 6 months after the transplant (**c**). Observe the complete transparency recovery and the peripheral partial-thickness donor rim tucked into the host cornea

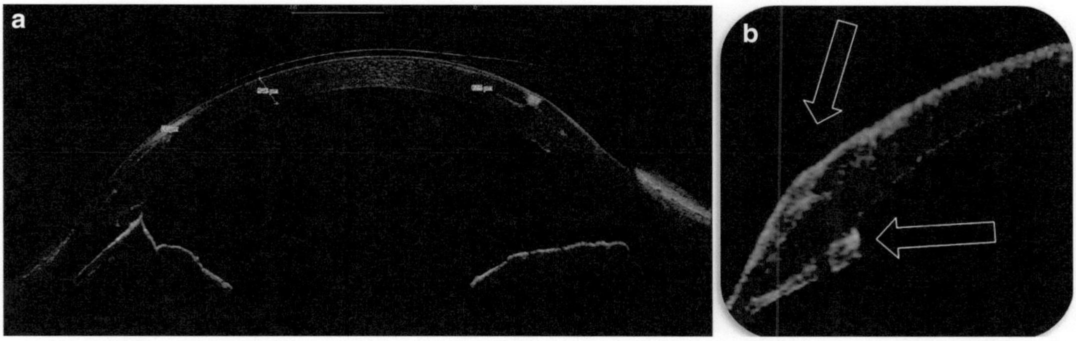

Fig. 9.3 Anterior segment optical coherence tomography (OCT) pictures (**a**, **b**). The peripheral donor partial-thickness rim is tucked into the host stromal pocket ((**b**), white arrows). In those areas not covered by the peripheral donor rim, the thickness remains low (**a**)

Conclusions

When severe keratoglobus associates with previous corneal hydrops and severe endothelial damage, routine PKP with an almost limbus to limbus diameter graft associates with a poor visual outcome due to a high risk of rejection and secondary glaucoma [13]. Such cases were previously managed with a tuck-in or epikeratoplasty lamellar technique to first reinforce the peripheral corneal thickness, followed by a PKP several months later for visual rehabilitation [10]. However, this approach requires two surgical procedures and the use of two donor corneas. On the other hand, femtosecond laser-assisted tuck-in PKP offers an alternative option to rehabilitate these patients but with a single surgical procedure and only one donor cornea.

Tuck-in PKP in keratoglobus eyes with previous corneal hydrops combines the advantages of PKP (the central full-thickness graft rehabilitates the stroma and the endothelium) and lamellar tuck-in techniques (the peripheral partial-thickness rim tucked into the intrastromal host pocket integrates perfectly and provides tectonic support to the recipient tissue). Simultaneously, damage to the recipient's limbal stem cells is avoided as the limbal region is not manipulated. The addition of the femtosecond laser to assist the host and donor cornea partial-thickness trephinations is not essential, but it reduces the risk of a full-thickness cut that may happen with manual suction trephines in these extremely thin corneas,

and it is more accurate than a free-hand manual technique with surgical blades. Also, the short ring lamellar cut assists the depth of the peripheral dissection that is performed up to the limbal area.

Take Home Notes
- Femtosecond laser-assisted tuck-in PKP ensures tectonic support and optimal thickness to the thinned peripheral cornea, in addition to replace the damaged endothelium.
- The addition of the femtosecond laser to assist the host and donor cornea partial-thickness trephinations is not essential, but it reduces the risk of a full-thickness cut that may happen with manual suction trephines in these extremely thin corneas, and it is more accurate than a free-hand manual technique with surgical blades.

Conflict of Interest None of the authors have any conflict of interest to disclose.

References

1. Wallang B, Das S. Keratoglobus. Eye. 2013;27:1004–12.
2. Javadi MA, Kanavi MR, Ahmadi M, Yazdani S. Outcomes of epikeratoplasty for advanced keratoglobus. Cornea. 2007;26:154–7.
3. Verrey F. Keratoglobe aigu. Ophthalmologica. 1947;114:284–8.

4. Cavara V. Keratoglobus and keratoconus. A contribution to the nosological interpretation of keratoglobus. Br J Ophthalmol. 1950;34(10):621–6.
5. Cameron J, Al-Rajhi A, Badr I. Corneal ectasia in vernal keratoconjunctivitis. Ophthalmology. 1989;96:1615–23.
6. Jacobs D, Green W, Maumenee A. Acquired keratoglobus. Am J Ophthalmol. 1974;77:393–9.
7. Koenekoop R. An overview of Leber congenital amaurosis: a model to understand human retinal development. Surv Ophthalmol. 2004;49:379–98.
8. Cameron J. Corneal abnormalities in Ehlers-Danlos syndrome type VI. Cornea. 1993;12:54–9.
9. Nelson M, Talbot J. Keratoglobus in Rubinstein Taybi syndrome. Br J Ophthalmol. 1989;73:385–7.
10. Jones DH, Kirkness CM. A new surgical technique for keratoglobus-tectonic lamellar keratoplasty followed by secondary penetrating keratoplasty. Cornea. 2001;20:885–7.
11. Grewal S, Laibson P, Cohen E, Rapuano C. Acute hydrops in the corneal ectasias: associated factors and outcomes. Trans Am Ophthalmol Soc. 1999;97:187–98.
12. Baillif S, Garweg J, Grange J, Burillon C, Kodjikian L. Keratoglobus: review of the literature. J Fr Ophthalmol. 2005;28:1145–9.
13. Cowden J, Copeland R, Schneider M. Large diameter therapeutic penetrating keratoplasties. Refract Corneal Surg. 1989;5:244–8.
14. Alió Del Barrio J, Al-Shymali O, Alió J. Femtosecond laser-assisted tuck-in penetrating keratoplasty for advanced keratoglobus with endothelial damage. Cornea. 2017;36(9):1145–9.
15. Kaushal S, Jhanji V, Sharma N, Tandon R, Titiyal JS, Vajpayee RB. " Tuck In" lamellar keratoplasty (TILK) for corneal ectasias involving corneal periphery. Br J Ophthalmol. 2008;92:286–90.
16. Vajpayee RB, Bhartiya P, Sharma N. Central lamellar keratoplasty with peripheral intralamellar tuck: a new surgical technique for keratoglobus. Cornea. 2002;21:657–60.

Rescuing Failed Penetrating Keratoplasty Grafts

Jorge L. Alió del Barrio, Scott Robbie, Marcus Ang, Andrea Montesel, and Jorge L. Alió

Key Points

- Corneal transplantation is the world's most frequent type of human tissue graft but still remains a critical shortage of corneal graft tissue.
- The global shortage of corneal tissue is likely to grow as the cumulative number of transplanted patients increases over time, making corneal graft failure one of the most common indications for corneal transplantation today.
- PK is one of the commonest forms of corneal transplantation and remains the procedure of choice for selected indications.
- Options for managing a failed PK depend on the clinical context, the failure mechanism, and any comorbidity.

J. L. A. del Barrio (✉) · J. L. Alió
Vissum Miranza, Miguel Hernández University, Alicante, Spain
e-mail: jlalio@vissum.com

S. Robbie
Cornea Unit, Guy's and St Thomas' Hospital, London, UK
e-mail: s.robbie@ucl.ac.uk

M. Ang
Singapore Eye Research Institute, Singapore National Eye Centre, Singapore, Singapore

Department of Ophthalmology and Visual Science, Duke-NUS Graduate Medical School, Singapore, Singapore
e-mail: Marcus.Ang@Singhealth.com.sg

Introduction

Corneal transplantation is the world's most frequent type of human tissue graft, with more than 180,000 corneal grafts performed every year worldwide [1]. Corneal transplantation aims to restore visual function when it is severely and irreversibly impaired by end-stage corneal disease after conservative surgical or medical treatment options have failed. Corneal transplantation techniques have evolved considerably over the last two decades, specifically with regard to lamellar techniques and the optimization and standardization of endothelial keratoplasty techniques in particular; however, there remains a critical shortage of corneal graft tissue, and it has been estimated that there is only 1 corneal donor available for every 70 needed [1]. The global shortage of corneal tissue is likely to grow as the cumulative number of transplanted patients increases over time, making corneal graft failure

A. Montesel
Cornea, Cataract and Refractive Surgery Unit, Vissum (Miranza Group), Alicante, Spain

Jules Gonin Eye Hospital, University of Lausanne, Lausanne, Switzerland

one of the most common indications for corneal transplantation today [2].

Corneal graft failure is defined as the failure of the corneal transplant to adequately restore the visual function of the patient in the absence of concomitant pathology and is typically classified into [2]:

- Primary graft failure (PGF) is defined as the presence of a diffusely edematous corneal graft on the first postoperative day that fails to clear at any time postoperatively, with a lack of an identifiable cause of corneal graft failure within three months from the transplant [2]. It is the result of inadequate donor endothelial cell function, inadequate tissue preservation, or surgical trauma from harvesting or the procedure.
- Secondary graft failure (SGF) involves the deterioration of vision as a consequence of the loss of corneal transparency in a previously functional corneal graft, usually due to the presence of diffuse and irreversible corneal edema in a previously functional transplant as a consequence of endothelial failure from immunological (rejection) or nonimmunological (chronic late endothelial loss) events. It may also refer to cases of transparency loss in the absence of endothelial failure, such as corneal stromal scarring (herpetic disease, trauma) or surface opacification (limbal stem cell deficiency). The latter causes will not be discussed in the current review.
- Morphological graft failure refers to clear grafts without transparency loss but conferring poor visual function as a result of severe irregular astigmatism (such as severe recurrent ectasia). It may be considered a subtype of SGF.

Despite the rise of lamellar keratoplasty techniques in the last two decades, PK remains one of the commonest forms of corneal transplantation and remains the procedure of choice for selected indications [3]. Options for the management of a failed PK depend on the clinical context, the mechanism of failure, and any comorbidity.

The first question one should pose when considering a repeat PK is, as always, whether surgery is indicated at all. Even for an eye that is blind—either from corneal or noncorneal pathology—corneal transplantation may still provide significant benefits in terms of making the eye more comfortable and reducing the risk of infection (although a conjunctival flap may be a more suitable alternative in this situation while not necessarily precluding subsequent corneal transplantation) [4]. Immunological graft failure may usually be diagnosed with confidence 2–3 months after the onset of treatment for endothelial rejection. Management for any acute (or suspected) endothelial rejection should, therefore, have already proceeded according to local practice patterns prior to considering further options, with topical corticosteroids the mainstay and the use of subconjunctival steroids, systemic steroids (in the form of either oral prednisone or pulsed intravenous methylprednisolone) and other immunosuppressive therapy instituted as appropriate. Rates of reversibility of severe endothelial rejection are between 51% and 64% [5–8].

The second question to consider is whether an endothelial keratoplasty might be performed. This confers a number of advantages discussed below and should not be discounted, even in the context of a chronically decompensated PK, because of the capacity for remodeling of any stromal opacification that might take a year or more [9]. Third, consideration should be given to the surgical aim and whether the existing graft, at its best, ever provided the patient with useful vision. For example, if the graft profile was excellent (low/moderate and regular corneal astigmatism), affording the patient a high level of unaided, spectacle-corrected, or contact lens-corrected visual acuity prior to failure, then every effort should be made to maintain this with endothelial keratoplasty. At the other extreme, if the profile of the graft was highly irregular even before failure, and the patient had been unable to tolerate a contact lens to correct for this, then it may be more advantageous to attempt a redo PK and improve on the existing levels of astigmatism.

PK Graft Failure: Incidence and Risk Factors

The survival rate for PK has been reported recently to be between 52% and 98.8% at 10-year follow-ups [3, 10–15]. This extended range derives from highly variable methods of data collection and reporting by investigators from different parts of the world [3, 16]. Furthermore, datasets published before the advent of endothelial keratoplasty likely provide a more comprehensive overview of the risks and benefits of repeat PK. PK is now less commonly performed for low-risk indications such as keratoconus or Fuchs dystrophy, where lamellar techniques are now generally regarded as the gold standard. PK is increasingly being reverted to in more complex cases where the technical difficulty inherent to lamellar techniques preclude their success [17]. Outcomes with PK are strongly related to the primary diagnosis—the indication for transplantation being the strongest predictor of survival [18]. Transplantation performed for keratoconus and stromal dystrophies have a better prognosis than grafts performed for endothelial diseases, bullous keratopathy, and postinfective corneal scars, for example [15, 17, 19]. Moreover, when a PK is performed for therapeutic and tectonic indications, as opposed to optical rehabilitation, the prognosis is even poorer [13, 20]. Other well-established risk factors for PK failure include a history of previous failed PK, the presence of active ocular inflammation (including surface inflammation), corneal neovascularization, other ocular comorbidities (such as herpetic eye diseases or glaucoma), aphakia, larger graft diameter, and the undertaking of combined surgical procedures [15, 18, 21–25].

Repeat PK

As a consequence of the recent introduction of posterior lamellar grafts, repeat PK remains the only surgical option for PK grafts that have failed and where the functional potential of the existing transplant has been fundamentally compromised

(e.g., where there is severe stromal opacification in addition to endothelial dysfunction). While there has been a progressive reduction in the volumes of primary PKs undertaken, the number of PKs constituting regrafts has remained relatively stable in recent years, accounting for 11.3–19.0% of the total PKs performed in the US from 2005 to 2019 [26, 27]. Mattahei and coworkers, in a systematic review of the global indications for PK surgery, found that between 1980 and 2014, PK regrafts represented 9.3–18.8% of the total number of PK performed in developed countries [16].

Preoperative medical management and planning are fundamental to success. Subsequent PKs usually carry all the risks of the first transplant plus the increased risk of allograft rejection, as well as cumulative comorbidities such as glaucoma [22, 28]. Consequently, every effort should be made to optimize the condition of the ocular surface, control intraocular pressure, address inflammation (including systemic inflammatory diseases), and manage other pathologies that might impact the risk of rejection such as corneal neovascularization and herpetic eye disease [22, 29]. Preoperative imaging, including anterior segment optical coherence tomography, may be helpful in anticipating and planning for additional procedures that may be indicated more frequently with repeat transplantation, including synechiolysis, iridectomy, and pupilloplasty [30]. For grafts at high risk of rejection—usually defined as one where there are two or more quadrants of neovascularization or where previous rejection has occurred—there is some, albeit limited, evidence to support the use of both pre- and postoperative systemic immunosuppression [31]. Management varies widely, but presurgical systemic corticosteroid treatment improves corneal transplant survival in murine models and courses of pre- and postoperative oral prednisone (1 mg/ kg) or intravenous methylprednisolone are often prescribed in this context, usually in combination with topical steroid treatment and, less commonly, steroid-sparing agents such as mycophenolate mofetil, cyclosporin A, tacrolimus, sirolimus, and topical cyclosporin [6, 31–33]. A significant proportion of surgeons in one study prescribe topical steroids for use indefinitely in high-risk cases and oral acyclovir for a median of 6 months in those cases involving *Herpes simplex* keratopathy [33]. There is moderate evidence for the benefit of mycophenolate mofetil on corneal transplant survival, but evidence for the effectiveness of other noncorticosteroid immunosuppressive agents is less conclusive [31, 34, 35]. The case for human leukocyte antigen (HLA) matching of tissue to the recipient has yet to be demonstrated in studies determining whether this results in a reduction in the risk of allograft rejection compared with random tissue allocation; equally, there some evidence to suggest a role for the indirect presentation of minor histocompatibility antigens (such as male H-Y antigen) in modulating the risk of corneal transplant rejection and graft survival, but this has yet to inform practice widely, and the effect may not be significant in high-risk cases [36, 37].

Given the risks of allograft rejection in eyes that have undergone multiple PKs, these may ultimately be better candidates for a keratoprosthesis, such as the Boston type 2 keratoprosthesis (BKPro), if the ocular surface is not compromised by dryness or a lack of blinking [28]. Refinements to the device itself and the management of eyes implanted with it have led to an expansion of the indications for the BKPro in recent years. There is some evidence to support the use of the BKPro earlier in the pathway of eyes at risk of further failed PKs, with one study demonstrating that the likelihood of maintaining 20/200 or better vision at 2 years and a clear graft at 5 years was significantly higher with the BKPro than PK in eyes with a previously failed PK (without a higher risk of postoperative glaucoma) [38–40].

Surgical Considerations

Basic surgical principles apply when undertaking a repeat PK. Particular care in surgical planning should be undertaken when the original transplant was a therapeutic keratoplasty for microbial keratitis, because disruption of the anterior segment anatomy, eccentrically-sited transplants, and

comorbidities such as glaucoma and cataract are more common in such cases [41, 42]. With regard to host trephination, consideration should be given to the indications for the transplant and the reasons for failure. The capacity to heal varies considerably between patients and eyes, and this is further affected by the duration of any steroid treatment and even whether the wound interface is that of a primary PK or a regraft, with evidence for a stronger wound-healing response in the latter [43]. It might be assumed, at the point where one might consider suture removal (usually ≥1 year after surgery), that the graft-host interface is sufficiently healed as to make re-trephination a more obvious choice but, in fact, the strength of the graft-host interface is never much more than that afforded by the endothelium and epithelium—this is what makes PKs particularly vulnerable to traumatic injury and, while most traumatic wound dehiscence occurs within 18–24 months of transplantation, this can occur even decades after the surgery [44–46]. Consequently, most PKs may be replaced by simply accessing the graft-host junction, peeling out the original graft, and suturing in a transplant of the same diameter [46, 47]. The appearance on slit lamp examination preoperatively of vessels and stromal opacification at the graft-host interface may give some indication as to the degree of healing that has already taken place and, if significant, a little more resistance might be expected with this approach, but remains the favored option in most cases.

As a general rule, the transplant should be as "large as possible and as small as necessary"—that is to say, a balance should be struck, in terms of the optical advantages conferred by a larger graft and the reduced risks of allograft rejection associated with smaller diameter transplants [17, 18]. While peeling out the original donor is relatively easily performed, repeat PK does afford the opportunity to excise the old transplant together with a rim of host cornea by performing a slightly larger trephination—if this can be accomplished while maintaining sufficient clearance from the limbus, ideally at least 1.5 mm. This may be preferred if decentration, high levels of astigmatism, or irregularity have been a problem with the original transplant. Otherwise, greater weight should be afforded to the risks of allograft rejection in the context of a repeat PK [28]. A "peephole" transplant, sited within a larger diameter, failed transplant, may offer considerable functional benefit while minimizing the risks of further failure, albeit with a flatter profile and higher levels of irregular astigmatism [48]. Conversely, a graft that has failed due to infection or a corneal melting disorder may require excision of diseased or thinned tissue far outside of the existing transplant, sometimes up to the limbus—with the caveat that it is almost always worth considering a tectonic anterior lamellar keratoplasty in an acute setting rather than a penetrating keratoplasty [20, 49]. Where a large diameter keratoplasty, such as a total corneal transplant, is indicated, every effort should be made to ensure that the underlying cause has been managed appropriately, that inflammation has settled, and that the host limbal stem cell populations are spared by undermining and retracting the corneal limbus prior to trephination [20, 50]. Some vacuum trephines may not be available in size required or even suitable for application in these circumstances—in which case marking of the surface, or partial trephination, with a hand-held trephine, followed by a freehand dissection may permit more controlled excision of the host button [49].

Given the increased risk of allograft rejection attached to repeat PK, any advantages of a continuous suture are usually outweighed by those conferred by the use of interrupted sutures. Interrupted sutures may permit the early removal of a combined continuous suture, a loose suture, a suture driving a foreign body response, or corneal neovascularization but also facilitate the management of astigmatism postoperatively [51]. The application of a Flieringa ring for scleral support is advisable when performing PK in aphakic eyes [51]. Transplants at high risk of rejection and any transplant performed in the context of ocular surface disease will likely benefit from a central temporary tarsorrhaphy at the end of the procedure [52]. This may afford a sufficient view of the transplant during the immediate postoperative period while facilitating corneal protection and epithelialization [52]. Repeat PK merits frequent and careful postoperative follow-up with particular attention to optimizing the ocular surface and managing postoperative inflammation.

Outcomes

Repeat PKs have a higher risk of failure compared with primary PK, with a worse prognosis and poorer visual outcomes. The 5-year graft failure rate for repeat PK is between 34% and 70% [41, 53–56], with numerous factors playing a role in the survival of the transplant. Repeated PKs share the same risk factors as primary PK, but there is a higher risk of immunological allograft rejection associated with violation of the immune-privileged status of the cornea. This risk increases with the number of prior corneal grafts performed, especially if they have failed as a result of allograft rejection [25, 53, 57]. In addition, the host corneal bed is usually suboptimal, with high rates of altered iridocorneal angle anatomy, peripheral anterior synechiae (PAS), and corneal surface disease. Moreover, when compared with patients receiving primary PK, PK regraft patients are slightly older, have higher use of IOP-lowering drugs, and are more prone to develop postoperative corneal neovascularization, all of which are associated with poor graft survival [56]. Finally, as for primary PK, the risk of a failed graft is closely associated with the original graft indication, with the best rates of survival reported for eyes with a primary diagnosis of keratoconus and stromal dystrophies [54].

With regard to visual outcomes, repeat PK is generally effective in improving the preoperative best-corrected visual acuity (BCVA), but the results achieved are usually worse than those for primary PK. In fact, a BCVA of 20/40 or better has been reported as being only 4.8–43.1% of clear PK regrafts at the last follow-up visit [54, 58–65]. In addition, the standard of final visual acuity achieved is inversely proportional to the number of corneal regrafts performed [59]. Despite this, a recent meta-analysis performed by Wang and coworkers found that visual outcomes in PK regrafts were not inferior to the ones for secondary endothelial grafts [66].

Descemet Stripping Endothelial Keratoplasty (DSEK) after Failed PK

Endothelial keratoplasty (EK) has essentially replaced PK for the treatment of end-stage corneal endothelial disease [67]. The advantages of Descemet stripping EK (DSEK) over that of a primary PK include a reduced need for sutures, resulting in a tectonically stronger eye, mitigated effects of ocular surface disease, and more rapid postoperative visual rehabilitation [68–71]. In cases of failed PK, however, positioning of a DSEK under the failed transplant may still be performed (Fig. 10.1), with the main theoretical advantage being a reduced risk of allograft rejection compared with a repeat PK [72, 73]. As such, patients with a failed PK who undergo a DSEK instead of a repeat PK are less likely to require systemic immunosuppression.

Surgical Considerations

Technically, performing a DSEK under a failed PK does not differ much from a standard DSEK case. Special attention should be paid to the posterior graft–host junction morphology (ideally imaged by anterior segment OCT) as significant steps between the donor and the host posterior surfaces may preclude correct graft adherence if the donor tissue is decentered or oversized compared to the PK posterior diameter. Subsequently, the diameter of the DSEK donor lenticule should ideally match that of the posterior diameter of the PK, and careful attention should be taken to center the DSEK graft within the PK graft-host junc-

tion and ensure that it will fit inside the area of the prior PK [74]. Finally, Descemet membrane (DM) stripping in these DSEK under PK cases can be more challenging and may also lead to inadvertent disruption of the graft-host junction [75]. Moreover, DM stripping has not been reported to reduce the graft dislocation rate in such cases [75], so surgeons may therefore choose not to perform DM stripping when performing a DSEK under a failed PK graft.

Outcomes

Noncomparative studies have reported 3-year graft survival rates of 69–81% for DSEK under PK, and 21–70% for repeat PK [14, 47, 56, 59, 62, 63, 76, 77]. Furthermore, a direct comparative long-term study found graft survival was prolonged significantly in eyes that underwent DSEK under a failed PK, compared with eyes undergoing repeat PK at up to 5 years follow-up (cumulative survival probability 86.4% versus 51.3%, respectively; log-rank P value = 0.013) [78]. Graft rejection episodes, specifically, were also reported to be more common in the repeat PK group compared with the DSEK under PK group, while the incidence of postoperative complications was no greater in the DSEK under PK group [78].

Another potential advantage of performing DSEK instead of PK in eyes with corneal decompensation is the promise of faster postoperative visual rehabilitation and possibly better long-term visual outcomes [79–81]. Most studies on DSEK after failed PK have reported significant

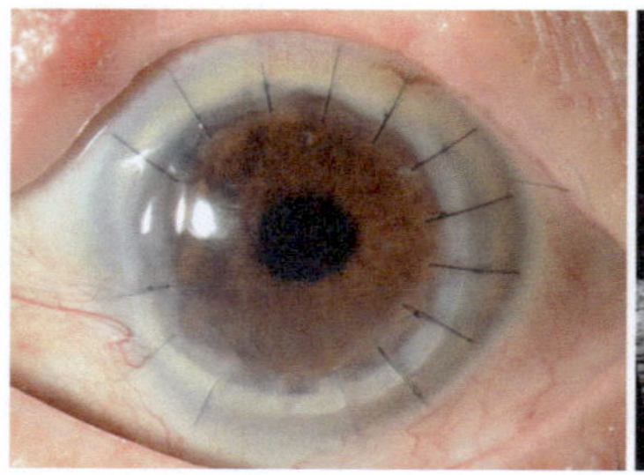
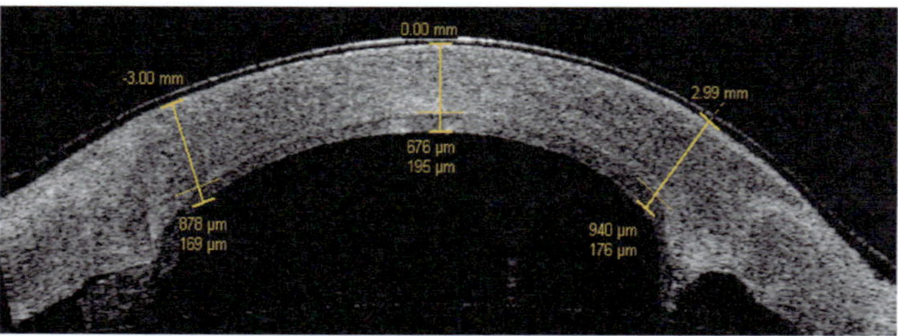

Fig. 10.1 Slit lamp picture and anterior segment OCT image (Visante, Zeiss, Germany) of a patient that received Descemet's stripping DSAEK under a previously failed PK

improvements in postoperative visual acuity [82–85]. Best-corrected visual acuity (BCVA) has been reported to increase from 1.00 logMAR preoperatively to 0.40 logMAR at 1 year postoperatively in 60 eyes ($P < 0.0001$) in one case series [86] and from 1.43 logMAR preoperatively to 0.55 logMAR at 1 year postoperatively in 22 eyes ($P = 0.001$) in another [84]; however, comparative case series of DSAEK under a failed PK and repeat PK have not found statistically significant differences in improvement in postoperative BCVA between the two techniques [61, 78]. This may be explained by the presence of stromal scarring or preexisting astigmatism of the failed PK in eyes that undergo DSEK under the PK [78]. In such cases, one may perform a DALK in the previous PK over the DSAEK graft [87].

Graft dislocation, which has a reported rate of 5.9–6.3%, remains the main concern when performing DSEK under failed PK [74, 85]. Suggested risk factors for this include the presence of a glaucoma drainage device, donor grafts that are smaller than the previous PK, and a mismatch of the posterior graft–host junction.

Descemet Membrane Endothelial Keratoplasty (DMEK) After Failed PK

EK in the form of Descemet Stripping Endothelial Keratoplasty (DSEK) has proven efficacy in restoring clarity to full-thickness grafts with endothelial decompensation. In the absence of significant scarring or surface irregularity, this has been the preferred surgical approach for the management of a decompensated PK over repeat PK for more than a decade because it affords a lower risk of rejection, prolongs graft survival, has greater safety in the presence of ocular surface disease, affords better intraocular pressure control (and therefore fewer cases of secondary glaucoma), and typically allows for faster visual recovery and a more acceptable refractive outcome [78, 82, 88, 89]; however, in recent years, Descemet membrane endothelial keratoplasty (DMEK) has been demonstrated to confer advantages over DSEK in terms of the speed of visual recovery, better visual outcomes, and a lower risk

of transplant rejection [73]. A recent comparative study demonstrated that DMEK delivers better visual outcomes than DSAEK for managing failed PK grafts [90]. This study found that, despite an overall failure rate in the medium-term that was similar between the two techniques (DMEK-43% vs. DSAEK-50%), the primary failure rate was higher in the DMEK group (due to persistent graft detachment), while the secondary failure rate was higher in the DSAEK group. The rejection rate was reported to be similar (DMEK-21% vs. DSAEK-29%) [90]. Thus, while grafting a DMEK under a failed PK is more technically challenging than DSAEK, with a higher risk of early failure, if successful, it confers better long-term visual outcomes and survival rates.

Descemet Stripping DMEK Under PK

Table 10.1 summarizes the reported outcomes of DMEK for the management of secondary failure of PK [91–100]. Performing DMEK in this scenario carries the additional intraoperative risk of dehiscence of the PK graft-host junction when performing descemetorhexis maneuvers. Consequently, it is recommended that the descemetorhexis is made 0.25–0.5 mm smaller than the PK diameter, thereby avoiding the graft-host junction. It is also recommended that the diameter of the DMEK is either matched or undersized (by 0.25 mm) compared with the PK diameter, noting that oversized DMEK grafts are associated with higher re-bubbling rates [93].

DMEK under a failed PK is also associated with a higher rate of re-bubbling—much higher than after primary DMEK cases—up to 60% in some series [91–96, 99]. This higher detachment rate and need to re-bubble is thought to be related to the DM tags and remnants associated with a more challenging descemetorhexis and the more irregular posterior corneal surfaces encountered (with pronounced gaps at the graft-host junction). Under these circumstances, gas tamponade with SF6 20% at the end of the surgery may be particularly advantageous, given that this has been demonstrated to reduce the need for re-bubbling compared with air tamponade [95].

Table 10.1 Reported outcomes of DMEK for failed PK management

Author	Year	N	Time	PK Descemetorhexis	Tamponade	Preop BCVA	Postop BCVA	ECC loss (time point)	Re-bubbling rate	Rejection rate	Graft failure
Anshu et al. [91]	2013	6	6 m	Yes	Air	20/70 Snellen	20/30 Snellen	33% (6 m)	50%	0%	17% PGF 0% SGF
Heinzelmann et al. [92]	2017	19	21.5 m (1–42 m)	Yes	Air	20/400 Snellen	20/200 Snellen	n/r	26%	10.5%	5% PGF 11% SGF
Lavy et al. [86]	2017	11	16 m	Yes	Air	Range HM-20/30	5 eyes ≥20/25 Snellen	59% (16 m)	36%	0%	9% PGF 18% SGF
Pasari et al. [93]	2019	93	21 m (1 m–7 y)	Yes	Air	20/100 (6 m) Snellen	20/30 (6 m) Snellen	31% (6 m) 44% (12 m) 47% (24 m)	53% (DMEK > PK) 27% (DMEK = PK) 33% (DMEK < PK)	2%	5% PGF 11% SGF
Pierné et al. [94]	2019	28	6 m	Yes	Air	1.34 LogMAR	0.54 LogMAR	24% (6 m)	50%	0%	0% PGF 0% SGF
Schrittenlocher et al. [95]	2020	52	12 m	Yes	Air/SF6 20%	1.07 LogMAR	0.56 (6 m) 0.38 (12 m) LogMAR	36% (6 m) 37% (12 m) 40% (24 m)	59.6%	13.5%	34.6%
Sorkin et al. [96]	2019	29	6 m	Yes	Air	0.97 LogMAR	0.51 LogMAR	38% (6 m)	58.6%	6.9%	27.6% PGF 6.9% SGF
Sorkin et al. [96]	2019	10	6 m	Yes (Femto)	Air	1.32 LogMAR	0.35 LogMAR	43.8% (6 m)	10%	10%	0% PGF 0% SGF
Alió del Barrio et al. [97]	2019	8	6 m	No	SF6 20%	20/800 Snellen	20/40 Snellen	50% (6 m)	25%	0%	0% PGF 0% SGF
Güell et al. [98]	2019	26	23.08m (6–48 m)	No	SF6 20%	20/80 (6 m) Snellen	20/32 (6 m) Snellen	27.7% (6 m) 34.4% (12 m)	11.53%	0%	0% PGF 7.7% SGF

N study sample, *BCVA* best-corrected visual acuity, *HM* hand movements, *ECC* endothelial cell count, *m* months, *y* years, *Femto* femtosecond laser-assisted descemetorhexis, *SF₆ 20%* sulfur hexafluoride, *DMEK>PK* DMEK graft diameter larger than PK graft diameter, *DMEK=PK* DMEK graft diameter equal than PK graft diameter, *DMEK<PK* DMEK graft diameter smaller than PK graft diameter, *PGF* primary graft failure, *SGF* secondary graft failure, *LogMAR* logarithm of the minimum angle of resolution, *Snellen* Snellen visual acuity.

A further concern is the relatively high rate of endothelial cell loss and graft failure observed following DMEK under PK. This may be accounted for by the higher rate of re-bubbling and additional manipulation of the DMEK donor required in such cases [93]. In contrast, known risk factors in repeat PK, such as the number of previous PKs, preexisting anterior synechiae, and corneal neovascularization, appear not to have a significant role in modulating the risk of failure for DMEK under PK [93]; however, previous glaucoma surgery in the operated eye has been shown to be an important risk factor for DMEK failure under PK. This relatively common situation may carry with it comorbidities that ultimately limit any visual gains [93]. In comparison with routine DMEK, visual recovery in eyes with preexisting PK is generally slower, with improvements in visual acuity observed up to 6 months postoperatively [94, 95].

To minimize any damage to the posterior PK surface during DMEK under PK surgery, femtosecond laser-assisted descemetorhexis has been attempted. This technique, which involves using the femtosecond laser to perform a side cut in the posterior surface of the PK and so facilitate the DMrhexis maneuvers, has shown encouraging results in reducing the rate of graft re-bubbling (10%) and failure (0%) [96, 100]; however, the study sample was limited ($n = 10$), and no differences in endothelial cell loss rates were observed in the short- or long-term compared to manual DMrhexis DMEK under PK (Table 10.1).

Recently, Steindor et al. published a case report where they stripped the DM starting from outside the failed PK and observed through a histopathologic analysis that the excised DM presented a continuous extracellular matrix connecting the host and donor DM, indicating that a primary intention wound healing after PK may occur in some cases at this tissue level, and so it could enable in such cases a DMrhexis outside the failed graft and the transplantation of a DMEK graft larger than the previous PK. Nevertheless, this finding is extracted from an isolated case report [101].

Non-Descemet Stripping DMEK Under PK

As it has been suggested previously with DSEK [85], another approach to minimizing posterior surface damage to the PK during descemetorhexis, and therefore reducing the risk of re-bubbling and DMEK failure, is to avoid this surgical step altogether—thereby making the surgery simpler, faster and less risky [97, 98]. Contrary to evidence supporting a role for descemetorhexis in routine DMEK [93], recent studies have demonstrated that nonstripping DMEK under a failed PK may be advantageous as long as the host DM is anatomically intact (no scarring or significant irregularities), with lower incidences of graft re-bubbling and failure reported compared with manual stripping techniques (Fig. 10.2 and Table 10.1) [97, 98].

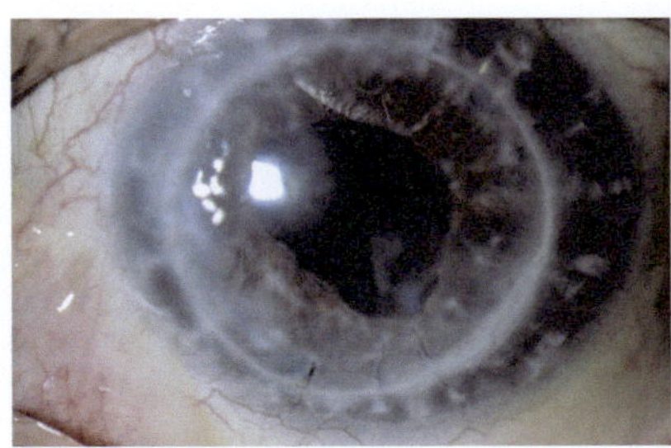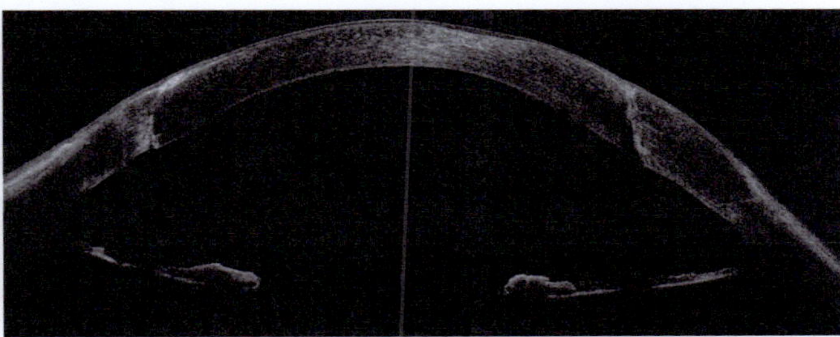

Fig. 10.2 Slit lamp picture and anterior segment OCT image (MS-39, CSO, Italy) of a patient that received non-Descemet's stripping DMEK under a previously failed PK. Images are taken 2 years after surgery. The inferior peripheral scar appeared as a consequence of microbial keratitis 1 year after surgery

Conclusion

Corneal graft failure is a growing medical challenge because of the constantly increasing volume of transplanted patients and the increase in life expectancy worldwide. The introduction of stromal and endothelial lamellar transplant techniques has brought specific complications and new forms of graft failure that will demand different approaches to those encountered with classical repeat PK. On the other hand, these novel and exciting lamellar techniques open new doors to rescuing failed PKs, helping overcome previous limitations linked to successive penetrating grafts and offering better and faster visual results with much-reduced intra- and postoperative risks. Corneal specialists should be aware of the modern surgical alternatives available to them for the rehabilitation of a patient's visual function when faced with a failed corneal transplant. A comprehensive understanding of the outcomes and limitations of these options is also critical.

Take Home Notes

- Corneal graft failure is a growing medical challenge because of the constantly increasing volume of transplanted patients and the increase in life expectancy worldwide.
- Endothelial keratoplasty techniques open new doors to rescuing failed PKs, helping overcome previous limitations linked to successive penetrating grafts and offering better and faster visual results with much reduced intra- and postoperative risks.

References

1. Gain P, Jullienne R, He Z, Aldossary M, Acquart S, Cognasse F, et al. Global survey of corneal transplantation and eye banking. JAMA Ophthalmol. 2016;134(2):167–73.
2. Alió JMA, El Sayyad F, Barraquer R, Arnalich-Montiel F, Alió del Barrio JL. Corneal graft failure: an update. Br J Ophthalmol. 2020;105(8):1049–58.
3. Patel SV. Graft survival after penetrating keratoplasty. Am J Ophthalmol. 2011;151(3):397–8.
4. Alino AM, Perry HD, Kanellopoulos AJ, Donnenfeld ED, Rahn EK. Conjunctival flaps. Ophthalmology. 1998;105(6):1120–3.
5. Qazi Y, Hamrah P. Corneal allograft rejection: immunopathogenesis to therapeutics. J Clin Cell Immunol. 2013;2013(9):6.
6. Kharod-Dholakia B, Randleman JB, Bromley JG, Stulting RD. Prevention and treatment of corneal graft rejection: current practice patterns of the Cornea Society (2011). Cornea. 2015;34(6):609–14.
7. Hudde T, Minassian DC, Larkin DF. Randomised controlled trial of corticosteroid regimens in endothelial corneal allograft rejection. Br J Ophthalmol. 1999;83(12):1348–52.
8. Yamazoe K, Yamazoe K, Shimazaki-Den S, Shimazaki J. Prognostic factors for corneal graft recovery after severe corneal graft rejection following penetrating keratoplasty. BMC Ophthalmol. 2013;13:5.
9. Pasari A, Price MO, Feng MT, Price FW Jr. Descemet membrane endothelial keratoplasty for failed penetrating keratoplasty: visual outcomes and graft survival. Cornea. 2018;38(2):151–6.
10. Borderie VM, Boëlle PY, Touzeau O, Allouch C, Boutboul S, Laroche L. Predicted long-term outcome of corneal transplantation. Ophthalmology. 2009;116(12):2354–60.
11. Fukuoka S, Honda N, Ono K, Mimura T, Usui T, Amano S. Extended long-term results of penetrating keratoplasty for keratoconus. Cornea. 2010;29(5):528–30.
12. Mannis MJ, Holland EJ, Gal RL, Dontchev M, Kollman C, Raghinaru D, et al. The effect of donor age on penetrating keratoplasty for endothelial disease: graft survival after 10 years in the cornea donor study. Ophthalmology. 2013;120(12):2419–27.
13. Tan DTH, Janardhanan P, Zhou H, Chan YH, Htoon HM, Ang LPK, et al. Penetrating keratoplasty in asian eyes. The Singapore Corneal Transplant Study. Ophthalmology. 2008;115(6):975–83.
14. Thompson RW, Price MO, Bowers PJ, Price FW. Long-term graft survival after penetrating keratoplasty. Ophthalmology. 2003;110(7):1396–402.
15. Williams KA, Lowe M, Bartlett C, Kelly T-L, Coster DJ. Risk factors for human corneal graft failure within the Australian Corneal Graft Registry. Transplantation. 2008;86(12):1720–4.
16. Matthaei M, Sandhaeger H, Hermel M, Adler W, Jun AS, Cursiefen C, et al. Changing indications in penetrating keratoplasty: a systematic review of 34 years of global reporting. Transplantation. 2017;101(6):1387–99.
17. Williams KA, Coffey NE, et al. The Australian corneal graft registry 2018 report. Adelaide: Flinders University; 2018.
18. Barraquer RI, Pareja-Aricò L, Gómez-Benlloch A, Michael R. Risk factors for graft failure after penetrating keratoplasty. Medicine. 2019;98(17):e15274.
19. Williams KA, Esterman AJ, Bartlett C, Holland H, Hornsby NB, Coster DJ. How effective is pen-

etrating corneal transplantation? Factors influencing long-term outcome in multivariate analysis. Transplantation. 2006;81(6):896–901.

20. Ang M, Mehta JS, Sng CC, Htoon HM, Tan DT. Indications, outcomes, and risk factors for failure in tectonic keratoplasty. Ophthalmology. 2012;119(7):1311–9.

21. Perera C, Jhanji V, Lamoureux E, Pollock G, Favilla I, Vajpayee RB. Clinical presentation, risk factors and treatment outcomes of first allograft rejection after penetrating keratoplasty in early and late postoperative period. Eye. 2012;26(5):711–7.

22. Price MO, Thompson RW Jr, Price FW Jr. Risk factors for various causes of failure in initial corneal grafts. Arch Ophthalmol. 2003;121(8):1087–92.

23. Sugar A, Gal RL, Kollman C, Raghinaru D, Dontchev M, Croasdale CR, et al. Factors associated with corneal graft survival in the cornea donor study. JAMA Ophthalmol. 2015;133(3):246–54.

24. Sugar A, Tanner JP, Dontchev M, Tennant B, Schultze RL, Dunn SP, et al. Recipient risk factors for graft failure in the cornea donor study. Ophthalmology. 2009;116(6):1023–8.

25. Wilson SE, Kaufman HE. Graft failure after penetrating keratoplasty. Surv Ophthalmol. 1990;34(5):325–56.

26. Park CY, Lee JK, Gore PK, Lim CY, Chuck RS. Keratoplasty in the United States: a 10-year review from 2005 through 2014. Ophthalmology. 2015;122(12):2432–42.

27. America EBAo. The 2019 EBAA statistical report: highlights, trends in eye banking and corneal transplantation. 2019.

28. Maguire MG, Stark WJ, Gottsch JD, Stulting RD, Sugar A, Fink NE, et al. Risk factors for corneal graft failure and rejection in the collaborative corneal transplantation studies. Collaborative Corneal Transplantation Studies Research Group. Ophthalmology. 1994;101(9):1536–47.

29. Hos D, Le VNH, Hellmich M, Siebelmann S, Roters S, Bachmann BO, et al. Risk of corneal graft rejection after high-risk keratoplasty following fine-needle vessel coagulation of corneal neovascularization combined with bevacizumab: a pilot study. Transplant Direct. 2019;5(5):e452.

30. Ang M, Baskaran M, Werkmeister RM, Chua J, Schmidl D, Aranha Dos Santos V, et al. Anterior segment optical coherence tomography. Prog Retin Eye Res. 2018;66:132–56.

31. Abudou M, Wu T, Evans JR, Chen X. Immunosuppressants for the prophylaxis of corneal graft rejection after penetrating keratoplasty. Cochrane Database Syst Rev. 2015;8:CD007603.

32. Kim HK, Choi JA, Uehara H, Zhang X, Ambati BK, Cho YK. Presurgical corticosteroid treatment improves corneal transplant survival in mice. Cornea. 2013;32(12):1591–8.

33. Koay PY, Lee WH, Figueiredo FC. Opinions on risk factors and management of corneal graft rejection in the United kingdom. Cornea. 2005;24(3):292–6.

34. Birnbaum F, Mayweg S, Reis A, Bohringer D, Seitz B, Engelmann K, et al. Mycophenolate mofetil (MMF) following penetrating high-risk keratoplasty: long-term results of a prospective, randomised, multicentre study. Eye. 2009;23(11):2063–70.

35. Sinha R, Jhanji V, Verma K, Sharma N, Biswas NR, Vajpayee RB. Efficacy of topical cyclosporine A 2% in prevention of graft rejection in high-risk keratoplasty: a randomized controlled trial. Graefes Arch Clin Exp Ophthalmol. 2010;248(8):1167–72.

36. Böhringer D, Grotejohann B, Ihorst G, Reinshagen H, Spierings E, Reinhard T. Rejection prophylaxis in corneal transplant. Dtsch Arzteblatt Int. 2018;115(15):259–65.

37. Hopkinson CL, Romano V, Kaye RA, Steger B, Stewart RM, Tsagkataki M, et al. The influence of donor and recipient gender incompatibility on corneal transplant rejection and failure. Am J Transplant. 2017;17(1):210–7.

38. Hager JL, Phillips DL, Goins KM, Kitzmann AS, Greiner MA, Cohen AW, et al. Boston type 1 keratoprosthesis for failed keratoplasty. Int Ophthalmol. 2016;36(1):73–8.

39. Ahmad S, Mathews PM, Lindsley K, Alkharashi M, Hwang FS, Ng SM, et al. Boston type 1 keratoprosthesis versus repeat donor keratoplasty for corneal graft failure: a systematic review and meta-analysis. Ophthalmology. 2016;123(1):165–77.

40. Fadous R, Levallois-Gignac S, Vaillancourt L, Robert MC, Harissi-Dagher M. The Boston keratoprosthesis type 1 as primary penetrating corneal procedure. Br J Ophthalmol. 2015;99(12):1664–8.

41. Ramamurthy S, Reddy JC, Vaddavalli PK, Ali MH, Garg P. Outcomes of repeat keratoplasty for failed therapeutic keratoplasty. Am J Ophthalmol. 2016;162(83-8):e2.

42. Srujana D, Kaur M, Urkude J, Rathi A, Sharma N, Titiyal JS. Long-term functional and anatomic outcomes of repeat graft after optically failed therapeutic keratoplasty. Am J Ophthalmol. 2018;189:166–75.

43. Abdelkader A. Changes in corneal wound healing and graft biomechanics after primary penetrating keratoplasty versus repeat penetrating keratoplasty. Cornea. 2019;38(8):1006–10.

44. Raber IM, Arentsen JJ, Laibson PR. Traumatic wound dehiscence after penetrating keratoplasty. Arch Ophthalmol. 1980;98(8):1407–9.

45. Binder PS, Abel R Jr, Polack FM, Kaufman HE. Keratoplasty wound separations. Am J Ophthalmol. 1975;80(1):109–15.

46. Pettinelli DJ, Starr CE, Stark WJ. Late traumatic corneal wound dehiscence after penetrating keratoplasty. Arch Ophthalmol. 2005;123(6):853–6.

47. Kirkness CM, Ezra E, Rice NS, Steele AD. The success and survival of repeat corneal grafts. Eye. 1990;4(1):58–64.

48. Seitz B, Langenbucher A, Kuchle M, Naumann GO. Impact of graft diameter on corneal power and the regularity of postkeratoplasty astigmatism

before and after suture removal. Ophthalmology. 2003;110(11):2162–7.

49. Bessant DA, Dart JK. Lamellar keratoplasty in the management of inflammatory corneal ulceration and perforation. Eye. 1994;8(1):22–8.

50. Jones DH, Kirkness CM. A new surgical technique for keratoglobus-tectonic lamellar keratoplasty followed by secondary penetrating keratoplasty. Cornea. 2001;20(8):885–7.

51. Lee RM, Lam FC, Georgiou T, Paul B, Then KY, Mavrikakis I, et al. Suturing techniques and post-operative management in penetrating keratoplasty in the United Kingdom. Clin Ophthalmol. 2012;6:1335–40.

52. Koenig SB, Harris GJ. Temporary suture tarsor-rhaphy after penetrating keratoplasty. Cornea. 1991;10(2):121–2.

53. Aboshiha J, Jones MNA, Hopkinson CL, Larkin DFP. Differential survival of penetrating and lamellar transplants in management of failed corneal grafts. JAMA Ophthalmol. 2018;136(8):859–65.

54. Al-Mezaine H, Wagoner MD. Repeat penetrating keratoplasty: indications, graft survival, and visual outcome. Br J Ophthalmol. 2006;90(3):324–7.

55. Kitazawa K, Wakimasu K, Kayukawa K, Yokota I, Inatomi T, Hieda O, et al. Moderately long-term safety and efficacy of repeat penetrating keratoplasty. Cornea. 2018;37(10):255–9.

56. Weisbrod DJ, Sit M, Naor J, Slomovic AR. Outcomes of repeat penetrating keratoplasty and risk factors for graft failure. Cornea. 2003;22(5):429–34.

57. Jabbehdari S, Rafii AB, Yazdanpanah G, Hamrah P, Holland EJ, Djalilian AR. Update on the management of high-risk penetrating keratoplasty. Curr Ophthalmol Rep. 2017;5(1):38–48.

58. Beckingsale P, Mavrikakis I, Al-Yousuf N, Mavrikakis E, Daya SM. Penetrating keratoplasty: outcomes from a corneal unit compared to national data. Br J Ophthalmol. 2006;90(6):728–31.

59. Bersudsky V, Blum-Hareuveni T, Rehany U, Rumelt S. The profile of repeated corneal transplantation. Ophthalmology. 2001;108(3):461–9.

60. Keane MC, Galettis RA, Mills RAD, Coster DJ, Williams KA. A comparison of endothelial and penetrating keratoplasty outcomes following failed penetrating keratoplasty: a registry study. Br J Ophthalmol. 2016;100(11):1569–75.

61. Kitzmann AS, Wandling GR, Sutphin JE, Goins KM, Wagoner MD. Comparison of outcomes of penetrating keratoplasty versus Descemet's stripping automated endothelial keratoplasty for penetrating keratoplasty graft failure due to corneal edema. Int Ophthalmol. 2012;32(1):15–23.

62. Patel NP, Kim T, Rapuano CJ, Cohen EJ, Laibson PR. Indications for and outcomes of repeat penetrating keratoplasty, 1989-1995. Ophthalmology. 2000;107(4):719–24.

63. Rapuano CJ, Cohen EJ, Brady SE, Arentsen JJ, Laibson PR. Indications for and outcomes of repeat penetrating keratoplasty. Am J Ophthalmol. 1990;109(6):689–95.

64. Yalniz-Akkaya Z, Nurozler AB, Yildiz EH, Onat M, Budak K, Duman S. Repeat penetrating keratoplasty: indications and prognosis, 1995-2005. Eur J Ophthalmol. 2009;19(3):362–8.

65. Barut Selver O, Karaca I, Palamar M, Egrilmez S, Yagci A. Graft failure and repeat penetrating keratoplasty. Exp Clin Transplant. 2018;19(1):72–6.

66. Wang F, Zhang T, Kang YW, He JL, Li SM, Li SW. Endothelial keratoplasty versus repeat penetrating keratoplasty after failed penetrating keratoplasty: a systematic review and meta-analysis. PLoS ONE. 2017;12(7):1–11.

67. Lee WB, Jacobs DS, Musch DC, Kaufman SC, Reinhart WJ, Shtein RM. Descemet's stripping endothelial keratoplasty: safety and outcomes: a report by the American Academy of Ophthalmology. Ophthalmology. 2009;116(9):1818–30.

68. Ang M, Htoon HM, Cajucom-Uy HY, Tan D, Mehta JS. Donor and surgical risk factors for primary graft failure following Descemet's stripping automated endothelial keratoplasty in Asian eyes. Clin Ophthalmol. 2011;5:1503–8.

69. Ang M, Mehta JS, Anshu A, Wong HK, Htoon HM, Tan D. Endothelial cell counts after Descemet's stripping automated endothelial keratoplasty versus penetrating keratoplasty in Asian eyes. Clin Ophthalmol. 2012;6:537–44.

70. Ang M, Mehta JS, Lim F, Bose S, Htoon HM, Tan D. Endothelial cell loss and graft survival after Descemet's stripping automated endothelial keratoplasty and penetrating keratoplasty. Ophthalmology. 2012;119(11):2239–44.

71. Ang M, Soh Y, Htoon HM, Mehta JS, Tan D. Five-year graft survival comparing descemet stripping automated endothelial keratoplasty and penetrating keratoplasty. Ophthalmology. 2016;123(8):1646–52.

72. Ezon I, Shih CY, Rosen LM, Suthar T, Udell IJ. Immunologic graft rejection in descemet's stripping endothelial keratoplasty and penetrating keratoplasty for endothelial disease. Ophthalmology. 2013;120(7):1360–5.

73. Anshu A, Price MO, Price FW Jr. Risk of corneal transplant rejection significantly reduced with Descemet's membrane endothelial keratoplasty. Ophthalmology. 2012;119(3):536–40.

74. Straiko MD, Terry MA, Shamie N. Descemet stripping automated endothelial keratoplasty under failed penetrating keratoplasty: a surgical strategy to minimize complications. Am J Ophthalmol. 2011;151(2):233–7 e2.

75. Clements JL, Bouchard CS, Lee WB, Dunn SP, Mannis MJ, Reidy JJ, et al. Retrospective review of graft dislocation rate associated with descemet stripping automated endothelial keratoplasty after primary failed penetrating keratoplasty. Cornea. 2011;30(4):414–8.

76. Al-Mezaine H, Wagoner MD, King Khaled Eye Specialist Hospital Cornea Transplant Study G. Repeat penetrating keratoplasty: indications, graft survival, and visual outcome. Br J Ophthalmol. 2006;90(3):324–7.

77. Williams KA, Roder D, Esterman A, Muehlberg SM, Coster DJ. Factors predictive of corneal graft survival. Report from the Australian Corneal Graft Registry. Ophthalmology. 1992;99(3):403–14.

78. Ang M, Ho H, Wong C, Htoon HM, Mehta JS, Tan D. Endothelial keratoplasty after failed penetrating keratoplasty: an alternative to repeat penetrating keratoplasty. Am J Ophthalmol. 2014;158(6):1221–7.

79. Ang M, Lim F, Htoon HM, Tan D, Mehta JS. Visual acuity and contrast sensitivity following Descemet stripping automated endothelial keratoplasty. Br J Ophthalmol. 2016;100(3):307–11.

80. Fuest M, Ang M, Htoon HM, Tan D, Mehta JS. Long-term visual outcomes comparing descemet stripping automated endothelial keratoplasty and penetrating keratoplasty. Am J Ophthalmol. 2017;182:62–71.

81. Bose S, Ang M, Mehta JS, Tan DT, Finkelstein E. Cost-effectiveness of Descemet's stripping endothelial keratoplasty versus penetrating keratoplasty. Ophthalmology. 2013;120(3):464–70.

82. Anshu A, Price MO, Price FW Jr. Descemet's stripping endothelial keratoplasty under failed penetrating keratoplasty: visual rehabilitation and graft survival rate. Ophthalmology. 2011;118(11):2155–60.

83. Covert DJ, Koenig SB. Descemet stripping and automated endothelial keratoplasty (DSAEK) in eyes with failed penetrating keratoplasty. Cornea. 2007;26(6):692–6.

84. Heitor de Paula F, Kamyar R, Shtein RM, Sugar A, Mian SI. Endothelial keratoplasty without Descemet stripping after failed penetrating keratoplasty. Cornea. 2012;31(6):645–8.

85. Nottage JM, Nirankari VS. Endothelial keratoplasty without Descemet's stripping in eyes with previous penetrating corneal transplants. Br J Ophthalmol. 2012;96(1):24–7.

86. Anshu A, Lim LS, Htoon HM, Tan DT. Postoperative risk factors influencing corneal graft survival in the Singapore Corneal Transplant Study. Am J Ophthalmol. 2011;151(3):442–8.

87. Fuest M, Siregar SR, Farrag A, Htoon HM, Tan D, Mehta JS. Long-term follow-up of deep anterior lamellar keratoplasty after Descemet stripping automated endothelial keratoplasty. Graefes Arch Clin Exp Ophthalmol. 2018;256(9):1669–77.

88. Price FW Jr, Price MO. Endothelial keratoplasty to restore clarity to a failed penetrating graft. Cornea. 2006;25(8):895–9.

89. Mitry D, Bhogal M, Patel AK, Lee BS, Chai SM, Price MO, et al. Descemet stripping automated endothelial keratoplasty after failed penetrating keratoplasty: survival, rejection risk, and visual outcome. JAMA Ophthalmol. 2014;132(6):742–9.

90. Einan-Lifshitz A, Mednick Z, Belkin A, Sorkin N, Alshaker S, Boutin T, et al. Comparison of descemet stripping automated endothelial keratoplasty and descemet membrane endothelial keratoplasty in the treatment of failed penetrating keratoplasty. Cornea. 2019;38(9):1077–82.

91. Anshu A, Price MO, Price FW Jr. Descemet membrane endothelial keratoplasty and hybrid techniques for managing failed penetrating grafts. Cornea. 2013;32(1):1–4.

92. Heinzelmann S, Bohringer D, Eberwein P, Lapp T, Reinhard T, Maier P. Descemet membrane endothelial keratoplasty for graft failure following penetrating keratoplasty. Graefes Arch Clin Exp Ophthalmol. 2017;255(5):979–85.

93. Pasari A, Price MO, Feng MT, Price FW Jr. Descemet membrane endothelial keratoplasty for failed penetrating keratoplasty: visual outcomes and graft survival. Cornea. 2019;38(2):151–6.

94. Pierne K, Panthier C, Courtin R, Mazharian A, Souedan V, Gatinel D, et al. Descemet membrane endothelial keratoplasty after failed penetrating keratoplasty. Cornea. 2019;38(3):280–4.

95. Schrittenlocher S, Schlereth SL, Siebelmann S, Hayashi T, Matthaei M, Bachmann B, et al. Long-term outcome of descemet membrane endothelial keratoplasty (DMEK) following failed penetrating keratoplasty (PK). Acta Ophthalmol. 2020;98(7):e901–6.

96. Sorkin N, Mimouni M, Santaella G, Trinh T, Cohen E, Einan-Lifshitz A, et al. Comparison of manual and femtosecond laser-assisted descemet membrane endothelial keratoplasty for failed penetrating keratoplasty. Am J Ophthalmol. 2020;214:1–8.

97. Alio Del Barrio JL, Montesel A, Ho V, Bhogal M. Descemet membrane endothelial keratoplasty under failed penetrating keratoplasty without host descemetorhexis for the management of secondary graft failure. Cornea. 2020;39(1):13–7.

98. Güell JL, Morral M, Barbany M, Gris O, Elies D, Manero F. Descemet membrane endothelial keratoplasty after penetrating keratoplasty. J EuCornea. 2019;2:10–3.

99. Lavy I, Liarakos VS, Verdijk RM, Parker J, Muller TM, Bruinsma M, et al. Outcome and histopathology of secondary penetrating keratoplasty graft failure managed by descemet membrane endothelial keratoplasty. Cornea. 2017;36(7):777–84.

100. Sorkin N, Trinh T, Einan-Lifshitz A, Mednick Z, Santaella G, Telli A, et al. Outcomes of femtosecond laser-assisted Descemet membrane endothelial keratoplasty for failed penetrating keratoplasty. Can J Ophthalmol. 2019;54(6):741–5.

101. Steindor FA, Clemens AC, Herwig-Carl MC, et al. Wound healing of descemet membrane after penetrating keratoplasty and its relevance for descemet membrane endothelial keratoplasty surgeons. Cornea. 2021;40(7):910–3.

Excimer Laser-Assisted Keratoplasty: Penetrating Keratoplasty "Excimer-PKP" and Deep Anterior Lamellar Keratoplasty "Excimer-DALK"

11

Loay Daas, Loïc Hamon, Elias Flockerzi, Shady Suffo, and Berthold Seitz

Key Points

- A comparison between excimer laser-assisted, Femtosecond laser-assisted, and mechanical trephination regarding donor and recipient centration, the occurrence of "vertical tilt" and "horizontal torsion" of the graft in the recipient bed, all-sutures-out—keratometric astigmatism, and visual acuity.
- The Homburg/Erlangen technique of nonmechanical excimer laser-assisted trephination.
- Indication, technique, and contraindications for excimer laser-assisted deep anterior lamellar keratoplasty "excimer-DALK".

Supplementary Information The online version contains supplementary material available at https://doi.org/10.1007/978-3-031-32408-6_11.

L. Daas (✉) · L. Hamon · E. Flockerzi · S. Suffo
B. Seitz
Department of Ophthalmology, Saarland University Medical Center, Homburg, Germany
e-mail: loay.daas@uks.eu; loic.hamon@uks.eu; elias.flockerzi@uks.eu; shady.suffo@uks.eu; berthold.seitz@uks.eu

Excimer Laser-Assisted Penetrating Keratoplasty "Excimer-PKP" (Video 11.1)

Corneal transplantation is the oldest, most common, and most successful transplantation in humans. The first penetrating keratoplasty (PKP) was performed in 1905 by Eduard Zirm in Olmütz, now in the Czech Republic [1]. With the increasing expertise of the microsurgeon, the technique of PKP exceeds by far the simple replacement of two collagen discs and is crucial for achieving good postoperative visual acuity.

Visual acuity after successful PKP depends largely on the clarity of the graft and postoperative astigmatism after suture removal [2]. One of the most common causes of patient dissatisfaction after PKP is severe irregular astigmatism [3]. A clear transplant after PKP with high irregular astigmatism cannot be considered successful anymore. The following factors are the most important cause of unsatisfactory postoperative astigmatism [4, 5]:

1. Decentration of the recipient bed [6]
2. Vertical tilt [7]
3. Horizontal torsion [7]
4. Mechanical deformation of the incision edges

When performing PKP, every step, from donor selection to intraoperative trephination and suturing technique to careful postoperative follow-up, can affect the final refractive outcome [3, 8].

This includes horizontal positioning of the patient's head and the limbal plane, type of trephination, the correct placement of the cardinal sutures, and suture technique [9–13].

Horizontal positioning of the patient's head and the limbal plane is an indispensable requirement to avoid decentration, "vertical tilt" and "horizontal torsion" (Fig. 11.1). In cases of doubt, centering should be based on the corneal limbus and not on the pupil. An "optimal trephination" requires a full visual inspection, no contact, optimal centering of donor, and recipient, the identical shape of donor and recipient (usually circular), congruent cutting angles, symmetrical 360° alignment of donor and recipient, no completion of trephination with scissors, and no injury to intraocular structures (iris, lens). Donor and recipient trephination should be performed from the epithelial side with the same system, which is the prerequisite for congruent cutting surfaces and angles in both the donor and recipient. For this purpose, an artificial anterior chamber should be used for donor trephination. To avoid the increase of astigmatism after suture removal, decentration, "vertical tilt" and "horizontal torsion", a trephination for PKP that creates a tension-free systemic fit of a circular donor disc into a circular recipient bed with congruent unproblematic watertight fitting incision edges system should be used for PKP. Furthermore, the noncontact technique avoids inappropriate trephination in case of instable corneas, such as perforated ulcers, status postcorneal hydrops or iatrogenic keratectasia after LASIK (Fig. 11.2).

Currently, these requirements for optimal trephination are best met by nonmechanical excimer laser-assisted trephination, which presents many advantages in terms of topographic astigmatism and visual acuity after suture removal [14, 15]. Seitz et al. [15] prospectively

Fig. 11.1 Intraoperative determinants of astigmatism after penetrating keratoplasty. (**a**) "Decentration" = donor and/or recipient trephination, (**b**) "vertical tilt" = incongruent cutting angle between donor and recipient, (**c**) "horizontal torsion" = horizontal discrepancy between the donor and recipient form and/or asymmetrical graft fitting—"The second cardinal suture is crucial!"

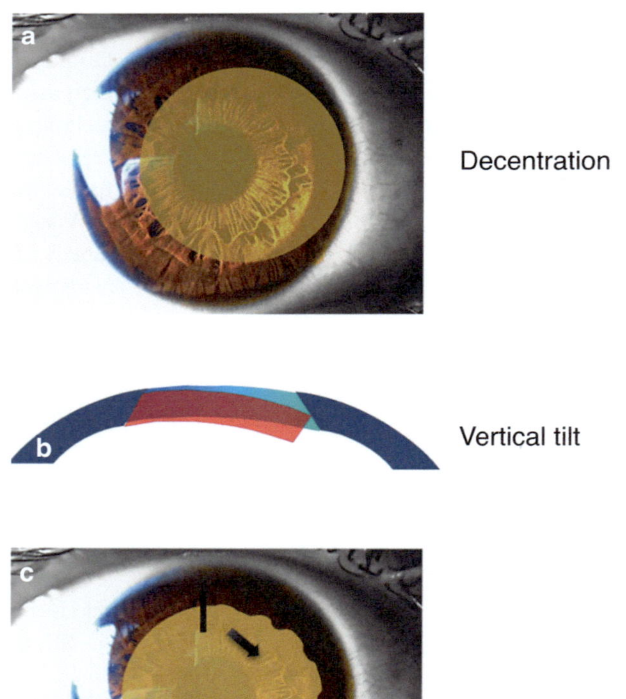

compared the nonmechanical excimer laser-assisted trephination and mechanical trephination using a hand-held motor trephine (Micorkeraton, Geuder). They showed that the former resulted in a significantly better postoperative visual acuity after suture removal (20/28 vs. 20/39, $p < 0.01$) as well as a significantly lower surface regularity index (SRI) (0.91 ± 0.45 vs. 1.05 ± 0.46, $P = 0.04$) after suture removal.

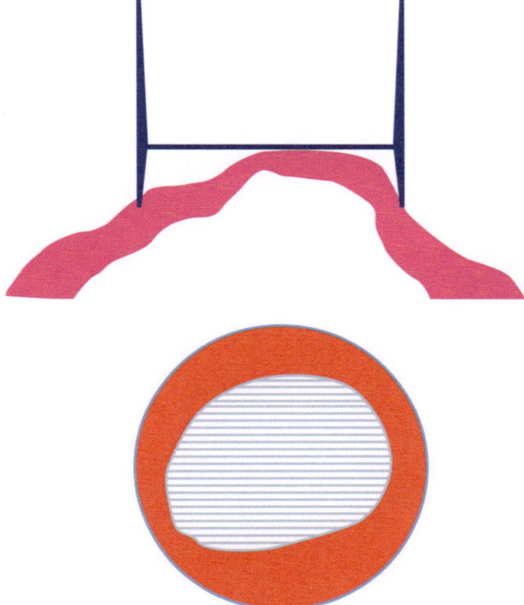

Fig. 11.2 Inappropriate mechanical trephination results in case of an unstable cornea due to tissue irregularities

The type of trephination also has a major impact on the proper placement of the primary four or eight cardinal sutures [11, 16]. For this aim, the Homburg/Erlangen technique of nonmechanical excimer laser-assisted trephination has a great advantage when compared to other trephination systems due to the presence of "orientation teeth and notches" along the metal masks. Using a curved donor mask on the corneoscleral disc in an artificial anterior chamber results in eight "orientation teeth" (Fig. 11.3). During the recipient trephination, eight corresponding "orientation notches" are lasered on the patient's cornea with the help of a recipient mask. The "orientation teeth" on the edge of the graft [14] and corresponding notches on the edge of the recipient support the symmetrical positioning of the first eight cardinal sutures, thus reducing the "horizontal torsion" (Fig. 11.4) and improve the optical quality after transplantation [5]. Furthermore, this procedure ensures donor and recipient centration [17]. These beneficial influences on the main intraoperative determinants of astigmatism after keratoplasty result in lower postoperative keratometric astigmatism (3.1 ± 2.1 vs. 6.2 ± 2.9, $P < 0.001$), higher topographic regularity, and improved spectacle-corrected visual acuity after suture removal [15, 16, 18]. Additional functions and benefits of these cardinal sutures include symmetrical horizontal distribution of the donor tissue in the recipient bed, stabilization of the anterior chamber to make sure that additional

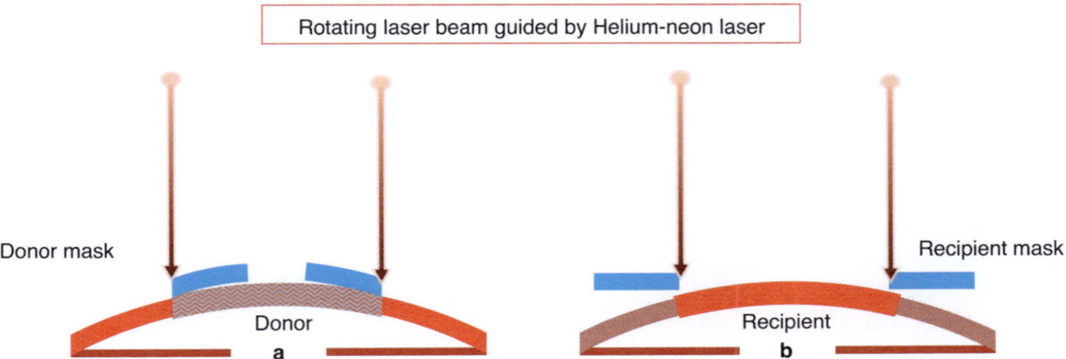

Fig. 11.3 Principle of excimer laser trephination using a 193 nm excimer laser along a metal mask, in the donor (**a**) and recipient (**b**) (schematic sketch, sagittal view)

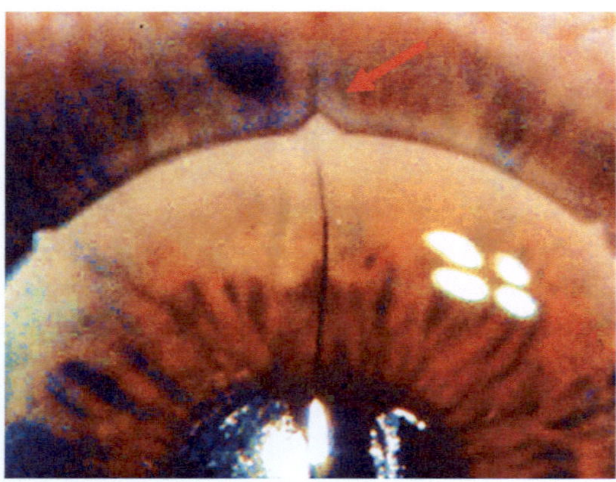

Fig. 11.4 The first cardinal suture: "orientation teeth" on the edge of the graft and corresponding notches on the edge of the recipient (arrow)

suturing is uniform and a good adaptation of the donor and recipient wound margins to the extent of Bowman's layer. Plus and minus steps (overriding or underriding of the donor, respectively) of the anterior corneal surface of the donor should be avoided. In contrast, the wound adaptation of the posterior corneal surface plays a subordinate role. Concerning the correct placement of the second cardinal suture, unintentional deviations from circular recipient openings can represent a challenge, even for an experienced keratoplasty surgeon.

Conventional mechanical trephination of the recipient is often associated with a deformation of corneal tissue layers, distortion of cutting edges, and irregular cutting surfaces due to the axial and radial forces that arise when using mechanical trephines [7, 16].

Prospective clinical studies have shown that the noncontact excimer laser-assisted PKP technique (1) improves donor and recipient trephination centering, (2) reduces vertical tilt, and (3) horizontal torsion of the graft in the recipient bed, resulting in significantly lower corneal astigmatism after removal of the corneal sutures, higher regularity of topography, and consequently, better vision when glasses are used for correction [15, 18–20]. Excimer laser-assisted trephination is also superior to femtosecond laser-assisted trephination in terms of postoperative refractive/pentacam/anterior segment-OCT astigmatism after removal of corneal sutures (4.3

$\pm$ 3.0 D/4.4 $\pm$ 3.1 D/4.0 $\pm$ 2.9 D vs. 6.2 $\pm$ 2.9 D/7.1 $\pm$ 3.2 D/7.4 $\pm$ 3.3 D, $p \leq 0.005$) [21]. The technical data of the excimer laser used in our center are summarized in Table 11.1. The masks used for the recipient/donor corneal incisions are

Table 11.1 Technical data of the SCHWIND-AMARIS excimer laser

Working laser	ArF-Excimer laser
Type	ArF-Excimer laser
Laser class	4
Wavelength	193 nm
Mode	Pulsed
Pulse energy (beam output)	14 mJ max.
Pulse frequency	500 Hz (AMARIS/AMARIS 500E)
	750 Hz (AMARIS 750S)
	1050 Hz (AMARIS 1050RS)
Pulse duration	3–15 ns
Pulse-to-pulse stability	<3%
Beam diameter (output)	6 × 3 mm
Beam divergence	1 × 2 mrad
Treatment parameter	
Energy	0.67–1.0 mJ (nominal)
Treatment area	App. 193 mm under beam output; Reference: lower edge of objective
Beam diameter (treatment area)	0.54 mm FWHM (full width half maximum)
Fluence (nominal)	Low fluence: 250 mJ/cm²
	High fluence: 500 mJ/cm²
Aiming laser	*Diode laser*
Laser class	1
Wavelength	650 nm
Power (middle, beam output)	<0.3 mW
Mode	cw (continuous wave)
Laser arm	90° swivelling
Cross laser (option)	*Diode laser*
(For AMARIS 750S/1050RS only)	
Laser class	1
Wavelength	635 nm
Power	<0.3 mW
Mode	cw
OCP laser (option for all AMARIS types)	
Laser class	1
Wavelength	1280–1360 nm
Energy/power	<1 mW
Mode	cw

Source: SCHWIND eye-tech-solutions GmbH Website, user manual for SCHWIND-AMARIS Excimer Laser (QR Code)

determined according to the indication for PKP and are available in the following sizes: 6.5/6.6, 7.0/7.1, 7.5/7.6, 8.0/8.1, and 8.5/8.6 mm.

In summary, the Homburg/Erlangen technique of nonmechanical excimer laser-assisted trephination can significantly improve donor and recipient centration, reduce "vertical tilt" and "horizontal torsion" of the graft in the recipient bed, resulting in significantly less—all-sutures-out—keratometric astigmatism, more regular topography, and better visual acuity compared to conventional trephination [7, 15, 18–20].

Excimer Laser-Assisted Deep Anterior Lamellar Keratoplasty "Excimer-DALK"

In recent years, an increase in lamellar procedures in corneal surgery has been observed, especially in posterior lamellar keratoplasty ("Descemet membrane endothelial keratoplasty" (DMEK)). According to the German Keratoplasty Registry [22], 3.0% of all 9042 corneal transplants in 2020 in Germany were performed as deep anterior lamellar keratoplasty (DALK). This low percentage may be explained by a currently missing standardized surgical technique to perform DALK.

Especially young patients with advanced keratoconus who also suffer from atopic eczema and cannot be treated with a rigid, gas-permeable contact lens, riboflavin-ultraviolet A cross-linking (CXL), or implantation of intracorneal ring segments (ICRS) profit from this method. Prerequisites for performing DALK include an intact corneal endothelium with sufficient endothelial cell density, and an intact Descemet's membrane (DALK is not an option after corneal hydrops) [23–25]. DALK is contraindicated in endothelial corneal dystrophies and any form of herpetic keratitis—due to the possible reactivation of herpes in the patient's own endothelium [26].

Surgical Technique

The steps of a standardized excimer laser-assisted DALK procedure [27] are as follows:

1. *Donor*: In equivalence to excimer laser-assisted penetrating keratoplasty (excimer-PKP): Using excimer laser with mask, a complete trephination of the donor cornea with "orientation teeth" is performed [3].

2. *Recipient cornea*: An excimer laser trephination of the recipient with congruent "notches" to 80% of midperipheral corneal thickness at the trephination site is performed. The corneal thickness is measured by anterior segment optical coherence tomography (AS-OCT). Successful manual excision of this superficial stromal lamella is followed by intrastromal air injection using a 30-gauge needle according to the "big bubble" technique described by Anwar and Teichmann [28]. After performing the "big bubble", a paracentesis is performed, and air is injected into the anterior chamber. The formation of a kidney-shaped intracameral air bubble indicates the successful separation of the deep stromal tissue and Descemet's membrane, without perforation. After puncture and deflation of the "big bubble", the intracameral air bubble moves toward the center. If complete exposure of Descemet's membrane ("naked Descemet's") is successful, the surgical procedure can be continued as DALK. Otherwise, a "conversion" to excimer-PKP with full graft is mandatory.

3. *Donor lamella*: The donor cornea is fixed without Descemet's membrane ("anterior donor lamella") using two continuous sutures, according to Hoppenreijs et al. [9] (Fig. 11.5).

4. At the end of surgery, an air/gas bubble (approximately 80%) is routinely injected into the anterior chamber to ensure attachment of the patient's own Descemet's membrane to the donor lamella. This avoids the development of a so-called "double anterior

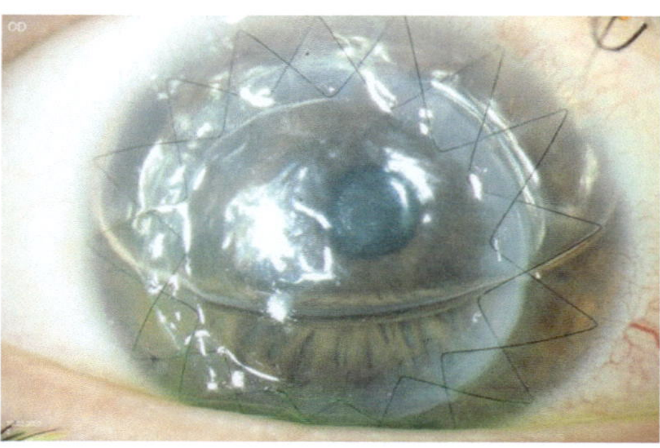

Fig. 11.5 Slit lamp biomicroscopy photography: 1 day after excimer laser-assisted DALK

chamber". To prevent a postoperative rise of intraocular pressure ("air block"), an Nd:YAG laser iridotomy at the 6 o'clock position should be routinely created preoperatively in analogy to the procedure prior to performing DMEK [29, 30].

In a review paper, the American Academy of Ophthalmology (AAO) evaluated DALK to be equivalent to PKP in terms of postoperative visual acuity outcomes [31]. Endothelial cell loss after successful DALK (without intraoperative perforation of Descemet's membrane) (12 months postoperatively: $-12.9\% \pm 17.6\%$) is lower than after PKP ($-27.7\% \pm 11.1\%$) [32]. Endothelial immune reaction of the graft is rarely observed after DALK [33]. Another significant advantage over PKP is that the globe remains intact and is not unroofed as in PKP.

The intraoperative conversion rate to PKP is at least 16.2%. Therefore, detailed informed consent for both surgeries is absolutely necessary [34]. However, the conversion rate decreases with the expertise of the surgeon.

The excimer laser-assisted technique allows for combining the advantages of DALK (fast visual recovery and less immune reaction) and excimer laser trephination (optimal visual recovery with low postoperative astigmatism) with a low intraoperative perforation rate. Moreover, excimer-DALK does not result in any disadvantages for the patient in case of conversion to excimer-PKP.

We believe excimer-DALK contributes to a certain standardization of deep anterior lamellar keratoplasty. Furthermore, the "big bubble" represents a safe and more controlled technique to finalize tissue dissection after the excision of about 80% of the superficial stromal lamella, especially in the absence of an intraoperative AS-OCT. Complete exposure of Descemet's membrane, so-called "naked Descemet's" with excision of the predescemetal stromal lamella [35], is an important prognostic factor with regard to postoperative visual acuity outcome (Figs. 11.6 and 11.7). If the residual thickness of the recipient bed is less than 80 µm and homoge-

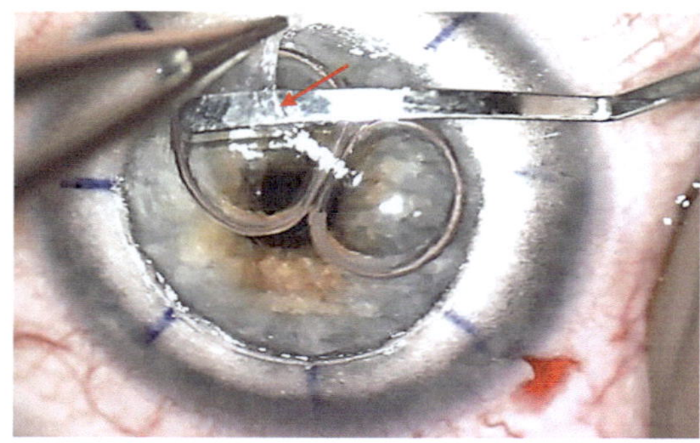

Fig. 11.6 Intraoperative imaging: complete exposure of Descemet's membrane in excimer laser-assisted DALK after successful "big bubble" dissection followed by manual excision of the superficial stromal lamina, but prior to excision of the predescemetal stromal lamina (arrow)

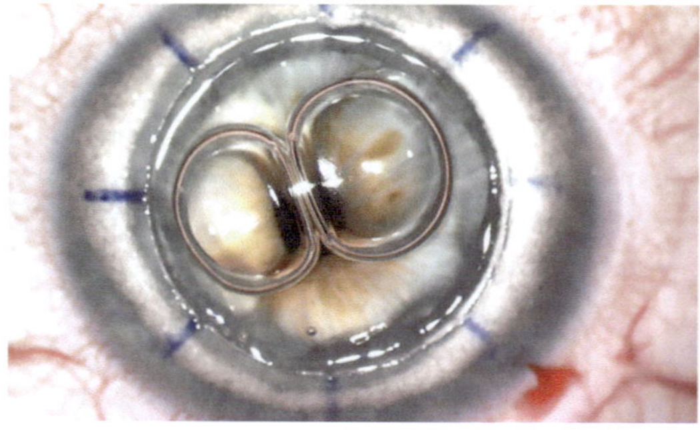

Fig. 11.7 Intraoperative imaging: complete exposure of Descemet's membrane (so-called "naked Descemet's") in excimer laser-assisted DALK with successful excision of the predescemetal stromal lamella and crystal clear view into the anterior chamber

neous in its thickness, the visual results are shown to be satisfactory. However, postoperative visual acuity development takes longer and may last between 2 and 5 years according to other studies [36].

Take Home Notes

- Compared to motor trephination, the Homburg/Erlangen technique of nonmechanical excimer laser-assisted trephination can significantly improve donor and recipient centration, reduce "vertical tilt" and "horizontal torsion" of the graft in the recipient bed, and results in significantly less all-sutures-out keratometric astigmatism, more regular topography, and better visual acuity.
- The recipient endothelium must be intact for DALK to be an option.
- Contraindications for DALK are acute corneal hydrops, any form of herpetic keratitis or endothelial corneal dystrophy.
- The surgeon should aim for a complete exposure of Descemet's membrane (so-called "naked Descemet's") to achieve the best postoperative visual acuity results.

Conflict of Interest All authors certify that they have no affiliation or interest in any organization or entity that has a financial or nonfinancial interest in the topics or materials covered in this chapter.

Funding No funding or support was received for this contribution.

References

1. Zirm E. A successful total keratoplasty. Graefes Arch Clin Exp Ophthalmol. 1906;64:580–93.
2. Naydis I, Klemm M, Hassenstein A, Richard G, Katz T, Linke SJ. Postkeratoplasty astigmatism. Comparison of three suturing techniques. Ophthamologe. 2011;108:252–9.
3. Seitz B, Daas L, Milioti G, Szentmáry N, Langenbucher A, Suffo S. Excimer laser-assisted penetrating keratoplasty: on 1 July 2019 excimer laser penetrating keratoplasty celebrates its 30th anniversary. Ophthalmologe. 2019;116:1221–30.
4. Artana LG. Computerized corneal topography in the treatment of high astigmatism after penetrating keratoplasty. Klin Monatsbl Augenheilkd. 1995;206:312–6.
5. Seitz B, Langenbucher A, Naumann GOH. The penetrating keratoplasty. A 100-year success story. Ophthamology. 2005;102:1128–36.
6. Riedel T, Seitz B, Langenbucher A, Naumann GOH. Morphological results after eccentric penetrating keratoplasty. Ophthalmologe. 2001;98:639–46.
7. Naumann GOH. Part II: corneal transplantation in anterior segment diseases. The Bowman Lecture (Number 56) 1994. Eye. 1995;9:395–421.
8. Seitz B, Szentmáry N, El-Husseiny M, Viestenz A, Langenbucher A, Naumann GOH. The penetrating keratoplasty (PKP) – a century of success. In: Hjortdal J, editor. Corneal transplantation. Berlin: Springer; 2016. p. 67–92.
9. Hoppenreijs VPT, Van Rij G, Beekhuis WH, Rijneveld WJ, Rinkel-Van DE. Causes of high astigmatism after penetrating keratoplasty. Doc Ophthalmol. 1993;85:21–34.
10. Naumann GOH, Sautter H. Surgical procedures on the cornea. In: Blodi FC, Mackensen G, Neubauer H, editors. Surgical ophthalmology. Berlin: Springer; 1991. p. 433–97.
11. Olson RJ. Modulation of postkeratoplasty astigmatism by surgical and suturing techniques. Int Ophthalmol Clin. 1983;23:137–51.
12. Van Rij G, Cornell FM, Waring GO III, Wilson LA, Beekhuis H. Postoperative astigmatism after central vs eccentric penetrating keratoplasties. Am J Ophthalmol. 1985;99:317–20.
13. Van Rij G, Waring GO. Configuration of corneal trephine opening using five different trephines in human donor eyes. Arch Ophthalmol. 1988;106:1228–33.
14. Behrens A, Seitz B, Küchle M, Langenbucher A, Kus MM, Rummelt C, Naumann GOH. "Orientation teeth" in non-mechanical laser corneal trephination for penetrating keratoplasty: 2.94 μm Er:YAGv 193 nm ArF excimer laser. Br J Ophthalmol. 1999;83:1008–12.
15. Seitz B, Langenbucher A, Kus MM, Küchle M, Naumann GOH. Nonmechanical corneal trephination with the excimer laser improves outcome after penetrating keratoplasty. Ophthalmology. 1999;106:1156–65.
16. Seitz B, Langenbucher A, Naumann GOH. Trephination in penetrating keratoplasty. In: Reinhard T, Larkin F, editors. Essentials in ophthalmology - corneal and external eye disease. Berlin: Springer; 2006. p. 123–52.
17. Lang GK, Naumann GOH, Koch JW. A new elliptical excision for corneal transplantation using an excimer laser. Arch Ophthalmol. 1990;108:914–5.
18. Seitz B, Hager T, Langenbucher A, Naumann GOH. Reconsidering sequential double running suture removal after penetrating keratoplasty – a prospective randomized study comparing excimer laser and motor trephination. Cornea. 2018;37:301–6.
19. Seitz B, Langenbucher A, Nguyen NX, Kus MM, Küchle M, Naumann GOH. Results of the first 1000 consecutive elective nonmechanical keratoplasties

with the excimer laser - a prospective study over more than 12 years. Ophthalmologe. 2004;101:478–88.

20. Szentmáry N, Langenbucher A, Naumann GOH, Seitz B. Intra-individual variability of penetrating keratoplasty outcome after excimer laser versus motorized corneal trephination. J Refract Surg. 2006;22:804–10.

21. Tóth G, Szentmáry N, Langenbucher A, Akhmedova E, El-Husseiny M, Seitz B. Comparison of excimer laser versus femtosecond laser assisted trephination in penetrating keratoplasty: a retrospective study. Adv Ther. 2019;36:3471–4382.

22. Flockerzi E, Maier P, Böhringer D, Reinshagen H, Kruse F, Cursiefen C, Reinhard T, Geerling G, Torun N, Seitz B. Trends in corneal transplantation from 2001 to 2016 in Germany: a report of the DOG-Section cornea and its keratoplasty registry. Am J Ophthalmol. 2018;188:91–8.

23. Cursiefen C, Schaub F, Bachmann B. Update: deep anterior lamellar keratoplasty (DALK) for keratoconus. Ophthalmologe. 2016;113:204–12.

24. Schaub F, Heindl LM, Enders P, Roters S, Bachmann BO, Cursiefen C. Deep anterior lamellar keratoplasty. Experiences and results of the first 100 consecutive DALK from the university eye hospital of cologne. Opthalmology. 2017;114:1019–26.

25. Seitz B, Cursiefen C, El Husseiny M, Viestenz A, Langenbucher A, Szentmary N. DALK and penetrating laser keratoplasty for advanced keratoconus. Ophthalmologe. 2013;110:839–48.

26. Holbach LM, Asano N, Naumann GO. Infection of the corneal endothelium in herpes simplex keratitis. Am J Ophthalmol. 1998;26:592–4.

27. Daas L, Hamon L, Ardjomand N, Safi T, Seitz B. Excimer laser-assisted DALK: a case report from the Homburg Keratoconus Center (HKC). Ophthalmologe. 2021;118:1245–8.

28. Anwar M, Teichmann KD. Big-bubble technique to bare Descemet's membrane in anterior lamellar keratoplasty. J Cataract Refract Surg. 2002;28:398–403.

29. Cursiefen C, Heindl LM. Perspectives of deep anterior lamellar keratoplasty. Ophthalmologe. 2011;108:833–9.

30. Seitz B, Daas L, Flockerzi E, Suffo S. Descemet membrane endothelial keratoplasty DMEK - donor and recipient step by step. Ophthalmologe. 2020;117:811–28.

31. Reinhart WJ, Musch DC, Jacobs DS, Lee WB, Kaufman SC, Shtein RM. Deep anterior lamellar keratoplasty as an alternative to penetrating keratoplasty: a report by the American Academy of Ophthalmology. Ophthalmology. 2011;118:209–18.

32. Cheng YYY, Visser N, Schouten JS, Wijdh RJ, Pels E, Cleynenbreugel H, Eggink CA, Zaal MJW, Rijneveld WJ, Nuijts RMMA. Endothelial cell loss and visual outcome of deep anterior lamellar keratoplasty versus penetrating keratoplasty: a randomized multicenter clinical trial. Ophthalmology. 2011;118:302–9.

33. Hos D, Matthaei M, Bock F, Maruyama K, Notara M, Clahsen T, Hou Y, Le VNH, Salabarria AC, Horstmann J, Bachmann BO, Cursiefen C. Immune reactions after modern lamellar (DALK, DSAEK, DMEK) versus conventional penetrating corneal transplantation. Prog Retin Eye Res. 2019;73:100768.

34. Myerscough J, Friehmann A, Bovone C, Mimouni M, Busin M. Evaluation of the risk factors associated with conversion of intended deep anterior lamellar keratoplasty to penetrating keratoplasty. Br J Ophthalmol. 2020;104:764–7.

35. Dua HS, Faraj LA, Said DG, Gray T, Lowe J. Human corneal anatomy redefined: a novel pre-Descemet's layer (Dua's layer). Ophthalmology. 2013;120:1778–85.

36. Sarnicola E, Sarnicola C, Cheung AY, Holland EJ, Sarnicola V. Surgical corneal anatomy in deep anterior lamellar keratoplasty: suggestion of new acronyms. Cornea. 2019;38:515–22.

Part III

Epithelial Lamellar Keratoplasty

Keratolimbal Grafts: Outcomes, Innovations and Alternatives

Rafael I. Barraquer and Juan Alvarez de Toledo

Key Points

- Limbal stem cell deficiency is one of the leading causes of corneal graft failure, with very difficult clinical and surgical management
- Limbal graft is the only viable way today available for the treatment of corneal stem cell deficiency
- Different types of corneal limbal graft transplants have been proposed with variable success
- In this chapter, the reader will find a description of the different alternatives today available for limbal stem cell transplantation and how to choose each, with a description of relevant technical surgical details and the postoperative clinical management essential for the success of the technique

Supplementary Information The online version contains supplementary material available at https://doi.org/10.1007/978-3-031-32408-6_12.

R. I. Barraquer (✉)
Centro de Oftalmologia Barraquer, Barcelona, Spain

International University of Catalonia,
Barcelona, Spain

Institut Universitari Barraquer, Univestitat Autònoma de Barcelona, Barcelona, Spain

J. A. de Toledo
Institut Universitari Barraquer, Univestitat Autònoma de Barcelona, Barcelona, Spain

Centro de Oftalmologia Barraquer, Barcelona, Spain

Introduction and Historical Background

The tissue-specific, layer-by-layer approach to the treatment of corneal disease characterizes the most relevant trends in keratoplasty during the first quarter of our century. Increased awareness of the different origins and varying involvement of the corneal layers in a particular condition led to question the rationale for a penetrating keratoplasty (PK)—no matter how successful its record- and naturally called for the development and application of the progressively dominant lamellar techniques.

However, in the case of the ocular surface, the importance of the regeneration dynamics of the epithelium and the role of the limbus had been recognized at least since the mid-twentieth century, long before the concept of "limbal stem cell deficiency" (LSCD) was formulated. In 1964, during a discussion at the first World Cornea Congress [1], José I. Barraquer described the use "epithelial conjunctivo-corneal limbus taken from the other eye" for the treatment of superficial burns of a single affected eye. In 1966, Strampelli et al. published a case of an opaque and highly vascularized cornea treated by the transplantation of a complete limbal ring from the fellow eye [2]. The following year, Strampelli presented a second case and described his technique in more detail at the 2nd International Corneo-Plastic Conference in London [3]. During the 1970 and

1980s, Joaquin Barraquer performed in Barcelona similar cases of 360° ring limbal transplants (Fig. 12.1) and later published his technique (Figs. 12.2 and 12.3) [4].

While relevant research on corneal epithelial regeneration and homeostasis can be traced back to the 1940s [5], the crucial role of the "limbal stem cells"—or, more precisely, corneal epithelial stem cells (CESC)—was understood only during the 1970s and 1980s [6, 7]. Richard Thoft was most likely unaware of this when he tried "conjunctival transplantation" for unilateral chemical burns (published in 1977) [8], which failed to obtain a functional corneal surface – as the donor tissue probably did not include CESC. He later described, in 1984, a "kerato-epithelioplasty" procedure [9]—subsequently modified by Turgeon et al. in 1990 [10], which

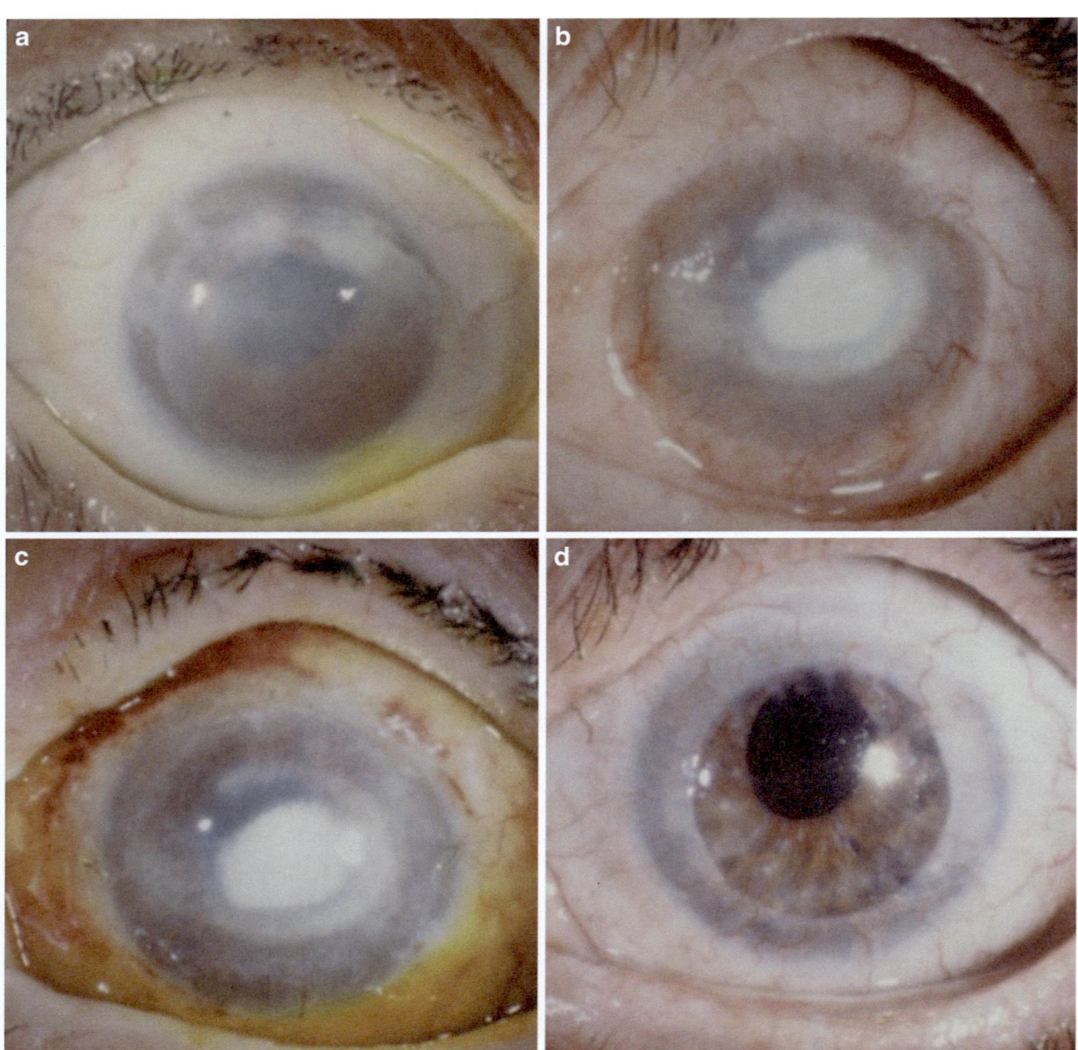

Fig. 12.1 (**a**) Right eye (RE) of a patient who had a chemical burn in her left eye. This RE was amblyopic due to childhood unilateral aphakia. The image shows the status of the ocular surface two months after the removal of a 360° ring of limbal conjunctiva. (**b**) Left eye (LE) of the patient affected by a chemical burn, before the autologous limbal ring transplantation. (**c**) The immediate postoperative result, 15 days after surgery. (**d**) One year after a PK rehabilitate the visual function. (Courtesy of Prof. Joaquin Barraquer, performed in 1981)

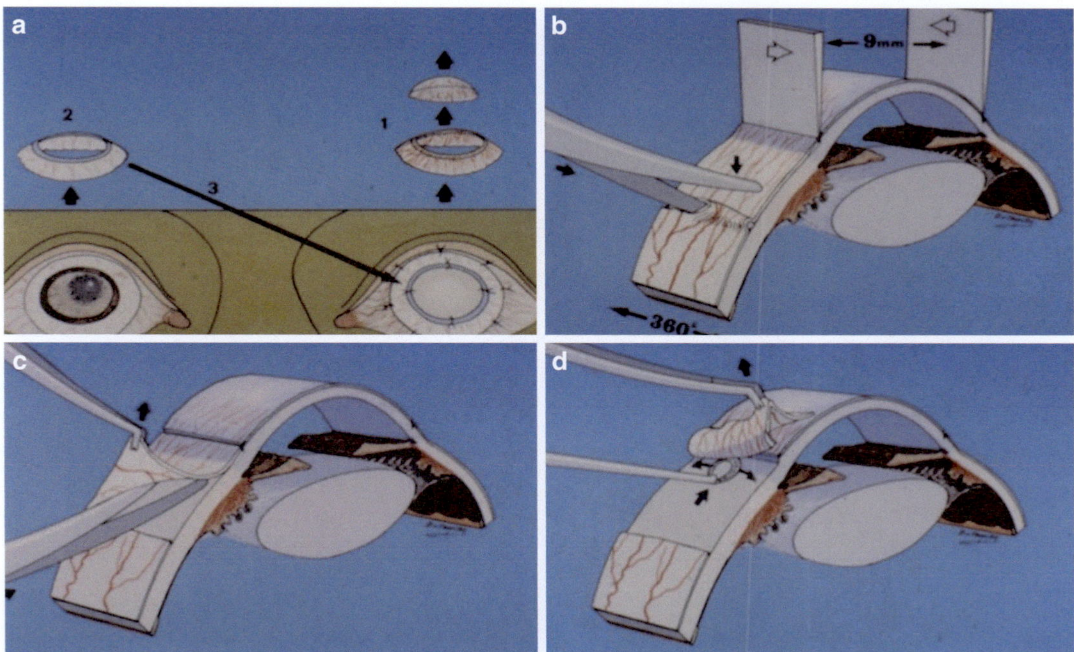

Fig. 12.2 (**a**) Schematic design of a ring-shaped autologous limbal transplant according to J. Barraquer. A ring of limbal tissue including 5 mm. of limbal conjunctiva and peripheral corneal epithelium is obtained from the donor eye and then anchored in the recipient eye, which has previously been subjected to a complete peritomy (**b**), a peripheral keratectomy marked with a superficial 9 mm. partial trephination (**c**), and dissection of the anomalous tissue at the limbus with a crescent blade (**d**). (Art by Emilio Iglesias MD, PhD, 1981, from [4])

involved the application of several thin disks or lenticles from cadaveric peripheral cornea. Although these grafts probably included only a scarce quantity of donor CESC, they represent the first attempt at using allografts for ocular surface reconstruction, which would allow treating bilateral diseases.

In 1989, Kenyon and Tseng were the first to publish a series of limbal transplantations acknowledging the CESC theory [11]. They employed two arcuate segments of conjunctival and peripheral corneal tissue from the fellow eye to treat unilateral LSCD. Their technique remains a standard treatment for most unilateral severe ocular surface disease, especially where ex vivo expansion techniques are not available. In 1994, Tsai and Tseng first described a proper limbal allograft technique using cadaveric donor tissue [12]. One year later, Kwitko et al. reported the use of conjunctiva from a living-related donor—siblings or other living relatives—for treating bilateral LSCD [13]. Their technique was modified by Kenyon and Rapoza to include limbus and conjunctiva from the living relative, being the first description of a living-related conjunctivo-limbal autograft (lr-CLAL) procedure [14]. This chapter will review the classical (nontissue engineered) techniques of limbal transplantation, especially the keratolimbal and their outcomes, innovations and alternatives.

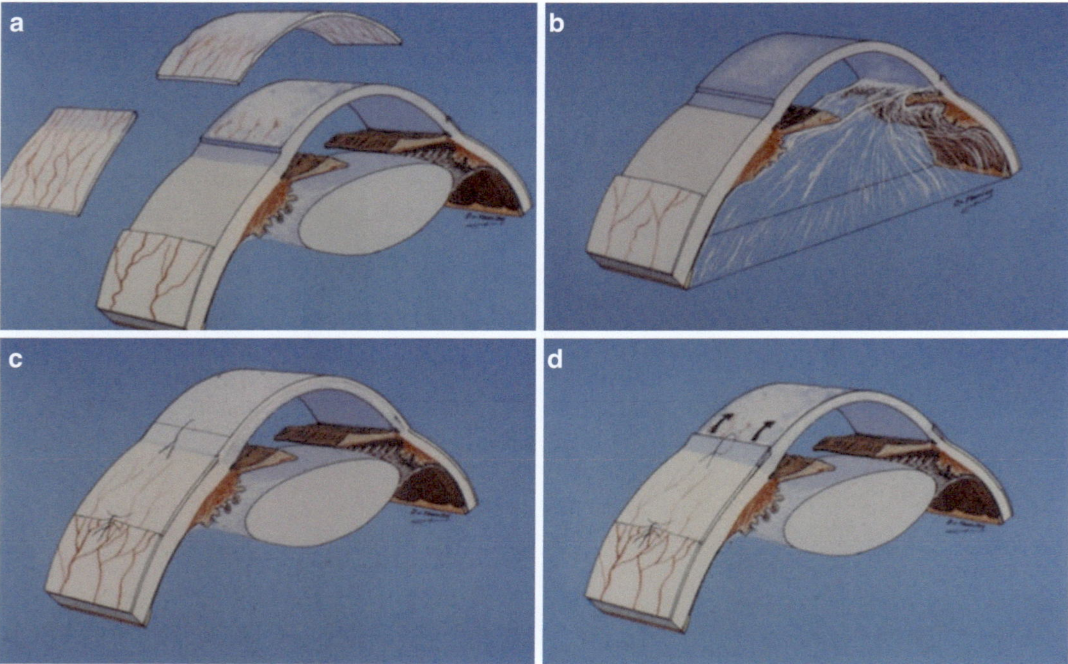

Fig. 12.3 (**a**) Complete removal of the fibro-vascular tissue covers recipient cornea and limbus. (**b**) Recipient's eye is prepared with a bare ocular surface. (**c**) The ring autograft is then anchored with sutures in the conjunctival and corneal circumferences. (**d**) Limbal area starts repopulating the epithelial layer from the stem cells present in this area. (Art by Emilio Iglesias MD, PhD, 1981, from [4])

Classification of Ocular Surface Transplantation Procedures

The transplantation procedures for ocular surface reconstruction were named as they emerged along several decades, increasingly since the 1980s. As this generated a varied terminology using different criteria, which was prone to cause confusion, Holland and Schwartz proposed in 1996 to classify these techniques according to the anatomical location of the donor tissue and whether the source was the same individual or not [15]. This was further developed by a committee from the Cornea Society into a classification published in 2011 (Table 12.1) [16], which defined the possible procedures according to three features:

1. The histological type of the transplanted tissue: conjunctiva, limbus/conjunctiva, limbus/cornea and other mucosal tissues.

2. The type of donor: either autologous (fellow eye, etc.) or homologous (cadaveric, living-related or living nonrelated).
3. Whether the tissue was transplanted directly or previously cultivated (or otherwise tissue engineered) ex vivo.

This classification established a framework that could eventually incorporate novel techniques and introduced a series of standard abbreviations or acronyms. It favored a better understanding of each technique and clarified the communication between surgeons, allowing a more accurate comparison of the outcomes. In the case of tissue-engineered procedures, despite the specific terms and acronyms proposed by this classification, the general term "cultivated limbal epithelial transplantation" (CLET) still dominates in the literature.

Table 12.1 Classification of ocular surface transplantation procedures, according to the Cornea Society 2011 [16]

Procedure	Abbreviation	Donor	Transplanted tissue
Conjunctival transplantation			
Conjunctival autograft	CAU	Fellow eye	Conjunctiva
Cadaveric conjunctival allograft	c-CAL	Cadaveric	Conjunctiva
Living related conjunctival allograft	Ir-CAL	Living relative	Conjunctiva
Living nonrelated conjunctival allograft	Inr-CAL	Living non-relative	Conjunctiva
Limbal transplantation			
Conjunctival limbal autograft	CLAU	Fellow eye	Limbus/conjunctiva
Cadaveric conjunctival limbal allograft	c-CLAL	Cadaveric	Limbus/conjunctiva
Living related conjunctival limbal allograft	Ir-CLAL	Living relative	Limbus/conjunctiva
Living nonrelated conjunctival limbal allograft	Inr-CIAL	Living non-relative	Limbus/conjunctiva
Keratolimbal autograft	KLAU	Fellow eye	Limbus/cornea
Keratolimbal allograft	KLAL	Cadaveric	Limbus/cornea
Other mucosal transplantation			
Oral mucosa autograft	DMAU	Recipient	Oral mucosa
Nasal mucosa autograft	NMAU	Recipient	Nasal mucosa
Intestine mucosa autograft	IMAU	Recipient	Intestinal mucosa
Peritoneal mucosa autograft	PMAU	Recipient	Peritoneum
Ex vivo cultivated conjunctival transplantation			
Ex vivo cultivated conjunctival autograft	EVCAU	Recipients eye(s)	Conjunctiva
Ex vivo cultivated cadaveric conjunctival allograft	EVc-CAL	Cadaveric	Conjunctiva
Ex vivo cultivated living-related conjunctival allograft	EVIr-CAL	Living relative	Conjunctiva
Ex vivo cultivated living nonrelated conjunctival allograft	EVInr-CAL	Living non-relative	Conjunctiva
Ex vivo limbal transplantation			
Ex vivo cultivated limbal autograft	EVLAU	Recipients eye(s)	Limbus/cornea
Ex vivo cultivated cadaveric limbal allograft	EVc-LAL	Cadaveric	Limbus/cornea
Ex vivo cultivated living-related limbal allograft	EVIr-LAL	Living relative	Limbus/cornea
Ex vivo cultivated living nonrelated limbal allograft	EVInr-LAL	Living non-relative	Limbus/cornea
Other ex vivo cultivated mucosal transplantation			
Ex vivo cultivated oral mucosa autograft	EVOMAU	Recipient	Oral mucosa

Tissue Options

Regarding the procedures for ocular surface rehabilitation, the first feature to be considered is the possible histological components of the graft. The main options include conjunctiva alone or reaching to the limbus, peripheral superficial cornea including the limbus, and other mucous membranes.

While conjunctiva is commonly framed as "the invading tissue" in cases of LSCD, healthy conjunctiva is nonetheless necessary as it is an important contributor to ocular surface homeostasis. This includes its crucial role in the production of mucins—from the goblet cells—and of cytokines, among other (patho-)physiological roles.

Conjunctival tissue for transplantation can be obtained from the same eye, from the patient's fellow eye, or from a donor. It can be harvested from either the bulbar or fornix conjunctiva. The latter has been reported as a greater source of conjunctival stem cells [17]. However, bulbar conjunctiva—especially the superior quadrant—

is more often used due to easier access and faster healing. In any case, a conjunctival graft will not provide CESC if it does not extend to include the limbus.

The CESC is known to be present around the limbus at the epithelial basal cell layer. As the corneal epithelium is continuous with that of the conjunctiva, the precise location of the CESC is not anatomically obvious. Furthermore, their distribution is not uniform around the cornea, especially in several discrete crypts or "niches" related to Vogt's palisades [18]. This creates variability regarding the actual amount of CESC transplanted by a particular technique.

Under the "limbal transplantation" heading in Table 12.1, we actually find two different modalities: "conjunctival limbal" and "keratolimbal" grafts. The former will include a variable amount of CESC depending on how close-cropped to the cornea it has been harvested, which is surgeon dependent. If the tissue is mostly conjunctival, a conjunctival limbal graft may include a few CESC. Conversely, a keratolimbal graft typically comprises a superficial layer of the peripheral cornea up to the limbus, including some conjunctiva and superficial sclera. It will, therefore, contain most of the CESC present in the collected sector.

Conjunctival limbal grafts are mainly used for the reconstruction of a conjunctival defect adjacent to the cornea, as in pterygium or limbal tumor surgery, or in cases with localized LSCD in which there is healthy and functional limbus in the wider remaining sectors. On the other hand, including few CESC in the graft also means lesser aggression to the donor site.

The keratolimbal tissue is preferred in cases with severe or complete LSCD, as it not only provides the lacking CESC but the normal supporting limbal stroma from the donor site as well. This probably favors the recreation of the limbal niches, promoting the long-term maintenance of CESC. Additionally, this kind of

graft also contributes to the repopulation of the corneal surface supplying new epithelial corneal cells. Although most of these will be late transient and postmitotic cells, it has been argued that oligopotent stem cells capable of generating either conjunctival or corneal phenotypes depending on the environment can be found dispersed throughout the entire ocular surface, including the cornea [19]. A downside of a keratolimbal graft is the greater impact on the (living) donor eye as more CESC are harvested.

Among other tissues, oral mucosa is probably the most frequently used for ocular surface reconstruction. It is commonly applied as a substitute for conjunctiva, especially when the latter is not available from the same individual due to bilateral disease, multiple surgeries or when a large surface graft is required. This includes treatment of symblepharon and reconstruction of the conjunctival fornixes, in recalcitrant pterygia and in association with biological keratoprosthesis. Alternatively, other mucous membrane tissues such as nasal, peritoneal and intestinal (rectal) have been used in some cases. While oral and other mucosa lack CESC and normally show a different phenotype, the advantage of being autologous can be an attractive feature in some situations, especially as a source for cultivated grafts [20].

Donor Options

A key parameter for the success and long-term prognosis in ocular surface transplantation is the relationship between donor and recipient, as can be represented by the degree of histocompatibility. The preferred tissue source is—in principle—the autologous, as no immune homograft reaction can occur. Unfortunately, this is not an option in cases with bilateral disease, at least for the same tissue from the fellow eye.

The second-best source is a compatible living donor: a parent or sibling with at least half of the major histocompatibility antigens identical. In this scenario, HLA types I and II should be determined for all the relatives and potential family donors.

In cases of nonrelated living or cadaveric donors, some degree of tissue matching should be attempted to improve the results. Tissue engineering techniques might offer the possibility of modifying the immunogenicity of cultivated cells, to decrease the immune rejection to homologous ex vivo amplified grafted cells.

Limbal Autograft Techniques

Limbal autografts, including conjunctival limbal and keratolimbal (respectively CLAU and KLAU) remain the corneal surface rehabilitation procedures with the largest record of success and best prognosis [21, 22]. Apart from avoiding the risk of immune rejection, autologous tissue generally offers better viability than the cadaveric, as the latter involves some degree of postmortem decay, somewhat more traumatic harvesting, and preservation methods that are only partially physiologic. The living-related sources do not have these last limitations but are relatively rare.

The donor tissue in CLAU comprises conjunctiva with some peripheral limbal epithelial cells (Fig. 12.4a, b), while in KLAU, it includes the limbal conjunctiva and peripheral superficial corneal—stroma and epithelium—including Vogt's palisades (Fig. 12.4c, d). As discussed above, this has an impact in the amount of CESC harvested.

In CLAU, donor conjunctiva is dissected carefully, separating Tenon's capsule up to its limbal insertion, and a superficial sheet of limbal (peripheral corneal) epithelium is cut with scissors, without including Bowman's membrane. This technique is mainly used for pterygium surgery (Fig. 12.5). However, there is little hard evidence on whether the limbal component of these grafts—which may be variable depending on a particular surgeon's technique—represents any significant benefit compared to a standard conjunctival graft.

In KLAU (Video 12.1), a portion of the peripheral superficial corneal stroma and the epithelium is included in the donor tissue. After dissecting the conjunctiva centripetally, a 0.15–0.20 mm groove is performed with a blade at the limbal sclera; lamellar dissection of the peripheral superficial corneal stroma is then performed, dissecting approximately 1.0–1.5 mm of the peripheral cornea. This donor tissue will include most of the CESC niches present at the local Vogt's palisades. In cases with severe unilateral LSCD, the KLAU grafts are usually obtained from the fellow eye-one or two limbal segments of up to 90° width each (Fig. 12.6). For treating a localized LSCD, a "translocation of the limbus" technique can be used, which corresponds to a KLAU from the same eye (Fig. 12.7).

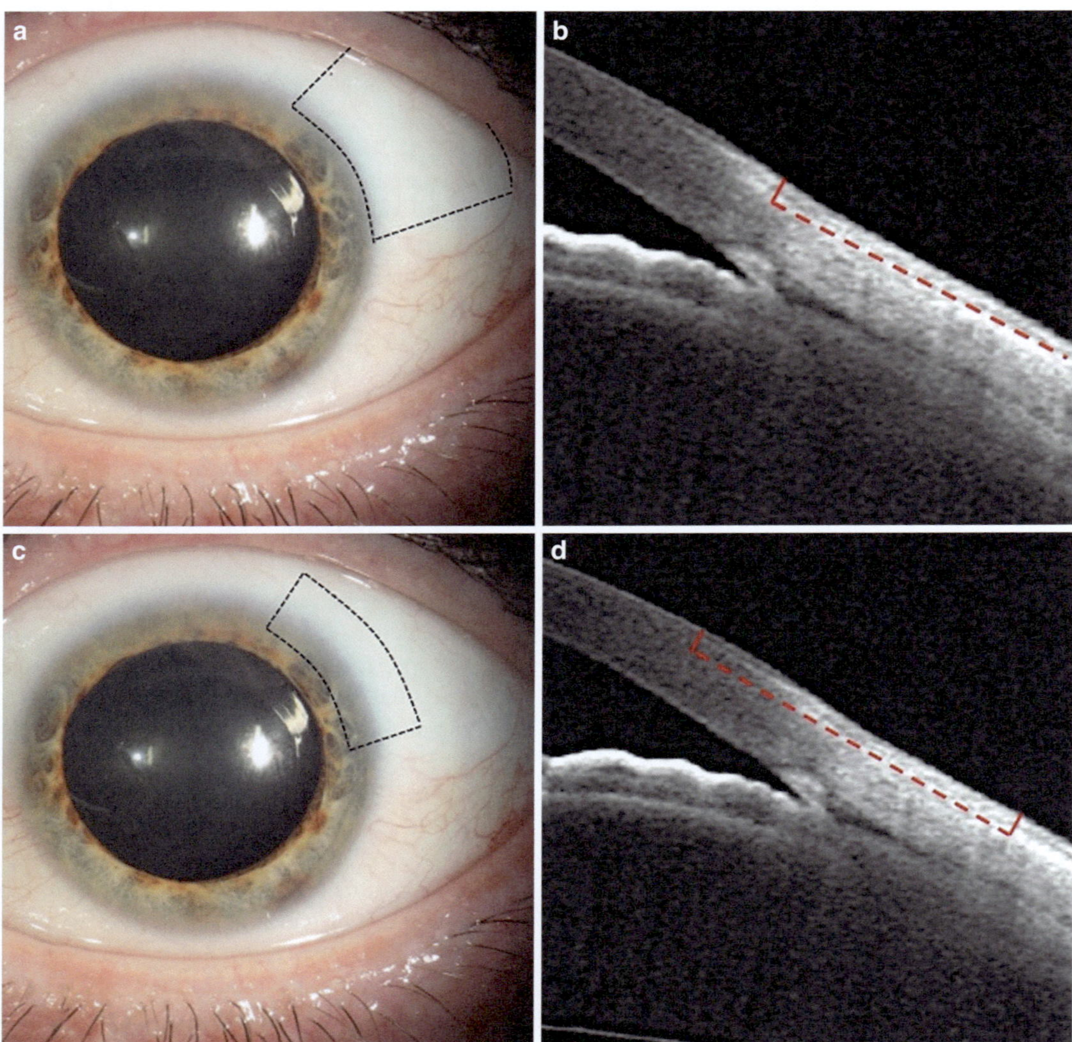

Fig. 12.4 (**a**) Delimitation of the area of a CLAU. Only an epithelial part of the limbal area is removed. (**b**) Dissection of the conjunctiva is done by splitting Tenon's capsule, which would induce retraction of the graft if included. (**c**, **d**) KLAU dissection includes peripheral superficial corneal stroma, epithelium and superficial limbal sclera to ensure the inclusion of all the niches of the CESC

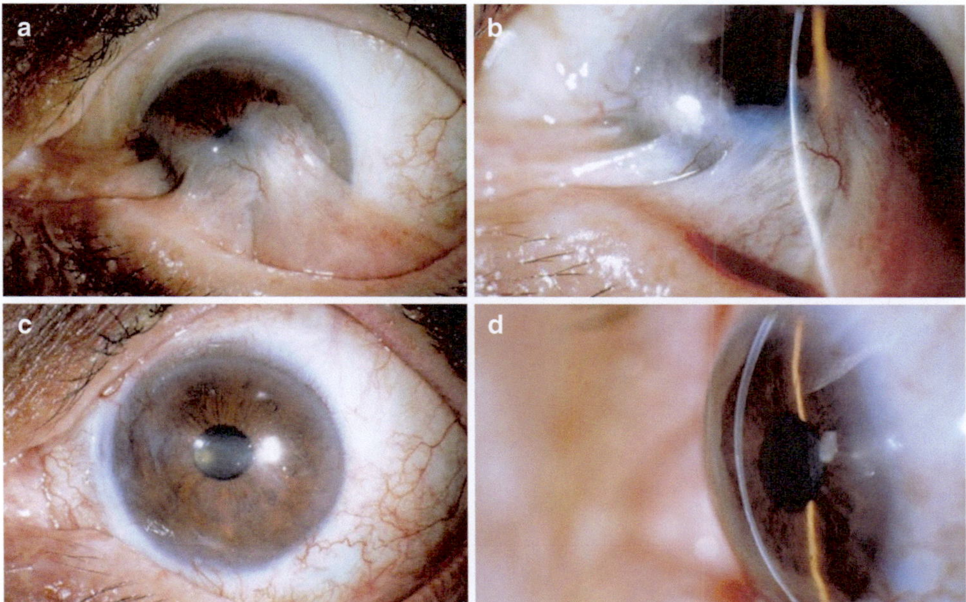

Fig. 12.5 (**a**) Recurrent pterygium after four surgeries with multiple corneal adherences and inferior-nasal symblepharon (detail in **b**). (**c**) Result after careful removal of the recurrent pterygium, symblepharon, superficial keratectomy and CLAU. (**d**) Slit lamp appearance of the result. The clear and re-epithelialized cornea shows some thinning of the inferior due to the keratectomy

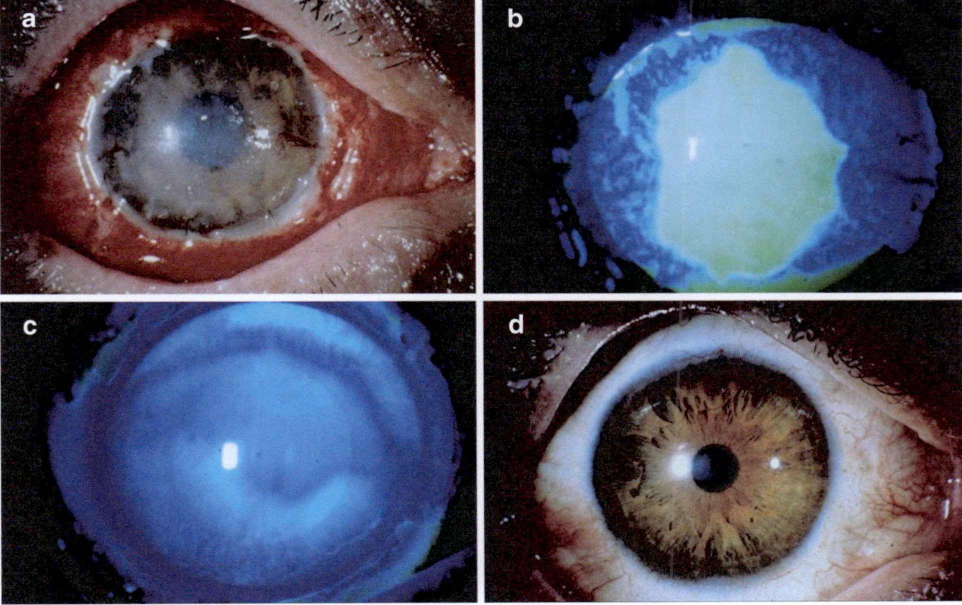

Fig. 12.6 (**a**) Keratolimbal autograft (KLAU) in a patient with a unilateral chemical burn in his RE. Two autografts were positioned in the superior and inferior limbus one day after surgery. (**b**) Centripetal re-epithelialization from the limbal autografts at day 2 postoperative (fluorescein staining). (**c**) Complete epithelial layer with no staining, 6 days after the surgery. (**d**) Stable ocular surface and improvement in corneal transparency 9 years after KLAU. Patient's BCVA reached 0.9 with RGP CL

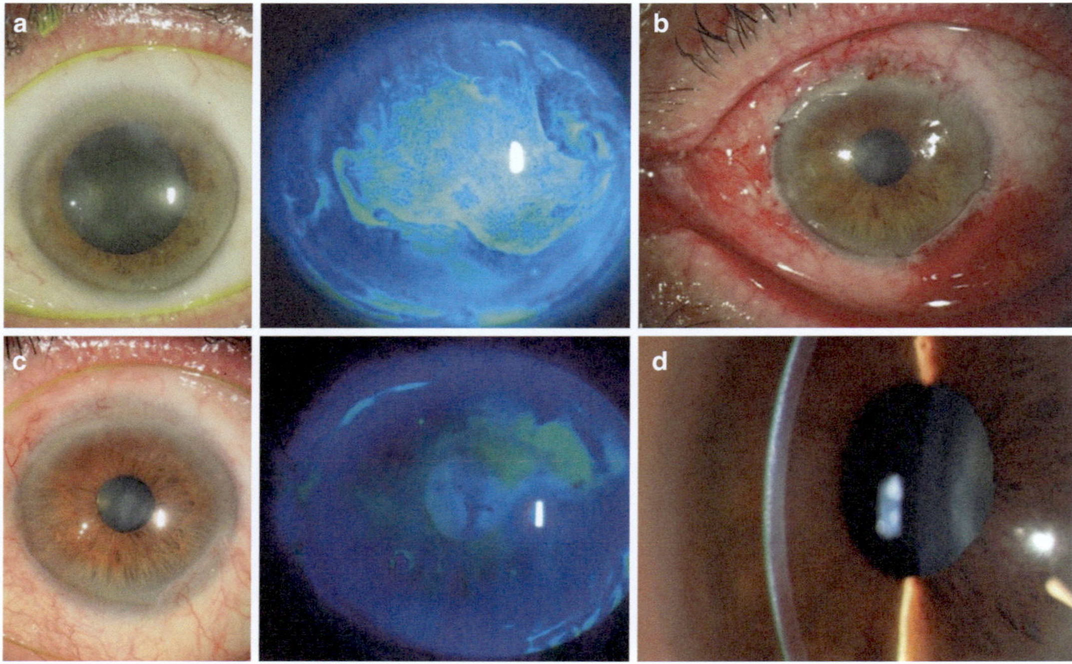

Fig. 12.7 (**a**) Limbal stem cell deficiency (LSCD) in the only eye of a patient after more than 20 intravitreal anti-VEGF injections through the upper nasal sclera. LSCD may be due to toxicity from the antiseptic or anaesthetic drugs applied during repeated procedures. (**b**) Single sector-KLAU from the inferior quadrant of this only eye (limbal translocation) and grafted in the superior nasal zone. (**c**) Two months later, a complete and healthy epithelium covers the cornea. (**d**) Corneal superficial stroma still shows a tenuous opacity, but BCVA and subjective symptomatology improved

Limbal Allograft Techniques

In cases with total bilateral LSCD, allogeneic limbal transplantation is the best option—short of a keratoprosthesis—to repopulate the affected ocular surface with CESC. Initial series of successful limbal allografts were published in the 1990s. Turgeon et al. reported on 13 patients in which Thoft's technique (kerato-epithelioplasty) was performed to stabilize the ocular surface affected with persistent epithelial defects [10]. Tsai and Tseng reported a series of 16 eyes with several causes of LSCD (chemical burns, Stevens-Johnson syndrome, congenital sclerocornea, Terrien's degeneration and chronic conjunctivitis) in which a limbal ring-shaped allograft was grafted as a source of CESC [12].

Donor age does not seem to be a critical factor for a successful clinical result. CESC cultures obtained from older donors showed >3% of p63+ cells, considered as the minimum value to predict a favorable outcome [23]. Routine hypothermic storage in liquid media at 4 °C is generally used to preserve the donor limbal tissue, but novel methods of preservation like hypothermic air-lifted conditions have demonstrated better maintenance of the epithelial structure, cell phenotype and higher viability of the stem cell pool [24].

Limbal allotransplants can be performed in different modalities. Isolated allografts are usually of the keratolimbal type (KLAL). Conjunctival limbal allografts (CLAL) combine the disadvantages of a high risk of rejection due to the vascularized tissue and low yield of CESC and are rarely performed. KLAL can be sectorial or ring-shaped (especially from cadaveric donors) as the latter can supply more CESC. All of these can also be combined with keratoplasty, as discussed below.

Ring-shaped KLAL is the most widely used technique to treat bilateral LSCD (Fig. 12.8). A 360° ring of keratolimbal tissue is obtained from a fresh cadaver eye (Fig. 12.9), with the inner and outer diameters appropriately marked with different trephines. Ring width and thickness should be enough to include the whole corneoscleral limbal zone including the CESC niches.

In the recipient's eye, a complete limbal peritomy and removal of the superficial corneal vascular pannus and scarring, including any perilimbal fibrosis, is mandatory. When the recipient Bowman's membrane is absent, the human amniotic membrane (hAM) can be fixated under the limbal allograft, covering the corneal stroma to promote epithelial repopulation, decrease the stromal inflammation and inhibit the neovascularization. A stable tear film and good eyelid function are paramount to achieving long-term success (Fig. 12.10).

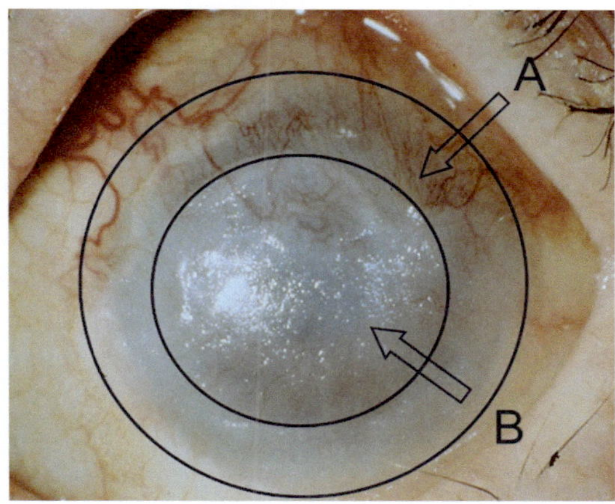

Fig. 12.8 Schematic representation of a ring-shaped KLAL. After removal of the pannus and fibrovascular tissue in the recipient's cornea and limbal area, a ring-shaped limbal allograft including limbal conjunctiva, superficial sclera and cornea is placed in the limbal area and secured with sutures

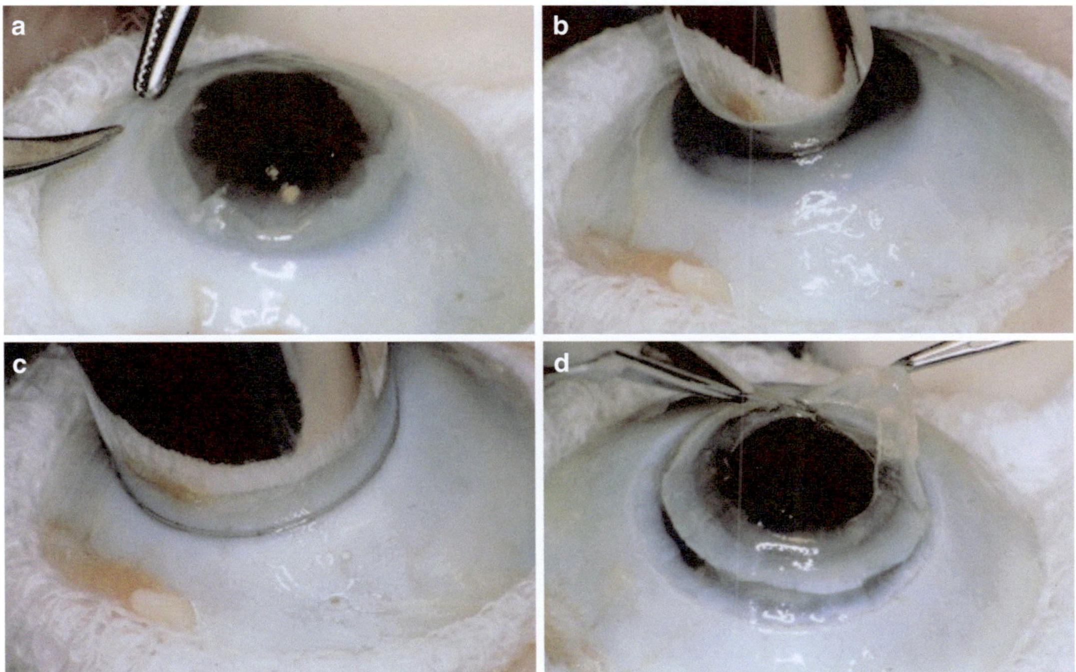

Fig. 12.9 (a) Harvesting of a ring-shaped KLAL from a fresh cadaveric eye. Conjunctiva is cut 3–5 mm. from the limbus and reflected over the corneal surface. (b) The inner diameter of the ring is marked with an 8–9 mm. trephine, which penetrates 0.15–0.20 mm in the corneal stroma. (c) The outer scleral diameter is also marked and trephined with a 13–14 mm. trephine. (d) A careful lamellar dissection is performed to obtain a ring of limbal tissue containing all the pool of the donor's CESC

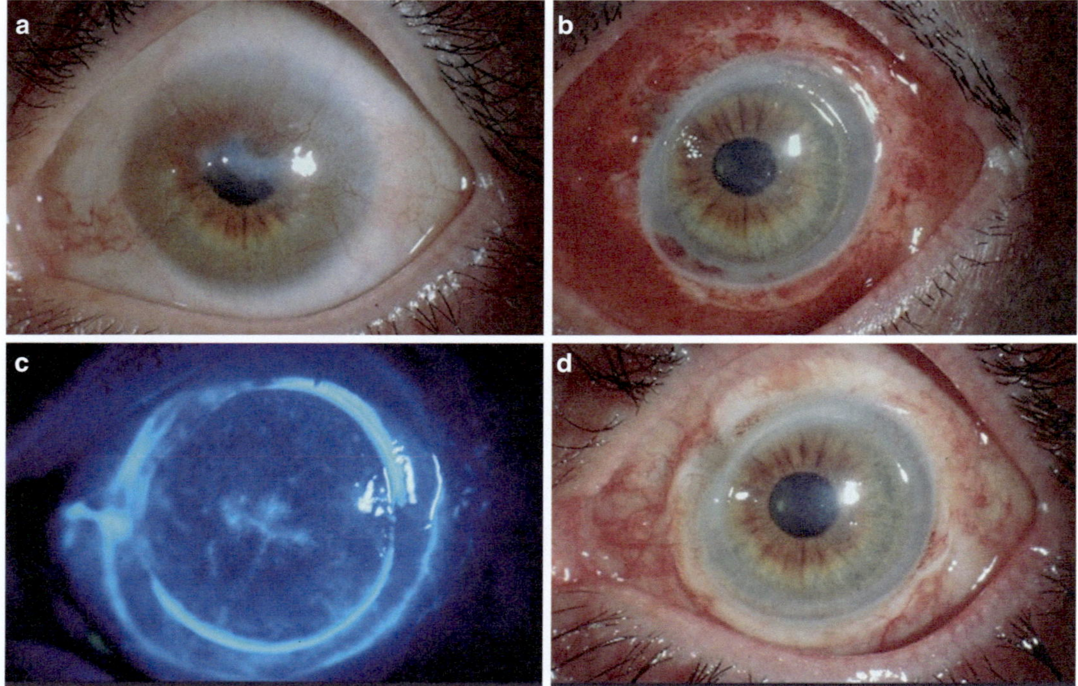

Fig. 12.10 (**a**) Bilateral chemical burn with superficial pannus and central corneal leukoma. (**b**) Ring-shaped KLAL four days after surgery. Only the outer border of the graft was sutured with 8-0 vicryl sutures, and no suture was placed at the inner circle. (**c**) Complete re-epithelialization, still with closure lines that are visible with fluorescein in the central cornea. (**d**) Final result one year after surgery with a stable epithelium and clear cornea. The patient is maintained under oral cyclosporine A

Sectorial KLAL (Fig. 12.11) consists in fixating two arcuate segments of limbal tissue from a donor (living-related or cadaveric) over the recipient limbus—typically at the vertical meridians, after removing the abnormal superficial corneal and limbal tissue. It is indicated in cases with total bilateral LSCD with less extensive or without vascularization and scarring of the ocular surface (Fig. 12.12). hAM can also be applied under the sectorial grafts to promote re-epithelialization.

Clear information of the advantages and possible complications of the different options should be given to the patients and to the potential living-related donors, highlighting the benefits of being the source of tissue for their affected relatives.

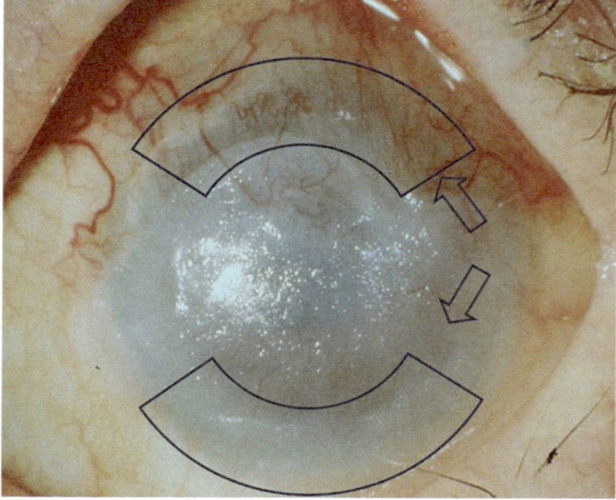

Fig. 12.11 Schematic representation of a sectorial KLAL. After the removal of the pannus and fibrovascular tissue in the recipient's cornea and limbal area, two wide limbal allografts of 90° width are placed at the superior and inferior limbus

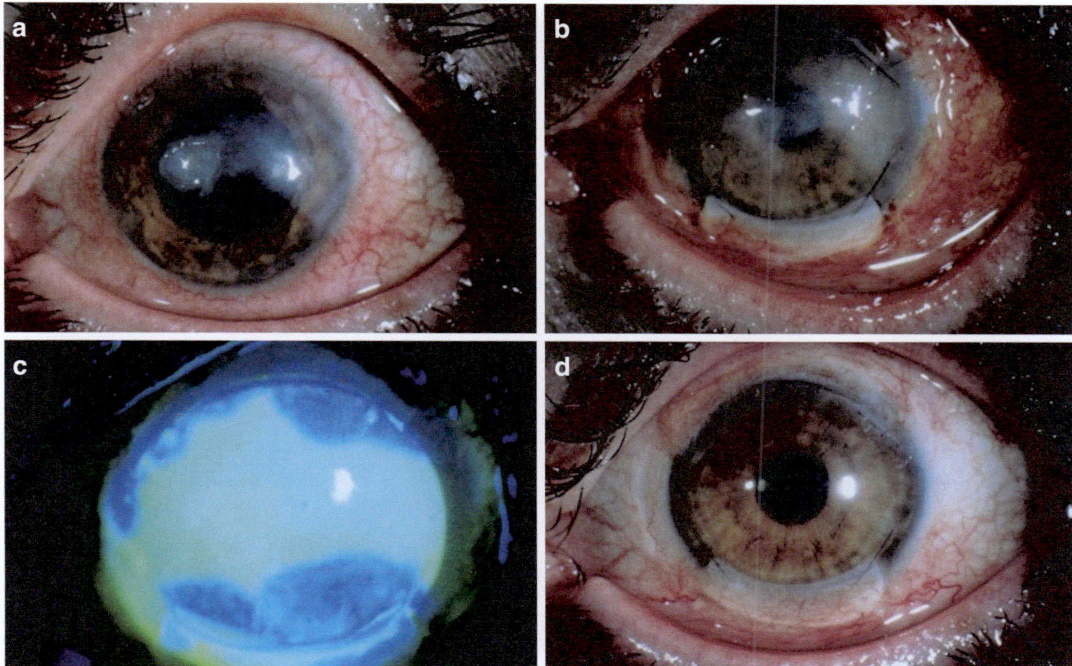

Fig. 12.12 (**a**) Bilateral LSCD in a patient due to chronic contact lens abuse. Persistent epithelial defects and superficial stromal scarring. (**b**) Sectorial KLAL with two limbal grafts placed in the vertical meridian of the limbus. (**c**) New epithelial centripetal growth from the two limbal allografts. (**d**) Complete reepithelialization and recovery of the corneal transparency observed one year after the surgery

Combined Techniques

A combined conjunctival autograft and kerato-limbal allograft (CLAU + KLAL), sometimes referred as "the modified Cincinnati procedure" [25], uses two fragments of recipient's conjunctiva obtained from the fellow eye and two sectors of a cadaveric donor keratolimbal ring. The conjunctival grafts are placed superior and inferiorly, while the keratolimbal allograft sectors are placed nasally and temporally.

In cases of LSCD associated with opacity and/or substance loss affecting the central corneal stroma, limbal transplantation (KLAU, CLAU or KLAL) can be combined with keratoplasty—either DALK (Fig. 12.13) or PK (Fig. 12.14) (Video 12.2). The addition of CESC will improve ocular surface stability and reduce the risk of neovascularization of the corneal graft. In unilateral cases where the fellow eye can be the donor (KLAU), a DALK or PK is performed following the standard techniques after all the superficial tissue invading the cornea has been removed. Once the corneal suture is completed, one or two autografts of up to 3 clock hours (90°) each are obtained from the fellow eye and anchored at the recipient limbus with monofilament sutures (10-0 nylon or 11-0 polyester), usually at the vertical sectors – most commonly the upper when a single graft is placed.

In bilateral LSCD with central corneal stromal opacity and/or substance loss, a ring-shaped KLAL can also be combined with simultaneous DALK or PK plus superficial keratectomy (Fig. 12.15). This procedure may also be indicated in cases where the depth and removability of the corneal opaque tissue are in doubt, and an isolated KLAL may not provide the rapid visual recovery required (or demanded) by the patient (Fig. 12.16). The inner diameter of the KLAL ring is the same as that of the central corneal

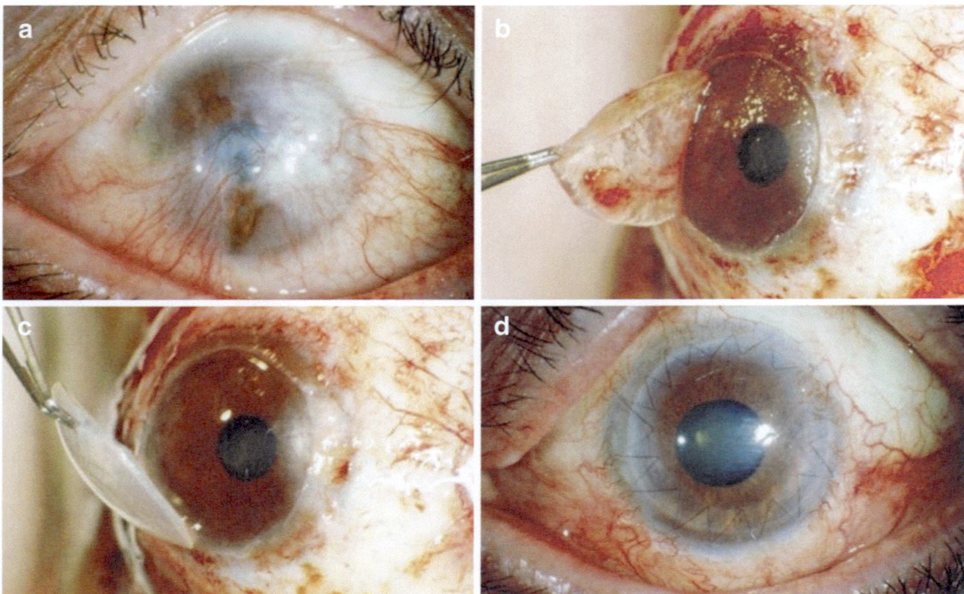

Fig. 12.13 (**a**) Corneal opacity and neovascularization after previous failed pterygium surgery. (**b**) Lamellar keratectomy was performed manually until reaching a transparent corneal stromal plane. (**c**) After reconstructing the limbal conjunctiva with a CLAU from the fellow eye, a lamellar corneal graft was sutured in the corneal bed. (**d**) Result 6 months after the procedure with a stable ocular surface and a transparent corneal graft

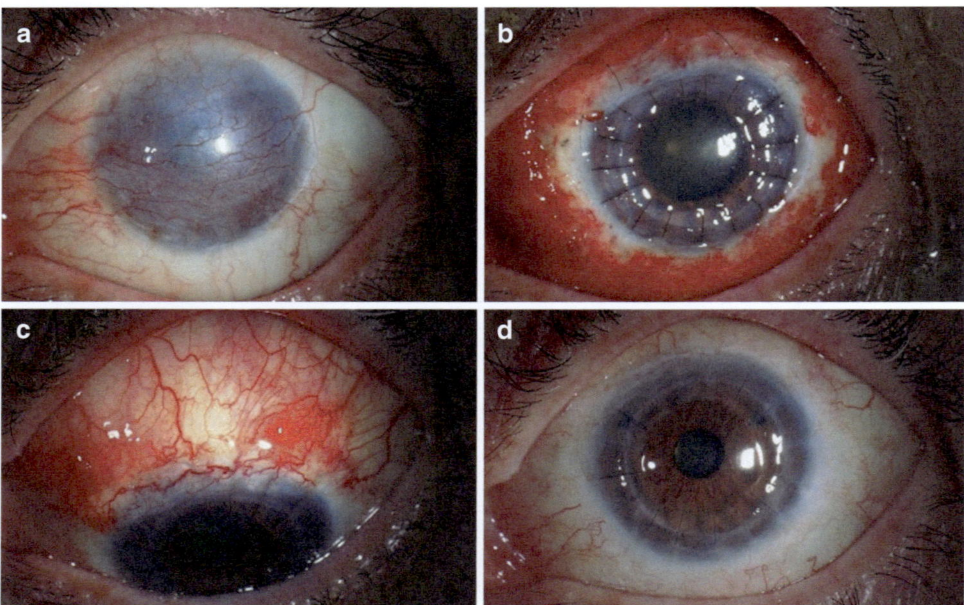

Fig. 12.14 (**a**) Total superficial corneal neovascularization after a previous conjunctival flap performed to treat bacterial keratitis with risk of perforation. (**b**) Combined PK with KLAU in the superior limbus. (**c**) KLAU is fixed in position with good revascularization. (**d**) Transparent corneal graft and stable ocular surface 1 year after the procedure

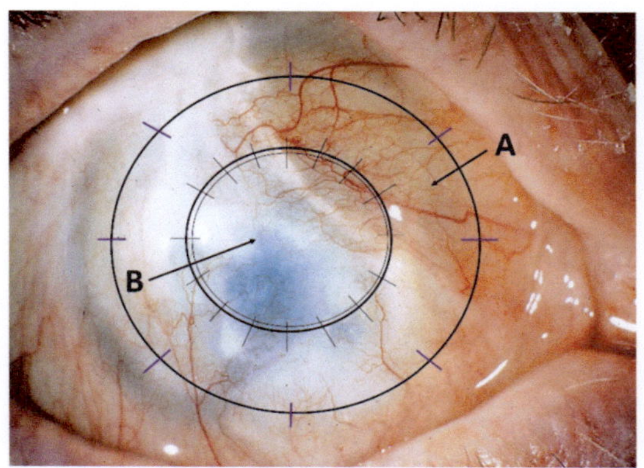

Fig. 12.15 Schematic representation of a ring-shaped KLAL combined with central lamellar or penetrating keratoplasty. After the removal of the pannus and fibrovascular tissue in the recipient's cornea and limbal area, a central keratoplasty is performed and fixed with eight temporary monofilament sutures. Then, a ring-shaped limbal allograft (**a**) including limbal conjunctiva, superficial sclera, and cornea is placed in the limbal area and fixed to the sclera with eight vicryl sutures at the outer edge. The central circle of the ring is sutured to the keratoplasty with eight additional monofilament sutures (**b**), while the initial temporary sutures are replaced with eight additional that include the three tissues

graft. After this has been fixated with eight temporary 10-0 nylon or 11-0 polyester interrupted sutures, the ring-shaped KLAL is placed on top of the peripheral recipient cornea, and its outer perimeter fixated to the sclera with 10-0 nylon or 9-0 vicryl sutures. The inner circle of the KLAL is secured to the corneal graft with eight additional monofilament sutures of the same material used for the temporary fixation, which is then replaced by other sutures including the three tissues in their bites. Finally, 8-0 or 9-0 vicryl is used to secure the conjunctiva included in with the donor tissue and that of the recipient.

A single large diameter DALK or PK, trephined eccentrically in the donor (Fig. 12.17), will include a sector of the donor's limbal area with its CESC. This procedure, named "limbo-keratoplasty" by Sundmacher et al. in 1997 [26] is technically less demanding that the previously described but has a higher risk of epithelial failure due to the smaller proportion (up to 40%) of the limbal zone included in the graft. With the recent advances in immunosuppression, better

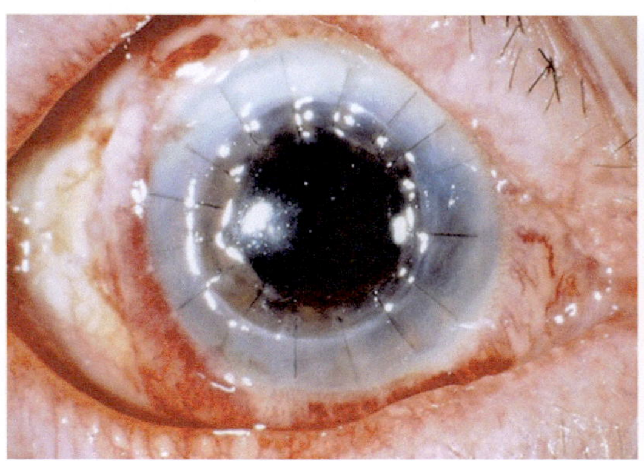

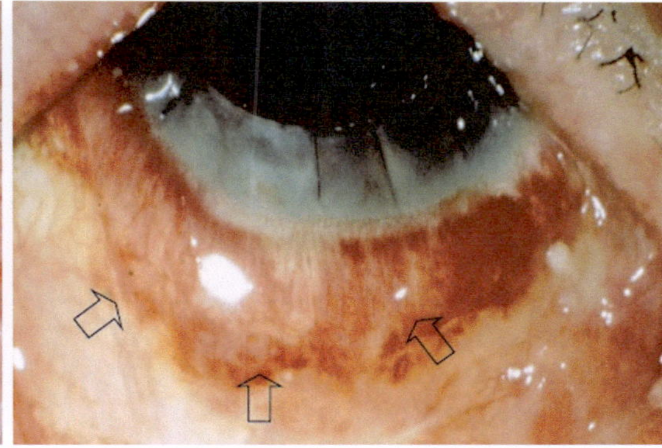

Fig. 12.16 Combined ring-shaped KLAL with PK in a case of Stevens-Johnson syndrome. The limits of the donor conjunctiva is highlighted (arrows). Typical postop-erative intra-tissular hemorrhage that occurs before re-connection of the blood microcirculation has been completed

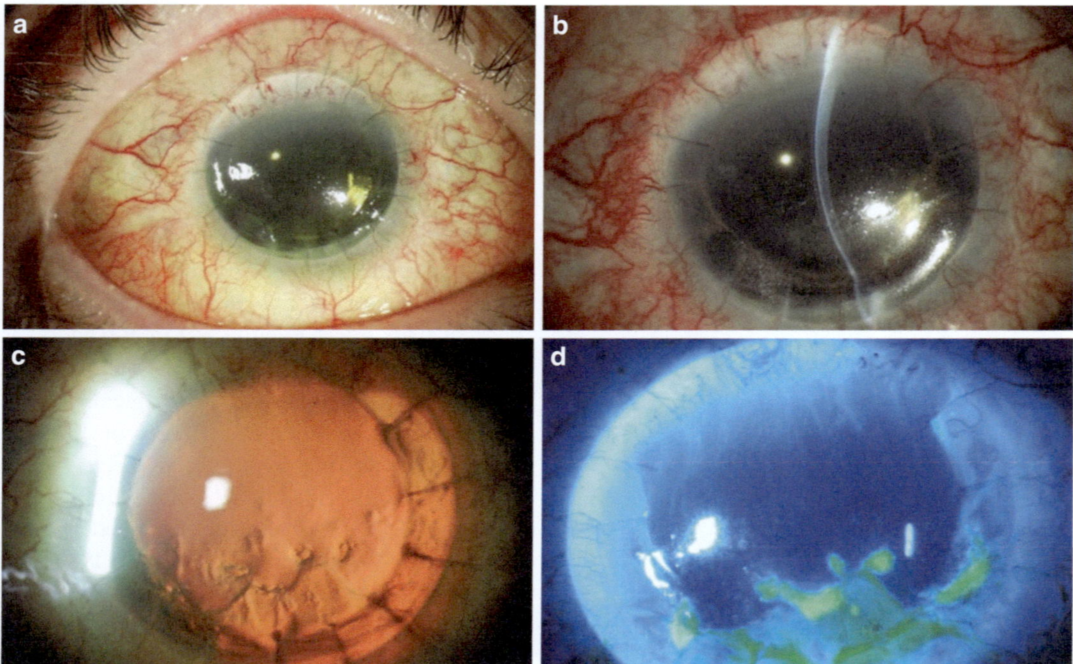

Fig. 12.17 (**a**) Limbokeratoplasty of 9 mm of diameter performed in the single eye of a congenital aniridia affected patient. (**b**) Around 40% of the donor limbus is included in the graft when trephined eccentrically. (**c**) Epithelial irregularities in the inferior cornea are seen under retroillumination. (**d**) Normal corneal epithelium pattern with fluorescein in the superior and central cornea; epithelial defects and conjunctival cell staining pattern in the inferior cornea, demonstrating that LSCD is present in the inferior limbus. Graft failed 3 years after surgery due to recurrence of LSCD

long-term results have been reported with this procedure in less severe special indications like gelatinous drop-like corneal dystrophy [27].

Postoperative Management, Outcomes and Complications After Limbal Autografts

In order to achieve an optimal outcome, ocular surface reconstruction procedures must be rationally planned and staged. The main issues after a limbal autograft relates to the healing process in both the donor and recipient eyes.

For a CLAU, the preferred area to obtain the donor tissue is the superior or superior-temporal conjunctival quadrant—of either the fellow or the same eye—due to the protection offered by the upper lid in the postoperative period. Scarring and fibrosis of the donor area, even granuloma and symblepharon in the upper fornix can occur when the donor area is not properly repaired, especially in individuals predisposed to scarring or poorly compliant of the postoperative steroid treatment.

One possible concern in cases of autografts is to induce LSCD in the donor eye, which has been rarely reported, even after CLAU [28]. Although LSCD has never been described in a healthy donor eye when at least half of the limbal circumference had been respected, any subclinical LSCD must be ruled out in the potential donor eye. One case of Mooren's ulcer has been reported after a CLAU procedure for recurrent pterygium [29].

KLAU are as a rule very successful, provided some guidelines are strictly followed. Rare and relatively minor complications have been reported after KLAU [30], including infections of the donor site, filamentary keratitis, negative fluorescein staining and subconjunctival hemorrhage. Astigmatism can be induced if the corneal stroma is removed too deep or too centrally. It has been documented that the CESC completely repopulate the donor limbal area within 1 year after the procedure [31].

However, autologous limbal transplantation (CLAU or KLAU) will not work if the ocular surface and cornea of the recipient's eye (including the stroma) are severely inflamed, and there is a tear film deficiency or eyelid malposition. All these factors should be medically or surgically corrected in advance. Postoperative treatment to ensure the survival of the CESC and a promote the correct regrowth of a stable corneal epithelial layer usually includes from a judicious use of steroids and unpreserved lubricants to advanced topical treatments such as carboxyl-methyl-glucose polysulfate, autologous serum or growth factors-enriched plasma drops and amniotic membrane extracts.

Postoperative Management, Outcomes and Complications after Limbal Allografts

Limbal allografts are at high risk of immune rejection due to the vascularity of the limbus, which negates the immune privilege of the central cornea, and because their antigen load is much larger than that of a standard PK, due to the presence of different cell types including Langerhans'.

Initial reports on lr-CLAL showed increased graft survival when performed with high HLA matching (0-1 mismatches) [32]. An early deep review of the evidence-based published results of limbal transplantations [33] found significantly better results with autologous tissue but no differences between KLAL and lr-CLAL ($p = 0.328$). Patients with Stevens-Johnson syndrome (SJS) and those with concurrent hAM transplantation had poorer prognosis and long-term surface improvement. The use of living-related tissue has

been confirmed as beneficial in more recent reports [34].

While oral immunosuppression is a key factor in the long-term success of limbal allografts, most ophthalmologists not specialized in this field are not familiar with the required protocols and their general side effects. Even though these are not serious in most cases [35], specific knowledge and experience is required for proper management. According to the postoperative evolution of each patient, these treatments must be frequently adjusted, which requires the participation of a specialist in immunosuppression—usually an internist—in their monitoring.

Holland et al. published in 2012 their 10-year results with a protocol involving two oral immunosuppressants (mycophenolate mofetil and tacrolimus) combined with 1 mg/kg oral prednisone, all of which should be started 1 week before surgery. Tacrolimus levels are adjusted to 8–10 ng/ml the first month postoperative and to 5–8 ng/ml at 6 months postoperative. Oral prednisone is slowly tapered and discontinued after 3 months [36]. One year after the procedure, monotherapy can be considered, and 3 years after surgery, oral medication can be stopped if the ocular surface is stable. Other protocols consist in combinations of azathioprine and cyclosporine A with prednisone.

In Holland's protocol, absolute contraindications for oral immunosuppression include patients with a history of previous malignancy 5 years before, nonadherence to a strict clinical or laboratory follow up or medications, and significant health issues like diabetes, uncontrolled hypertension, renal insufficiency, severe heart diseases or other organ failures. Age over 70 is also a contraindication, and patients between 60 and 70 years are selected for immunosuppression depending on their general health.

A further report from the Holland group in 2017 found KLAL to achieve a true ocular surface stability in 72.7% of cases with a mean follow up of 9.1 years, provided the appropriate selection criteria and proper immunosuppression were applied "and the procedure repeated as needed" [37]. Obviously, including this last option conditions the meaning "long-term success", as the actual survival of a particular transplant is frequently shorter.

The topical measures previously commented regarding the postoperative management of autologous limbal grafts also apply to allografts, plus the possible role of topical immunosuppressives [38].

Discontinuation of oral immunosuppression remains a controversial issue. Acute rejection has been described [39] in a series of six patients more than 3 years after a KLAL procedure, suggesting that donor cells are still present, thus at risk of acute rejection. Therefore, long-term or indefinite immunosuppression should be considered despite a good mid-term result. Rare complications of a limbal allograft include the possible transmission of a donor infection [40], a conjunctival neoplasia [41], and even a systemic malignancy [42].

Simple Epithelial Limbal Transplantation (SLET): A Real Innovation?

In 2012, Sangwan et al. presented a novel surgical technique for transplanting CESC that they called "Single Epithelial Limbal Transplantation" (SLET) [43]. This was initially described as an autograft from the fellow eye limbus and later as an allograft from a fresh cadaveric coneo-scleral rim [44]. It involves first fixating an hAM graft with fibrin glue over the ocular surface – previously bared by a superficial keratectomy to remove the abnormal tissue. A small piece from the donor limbus is harvested, cut into tiny fragments and placed over the hAM in a circular fashion – avoiding the visual axis. A layer of fibrin glue is applied to fixate these small tissue "explants", and finally, a bandage soft contact lens is fitted over the cornea. These multiple fragments of CESC-containing tissue will originate a new epithelial multilayer, favored by the known beneficial effects of hAM on cell growth.

The minimal amount of tissue needed for assure a correct growth of epithelial cells has been established by in vitro studies in about

0.3 mm^2 of a live limbal fragment including a CESC niche [45]. Depending of the donor source (cadaver or live tissue) the growth potential is different, being necessary a larger amount of cadaveric tissue (0.5 mm^2) to obtain a similar proliferative rate as with the live tissue.

A large series of 125 eyes treated with autologous SLET found an overall success of 76% after 1.5 years of follow-up, with progressive conjunctivalization in 18.4% of treated eyes [46]. The main factors of failure were acid injury, severe symblepharon, SLET combined with keratoplasty and postoperative loss of the transplants, which highlights the importance of performing the procedure in quiet eyes without inflammation and with previously repaired eyelid or conjunctival malposition. Success with allogeneic SLET has also been reported by the same group [47].

Since its description, SLET has been applied to a variety of conditions—from chemical injuries to ocular surface tumors, among many others, with a success comparable to both CLAU and CLET, with the restoration of the corneal epithelium in 83% of operations and improvement in visual acuity in 69% of reported cases [48]. Successful SLET has been reported after failed CLET for unilateral chronic ocular burns [49]. SLET has been combined with CLAU for severe chemical burn [50], with pre-descemetic DALK in a case of a massive corneal epibulbar dermoid [51], and with PK for keratolysis after chemical burn [52], or in severe congenital corneal opacities [53]. Several modifications have been proposed, including a "mini-SLET" for pterygium surgery [54] or in pediatric cases [55], a glueless technique [56], and a SLET variant using autologous fornix conjunctiva for the explants instead of limbus [57].

SLET has been described as "an ingenious, low cost and effective technique for limbal stem cell transplantation" [58], and "a paradigm shift in limbal transplantation" [59]. It represents an in vivo or in situ CESC expansion, which employs a small piece of the donor limbus, thus protecting the donor eye in autologous cases. This would extend the indications to those with partial bilateral involvement, as an eye with partially damaged limbus—thus not eligible as donor CLAU/

KLAU—could still donate the small biopsy for SLET. Moreover, SLET bypasses the need for sophisticated and expensive ex vivo cell expansion technology. This may be particularly relevant in countries where these are not available.

Prior to the description of SLET, Kim et al. presented in 2008 another very ingenious and somewhat related technique in which the small limbal biopsy was subjected to "in vivo" expansion over an hAM placed for two weeks on the cornea of a patient's relative. After this time, the hAM with the expanded donor CESC was grafted on the patient's cornea [60].

Conclusion

The management of LSCD is a complex and challenging field, where the many causes and factors involved, together with the heterogeneity of specific situations and the multiple options available, make it difficult to choose the best treatment. As a result, the decision in a particular case will be highly influenced by the preferences of the surgeon and the patient. Nevertheless, a few fundamental factors can be selected in an attempt at establishing a useful and simple decision tree, as shown in Fig. 12.18.

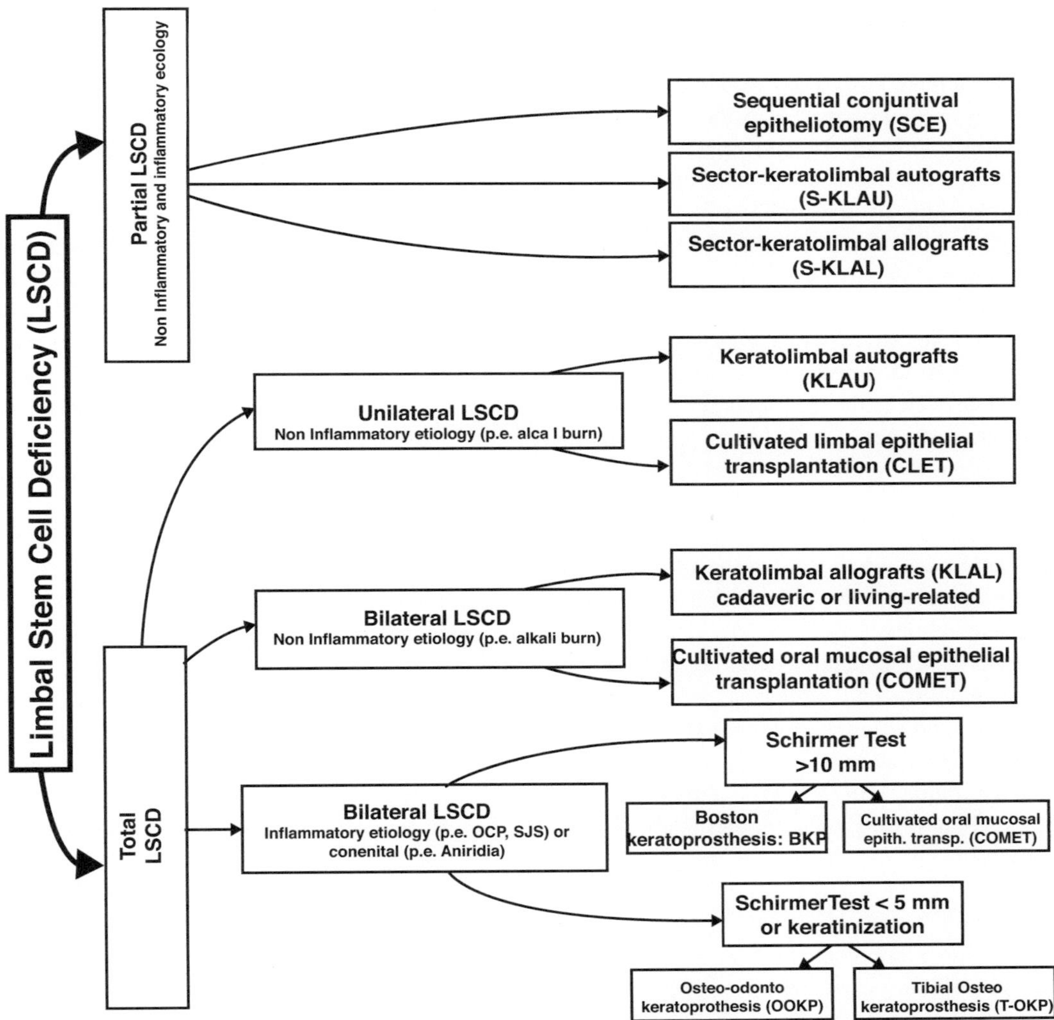

Fig. 12.18 Author's proposed decision tree for the selection of the different surgical procedures for LSCD

In summary, Keratolimbal transplants are established effective and safe techniques for ocular surface reconstruction in many conditions involving moderate to severe LSCD. In unilateral cases, KLAU offers the best combination of efficacy, safety, availability and low cost. This is being challenged by autologous SLET, especially in cases with partial bilateral involvement. In bilateral noninflammatory total LSCD, the different variants of KLAL (preferably living-related if available and with good histocompatibility) and its combinations with other techniques are preferable unless CLET (or COMET) is available and its cost not an issue. Allogeneic SLET may be another option, as well as a KP. These become the preferred alternative in bilateral total LSCD of inflammatory origin.

An adequate knowledge of the pathology and pathophysiology of the condition, together with familiarity with all surgical options and armamentarium, are requisites for the selection of the best procedure. Even techniques like oral mucosa transplantation, which may have been considered old-fashioned at a certain point in time, can be very useful to solve some complex situations. Paramount for success is attention to the preoperative preparation of the ocular environment and adnexa, as well as the postoperative management to promote surface stability and avoid complications. When allografts are required, establishing a close collaboration with the specialist in systemic immunosuppression remains crucial, as the application and monitoring of the adequate treatment protocol appear to substantially improve the long-term results.

As long as the technological complexity, limited availability and high cost of ex vivo cell expansion and regeneration methods hinder their practical application, the classical limbal transplant techniques will remain a valid option offering excellent results when properly indicated and performed.

Take Home Notes

1. The initial approach to the selection of the adequate surgical technique is based on the observation whether the LSCD is partial or total.

 a. In partial LSCD, the milder cases might be manageable with medical measures alone or combined with nontransplant interventions such as the sequential conjunctival epitheliectomy of Dua.

 b. Moderate partial LSCD may require a limited CESC transplant, which could be a sector-KLAU or a mini-SLET (rarely justifying the cost of a CLET or the risks associated with KLAL).

 c. In cases with partial LSCD associated with a conjunctival defect, the techniques in the previous item may be substituted or combined with sector-CLAU.

2. In cases of total LSCD, whether the condition is unilateral or bilateral.

 a. In unilateral total LSCD (typically after a chemical burn), the options include KLAU, CLET and now also autologous SLET.

3. In bilateral total LSCD the main decision factor might be whether the cause is or not inflammatory.

 a. Noninflammatory bilateral total LSCD can be treated with KLAL, allogeneic CLET, and possibly with autologous cultivated oral mucosa epithelial transplantation (COMET) or allogeneic SLET. Keratoprosthesis (KP, including the simpler, allogeneic tissue haptic as in the Boston-KP) becomes an option to consider.

4. In bilateral total LSCD with inflammatory cause (as in SJS and mucous membrane pemphigoid), the preferred treatment are the different types of KP. A fourth decision factor is whether there is or not a severe dry eye.

 a. In a relatively preserved wet ocular surface (Schirmer test >10 mm), the best option for a total bilateral LSCD with (chronic) inflammatory cause is a KP (i.e., Boston-KP, although there may be a role for COMET.

 b. In cases with severe dry eye (Schirmer <5 mm and/or keratinization 9), the options become progressively limited to the autologous tissue-supported KPs, such as the osteo-odonto-KP, the tibia-KP, or a transmucosal Boston-KP [61].

References

1. Barraquer JI. Panel three discussion. In: King JH, McTigue JW, editors. The world cornea congress I. Washington: Butterworths; 1965. p. 354.
2. Strampelli B, Restivo Manfredi ML. Total keratectomy in leukomatous eye associated with autograft of a keratoconjunctival ring removed from the contralateral eye. Ann Ottalmol Clin Ocul. 1966;92:778–86.
3. Strampelli B. Ring autokeratoplasty. In: Rycroft PV, editor. Corneoplastic surgery. Oxford: Pergamon Press; 1969. p. 253–75.
4. Barraquer J, Rutllán J. Microsurgery of the cornea: an atlas and textbook. Barcelona: Ediciones Scriba; 1984. p. 160–2.
5. Buschke W, Friedenwald JS, Fleischmann W. Studies on the mitotic activity of the corneal epithelium; methods; the effects of colchicine, ether, cocaine and ephedrin. Bull Johns Hopkins Hosp. 1943;73:143–67.
6. Davanger M, Evensen A. Role of the pericorneal papillary structure in renewal of corneal epithelium. Nature. 1971;229:560–1.
7. Schermer S, Galvin S, Sun TT. Differentiation-related expression of a major 64K corneal keratin in vivo and in culture suggests limbal location of corneal epithelial stem cells. J Cell Biol. 1986;103:49–62.
8. Thoft RA. Conjunctival transplantation. Arch Ophthalmol. 1977;95:1425–7.
9. Thoft RA. Keratoepithelioplasty. Am J Ophthalmol. 1984;97:1–6.
10. Turgeon PW, Nauhein RC, Roat MI, et al. Indications for keratoepitelioplasty. Arch Ophthalmol. 1990;108:33–6.
11. Kenyon KR, Tseng SCG. Limbal autograft transplantation for ocular surface disorders. Ophthalmology. 1989;96:709–23.
12. Tsai RJF, Tseng SCG. Human allograft limbal transplantation for corneal surface reconstruction. Cornea. 1994;13:389–400.
13. Kwitko S, Raminho D, Barcaro S, et al. Allograft conjunctival transplantation for bilateral ocular surface disorders. Ophthalmology. 1995;102:1020–5.
14. Kenyon KR, Rapoza PA. Limbal allograft transplantation for ocular surface disorders. Ophthalmology. 1995;102(suppl):101–2.
15. Holland EJ, Schwartz OS. The evolution of epithelial transplantation for severe ocular surface disease and a proposed classification system. Cornea. 1996;15:549–56.
16. Daya SM, Chan CC, Holland EJ. Cornea Society nomenclature for ocular surface rehabilitative procedures. Cornea. 2011;30:1115–9.
17. Wei ZG, Cotsarelis G, Sun TT, et al. Label-retaining cells are preferentially located in fornical epithelium: implications on conjunctival epithelial homeostasis. Invest Ophthalmol Vis Sci. 1995;36:236–46.
18. Dua HS, Shanmuganathan VA, Powell-Richards AO, et al. Limbal epithelial crypts: a novel anatomical structure and a putative limbal stem cell niche. Br J Ophthalmol. 2005;89:529–32.
19. Majo F, Rochat A, Nicolas M, et al. Oligopotent stem cells are distributed throughout the mammalian ocular surface. Nature. 2008;456:250–4.
20. Prabhasawat P, Ekpo P, Uiprasertkul M, et al. Long-term result of autologous cultivated oral mucosal epithelial transplantation for severe ocular surface disease. Cell Tissue Bank. 2016;17:491–503.
21. Daya SM. Conjunctival-limbal autograft. Curr Opin Ophthalmol. 2017;28:370–6.
22. Kate A, Basu S. A review of the diagnosis and treatment of limbal stem cell deficiency. Front Med. 2022;25(9):836009.
23. Nieto-Nicolau N, Martínez-Conesa EM, Casaroli-Marano RP. Limbal stem cells from aged donors are a suitable source for clinical application. Stem Cells Int. 2016;2016:3032128.
24. Li C, Dong N, Wu H, et al. A novel method for preservation of human corneal limbal tissue. Invest Ophthalmol Vis Sci. 2013;54:4041–7.
25. Chan CC, Biber JM, Holland EJ. The modified Cincinnati procedure: combined conjunctival limbal autografts and keratolimbal allografts for severe unilateral ocular surface failure. Cornea. 2012;31:1264–72.
26. Sundmacher R, Reinhard T, Althaus C. Homologous central limbo-keratoplasty in limbus stem cell damage. Retrospective study of 3 years' experience. Ophthalmologe. 1997;94:897–901.
27. Lang SJ, Böhringer D, Reinhard T. Penetrating limbokeratoplasty for gelatinous dorneal dystrophy. Klin Monatsbl Augenheilkd. 2019;236:169–72.
28. Cheung AY, Sarnicola E, Holland EJ. Long-term ocular surface stability in conjunctival limbal autograft donor eyes. Cornea. 2017;36:1031–5.
29. Kim EC, Jun AS, Kim MS, et al. Mooren ulcer occurring at donor site after contralateral conjunctivolimbal autograft for recurrent pterygium. Cornea. 2012;31:1357–8.
30. Miri A, Said DG, Dua HS. Donor site complications in autolimbal and living-related allolimbal transplantation. Ophthalmology. 2011;118:1265–71.
31. Busin M, Breda C, Bertolin M, et al. Corneal epithelial stem cells repopulate the donor area within 1 year from limbus removal for limbal autograft. Ophthalmology. 2016;123:2481–8.
32. Daya SM, Ilari FA. Living related conjunctiva limbal allograft for the treatment of stem cell deficiency. Ophthalmology. 2001;108:126–33; discussion 133–4.
33. Health Quality Ontario. Limbal stem cell transplantation: an evidence-based analysis. Ont Health Technol Assess Ser. 2008;8(7):1–58.
34. Titiyal JS, Sharma N, Agarwal AK, et al. Live related versus cadaveric limbal allograft in limbal stem cell deficiency. Ocul Immunol Inflamm. 2015;23:232–9.
35. Krakauer M, Welder JD, Pandya HK, et al. Adverse effects of systemic immunosuppression in keratolimbal allograft. J Ophthalmol. 2012;2012:576712.

36. Holland EJ, Mogilishetty G, Skeens HM, et al. Systemic immunosuppression in ocular surface stem cell transplantation: results of a 10-year experience. Cornea. 2012;31:655–61.
37. Movahedan A, Cheung AY, Eslani M, et al. Long-term outcomes of ocular surface stem cell allograft transplantation. Am J Ophthalmol. 2017;184:97–107.
38. Pfau B, Kruse FE, Rohrschneider K, et al. Comparison between local and systemic administration of cyclosporin A on the effective level in conjunctiva, aqueous humor and serum. Ophthalmologe. 1995;92:833–9.
39. Eslani M, Haq Z, Movahedan A, et al. Late acute rejection after allograft limbal stem cell transplantation: evidence for long-term donor survival. Cornea. 2017;36:26–31.
40. Cheung AY, Govil A, Friedstrom SR, et al. Probable donor-derived cytomegalovirus disease after keratolimbal allograft transplantation. Cornea. 2017;36:1006–8.
41. Sepsakos L, Cheung AY, Nerad JA, et al. Donor-derived conjunctival-limbal melanoma after a keratolimbal allograft. Cornea. 2017;36:1415–8.
42. Miller AK, Young JW, Wilson DJ, et al. Transmission of donor-derived breast carcinoma as a recurrent mass in a keratolimbal allograft. Cornea. 2017;36:736–9.
43. Sangwan VS, Basu S, MacNeil S, et al. Simple limbal epithelial transplantation (SLET): a novel surgical technique for the treatment of unilateral limbal stem cell deficiency. Br J Ophthalmol. 2012;96:931–4.
44. Bhalekar S, Basu S, Sangwan VS. Successful management of immunological rejection following allogeneic simple limbal epithelial transplantation (SLET) for bilateral ocular burns. BMJ Case Rep. 2013;2013:bcr2013009051.
45. Kethiri AR, Basu S, Shukla S, et al. Optimizing the role of limbal explant size and source in determining the outcomes of limbal transplantation: an in vitro study. PLoS One. 2017;12(9):e0185623.
46. Basu S, Sureka SP, Shanbhag SS, et al. Simple limbal epithelial transplantation: long-term clinical outcomes in 125 cases of unilateral chronic ocular surface burns. Ophthalmology. 2016;123:1000–10.
47. Vasquez-Perez A, Nanavaty MA. Modified allogenic simple limbal epithelial transplantation followed by keratoplasty as treatment for total timbal stem cell deficiency. Ocul Immunol Inflamm. 2018;26:1189–91.
48. Shanbhag SS, Patel CN, Goyal R, et al. Simple limbal epithelial transplantation (SLET): review of indications, surgical technique, mechanism, outcomes, limitations, and impact. Indian J Ophthalmol. 2019;67:1265–77.
49. Basu S, Mohan S, Bhalekhar S, et al. Simple limbal epithelial transplantation (SLET) in failed cultivated limbal epithelial transplantation (CLET) for unilateral chronic ocular burns. Br J Ophthalmol. 2018;102:1640–5.
50. Panthier C, Bouvet M, Debellemaniere G, et al. Conjunctival limbal autografting (CLAU) combined with customised simple limbal epithelial transplantation (SLET) in a severe corneal chemical burn: Case report. Am J Ophthalmol Case Rep. 2020;20:100906.
51. Choudhary DS, Agrawal N, Hada M, et al. Massive corneal-epibulbar dermoid managed with pre-descemetic DALK and SLET. GMS Ophthalmol Cases. 2021;11:Doc05. https://doi.org/10.3205/oc000178.
52. Kunapuli A, Fernandes M. Successful outcome of simultaneous allogeneic simple limbal epithelial transplantation with therapeutic penetrating keratoplasty (PKP) for limbal stem cell deficiency and sterile keratolysis after chemical injury. Cornea. 2021;40:780–2.
53. Showail M, Mireskandari K, Ali A. Simple limbal epithelial transplantation (SLET) in conjunction with keratoplasty for severe congenital corneal opacities. Can J Ophthalmol. 2021;56(3):e78–82.
54. Hernández-Bogantes E, Amescua G, Navas A, et al. Minor ipsilateral simple limbal epithelial transplantation (mini-SLET) for pterygium treatment. Br J Ophthalmol. 2015;99:1598–600.
55. Pannu A, Sati A, Mishra SK, et al. Innovative technique of mini-simple limbal epithelial transplantation in pediatric patients. Indian J Ophthalmol. 2021;69:2222–4.
56. Malyugin BE, Gerasimov MY, Borzenok SA. Glueless simple limbal epithelial transplantation: the report of the first 2 cases. Cornea. 2020;39:1588–91.
57. Sakimoto T, Sakimoto A, Yamagami S. Autologous transplantation of conjunctiva by modifying simple limbal epithelial transplantation for limbal stem cell deficiency. Jpn J Ophthalmol. 2020;64:54–61.
58. Singh A, Virender, Sangwan VS. Mini-review: regenerating the corneal epithelium with simple limbal epithelial transplantation. Front Med. 2021;8:673330.
59. Vazirani J. Commentary: SLET - A paradigm shift in limbal transplantation. Indian J Ophthalmol. 2019;67:1277–8.
60. Kim JT, Chun YS, Song KY, et al. The effect of in vivo grown corneal epithelium transplantation on persistent epithelial defects with limbal stem cell deficiency. J Korean Med Sci. 2008;23:502–8.
61. Camacho L, Soldevila A, de la Paz MF. Transmucosal Boston keratoprosthesis type I in a patient with advanced ocular cicatricial pemphigoid. Cornea. 2020;39:1563–5.

Simple Limbal Epithelial Transplantation

Anahita Kate and Sayan Basu

Key Points

- The chapter will cover the indications and the process of case selection for simple limbal epithelial transplantation (SLET).
- A detailed description of the surgical technique of SLET has been presented.
- The normal postoperative course with the modalities for monitoring the outcomes has been described.
- The common complications that can occur after SLET along with the management of the same, have been discussed.

Supplementary Information The online version contains supplementary material available at https://doi.org/10.1007/978-3-031-32408-6_13.

A. Kate
Shantilal Shanghvi Cornea Institute, LV Prasad Eye Institute, Vijayawada, India

S. Basu (✉)
Shantilal Shanghvi Cornea Institute, LV Prasad Eye Institute, Hyderabad, Telangana, India

Center for Ocular Regeneration (CORE), LV Prasad Eye Institute, Hyderabad, Telangana, India

Prof. Brien Holden Eye Research Centre, Champalimaud Translational Centre for Eye Research, LV Prasad Eye Institute, Hyderabad, India
e-mail: sayanbasu@lvpei.org

Introduction

The functional integrity of the corneal epithelium is maintained by the migration and turnover of epithelial cells from the limbal palisades [1, 2]. Deficiency of these stem cells or damage to the surrounding microenvironment can result in epithelial instability, defects, corneal vascularization, and eventual scarring [1, 2]. Management of this entity usually requires surgical intervention, and over the years, several different procedures have emerged which aim to reestablish the corneal epithelium. These include conjunctival limbal autograft /allograft (CLAu/CLAL), keratolimbal allograft (KLAL), cultivated limbal epithelial transplantation (CLET), etc. [3–5]. In conjunctival limbal grafts, a large area of the limbus is harvested, and thus there exists a risk of inducing iatrogenic limbal stem cell deficiency (LSCD) in the healthy eye [6, 7]. This risk is circumvented in CLET as only 3–4 mm of limbal biopsy is obtained [8]. However, the surgery is a two-stepped procedure and requires extensive laboratory support and regulatory approval. Thus, to overcome these limitations, Sangwan et al proposed a single-stage surgery involving in vivo expansion of corneal epithelial cells from a small harvest of limbal stem cells [9]. This novel procedure, simple limbal epithelial transplantation (SLET), has been gaining popularity because of its relatively simple technique and its efficacy in restoring the normal corneal epithelial phenotype. This chapter will focus on the indications, surgical steps, complications, and outcomes of SLET.

Indications

SLET can be autologous (auSLET) or allogeneic (alloSLET), depending on the source of the limbal epithelial stem cells (LESCs). In the latter case, the LECS can be harvested from a living or a cadaveric donor. AuSLET is performed in eyes with unilateral LSCD while alloSLET is reserved for bilateral LSCD. Since ocular burns are the most common causes of unilateral and bilateral LSCD, SLET is most commonly performed in eyes with this pathology. Table 13.1 details the indications for SLET. Although SLET is indicated in eyes with established LSCD, the surgery has also been carried out in eyes with acute ocular burns to promote epithelialization and decrease the inflammation associated with a persistent defect [10]. In this scenario, an alloSLET is carried out while reserving the autologous tissue for addressing the ensuing LSCD. The concurrent presence of LSCD in eyes with congenital corneal opacities has prompted the combination of SLET with corneal transplantation in these eyes, and stable outcomes have been reported with the same [11]. SLET can also be performed in patients with prior failed limbal stem cell transplantation (LSCT) and this includes eyes wherein a limbal biopsy has been previously harvested [12]. Obtaining multiple biopsies from the

Table 13.1 Indications for simple limbal epithelial transplantation

Unilateral
Ocular chemical burns
Postsurgical (ocular surface neoplasia)
Pterygia
Bilateral
Ocular chemical burns
Vernal keratoconjunctivitis
Stevens–Johnson syndrome
Mucous membrane pemphigoid
Sjogren's syndrome (primary/secondary)
Congenital corneal opacities

same eye has not been associated with adverse outcomes to the donor eye [12].

Preoperative Workup

Case Selection

A stepwise approach with meticulous ocular examination to ensure proper case selection is of utmost importance in order to achieve ideal postoperative outcomes (Fig. 13.1). Several disorders with corneal scarring and vascularization may mimic LSCD and identifying the true cases is essential to avoid unwarranted stem cell transplantation. Ancillary tests such as confocal microscopy and impression cytology can confirm the presence of LSCD by identifying the conjunctival epithelial cells within the cornea [13–15]. An anterior segment optical coherence tomography (AS-OCT) is now a commonly available device and can also be used to differentiate true LSCD from its masquerades. The normal corneal epithelium is hyporeflective with a uniform thickness, and a reversal of this pattern is seen in LSCD. Varma et al have described a ratio of the epithelial to stromal reflectivity on the AS-OCT line scans and have reported good sensitivity and specificity of this parameter in the diagnosis of LSCD [16]. The next step in the evaluation of these cases is the assessment of visual potential, and typically no intervention is carried out in cases where visual recovery is not expected. The last prerequisite for performing SLET is the presence of a wet ocular surface, and thus SLET is contraindicated in eyes with aqueous deficiency dry eye or a dermalised surface. Evaluation of the stromal thickness on the AS-OCT line scan is also important, as eyes with thinned-out corneas are at risk for perforation during the intraoperative dissection of the pannus. Shanbhag et al. have detailed a grading system based on the preoperative clinical features that assess the likely prognosis and outcomes following SLET [17]. Table 13.2 enlists the parameters to help prognosticate the outcomes of SLET based on the presenting characteristic.

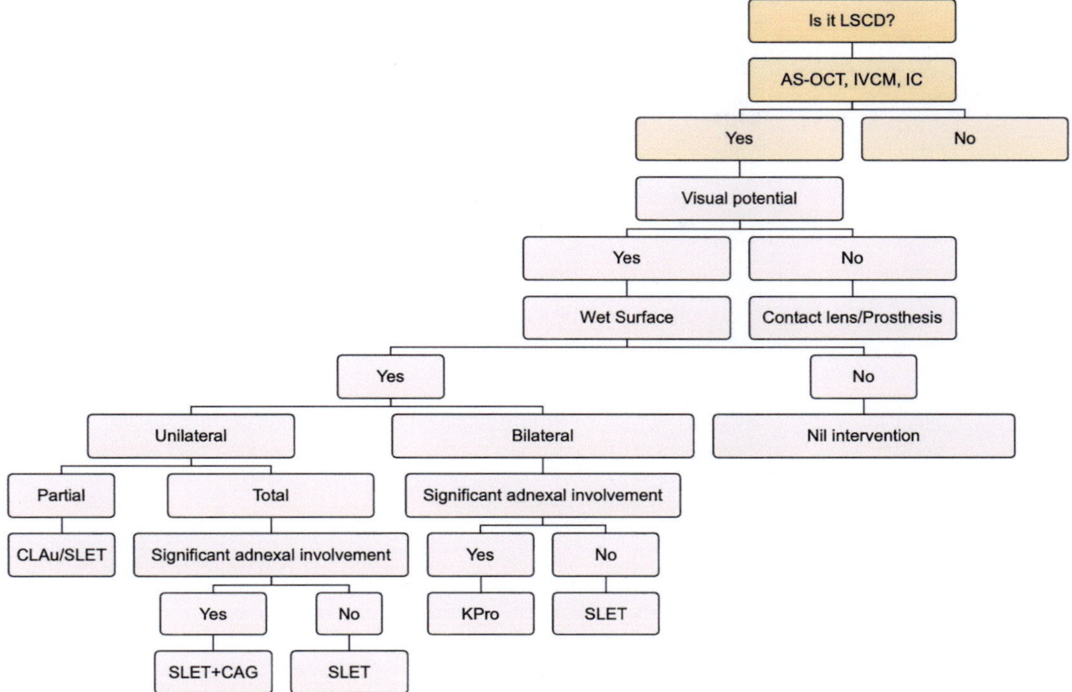

Fig. 13.1 Algorithmic approach to case selection for cases suitable for simple limbal epithelial transplantation (SLET). *LSCD* limbal stem cell deficiency, *AS-OCT* anterior segment optical coherence tomography, *IVCM* in vivo confocal microscopy, *IC* impression cytology, *CAG* conjunctival autograft, *CLAu* conjunctival limbal autograft, *KPro* keratoprosthesis

Sequence of Surgeries

Most disorders that result in LSCD usually have significant ocular comorbidities that must be addressed to reestablish a stable ocular surface and for visual rehabilitation. Adnexal involvement in the form of malposed lids or lashes is common, and correction of these entities prior to SLET is vital. Conjunctival cicatrization, when present, can not only affect the outcome of the surgery but also hamper the placement of contact lenses [17]. The symblephara can be addressed before SLET or in conjunction with the same. In unilateral cases, a conjunctival graft can be harvested from the ipsilateral or fellow eye, whereas in bilateral cases, a mucous membrane graft can be used to cover the bare area.

Corneal stromal scarring can occur due to the underlying disease or secondary to the LSCD itself. Assessment of the grade of scarring can be difficult as the fibrovascular pannus obscures the underlying corneal stroma. The enface infrared image of the cornea that is given with the AS-OCT line scan can provide insight into corneal clarity [18]. This is based on the extent to which the structures of the anterior chamber can be visualized through the corneal scarring, and SLET can be performed in isolation if iris details are discernible. Cases with significant scarring will require simultaneous or sequential keratoplasty to restore a clear visual axis. However, restraint must be exercised before deciding to surgically intervene, as stromal remodeling with a reduction in the scar density may continue to occur several years after SLET. With rigid contact lenses, a significant improvement in visual acuity is often noted, and keratoplasty can be deferred in these cases.

Table 13.2 Features prognosticating the outcomes after simple limbal epithelial transplantation

	Parameter	Excellent	Good	Fair	Poor
Prior history	Corneal perforation	No	No	Yes	Yes
	AMG	Yes	Yes	No	No
	LK/PK	No	No	Yes	Yes
	SLET/LSCT	No	Yes	Yes	Yes
	Multiple surgeries	No	No	Yes	Yes
	Glaucoma	No	No	No	Yes
Clinical features	Eyelids	No	No	No	Yes
	Entropion/	No	No	No	Yes
	ectropion	No	No	Yes (good Bell's)	Yes (poor Bell's)
	Irregular margin/	Complete	Complete	Incomplete	Poor blink rate
	keratinization				
	Lagophthalmos				
	Blink				
	Conjunctiva	Minimal	Mild	Moderate	Severe
	Inflammation	Grade 0	Grade 1	Grade 2	Grade 3
	Symblephara				
	Ocular wettability	Good	Good	Good	Dry ocular surface
	Cornea	>400 μ	300–400 μ	200–300 μ	<200 or >600 μ
	Stromal thickness	Anterior chamber	Anterior chamber	Hazy view of	No view of
	Clarity	details clearly	details discerned	anterior chamber	anterior chamber
		visible on infrared	on infrared image	details on infrared	structures
		image		image	
	Anterior segment	Organized	Organized	Disorganized	Disorganized

AMG amniotic membrane grafting, *LK* lamellar keratoplasty, *PK* penetrating keratoplasty, *SLET* simple limbal epithelial transplant, *LSCT* limbal stem cell transplant. Adapted from Shanbhag et al. [17]

Presurgical Care

Management of the underlying systemic and ocular pathology prior to SLET is important to achieve ideal postoperative outcomes. This includes control of the ocular allergy in eyes with vernal keratoconjunctivitis, decreasing the surface inflammation in eyes with ocular burns, cicatrizing conjunctivitis, etc. Additionally, systemic immunosuppression may be required perioperatively in patients with underlying autoimmune disorders such as Stevens–Johnson Syndrome, mucous membrane pemphigoid, etc. The use of topical brimonidine tartrate 0.15% is recommended as it induces localized vasoconstriction and decreases bleeding intraoperatively [17]. The medication is instilled in both the donor and the recipient eyes 10–15 min before commencing the surgery.

Technique

Anesthesia

General anesthesia is required when SLET is performed in children. In adults, harvesting the limbal biopsy can be done under topical anesthesia while SLET is performed under a peribulbar block.

Donor Eye

In autologous SLET, the limbal graft is usually obtained from the superior limbus. Caution must be exercised while choosing this site, and relying solely on limbal pigmentation is not recommended as they do not confirm the location of the LESC. A subconjunctival bleb is created with preservative-free lignocaine following which a limbus-based conjunctival flap is fashioned by dissecting between the conjunctiva and the Tenon's layer. This flap extends across one clock hour (3–4 mm) of the limbus. Further dissection of the limbal tissue is carried out using a 15-number blade, and care is taken to proceed in a horizontal manner to remain in the superficial plane of the limbus. The onset of bleeding marks the posterior border of the limbus. The dissection is continued until the clear gray cornea is visible. The conjunctival tissue is then excised carefully so as to not leave any remanent tissue abutting the limbal biopsy, which is then harvested flush to the cornea. A nontoothed forceps is used to handle the limbal tissue to avoid traumatizing the LESC. The biopsied tissue is then placed in a bowl of balanced salt solution until it is utilized.

In eyes requiring alloSLET, the biopsy is obtained from a donor aged 60 or less, with visible palisades of Vogt and an intact epithelium. The donor tissue should be utilized within 48 h of procurement. The limbal tissue is harvested using a pinch biopsy technique wherein the tissue is grasped with Lims's forceps and then excised. The size of the biopsy is similar to that of auS-LET, as a longer biopsy may result in a greater antigenic load [17].

Recipient Eye

A 360-degree peritomy is carried out 2–3 mm away from the limbus in the subtenon space. The dissection is advanced using both blunt and sharp dissection in a similar circumferential pattern until the entire pannus has been removed. This allows the pannus to be removed in toto and reduces the intraoperative risk of perforation. This is followed by a blunt tenotomy and removal of a frill of Tenon's tissue from beneath the conjunctiva. This allows the surrounding conjunctiva to recess and creates space for laying down the human amniotic membrane (hAM). Additionally, this step aids in creating an area of the bare sclera, which will prevent early degradation of the hAM and rapid postoperative conjunctivalization. The hAM is then placed over the corneal surface with

its basement side up and secured with fibrin glue (Tisseel Kit, Baxter AG, Vienna, Austria). The edges of the membrane are then tucked underneath the free conjunctiva, and the excess tissue is excised. Care is taken to ensure that there are no redundant or loose folds within the membrane.

The limbal biopsy is retrieved with nontoothed forceps and cut into 6–10 pieces. Triangular sections are made with the middle part of the blades of the scissors to avoid placing tentative cuts. The transplants are placed in the mid-periphery and concentrically with their epithelial side up, which is identified by their smooth, shiny, and pigmented surface. Fibrin glue is used to affix the biopsied bits. After the glue has polymerized, which typically takes around a minute, a bandage contact lens (BCL) is placed. Any excess glue that is present must be carefully removed by sharp dissection to avoid displacement of the transplants. A suture tarsorrhaphy is carried out in children to protect the transplants from inadvertent trauma (Video 13.1).

Postoperative Care

Both the donor and the recipient eye receive topical antibiotics (moxifloxacin 0.5%) until the corneal and conjunctival epithelial defects heal. The status of healing is monitored at each visit with fluorescein stain and a BCL is maintained in the recipient eye until the surface is completely epithelialized. A tapering dose of topical corticosteroids (prednisolone acetate 1%) is administered in conjunction with the antibiotics. The steroids are started at a six times/day dose and tapered over 6 weeks in auSLET while a maintenance dose of one to two times a day is continued in eyes with alloSLET. The latter group of patients also requires systemic immunosuppression to stave off rejection episodes. This is given in the form of a staggered regimen of pulse doses of intravenous methylprednisolone in isolation or in combination with oral cyclosporine and prednisolone. A standardized protocol for the same has been described Shanbhag et al. [17].

SLET Modifications

Sandwich Technique

Amescua et al. have described a technique where two layers of the cryopreserved amniotic membrane are used, and the limbal biopsies are sandwiched between these layers [19]. The double layer offers additional protection to the transplants and is a viable alternative if fresh AM is not available. Also, in pediatric cases where retaining the BCL is a concern, the sandwich technique can be used to prevent displacement of the transplants. However, these membranes are associated with a higher risk of detachment and subsequent loss of the limbal transplants [17].

Minor Ipsilateral SLET (Mini-SLET)

This technique has been adopted to address pterygia in eyes where harvesting a conjunctival autograft may not be feasible or desirable such as eyes with multiple prior surgeries or those with glaucoma [20, 21]. In such cases, a mini-SLET is performed where the biopsy is harvested from the same eye, and the transplants are placed over the affected area alone. The rate of recurrence of mini-SLET is comparable to that of conjunctival autograft [21, 22]. The procedure has also been described in eyes with partial LSCD [23].

Glueless SLET

Here the SLET transplants are inserted within stomal pockets created in the donor cornea [24]. The procedure can be considered in low-resource settings where the availability of fibrin glue availability is a concern. However, embedding the LESCs in the intrastromal area may be associated with a risk of epithelial ingrowth due to the misdirected proliferation of the stem cells.

Mechanism of Action

The corneal epithelial cells arise from within the limbal harvests and spread circumferentially around each transplant. This multidirectional growth of the epithelial sheet is a significant difference between SLET and other in vivo options of stem cell transplantation such as CLAu, CLAL, and KLAL where the epithelial cells migrate in a unidirectional and centripetal pattern. As a result, the center of the cornea is the last area to epithelialize, rendering this area susceptible to healing issues. This is in contrast to SLET where the rate of epithelialization is similar in both the center and the periphery of the cornea. Factors such as the age of the donor, number of transplants from a single biopsy, and size of the transplants may also affect the speed of epithelial sheet formation, especially in eyes with cadaveric alloSLET [25, 26]. Slower growth rates from transplants from the same source are attributed to intraoperative tissue handling and the use of excessive fibrin glue [25].

The AM acts as a substrate for epithelial cell proliferation and helps keep the conjunctival cells at bay until complete corneal epithelialization has occurred. This process typically takes up to 2 weeks though stratification and epithelial thickening may continue to occur in the 3–4 weeks after SLET [25, 27]. Long-term retention of the AM with its eventual thinning has been noted in different studies [19, 27, 28]. Confocal microscopy studies following SLET have demonstrated the resorption of the limbal biopsy fragment after 6 months of the surgery [29]. However, despite the lack of visible biopsied tissues, the stemness is preserved. This has been demonstrated by immunohistochemistry for stem cell markers in eyes that underwent keratoplasty after SLET, thus underscoring the potential of SLET in creating a self-sustaining milieu for epithelial cell turnover [28, 30]. This aspect has also been highlighted by the ability of a post-SLET eye to re-epithelize a large area of defect within a time frame similar to that of a normal eye [31].

Outcomes

Monitoring Outcomes

Epithelialization after SLET begins within 48 h of the surgery and is completed by the second postoperative week [25]. However, the healing of the corneal surface following SLET is a complex process that extends beyond mere epithelialization of the cornea. Several tools can be used to monitor this course postoperatively, which in turn may help in the early identification and prompt management of recurrences of LSCD. The replacement of the hyperreflective thick conjunctival epithelium by the hyporeflective corneal epithelium can be assessed with the AS-OCT line scan (Figs. 13.2 and 13.3). The thickness of the corneal epithelium reverts to normal within 3 months of the surgery postoperative period [32].

Although the reflectivity patterns of the epithelium and stroma approach near normal levels in the first postoperative year, remodeling within these layers continues to occur beyond this period [32]. Histopathological differences have also been reported in the pattern of wound healing when compared to the normal corneal epithelium [33]. These factors probably account for the changes in the stromal scar density, and the progressive nature of this change must be considered before planning keratoplasty for visual rehabilitation. The use of impression cytology and confocal microscopy has also been described for the assessment of outcomes after SLET [30, 33]. The presence of pure corneal epithelial phenotype is ideal; however, a mixed phenotype with both conjunctival and corneal epithelial cells can also occur. In such cases, the degree to which conjunctival cells predominate the phenotype often determines the outcomes [33]. Serial monitoring of post-SLET eyes is feasible with confocal microscopy, which can reveal the development of the multilayered corneal epithelium along with a transition zone between the corneal and conjunctival epithelial cells [29]. This device can also be used to identify eyes with partial success as they present with activated nuclei and dysmorphic epithelial patterns [29].

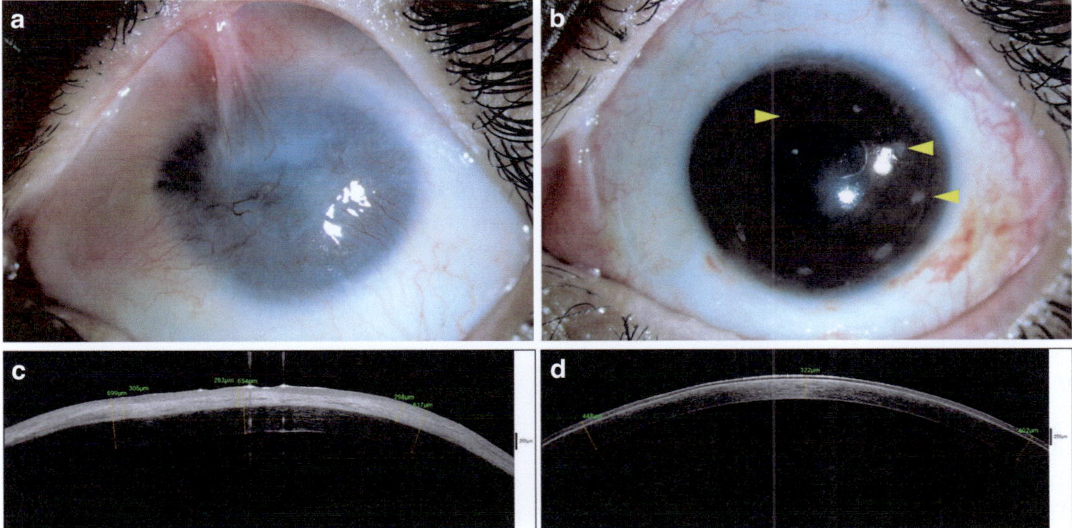

Fig. 13.2 (**a**, **c**) Preoperative image of a case of unilateral total limbal stem cell deficiency with a superior symblepharon. Optical coherence tomography (OCT) line scan of the same eye depicting a hyperreflective thickened epithelium with a relatively spared underlying corneal stroma. (**b**, **d**) Clinical photograph of the same eye after autologous simple limbal epithelial transplantation (SLET) showing a stable ocular surface and a clear visual axis. The SLET transplants are also visible (yellow arrowheads). Postoperative OCT line scan showing a normal hyporeflective corneal epithelium with a compact underlying stroma

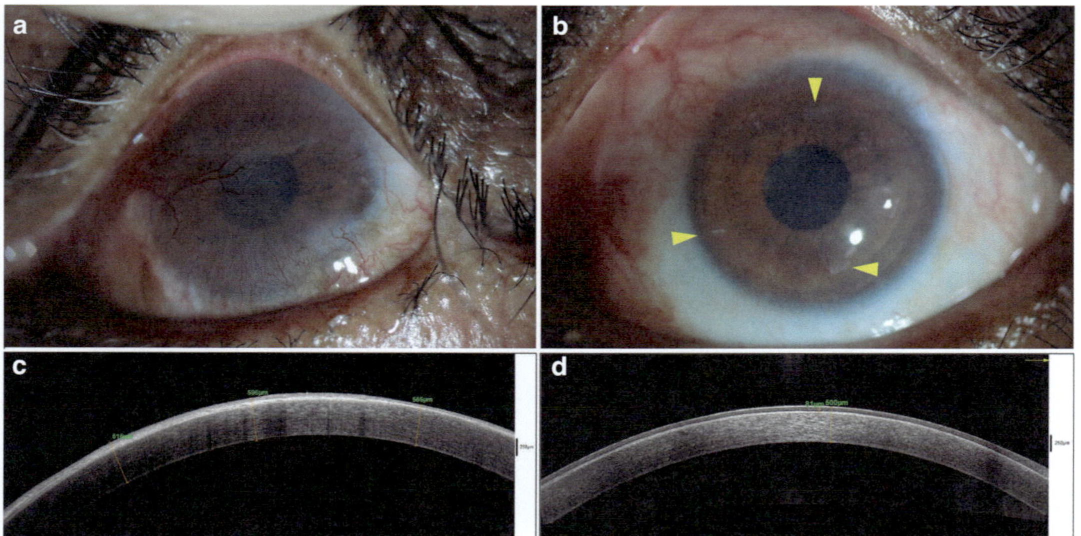

Fig. 13.3 (**a**, **c**) Preoperative image of a case of total limbal stem cell deficiency with a lateral permanent tarsorrhaphy. A hyperreflective pannus is seen on the optical coherence tomography (OCT) line scan of the same eye. No thinning of the underlying corneal stroma is noted. (**b**, **d**) Clinical photograph of the same eye after allogeneic simple limbal epithelial transplantation (SLET) depicting a well-epithelized corneal surface with visible SLET transplants (yellow arrowheads) Reversal of the epithelial reflectivity with a normal hyporeflective pattern of the corneal epithelium is seen on the postoperative OCT line scan

Clinical Efficacy

Anatomical success following SLET is typically defined as the restoration of a well-epithelialized avascular corneal surface. Several studies have determined the anatomic success rate to be around 80% in cases of both partial and total LSCD [17, 28, 33–39]. This rate is higher than the success rate of CLET, which is around 70% [40, 41]. On comparing the outcomes of SLET with CLAU, the outcomes were found to be similar, and since the quantity of harvested limbal tissue is significantly less in SLET versus CLAU, the former procedure is considered superior to latter [42]. The outcomes of alloSLET are similar to that of auSLET, with a success rate ranging from 71–83% (Figs. 13.2 and 13.3) [17, 33, 43]. These results were not affected by the source of the donor LESC, i.e., if they were obtained from a living-related or a cadaveric donor [17]. Furthermore, they are comparable to other modalities of allogeneic LSCT such as CLET, KLAL, and CLAL [44–46].

Although the success rate of SLET drops to around 71% when performed in pediatric cases of LSCD, it is still higher than the success rate of CLET in pediatric eyes, which is around 47% [28, 47]. The repeatability of this outcome by surgeons of varying experience has also been demonstrated, highlighting the relative ease of the surgical learning curve [28]. The ability of SLET to maintain a stable ocular surface ranges from 75–80% at the end of the first year after surgery in both adults and children [28, 35]. Good functional outcomes have also been reported after SLET, with a two-line improvement in visual in nearly 70% of both adult and pediatric cases [28, 34, 35]. Causes of suboptimal visual recovery include the presence of stromal scarring, amblyopia, etc., and hence, careful case selection for SLET is crucial to obtain good outcomes.

Approach to Keratoplasty

Keratoplasty in cases of LSCD is required in eyes with significant stromal opacification in order to visually rehabilitate them. Depending upon the depth of the stromal scarring, a lamellar (LK) or penetrating keratoplasty (PK) can be planned. However, every attempt should be made to perform an LK as it is associated with lower rejection rates. Although SLET and PK/LK can be performed sequentially or in combination, the latter has been consistently associated with poorer outcomes and a higher risk of failure of SLET [28, 34, 48]. Hence performing the keratoplasty following the SLET is recommended. An additional benefit of deferring the keratoplasty is that it provides time for stromal remodeling to occur. This process can decrease scar density, and a significant proportion of these cases have good visual outcomes with rigid contact lenses [49]. Retention of clarity of the graft for greater than a year, along with good visual outcomes, has been reported in keratoplasties performed after SLET [50, 51].

Complications

Intraoperative Complications

1. Perforation of the cornea can occur during dissection of the pannus. Judicious use of the AS-OCT will help identify the cases which have a higher risk of the same. Careful removal of the pannus has to be performed in such eyes while reserving the dissection over the thinned-out cornea for the last.
2. The amniotic membrane and the transplants may get displaced while removing the speculum due to the presence of tags of fibrin glue between the two. Isolating such attachments and separating them by sharp dissection can help prevent this complication.

Early Postoperative Complications

Loss of the limbal transplants may occur in the immediate postoperative period because of excess glue, the reverse orientation of the hAM, loss of BCL, or inadvertent trauma. Free edges of the hAM may also cause its displacement along with the transplants. Although most hematomas that collect beneath the hAM are self-limiting, they may become large enough to displace the hAM. In such cases, the bleed can be released from beneath the hAM with a 26-gauge needle.

Late Complications

Rejection

Acute episodes of rejection can occur following alloSLET, especially if the immunosuppression is not administered adequately. These cases present with congestion, epithelial haze, and stippled staining of the cornea and often have foci of cellularity around the limbal transplants. A rejection line can also be seen adjacent to the limbus, which takes up fluorescein stain [52]. They are managed by increasing the dose of topical steroids and by giving pulse doses of methylprednisolone [52, 53]. With timely intervention and appropriate immunosuppression, these episodes can typically be reversed.

Focal Recurrence

Partial failure of SLET with focal recurrence of LSCD can ensue in a small subset of cases who undergo the procedure. Several such cases have symblephara that abut the cornea or extend over it and are not addressed either prior to or in conjunction with SLET. These cases often require a conjunctival autograft after the excision of the fibrotic tissue to ensure optimal outcomes following SLET [17].

Primary Failure

Primary failure of SLET occurs when the surface fails to stabilize, and recurrence of the LSCD is noted. It is usually secondary to intraoperative technique-related issues such as superficial harvest of LESC or inadvertent trauma to the same. Other risk factors that can predispose these eyes to failure of SLET include simultaneous keratoplasty with SLET, causative etiologies such as acid injury, etc. [28, 34, 35]. These eyes typically require a repeat stem cell transplant for their management.

Miscellaneous

Iatrogenic LSCD and pyogenic granulomas can rarely be observed in the donor eye [28, 34, 38]. Infective or sterile keratitis, persistent epithelial defects leading to thinning, and eventual perforation can occur in the recipient eye [17]. Migration of the limbal transplants into the area of the visual axis has also been reported [43]. Excessive proliferation of the epithelial cells can cause a build-up of the cells over the bandage contact lenses [54]. And so, long-term retention of BCL must be avoided, especially in young patients.

Conclusion

SLET is a simple and novel approach for the management of LSCD, especially in eyes with unilateral disease. Proper case selection is vital to ensure optimal outcomes. Ideal candidates for SLET include unilateral cases of LSCD with wet eyes, minimal adnexal, and corneal stromal involvement. By following the established set of intraoperative steps, a successful outcome with a well-epithelialized avascular corneal surface is ensured in a majority of cases. Preexisting symblephara, which are not adequately addressed, concurrent keratoplasties, and underlying causes such as acid injuries are associated with a higher risk of failure of the surgery.

Although allogeneic SLET also has stable long-term outcomes, the subgroup of patients who are suitable for the procedure is small, which restricts its widespread utility. It requires long-term topical and systemic immunosuppression to ensure the viability of the transplants. The surgical technique of SLET has a quick learning curve and is not dependent on sophisticated equipment or laboratory support. This in combination with the single-staged nature of the surgery, has eased the logistics associated with a stem cell transplant and has also reduced the cost incurred for the same. These factors have facilitated the global adoption of the procedure for the management of stem cell deficiency across different etiologies.

Take Home Notes

- Simple limbal epithelial transplantation (SLET) is a novel and effective technique of restoring a stable ocular surface in eyes with limbal stem cell deficiency (LSCD).
- As the procedure is not dependent on specialized infrastructure or surgical instruments, it can be easily adopted by trained corneal surgeons.
- Ideal cases for SLET include wet eyes with unilateral LSCD, minimal adnexal stromal involvement, and a fairly clear corneal stroma.
- Systemic immunosuppression is required in cases of allogeneic SLET to ensure the viability of the stem cells.
- Failure of SLET due to loss of transplants and focal recurrences are the most common complications and can be prevented by meticulous preoperative and intraoperative surgical planning.

References

1. Tseng SCG. Concept and application of limbal stem cells. Eye. 1989;3:141–57.
2. Ordonez P, Di Girolamo N. Limbal epithelial stem cells: role of the niche microenvironment. Stem Cells. 2012;30:100–7.
3. Ganger A, Singh A, Kalaivani M, Gupta N, Vanathi M, Mohanty S, Tandon R. Outcomes of surgical interventions for the treatment of limbal stem cell deficiency. Indian J Med Res. 2021;154:51–61.
4. Vazirani J, Mariappan I, Ramamurthy S, Fatima S, Basu S, Sangwan VS. Surgical management of bilateral limbal stem cell deficiency. Ocul Surf. 2016;14:350–64.

5. Deng SX, Kruse F, Gomes JAP, et al. Global consensus on the management of limbal stem cell deficiency. Cornea. 2020;39:1291–302.

6. Miri A, Said DG, Dua HS. Donor site complications in autolimbal and living-related allolimbal transplantation. Ophthalmology. 2011;118:1265–71.

7. Baradaran-Rafii A, Eslani M, Jamali H, Karimian F, Tailor UA, Djalilian AR. Postoperative complications of conjunctival limbal autograft surgery. Cornea. 2012;31:893–9.

8. Pellegrini G, Traverso CE, Franzi AT, Zingirian M, Cancedda R, De Luca M. Long-term restoration of damaged corneal surfaces with autologous cultivated corneal epithelium. Lancet. 1997;349:990–3.

9. Sangwan VS, Basu S, MacNeil S, Balasubramanian D. Simple limbal epithelial transplantation (SLET): a novel surgical technique for the treatment of unilateral limbal stem cell deficiency. Br J Ophthalmol. 2012;96:931–4.

10. Iyer G, Srinivasan B, Agarwal S, Tarigopula A. Outcome of allo simple limbal epithelial transplantation (alloSLET) in the early stage of ocular chemical injury. Br J Ophthalmol. 2017;101:828–33.

11. Showail M, Mireskandari K, Ali A. Simple limbal epithelial transplantation (SLET) in conjunction with keratoplasty for severe congenital corneal opacities. Can J Ophthalmol. 2021;56:e78–82.

12. Basu S, Mohan S, Bhalekar S, Singh V, Sangwan V. Simple limbal epithelial transplantation (SLET) in failed cultivated limbal epithelial transplantation (CLET) for unilateral chronic ocular burns. Br J Ophthalmol. 2018;102:1640–5.

13. de Araújo AL, da Ricardo S, Sakai VN, de Barros JN, Gomes JAP. Impression cytology and in vivo confocal microscopy in corneas with total limbal stem cell deficiency. Arq Bras Oftalmol. 2013;76:305–8.

14. Banayan N, Georgeon C, Grieve K, Ghoubay D, Baudouin F, Borderie V. In vivo confocal microscopy and optical coherence tomography as innovative tools for the diagnosis of limbal stem cell deficiency. J Fr Ophtalmol. 2018;41:e395–406.

15. Chidambaranathan GP, Mathews S, Panigrahi AK, Mascarenhas J, Prajna NV, Muthukkaruppan V. In vivo confocal microscopic analysis of limbal stroma in patients with limbal stem cell deficiency. Cornea. 2015;34:1478–86.

16. Varma S, Shanbhag SS, Donthineni PR, Mishra DK, Singh V, Basu S. High-resolution optical coherence tomography angiography characteristics of limbal stem cell deficiency. Diagnostics. 2021;11:1130.

17. Shanbhag SS, Patel CN, Goyal R, Donthineni PR, Singh V, Basu S. Simple limbal epithelial transplantation (SLET): review of indications, surgical technique, mechanism, outcomes, limitations, and impact. Indian J Ophthalmol. 2019;67:1265–77.

18. Kate A, Basu S. Mini-conjunctival autograft combined with deep anterior lamellar keratoplasty for chronic sequelae of severe unilateral chemical burn: a case report. Int J Surg Case Rep. 2021;88:106508.

19. Amescua G, Atallah M, Nikpoor N, Galor A, Perez VL. Modified simple limbal epithelial transplantation using cryopreserved amniotic membrane for unilateral limbal stem cell deficiency. Am J Ophthalmol. 2014;158:469–75.

20. Hernández-Bogantes E, Amescua G, Navas A, Garfias Y, Ramirez-Miranda A, Lichtinger A, Graue-Hernández EO. Minor ipsilateral simple limbal epithelial transplantation (mini-SLET) for pterygium treatment. Br J Ophthalmol. 2015;99:1598–600.

21. Sati A, Banerjee S, Kumar P, Kaushik J, Khera A. Mini-simple limbal epithelial transplantation versus conjunctival autograft fixation with fibrin glue after pterygium excision: a randomized controlled trial. Cornea. 2019;38:1345–50.

22. Jha A, Simba A. Conjunctival autograft versus combined amniotic membrane and mini-simple limbal epithelial transplant for primary pterygium excision. J Ophthalmic Vis Res. 2022;17:4–11.

23. Pannu A, Sati A, Mishra SK, Kumar S, Dhar S. Innovative technique of mini-simple limbal epithelial transplantation in pediatric patients. Indian J Ophthalmol. 2021;69:2222–4.

24. Malyugin BE, Gerasimov MY, Borzenok SA. Glueless simple limbal epithelial transplantation: the report of the first 2 cases. Cornea. 2020;39:1588–91.

25. Mittal V, Jain R, Mittal R. Ocular surface epithelialization pattern after simple limbal epithelial transplantation: an in vivo observational study. Cornea. 2015;34:1227–32.

26. Kethiri AR, Basu S, Shukla S, Sangwan VS, Singh V. Optimizing the role of limbal explant size and source in determining the outcomes of limbal transplantation: an in vitro study. PLoS One. 2017;12:e0185623.

27. Kate A, Shanbhag SS, Goyal R, Basu S. Serial anterior segment optical coherence tomography post autologous simple limbal epithelial transplantation. BMJ Case Rep. 2020;13:e236692.

28. Basu S, Sureka SP, Shanbhag SS, Kethiri AR, Singh V, Sangwan VS. Simple limbal epithelial transplantation: long-term clinical outcomes in 125 cases of unilateral chronic ocular surface burns. Ophthalmology. 2016;123:1000–10.

29. Pedrotti E, Chierego C, Cozzini T, Merz T, Lagali N, De Gregorio A, Fasolo A, Bonacci E, Bonetto J, Marchini G. In vivo confocal microscopy of the corneal-conjunctival transition in the evaluation of epithelial renewal after SLET. J Clin Med. 2020;9:3574.

30. Prabhasawat P, Chirapapaisan C, Ngowyutagon P, et al. Efficacy and outcome of simple limbal epithelial transplantation for limbal stem cell deficiency verified by epithelial phenotypes integrated with clinical evaluation. Ocul Surf. 2021;22:27–37.

31. Kate A, Basu S. Amniotic membrane granuloma in a case of ocular chemical injury: clinical features, histopathology, and outcomes. Cureus. 2021;13:e19171.

32. Kate A, Mudgil T, Basu S. Longitudinal changes in corneal epithelial thickness and reflectivity following

simple limbal epithelial transplantation: an optical coherence tomography-based study. Curr Eye Res. 2021;2021:1–7.

33. Prabhasawat P, Luangaram A, Ekpo P, Lekhanont K, Tangpagasit W, Boonwong C, Inthasin N, Chirapapaisan C. Epithelial analysis of simple limbal epithelial transplantation in limbal stem cell deficiency by in vivo confocal microscopy and impression cytology. Cell Tissue Bank. 2019;20:95–108.

34. Vazirani J, Ali MH, Sharma N, et al. Autologous simple limbal epithelial transplantation for unilateral limbal stem cell deficiency: multicentre results. Br J Ophthalmol. 2016;100:1416–20.

35. Gupta N, Joshi J, Farooqui JH, Mathur U. Results of simple limbal epithelial transplantation in unilateral ocular surface burn. Indian J Ophthalmol. 2018;66:45–52.

36. Wang Y, Hu X, Yang K, Zhang Y, Deng S, Wang Z, Li S, Tian L, Jie Y. Clinical outcomes of modified simple limbal epithelial transplantation for limbal stem cell deficiency in Chinese population: a retrospective case series. Stem Cell Res Ther. 2021;12:259.

37. Shanbhag SS, Nikpoor N, Rao Donthineni P, Singh V, Chodosh J, Basu S. Autologous limbal stem cell transplantation: a systematic review of clinical outcomes with different surgical techniques. Br J Ophthalmol. 2020;104:247–53.

38. Mittal V, Jain R, Mittal R, Vashist U, Narang P. Successful management of severe unilateral chemical burns in children using simple limbal epithelial transplantation (SLET). Br J Ophthalmol. 2016;100:1102–8.

39. Queiroz AG, Barbosa MMO, Santos MS, Barreiro TP, Gomes JÁP. Assessment of surgical outcomes of limbal transplantation using simple limbal epithelial transplantation technique in patients with total unilateral limbal deficiency. Arq Bras Oftalmol. 2016;79:116–8.

40. Zhao Y, Ma L. Systematic review and meta-analysis on transplantation of ex vivo cultivated limbal epithelial stem cell on amniotic membrane in limbal stem cell deficiency. Cornea. 2015;34:592–600.

41. Mishan MA, Yaseri M, Baradaran-Rafii A, Kanavi MR. Systematic review and meta-analysis investigating autograft versus allograft cultivated limbal epithelial transplantation in limbal stem cell deficiency. Int Ophthalmol. 2019;39:2685–96.

42. Arora R, Dokania P, Manudhane A, Goyal JL. Preliminary results from the comparison of simple limbal epithelial transplantation with conjunctival limbal autologous transplantation in severe unilateral chronic ocular burns. Indian J Ophthalmol. 2017;65:35–40.

43. Riedl JC, Musayeva A, Wasielica-Poslednik J, Pfeiffer N, Gericke A. Allogenic simple limbal epithelial transplantation (alloSLET) from cadaveric donor eyes in patients with persistent corneal epithelial defects. Br J Ophthalmol. 2021;105:180–5.

44. Shanbhag SS, Saeed HN, Paschalis EI, Chodosh J. Keratolimbal allograft for limbal stem cell deficiency after severe corneal chemical injury: a systematic review. Br J Ophthalmol. 2018;102:1114–21.

45. Cheung AY, Eslani M, Kurji KH, Wright E, Sarnicola E, Govil A, Holland EJ. Long-term outcomes of living-related conjunctival limbal allograft compared with keratolimbal allograft in patients with limbal stem cell deficiency. Cornea. 2020;39:980–5.

46. Basu S, Fernandez MM, Das S, Gaddipati S, Vemuganti GK, Sangwan VS. Clinical outcomes of xeno-free allogeneic cultivated limbal epithelial transplantation for bilateral limbal stem cell deficiency. Br J Ophthalmol. 2012;96:1504–9.

47. Sejpal K, Ali MH, Maddileti S, Basu S, Ramappa M, Kekunnaya R, Vemuganti GK, Sangwan VS. Cultivated limbal epithelial transplantation in children with ocular surface burns. JAMA Ophthalmol. 2013;131(6):731–6. https://doi.org/10.1001/jamaophthalmol.2013.2308.

48. Kunapuli A, Fernandes M. Successful outcome of simultaneous allogeneic simple limbal epithelial transplantation with therapeutic penetrating keratoplasty (PKP) for limbal stem cell deficiency and sterile keratolysis after chemical injury. Cornea. 2021;40:780–2.

49. Basu S, Hertsenberg AJ, Funderburgh ML, et al. Human limbal biopsy–derived stromal stem cells prevent corneal scarring. Sci Transl Med. 2014;6:266ra172.

50. Singh D, Vanathi M, Gupta C, Gupta N, Tandon R. Outcomes of deep anterior lamellar keratoplasty following autologous simple limbal epithelial transplant in pediatric unilateral severe chemical injury. Indian J Ophthalmol. 2017;65:217–22.

51. Gupta N, Farooqui JH, Patel N, Mathur U. Early results of penetrating keratoplasty in patients with unilateral chemical injury after simple limbal epithelial transplantation. Cornea. 2018;37(10):1249–54. https://doi.org/10.1097/ICO.0000000000001681.

52. Vazirani J, Basu S, Sangwan VS. Allograft rejection after living-related simple limbal epithelial transplantation. Indian J Ophthalmol. 2021;69:433–5.

53. Bhalekar S, Basu S, Sangwan VS. Successful management of immunological rejection following allogeneic simple limbal epithelial transplantation (SLET) for bilateral ocular burns. BMJ Case Rep. 2013;2013:bcr2013009051.

54. Bhalekar S, Sangwan VS, Basu S. Growth of corneal epithelial cells over in situ therapeutic contact lens after simple limbal epithelial transplantation (SLET). BMJ Case Rep. 2013;2013:bcr2013009113.

Cultivated Limbal Epithelial Transplantation (CLET)

Paolo Rama

Key Points

- Limbal stem-cell transplantation (LSCT) is the surgical procedure indicated for the treatment of limbal stem-cell deficiency (LSCD).
- Cultivated limbal epithelial transplantation (CLET) is the latest advanced cell therapy applied to the treatment of limbal stem-cell deficiency.
- From a small limbal biopsy (1–2 mm^2) stem cells of the corneal epithelium can be expanded in vitro and cultivated on fibrin.
- CLET is a GMP-validated procedure that has recently been approved in Europe by the EMA Competent Authority and is now available for clinical use for the treatment of corneal burns.

Introduction

Limbal stem-cell transplantation is the surgical procedure indicated when the limbus has been irreversibly damaged [1]. The stem cells of the corneal epithelium (LSCs) reside in the basal layer of the limbus [2–5]. In limbal stem-cell deficiency (LSCD), impairment of the limbal stem-cell compartment causes a breakdown of the corneal epithelial turnover, resulting in damage to the corneal epithelial layer, which will ultimately repair due to conjunctival migration onto the cornea [6] (Fig. 14.1).

Limbal stem cells guarantee regular turnover and response to injuries of the corneal epithelium through differentiation and migration of cells from the limbal niches to the corneal surface. Conjunctival migration, or "conjuctivalization", is a compensatory repair mechanism that protects the cornea from infection, stromal ulceration, melting and perforation. While it provides a stable and protective superficial layer to the cornea, it is often accompanied by persistent inflammation and severe visual impairment. Lamellar and/or penetrating keratoplasty cannot be used suc-

P. Rama (✉)
Vita-Salute University, San Raffaele, Milan, Italy

Cornea and Ocular Surface Unit, San Raffaele Hospital, Milano, Italy
e-mail: rama.paolo@hsr.it

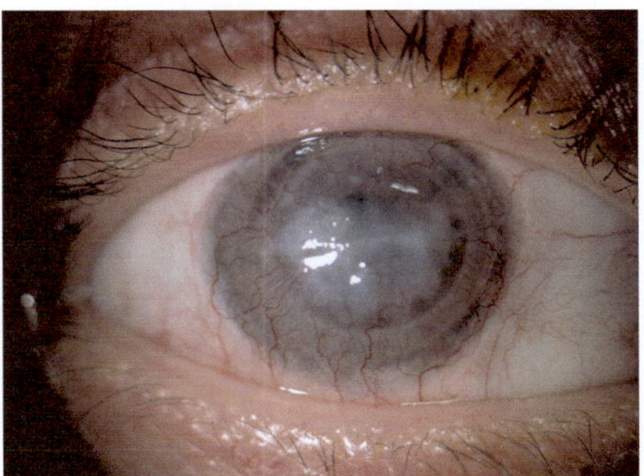

Fig. 14.1 Severe limbal stem-cell deficiency after chemical burn with graft failure after penetrating keratoplasty with recurrence of conjunctivalization

cessfully in these cases as donor corneal epithelium is replaced by that of the recipient within months. In the presence of corneal epithelial stem-cell compartment deficiency, donor graft reepithelialization will not take place, with subsequent epithelial defects and the ultimate recurrence of conjunctivalization, and the risk of rejection and failure (Fig. 14.1).

LSCD includes a group of heterogeneous diseases including congenital abnormalities, acquired diseases such as chemical and thermal injuries, immunological diseases, toxicity and infections [6]. Such diseases may damage not only the limbus but also the eyelids, conjunctiva, corneal nerves, stroma and lacrimal system.

Ocular surface disease is the most appropriate term for such a complex disorder. Scrupulous step-by-step reconstruction should be planned, treating the structures involved separately to prepare the best recipient bed for limbal stem-cell transplantation. Limbal stem-cell transplantation (LSCT) is, therefore, a step in the reconstruction of the ocular surface, while lamellar or penetrating corneal grafts will ultimately restore corneal transparency, leading to the recovery of visual capacity.

Eyelid malposition and malocclusion should first be treated. Conjunctival symblepharon should be then addressed using the appropriate procedures. Once the eyelids and conjunctiva have been treated, tear film and inflammation should be carefully evaluated. The minimum required tear film and the maximum amount of inflammation that allows the successful long-term survival of the grafted stem cells are not clear. In our previous clinical trials [7, 8], we excluded patients with the Schirmer test below 5 mm/5 min, but this was arbitrarily chosen, and one might suggest that the quality of tears might be even more important than the quantity. Unfortunately, at present, there is still no valid method for its assessment. In our clinical protocol for limbal transplantation, we exclude patients showing severe active inflammation. As for tear film, we are still far from having reproducible clinical assessment and inflammation grading, with the exception of redness scoring.

Cultivated Limbal Epithelial Transplantation (CLET)

Autologous CLET

To overcome risks for the donor eye, Pellegrini et al. [9] proposed to expand limbal stem cells in culture to treat LSCD secondary to burns. The pioneering work of Rheinwald and Green showed that it was possible to culture a layer of stratified squamous epithelium with stem cells taken from a small skin biopsy to prepare cultivated skin grafts for the treatment of severe-burn patients [10, 11]. The same procedure was used to prepare autologous grafts of corneal epithelium with stem cells from a 1–2 mm^2 limbal biopsy. Various protocols for the cultivation of limbal stem cells for transplantation have been proposed and recently reviewed by Shortt et al. and Joe and Yeung, including methods to extract cells from the biopsy (mechanical disruption or enzymatic dissociation), substrates and carriers (fibrin sheet, amniotic membrane, polymers, contact lenses, collagen), mediums with animal-derived components or xeno-free [12, 13]. Although good clinical outcomes have been reported with all of these different culture procedures, few studies have evaluated the clonal characteristics of the cultivated cells and their proliferative potential. When dealing with stem-cell-based therapies for diseases involving cell-renewing tissue, it should be mandatory to demonstrate the presence, survival, and concentration of stem cells in culture and in the graft and validate the procedure under GMP conditions [14, 15]. In February 2015, this therapy was approved by the European Medicine Agency (EMA) for the treatment of corneal burns (Holoclar®). Two recent publications summarize the history of CLET, from discovery to clinical approval, including the regulatory aspects [16, 17].

A pre-requisite for CLET is the presence of a small area of preserved limbus (2–3 mm), which is biopsied, expanded in culture and transplanted onto the LSCD-affected eye.

Ex vivo stem-cell expansion is a complex, time-consuming and expensive procedure, but with several advantages compared with traditional limbal grafting: fewer risks for the donor eye, the possibility to treat partial bilateral LSCD, and the possibility to re-graft following eventual failure.

Surgical Procedure of CLET

Biopsy

A 1–2 mm² wide, approximately 150–200 μm deep, limbal biopsy is taken from the contralateral eye, or from an unaffected portion of the limbus in partial bilateral cases (Fig. 14.2).

The procedure can be carried out under topical anaesthesia with oxybuprocaine, or para/retrobulbar anaesthesia with carbocaine or Marcaine without adrenaline depending on patient collaboration. The use of topical lidocaine should be avoided due to its toxicity. Limbal tissue is normally harvested in the superior quadrant, although harvesting can be carried out from any quadrant if necessary. We previously showed that there are no differences in the efficacy of stem-cell isolation and growth comparing different areas of the limbus [4]. The biopsy specimen is then inserted into a sterile tube containing the transport medium, and immediately sent to the laboratory where it will be processed within 24 hours. Sutures are not required, but we usually use two 10/0 nylon stitches to bring the conjunctiva over the area of the corneal biopsy to reduce risks and symptoms. Bandaging is generally not required.

Stem-Cell Expansion in Culture

Cells are enzymatically dissociated, characterized and expanded in vitro on a feeding layer of lethally irradiated 3T3-J2 cells to a size of approximately 2.2 cm² [4, 7, 8]. Limbal biopsies are processed within 24 h of withdrawal. Following dissociation with a solution of trypsin and EDTA, one aliquot of the cell suspension (10%) is plated on a lethally irradiated layer of 3T3-J2 cells for colony-forming efficiency analysis, while the remaining volume of the cell suspension (90%) is plated at high density on lethally irradiated layer of 3T3-J2 cells. When the culture reaches sub-confluence, cells are again dissociated using trypsin, divided into two aliquots and cryopreserved. Once the surgery is planned, one aliquot of cells is thawed and plated on a layer of lethally irradiated 3T3-J2 cells on a supportive fibrin layer. The fibrin disk carrying cultivated cells, 2.2 cm² in dimension, is packed in sterile stainless-steel containers with 4 ml of transport medium, placed in a sterile Petri dish, and inserted into a polystyrene box for transport. Once packaged, the graft has a shelf-life of 36 h. The second aliquot of frozen limbal cells cultivated from the original biopsy, when available after having prepared the graft, is kept cryopreserved to be used for a second application, if required.

Grafting

The anaesthesia can be para/retrobulbar, using a long-lasting drug such as naropine to prolong the

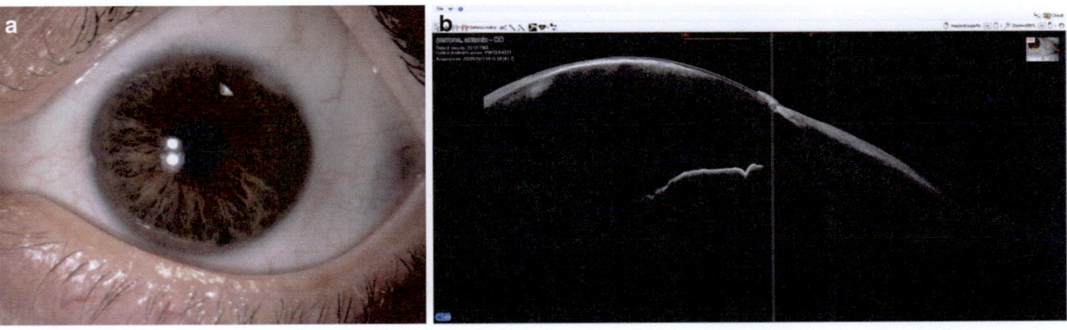

Fig. 14.2 2 mm² limbal biopsy, 160 μm deep, in the healthy fellow eye. Biopsy and grafting were performed twice after CLET failure for persistent severe inflammation

blocking of eye movement after surgery. When general anaesthesia is used, an associated para/retrobulbar injection will help prevent eye movement after surgery. Lidocaine and adrenaline must not be used due to their toxic effects on the cultivated cells.

The surgical procedure is as follows:

1. Limbal peritomy a few millimetres outside the limbus, with proper coagulation. A 4–5 mm pocket in the bulbar conjunctiva is created into which the fibrin-cultured epithelial sheet is inserted.
2. Pannectomy: removal of fibrovascular corneal layer of conjunctival origin; try to find the cleavage level between the pannus and the cornea to avoid, when possible, keratectomy.
3. Lavage with BSS, whilst checking for an absence of consistent blood loss that could form blood collections ('sacks') under the epithelial graft.
4. Transfer of the stem-cell graft on fibrin from the transport container to a suitable dish. It is best to use the protective film of the adhesive tab from surgical gowns, which is to be kept sterile; under the microscope, it is possible to recognize the fibrin "nude" side (smooth and translucent) from the cell-seeded side (rough). It is absolutely crucial to place the fibrin sheet with the cultivated cells outside and not upside down. The fibrin sheet is allowed to slide onto the recipient's prepared graft area, using BSS and slight traction with forceps at the edge of the graft as required.
5. The excess of the fibrin sheet is trimmed, and the edge is covered with the conjunctiva applying 2 or 3 stitches of vicryl or silk 8/0.
6. Close the eyelids with Steri-Strips.

Post-operative Management

We prefer systemic treatment for the first 2 weeks to avoid inadvertent trauma and local toxicity. Oral doxycycline 100 mg (or if allergic, amoxicillin 500 mg) twice a day for 2 weeks, oral prednisone 0.5 mg/kg/day for 2 weeks, tapering the dose after that to 0.25 mg/kg/day for 1 week and 0.125 mg/kg/day for 1 week, and then stopped. After 2 weeks, topical treatment is started: topical preservative-free dexamethasone 0.1% three times per day for 2 weeks, then reduced to one drop twice daily for 1 week and one drop once daily for a further week, and then stopped. The topical corticosteroid can be continued in the presence of persistent ocular inflammation. Topical preservative-free antibiotics are used only in the presence of epithelial defects.

Eye drops containing benzalkonium chloride should be avoided. Benzalkonium chloride (as well as other quaternary ammonium compounds) is cytotoxic, and eye drops containing this preservative might damage the newly regenerated corneal epithelium.

Allogeneic CLET

In total LSCD when the limbus is completely destroyed in both eyes, limbal tissue taken from a deceased donor or from a living relative can be used. In the literature, contrasting results have been reported on the use of allogeneic keratolimbal grafts, with an overall success rate of 73% [18]. Both clinical successes and failures have been observed in the presence of systemic immunosuppressive therapy [19–21] while positive clinical results have been reported in the absence of immunosuppression [22, 23] and/or in the absence of allogeneic cell survival [24, 25]. In most cases, however, the interpretation of results has been hampered, either by the lack of a proper genetic evaluation of the presumptive long-term engraftment of allogeneic limbal grafts or by the inadequate length of follow-up. In the absence of demonstrated surviving donor cells, a possible explanation for clinical success is that patients with non-total limbal stem-cell deficiency have been included, and the grafted allogeneic limbal cells might have induced modification of the microenvironment, and promoted proliferation of the patient's own dormant stem cells, whose progeny gradually replaces donor cells. While remaining in situ in the injured eye, these limbal cells are evidently unable to generate corneal epithelium, either because of the lack of a suitable microenvironment for multiplication or because of fibrotic obstruction to their migration over the cornea.

This would explain the mixed population of donor and recipient corneal cells observed at short-term follow-up. These findings are consistent with reports showing that clinical improvement observed following allogeneic keratolimbal grafts does not necessarily correlate with the long-term survival of donor cells [24, 25]. Similarly, cultured allogeneic epidermal keratinocytes do not engraft permanently but provoke epidermal regeneration in partial-thickness skin burns, presumably by stimulating residual hair follicle stem cells [26].

Conclusions

Autologous cultivated limbal epithelial transplantation is an effective and safe procedure to treat limbal stem-cell deficiency when there is an undamaged, even small, portion (1–2 mm^2 are sufficient) of the limbus that will provide donor cells to be expanded in vitro. Unilateral and partial bilateral limbal deficiency can thus be successfully treated with long-term survival and without the need for systemic immunosuppression (Figs. 14.3 and 14.4).

Limbal stem-cell deficiency is part of the complex disorder known as ocular surface disease, and scrupulous step-by-step reconstruction should be planned, treating the structures involved separately, to prepare the best recipient bed for the cultivated cells.

The procedure of ex vivo stem-cell expansion is crucial and mandatory to demonstrate the presence, survival, and concentration of stem cells in culture and in the graft, and validate the procedure under GMP conditions. We are still dependent on the presence of animal-derived products, such as 3T3 feeder layer and fetal calf serum. Even though all these ingredients have been proven to be safe and have been approved for human use by regulatory agencies, we hope to find a way to be free of them in the future.

We still lack a valid solution for total limbal stem-cell deficiency cases. Contrasting results have been reported on the use of allogeneic keratolimbal grafts, and in the absence of allogeneic cell survival, we cannot rely on this treatment for long-term success in total bilateral diseases.

Future perspectives include: (1) finding other sources of autologous stem cells able to function like the corneal epithelium to treat bilateral limbal stem-cell deficiency, (2) preparation of a "composite" graft with stem cells seeded with other cells, such as keratocytes, fibroblasts, melanocytes, and/or other cells, on a 3D scaffold that might reproduce the "niche" where stem cells normally reside, (3) improve tear substitutes and/or tissue engineering of the lacrimal gland to treat

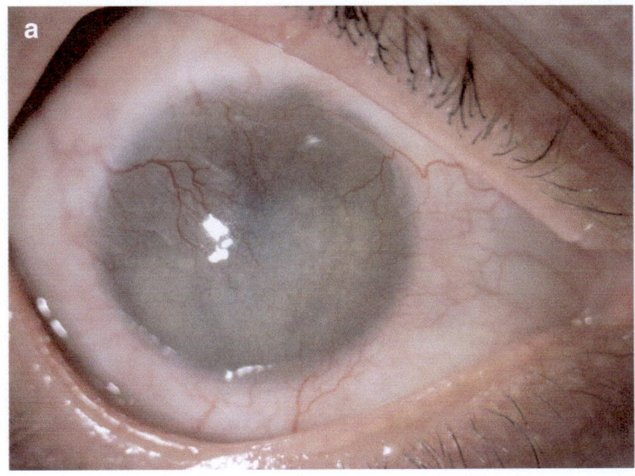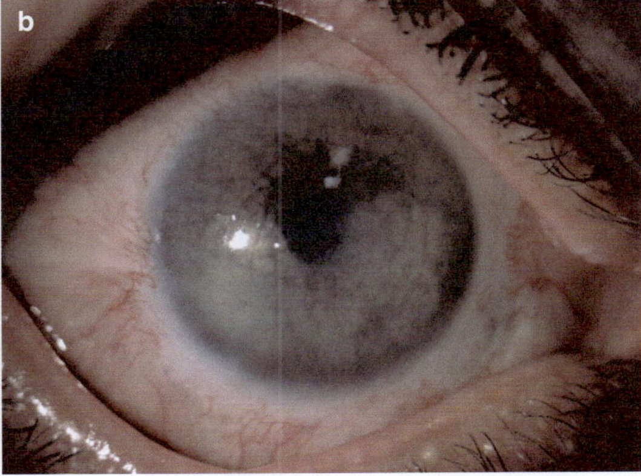

Fig. 14.3 (**a**) chemical burn with total corneal "conjunctivalization" due to severe LSCD; (**b**) one year after CLET, stable and avascular epithelium demonstrating successful epithelial regeneration. Lamellar keratoplasty has been planned for stromal scarring

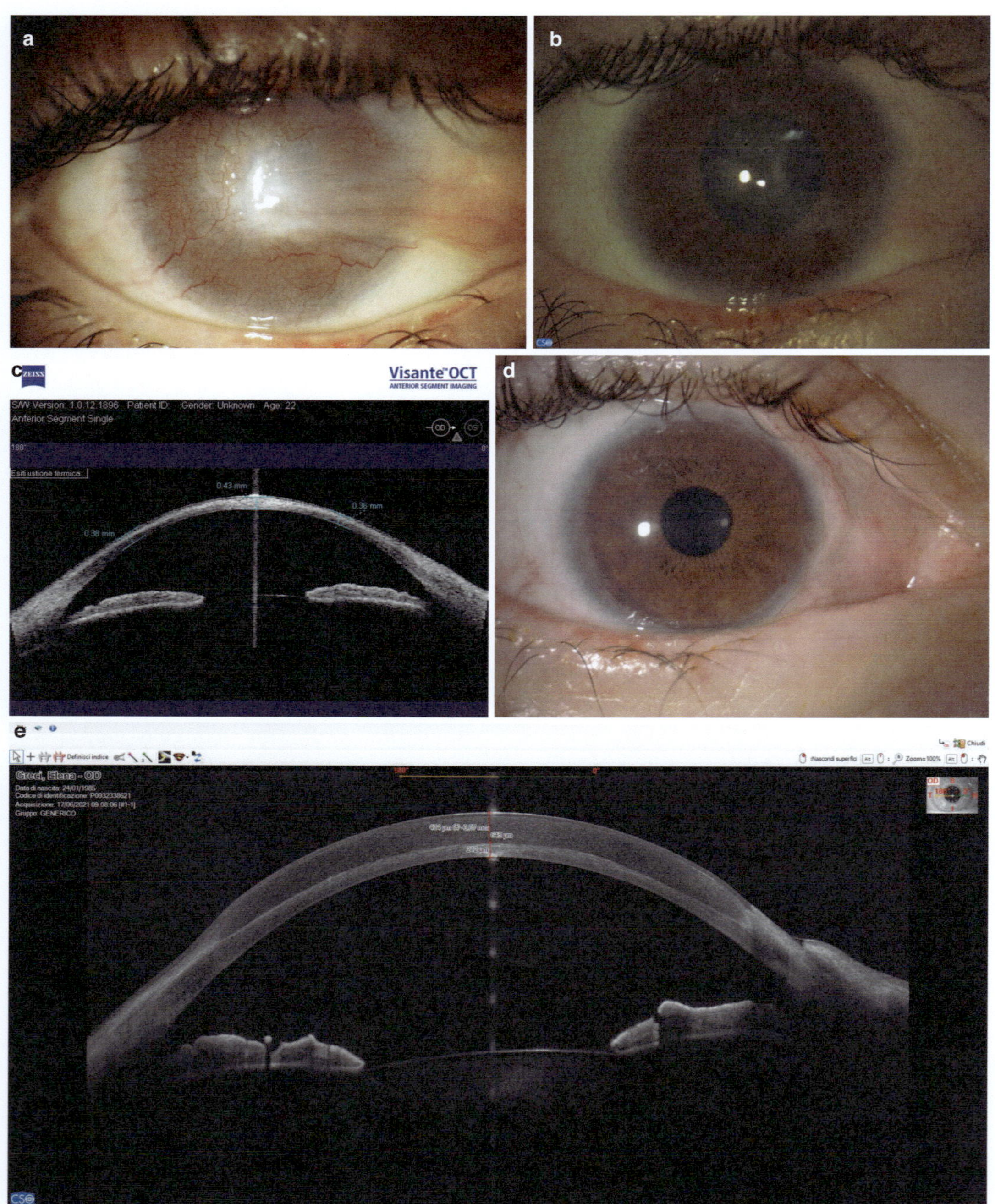

Fig. 14.4 (**a**) severe burn with total LSCD; (**b**, **c**) one year after CLET with a regular and avascular epithelial layer with hazy, thinned, and irregular stroma; (**d**, **e**) nine-teen years after large (10 mm) lamellar keratoplasty. Very stable epithelium with excellent visual recovery (0.8)

severe dry eye, (4) more accurate modulation of the inflammatory response before and after grafting.

Take Home Notes
- Limbal stem-cell deficiency is an ocular surface disease, and scrupulous step-by-step reconstruction, treating the structures involved separately, should be planned to prepare the best recipient bed for limbal stem-cell transplantation.
- Autologous cultivated limbal epithelial transplantation is an effective and safe procedure for the treatment of severe limbal stem-cell deficiency with a long follow-up (over 20 years).
- It has several advantages over direct limbal transplantation: (1) minimum risk for the donor's eye, (2) the procedure can be repeated due to the reduced size of the biopsy, (3) partial bilateral LSCDs can be treated.
- Conflicting long-term results have been reported on the use of allogeneic cells, and we need to find other sources of autologous stem cells capable of functioning as the corneal epithelium to treat bilateral totala limbal stem-cell deficiency.

References

1. Deng SX, Kruse F, Gomes JAP, Chan CC, Daya S, Dana R, et al. Global consensus on the management of limbal stem cell deficiency. Cornea. 2020;39(10):1291–302. https://doi.org/10.1097/ICO.0000000000002358. PMID: 32639314.
2. Schermer A, Galvin S, Sun TT. Differentiation-related expression of a major 64K corneal keratin in vivo and in culture suggests limbal location of corneal epithelial stem cells. J Cell Biol. 1986;103:49–62. https://doi.org/10.1083/jcb.103.1.49. PMID: 2424919.
3. Cotsarelis G, Cheng SZ, Dong G, Sun TT, Lavker RM. Existence of slow-cycling limbal epithelial basal cells that can be preferentially stimulated to proliferate: implications on epithelial stem cells. Cell. 1989;57:201–9. https://doi.org/10.1016/0092-8674(89)90958-6. PMID: 2702690.
4. Pellegrini G, Golisano O, Paterna P, Lambiase A, Bonini S, Rama P, De Luca M. Location and clonal analysis of stem cells and their differenti-
ated progeny in the human ocular surface. J Cell Biol. 1999;145(4):769–82. https://doi.org/10.1083/jcb.145.4.769. PMID: 10330405.
5. Tseng SC. Concept and application of limbal stem cells. Eye. 1989;3:141–57. https://doi.org/10.1038/eye.1989.22. PMID: 2695347.
6. Deng SX, Borderie V, Chan CC, Dana R, Figueiredo FC, Gomes JAP, et al. Global consensus on definition, classification, diagnosis, and staging of limbal stem cell deficiency. Cornea. 2019;38(3):364–75. https://doi.org/10.1097/ICO.0000000000001820. PMID: 30614902.
7. Rama P, Bonini S, Lambiase A, Golisano O, Paterna P, De Luca M, Pellegrini G. Autologous fibrin-cultured limbal stem cells permanently restore the corneal surface of patients with total limbal stem cell deficiency. Transplantation. 2001;72(9):1478–85. https://doi.org/10.1097/00007890-200111150-00002.PMID: 11707733.
8. Rama P, Matuska S, Paganoni G, Spinelli A, De Luca M, Pellegrini G. Limbal stem-cell therapy and long-term corneal regeneration. N Engl J Med. 2010;363(2):147–55. https://doi.org/10.1056/NEJMoa0905955. PMID: 20573916.
9. Pellegrini G, Traverso CE, Franzi AT, Zingirian M, Cancedda R, De Luca M. Long-term restoration of damaged corneal surfaces with autologous cultivated corneal epithelium. Lancet. 1997;349(9057):990–3. https://doi.org/10.1016/S0140-6736(96)11188-0. PMID: 9100626.
10. Rheinwald JG, Green H. Serial cultivation of strains of human epidermal keratinocytes: the formation of keratinizing colonies from single cells. Cell. 1975;6(3):331–43. https://doi.org/10.1016/s0092-8674(75)80001-8. PMID: 1052771.
11. Gallico GG, O'Connor NE, Compton CC, Kehinde O, Green H. Permanent coverage of large burn wounds with autologous cultured human epithelium. N Engl J Med. 1984;311(7):448–51. https://doi.org/10.1056/NEJM198408163110706. PMID: 6379456.
12. Shortt AJ, Secker GA, Notara MD, Limb GA, Khaw PT, Tuft SJ, Daniels JT. Transplantation of ex vivo cultured limbal epithelial stem cells: a review of techniques and clinical results. Surv Ophthalmol. 2007;52(5):483–502. https://doi.org/10.1016/j.survophthal.2007.06.013. PMID: 17719371.
13. Joe AW, Yeung SN. Concise review: Identification of limbals stem cells: classical concepts and new challenges. Stem Cells Transl Med. 2014;3(3):318–22. https://doi.org/10.5966/sctm.2013-0137. PMID: 24327757.
14. De Luca M, Pellegrini G, Green H. Regeneration of squamous epithelia from stem cells of cultured grafts. Regen Med. 2006;1(1):45–57. https://doi.org/10.2217/17460751.1.1.45. PMID: 17465819 Review.
15. Pellegrini G, Rama P, De Luca M. Vision from the right stem. Trends Mol Med. 2011;17(1):1–7. https://

doi.org/10.1016/j.molmed.2010.10.003. PMID: 21075055.

16. Pellegrini G, Rama P, Di Rocco A, Panaras A, De Luca M. Concise review: Hurdles in a successful example of limbal stem cell-based regenerative medicine. Stem Cells. 2014;32(1):26–34. https://doi.org/10.1002/stem.1517. PMID: 24038592.

17. Pellegrini G, Lambiase A, Macaluso C, Pocobelli A, Deng S, Cavallini GM, et al. From discovery to approval of an advanced therapy medicinal product-containing stem cells, in the EU. Regen Med. 2016;11(4):407–20. https://doi.org/10.2217/rme-2015-0051. PMID: 27091398.

18. Baylis O, Figueiredo F, Henein C, Lako M, Ahmad S. 13 years of cultured limbal epithelial cell therapy: a review of the outcomes. J Cell Biochem. 2011;112(4):993–1002. https://doi.org/10.1002/jcb.23028. PMID: 21308743 Review.

19. Djalilian AR, Mahesh SP, Koch CA, Nussenblatt RB, Shen D, Zhuang Z, Holland EJ, Chan CC. Survival of donor epithelial cells after limbal stem cell transplantation. Invest Ophthalmol Vis Sci. 2005;46(3):803–7. https://doi.org/10.1167/iovs.04-0575. PMID: 15728534.

20. Mills RA, Coster DJ, Williams KA. Effect of immunosuppression on outcome measures in a model of rat limbal transplantation. Invest Ophthalmol Vis Sci. 2002;43(3):647–55. PMID: 11867579.

21. Ilary L, Daya SM. Long-term oucomes of keratolimbal allografts for the treatment of severe ocular surface disorders. Ophthalmology. 2002;109(7):1278–84. https://doi.org/10.1016/s0161-6420(02)01081-3. PMID: 12093650.

22. Kwitko S, Marinho D, Barcaro S, Bocaccio F, Rymer S, Fernandes S, Neumann J. Allograft conjunctival transplantation for bilateral ocular surface disorders. Ophthalmology. 1995;102(7):1020–5. https://doi.org/10.1016/s0161-6420(95)30918-9. PMID: 9121746.

23. Rao SK, Rajagopal R, Sitalakshmi G, Padmanabhan P. Limbal allografting from related live donors for corneal surface reconstruction. Ophthalmology. 1999;106(4):822–8. https://doi.org/10.1016/S0161-6420(99)90173-2. PMID: 10201609.

24. Henderson TR, Coster DJ, Williams KA. The long term outcome of limbal allografts: the search for surviving cells. Br J Ophthalmol. 2001;85:604–9. https://doi.org/10.1136/bjo.85.5.604. PMID: 11316725.

25. Daya SM, Watson A, Sharpe JR, Giledi O, Rowe A, Martin R, James SE. Outcomes and DNA analysis of ex vivo expanded stem cell allograft for ocular surface reconstruction. Ophthalmology. 2005;112(3):470–7. https://doi.org/10.1016/j.ophtha.2004.09.023. PMID: 15745776.

26. De Luca M, Albanese E, Bondanza S, Megna M, Ugozzoli L, Molina F, et al. Multicentre experience in the treatment of burns with autologous and allogenic cultured epithelium, fresh or preserved in a frozen state. Burns. 1989;15(5):303–9. https://doi.org/10.1016/0305-4179(89)90007-7. PMID: 2686683.

Suggested Reading

Kenyon KR, Tseng SC. Limbal autograft transplantation for ocular surface disorders. Ophthalmology. 1989;96(5):709–22. https://doi.org/10.1016/s0161-6420(89)32833-8. PMID: 2748125.

Holland EJ. Epithelial transplantation for the management of severe ocular surface disease. Trans Am Ophthalmol Soc. 1996;94:677–743. PMID: 8981714.

Frucht-Pery J, Siganos CS, Solomon A, Scheman L, Brautbar C, Zauberman H. Limbal cell autograft transplantation for severe ocular surface disorders. Graefes Arch Clin Exp Ophthalmol. 1998;236(8):582–7. https://doi.org/10.1007/s004170050125. PMID: 9717653.

Jenkins C, Tuft S, Lui C, Buckley R. Limbal transplantation in the management of chronic contact lens-associated epitheliopathy. Eye. 1993;7:629–33. https://doi.org/10.1038/eye.1993.145. PMID: 8287983.

Sangwan VS, Basu S, Macneil S, et al. Simple limbal epithelial transplantation (SLET): a novel surgical technique for the treatment of unilateral limbal stem cell deficiency. Br J Ophthalmol. 2012;96(7):931–4. https://doi.org/10.1136/bjophthalmol-2011-301164. PMID: 22328817.

Sangwan VS, Sharp JAH. Simple limbal epithelial transplantation. Curr Opin Ophthalmol. 2017;28(4):382–6. https://doi.org/10.1097/ICU.0000000000000377. PMID: 28406800 Review.

Dietrich-Ntoukas T, Hofmann-Rummelt C, Kruse FE, Schlötzer-Schrehardt U. Comparative analysis of the basement membrane composition of the human limbus epithelium and amniotic membrane epithelium. Cornea. 2012;31(5):564–9. https://doi.org/10.1097/ICO.0b013e3182254b78. PMID: 22382594.

Mesenchymal Stem Cells for Regeneration of the Ocular Surface

15

Marina López-Paniagua, Sara Galindo,
Margarita Calonge, Inmaculada Pérez,
José M. Herreras, Ana de la Mata,
and Teresa Nieto-Miguel

Marina López-Paniagua, Sara Galindo, Ana de la Mata
and Teresa Nieto-Miguel contributed equally.

M. López-Paniagua · S. Galindo · M. Calonge
A. de la Mata
IOBA (Institute of Applied Ophthalmobiology),
University of Valladolid, Valladolid, Spain

CIBER-BBN (Biomedical Research Networking
Center in Bioengineering, Biomaterials and
Nanomedicine), Carlos III National Institute of
Health, Madrid, Spain

Castile and Leon Networking Center for Regenerative
Medicine and Cell Therapy, Valladolid, Spain
e-mail: marina@ioba.med.uva.es; sgalindor@ioba.
med.uva.es; calonge@ioba.med.uva.es;
adelamatas@ioba.med.uva.es

I. Pérez
IOBA (Institute of Applied Ophthalmobiology),
University of Valladolid, Valladolid, Spain

Castile and Leon Networking Center for Regenerative
Medicine and Cell Therapy, Valladolid, Spain

Department of Nursing. Faculty of Nursing,
University of Valladolid, Valladolid, Spain
e-mail: maku@ioba.med.uva.es

J. M. Herreras
IOBA (Institute of Applied Ophthalmobiology),
University of Valladolid, Valladolid, Spain

CIBER-BBN (Biomedical Research Networking
Center in Bioengineering, Biomaterials and
Nanomedicine), Carlos III National Institute of
Health, Madrid, Spain

Castile and Leon Networking Center for Regenerative
Medicine and Cell Therapy, Valladolid, Spain

University Clinic Hospital, Valladolid, Spain
e-mail: herreras@ioba.med.uva.es

T. Nieto-Miguel (✉)
IOBA (Institute of Applied Ophthalmobiology),
University of Valladolid, Valladolid, Spain

CIBER-BBN (Biomedical Research Networking
Center in Bioengineering, Biomaterials and
Nanomedicine), Carlos III National Institute of
Health, Madrid, Spain

Castile and Leon Networking Center for Regenerative
Medicine and Cell Therapy, Valladolid, Spain

Department of Cell Biology, Genetics, Histology and
Pharmacology, University of Valladolid, Valladolid,
Spain
e-mail: tnietom@ioba.med.uva.es

J. L. Alió, J. L. A. del Barrio (eds.), *Modern Keratoplasty*, Essentials in Ophthalmology,
https://doi.org/10.1007/978-3-031-32408-6_15

Abbreviations

CD	Cluster of differentiation
CK	Cytokeratin
CLET	Cultivated limbal epithelial transplantation
DED	Dry eye disease
EVs	Extracellular vesicles
GVHD	Graft-versus-host disease
HLA-DR	Human leukocyte antigen-DR
IL	Interleukin
LESCs	Limbal epithelial stem cells
LSCD	Limbal stem cell deficiency
MSCs	Mesenchymal stem cells
oGVHD	Ocular graft-versus-host disease
TNF-α	Tumour necrosis factor alpha
Treg	Regulatory T cells
TSG-6	Tumour necrosis factor-stimulated gene/protein-6

Key Points
- Mesenchymal stem cells (MSCs) have significant therapeutic potential to regenerate the ocular surface.
- Preclinical evidence demonstrates that MSCs can be used for the treatment of ocular surface diseases.
- MSCs have been successfully applied in clinical settings for the treatment of some ocular surface diseases.
- Work must continue to overcome the technical and scientific challenges that remain unsolved to establish the use of MSCs as a widely accepted treatment for ocular surface diseases.

Regeneration of the Ocular Surface by Mesenchymal Stem Cells

The integrity of the corneal epithelium is crucial for maintaining corneal transparency and visual function. Corneal damage due to different circumstances such as chemical or thermal burns, eye surgeries, cicatrizing-autoimmune pathologies, severe dry eye disease (DED), infections, transplant rejections, or congenital disorders can disrupt the integrity of the corneal epithelium. This type of loss is an important cause of visual impairment and blindness that affects millions of people worldwide [1]. The corneal epithelium has an extremely high turnover rate (4–7 days) that is mediated by the limbal epithelial stem cells (LESCs) located in the palisades of Vogt within the corneo-scleral limbal niche [2–4]. LESC deficiency or dysfunction and/or the destruction of the niche microenvironment produces a condition known as limbal stem cell deficiency (LSCD). LSCD reduces the regeneration and repair of the corneal epithelium, and the corneal surface is gradually replaced by conjunctival epithelium. This process is accompanied by chronic inflammation of the ocular surface, chronic pain, ulceration, and neovascularization, all of which result in corneal blindness due to the loss of corneal transparency [5].

At present, among the stem cell-based therapies, cultivated limbal epithelial cell transplantation (CLET) is the treatment of choice for LSCD. In unilateral cases of LSCD, treatment by autologous CLET is possible following acquisition of limbal tissue from the contralateral healthy eye [6–11]. However, bilateral cases of LSCD are more frequent; therefore, it is necessary to use allogeneic limbal tissue. Consequently, this requires one year of immunosuppression to avoid immune rejection, resulting in an increased risk of patient morbidity and associated medical costs [11]. To avoid this immunosuppression, it is necessary to seek either an extraocular autologous source of stem cells or a non-immunogenic allogeneic source.

In recent years, the use of mesenchymal stem cells (MSCs) has remarkably increased in the fields of cell therapy and regenerative medicine. Collectively, these stromal-derived cells retain some intrinsic developmental and differentiation features after they are derived from a variety of animal and human tissues, including bone marrow, adipose tissue, dental pulp, umbilical cord, and ocular limbal stroma, among others [12]. They are defined by their adherence to plastic substrates when cultured in standard conditions and their multipotent differentiation capacity to form bone, cartilage, and adipose tissue in vitro. Importantly, the MSCs exhibit expression of a characteristic set of specific surface antigens, including positive expression for the cluster of differentiation (CD) 73, CD90, and CD105 [13]. However, they do not express antigens CD34, CD45, CD11b or CD14, CD19 or CD79α, or human leukocyte antigen-DR (HLA-DR) markers [13].

Moreover, MSCs present four potential advantages over LESCs with regard to their utility in cell therapy and tissue regeneration. First, acquisition of MSCs is not restricted to deceased donors or healthy eyes of living donors as they can be easily obtained from several different living tissues [12]. Second, they can be cultured in vitro to clinical scales in a short period of time, thus overcoming the limitations of LESCs, which are difficult to isolate and culture [14, 15]. Third, the stem cell phenotype is maintained even during cryopreservation [16]. Fourth, they are not immunogenic; therefore, immunosuppression is not necessary after allogeneic transplantation [17, 18].

MSCs have additional advantages over LESCs, especially for ocular surface repair. For instance, the capacity of MSCs for differentiation following transplantation enables them to undergo integration, proliferation, and differentiation in the damaged tissues, and in many cases, facilitate tissue regeneration [19–21]. MSCs may also reduce inflammation, apoptosis, and fibrosis and improve tissue regeneration by activating endogenous progenitor cells [22]. MSCs also have immunomodulatory properties that enable the regulation of T cells, B-cells, and natural killer cells, thus mitigating the secretion of inflammatory cytokines [23, 24].

Considering all, MSCs have emerged as very attractive candidates for cell-based therapies in numerous and highly varied clinical applications including the treatment of some ocular surface diseases such as LSCD, DED, or even as a potential treatment to improve corneal allograft survival [11, 25]. This chapter summarizes the main existing preclinical and clinical evidence that currently supports MSC-based therapies as safe and effective for the regeneration of the ocular surface.

Preclinical Evidence of MSC Efficacy in Ocular Surface Regeneration

Currently, there are many published preclinical studies showing the potential restorative effects of MSCs for ocular surface pathologies in experimental models [26, 27]. These studies were conducted with MSCs obtained from different sources such as bone marrow, adipose tissue, limbal stroma, umbilical cord, and others, and they were administered by different routes. The most relevant therapeutic preclinical studies that support the use of MSCs for the treatment of ocular surface diseases are described below.

MSCs for the Treatment of LSCD and Corneal Epithelial Damage

CLET is the current treatment of choice among stem cell-based interventions for LSCD. This surgical procedure aims to replace the destroyed limbal stem cell population by an autologous or allogeneic cell population with full functionality [6, 7]. However, this treatment has some limitations such as the low availability of donor tissues, or the difficulty in culturing the limbal epithelial cells [11]. Nevertheless, in recent years MSCs have been shown to be safe and effective and, therefore, good candidates for the treatment of LSCD [8, 11].

In experimental models of corneal epithelial damage and LSCD, transplantation of both bone marrow- and adipose tissue-derived MSCs reduces the clinical signs of LSCD such as neovascularization, corneal opacity, and epithelial defects (Fig. 15.1). The cells can be administered using routes such as sub-conjunctival injection [29–37], topical administration [38, 39], application of MSC-bearing amniotic membrane [28, 40–43] or MSC-bearing biopolymers [44–47], or by intravenous [48–53] and intraperitoneal injection [51]. MSCs obtained from other cell sources

Superior limbus   Central cornea   Inferior limbus

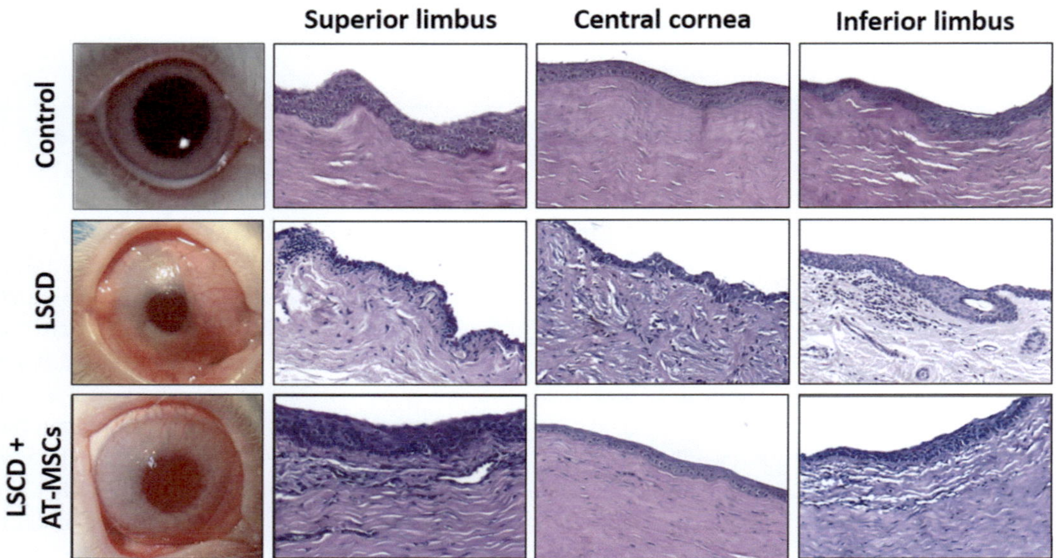

Fig. 15.1 Histological evaluation of ocular surface tissues from a rabbit model of total limbal stem cell deficiency (LSCD) treated with human adipose tissue-derived mesenchymal stem cells (AT-MSCs). Representative images of periodic acid-Schiff staining of ocular surface tissues obtained from healthy control eyes, untreated LSCD eyes, and LSCD eyes 8 weeks after being transplanted with AT-MSCs on amniotic membranes. Compared to healthy control eyes, untreated LSCD eyes had fewer epithelial layers, a disorganized corneal epithelium and stroma, and the presence of inflammatory cells (in dark purple) in the stroma of the central cornea. However, LSCD eyes transplanted with AT-MSCs showed fewer inflammatory cells and less disorganization in the epithelium and stroma of the central cornea than the untreated eyes. (Results from [28])

such as limbal stroma [35, 54, 55] or dental pulp [56] are also able to decrease these clinical signs in experimental models of LSCD. The preclinical data have also demonstrated that transplantation of MSCs to treat LSCD does not induce adverse events or toxicological effects, even with xenogeneic transplantation [28, 32, 38, 40, 41, 49, 51, 53, 54, 56, 57].

The molecular mechanism(s) of MSC-based tissue restoration is not yet fully understood. However, we do know that the transplanted cells reduce inflammation in the ocular surface of experimental models of corneal epithelial damage or LSCD, both by decreasing inflammatory infiltrates [28, 33, 38–40, 43, 57–59] and reducing proinflammatory cytokines such as tumour necrosis factor-alpha (TNF-α), IL-6, and IL-1β, among others [29–31, 34, 37, 53]. In addition, some authors have described the tumour necrosis factor-stimulated gene/protein-6 (TSG-6) as one of the molecules involved in the anti-inflammatory effect of MSCs in the cornea [29, 37, 51, 53].

Furthermore, other authors have also shown that MSCs have an antioxidant effect on the ocular surface of experimental models of corneal burns or LSCD [45–47, 49, 51]. Some authors have demonstrated migration and engraftment of the cells on the ocular surface after topical administration [28, 38–40, 42, 56], sub-conjunctival injection [29, 34, 35, 54], and intravenous injection [48, 50, 52, 58]. However, others did not observe the presence of MSCs at the area of damage after topical administration on amniotic membranes [55], or sub-conjunctival [30, 33, 37], intravenous, or intraperitoneal injections [51]. Therefore, the evidence suggests that MSCs can promote therapeutic effects at a distance from the target tissues by releasing trophic factors.

Additionally, some preclinical data showed recovery of the differentiated corneal epithelial cell markers cytokeratin (CK) 3 and CK12 [28, 41, 43, 47, 50, 56, 60] and the limbal epithelial stem cell markers p63, CK15, and ATP-binding cassette sub-family G member 2 [28, 29, 41, 50, 56, 58, 61] in the ocular surface of the MSC-transplanted experimental LSCD models. Although transdifferentiation of MSCs into corneal and limbal epithelial cells has not been demonstrated in vivo, MSCs seem to contribute to the recovery of the corneal and limbal phenotype by secreting factors and helping resident stem cells.

MSCs for the Treatment of DED

DED is a multifactorial and inflammatory-based pathology [62] that affects between 5.5% and 35% of the world population [63]. It presents with varying severity of symptoms such as pain and blurred vision, and the most severe cases can lead to corneal ulcers, infections, and even perforations [64, 65]. DED is also characterized by an increase of inflammatory molecules and reactive oxygen species and by a decrease of anti-inflammatory and growth factors in the ocular surface [66, 67].

In this context, MSCs have been proposed as a possible treatment for patients affected by the most severe forms of DED. MSCs isolated from bone marrow [68–72], adipose tissue [73–75], or umbilical cord [76] have been therapeutically administered in experimental in vivo DED models using different routes of delivery such as topical application through eye drops [69], intraorbital injection around or directly into lacrimal glands [70, 73–75], and intraperitoneal [71] or intravenous injections [68, 72, 76, 77]. These studies have shown that MSC therapy to treat DED improves tear volume and tear film stability [69–72, 74–76], maintains corneal epithelial integrity [72, 74], increases the number of conjunctival goblet cells [69, 70], and reduces ocular surface hyperemia [74–76]. Some studies also reported lacrimal gland regeneration [72, 77]. Moreover, several authors found decreased ocular surface inflammation following MSC treatment. The reduced inflammation was associated with decreased lymphocytic foci [71, 73] or CD4+ T cell infiltration [70], maintained or increased regulatory T cell (Treg) and Th2 presence [68, 71, 72], modulation of macrophage infiltration [77] or macrophage maturation [76], decreased proinflammatory factors such as TNF-α [72, 76], IL-1 [72], or IL-6 [76], and/or increased anti-inflammatory factors such as IL-10 [72, 76] or epidermal growth factor [72].

One of the most severe forms of DED occurs in the context of chronic graft-versus-host disease (GVHD) that can develop after allogeneic haematopoietic stem cell transplantation, appearing in 60% of patients [78]. GVHD with ocular damage (oGVHD) is caused by the immune response produced by the immunocompetent cells from the donor graft that "attack" the recipient ocular surface (conjunctiva, cornea, limbus, and tear film) and all of the glands that produce tear components. This attack produces chronic ocular inflammation and ocular tissue destruction [79–83].

Because of the high immunoregulatory and immunosuppressive capacity and the ocular anti-inflammatory and ocular tissue regenerative potential of MSCs, they have been successfully tested as therapy in vivo models of DED associated with oGVHD [83–86]. Sub-conjunctival injection of bone marrow-derived MSCs in a mouse model of GVHD decreased both the presence of CD3+ T cells in corneal tissues and corneal keratinization [84, 85]. In addition, other authors showed that for mice with GHVD, MSCs can engraft into lacrimal gland tissues and secrete collagen type I that reduces the pathogenic fibrosis of the gland [86]. All of these preclinical results suggest that MSCs are a promising cell therapy to treat DED, although more studies are needed to optimize it [87–89].

MSCs Promote Corneal Allograft Survival

Corneal transplantation or keratoplasty is the most frequent type of human tissue transplant [90]. In low-risk patients, the survival rate of full-thickness corneal grafts at 1 year is around 90% (even without donor-recipient major histocompatibility complex matching). However, in high-risk patients with corneal neovascularization and inflammation, the long-term prognosis is lower than 50% [91, 92]. Topical corticosteroids are currently the most common immunosuppressive drugs used in corneal transplantation. However, their effectiveness is lower in high-risk patients, and prolonged application can provoke numerous side effects [93, 94]. Therefore, alternative therapeutic strategies are required to improve the prognosis of long-term corneal transplantation and to diminish the adverse side effects of the current pharmacological treatments.

Preclinical studies have shown that systemic and sub-conjunctival administration of MSCs can prolong corneal allograft survival. Therefore, their administration in combination with or in the absence of immunosuppressive drugs could help prevent immune rejection of the corneal graft [95–97]. The mechanism by which MSCs modulate corneal allograft survival has not been fully elucidated yet; however, it has been associated with inhibition of antigen-presenting cell activation, change in Th1/Th2 balance, reduction of CD4$^+$ T cell infiltration, and induction of Treg proliferation [95, 96, 98, 99]. These immunomodulatory and immunosuppressive actions are related to the MSC-dependent secretion of soluble factors such as TSG-6, hepatocyte growth factor, nitric oxide, and prostaglandin E2 [100, 101]. Despite the encouraging preclinical results obtained so far, there are still many issues and challenges that need to be overcome before the clinical application of this therapeutic approach in humans is attempted. These include determination (1) if one or a few sources of MSCs produce better clinical results than others, (2) the best dose and route of administration, and also (3) the most effective frequency and timing of cell administration [95, 96].

Clinical Evidence of MSC Efficacy in Ocular Surface Pathology

Most studies of ocular surface stem cell functional failure have focused on the LESCs that reside in the corneoscleral limbal niche. However, there are several other potential stem cell niches in the ocular surface that could help maintain cellular homeostasis of the corneal stroma, conjunctiva, and meibomian glands [102]. And although the main stem cell deficiency at the ocular surface is the LSCD, causing corneal opacity, other pathologies are starting to be thought of as amenable to therapy with stem cells, as reviewed in a previous section on preclinical studies. The following are the most relevant ocular surface pathologies for which stem cell treatment, most specifically with MSCs, have already been translated into clinical practice and published.

MSCs for the Treatment of LSCD

The destruction or dysfunction of the stem cells residing in the limbal niche, leading to LSCD, can have several aetiologies: chemical injuries, immune-mediated cicatrizing diseases of the ocular surface (e.g., Stevens-Johnson syndrome and its spectrum, mucous membrane pemphigoid, atopic keratoconjunctivitis, ocular rosacea), sequelae of infectious keratitis, or primary causes such as congenital aniridia or ectodermal dysplasia. All of these conditions lead to neovascular pannus, an unstable corneal surface, and eventually, visual deficit and chronic nociceptive pain [11]. Diseases leading to LSCD are difficult to manage, requiring complex medical and surgical approaches. Upon the development of LSCD, the problem becomes unsolvable unless new stem cells can be provided in the correct location [103]. Since the first transplantations of autologous limbal tissue in 1989 [104] and the cultivated autologous limbal cells in 1997 [105] to the more recent techniques of delivering limbal tissue (simple limbal epithelial transplantation) in 2012 [106] or the cultivation of autologous and allogeneic stem cells (reviewed in [11]), many cases have been successfully treated.

There is still a big need for the development of safer, more accessible techniques that avoid the necessity of immunosuppression when the source of tissue or cells must be allogeneic, as it is often the case in bilateral diseases. This can be achieved with MSCs due to their many beneficial properties, especially the absence of immunogenicity. The use of allogeneic bone marrow-derived MSCs has already been applied in the clinic. A randomized controlled clinical trial demonstrated the benefits of this stem cell type, which was assessed to be comparable and slightly superior to CLET in the management of LSCD [8]. This methodology avoids the use of immunosuppression but can only be applied in places where a Cell Processing Unit that complies with the accepted standards of good manufacturing procedures [107] is available. Therefore, work must progress to find solutions that are more accessible and that perhaps can do more to replace the damage limbal niche instead of just providing stem cells.

MSCs for the Treatment of DED

The most severe forms of DED are still difficult to manage with current therapies. Undoubtedly, DED associated with chronic GVHD is one of the most, if not the most, severe form of DED. It can be devastating with unbearable pain, photophobia, and reduced quality of life [108]. The therapeutic efficacy of MSCs in the treatment of DED was first reported in a 2012 clinical study of 22 chronic GVHD patients with refractory DED. The patients were intravenously transfused with allogeneic MSCs, and 55% achieved clinical improvement that was attributed to the generation of CD8+CD28-Tcells [109].

In 2020, 7 patients with severe Sjögren's syndrome-associated DED were treated with adipose tissue-derived MSCs that were delivered by a single transconjunctival injection into the main lacrimal gland. The treatment was well tolerated, and patients showed great improvement that lasted up to 16 weeks [110].

In 2022, a clinical trial demonstrated the beneficial effects of exosomes from human umbilical cord MSCs that were administered as eye drops to treat DED associated with chronic GVHD in 14 patients [111]. Exosomes are a sub-type of extracellular vesicles (EVs) of endosomal origin with a size range of ~30 to ~200 nm in diameter. EVs are lipid-encapsulated membranous vesicles that are released by cells into the extracellular spaces and contain components (protein, DNA, and RNA) from the cells that release them. While that trial was run for only 14 days, the signs and symptoms of the GVHD-dependent DED were significantly mitigated. Thus, this cell-free approach for delivering MSC components to treat DED in general and specifically DED associated with chronic GVHD is promising. The long-term effects and safety remain to be demonstrated, and MSC exosome-based therapy still faces challenges such as determining the stability during storage and transport, and determination of the heterogeneity of the exosome composition.

Conclusions and Future Perspectives

MSC-based therapies for ocular surface pathology, from corneal blindness due to LSCD, to immune-based inflammatory diseases such as DED, or to corneal transplantation, show great potential to reduce the onset of vision loss. Current preclinical evidence has already been partially translated into clinical applications. These studies, of course, still need to be confirmed with larger controlled clinical trials, and some questions and technical problems remain to be solved. Among them, it should be elucidated if some MSC sources are better than others, and what are the safest and most clinically effective MSC doses and routes of administration. In addition, it is essential to develop standardized protocols for the culture and characterization of MSCs so that the results obtained in different preclinical and clinical centres can be properly compared. Despite all the challenges and unknowns that remain, the future of MSCs in the ocular surface is certainly promising (Fig. 15.2).

Over the last few years, EVs derived from MSCs have strongly emerged as a potential alternative to MSC treatment. EVs appear to replicate many of the therapeutic effects of MSCs but without most of the safety risks and

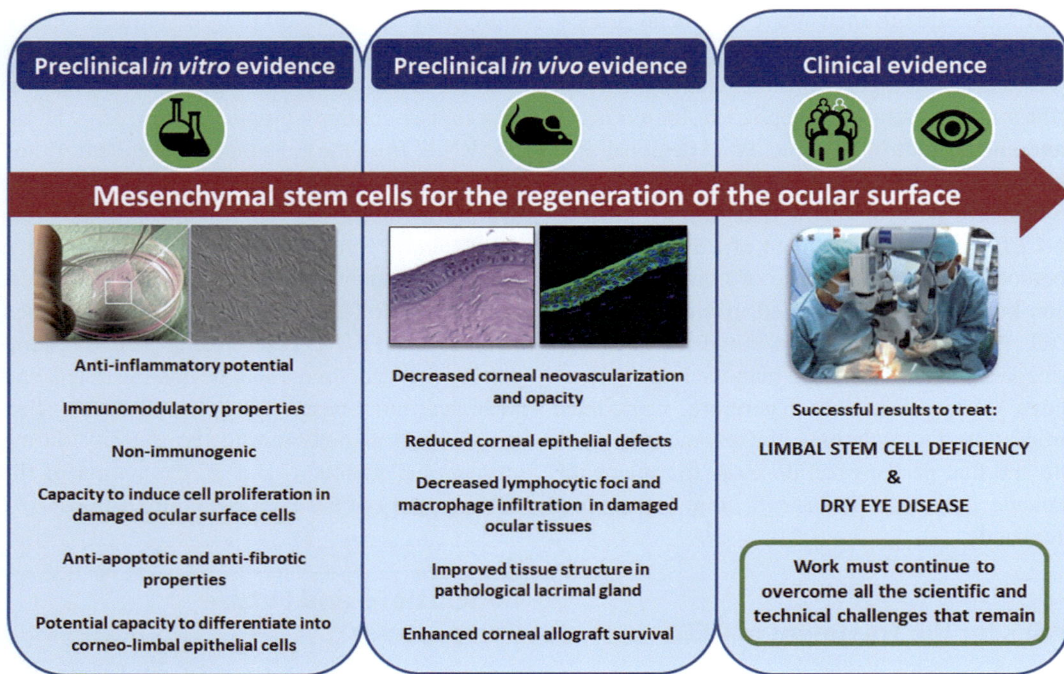

Fig. 15.2 Mesenchymal stem cells for the regeneration of the ocular surface: from preclinical to clinical evidence

regulatory issues related to live cell therapies [112, 113]. As a consequence, MSC-derived EVs could represent a safer and more cost-effective alternative than cell therapies with live MSCs. Currently, a lot of preclinical evidence supports the idea that MSC-derived EV application in corneal disease models induces anti-fibrotic, anti-apoptotic, and anti-inflammatory effects, and that it promotes corneal epithelial cell proliferation. These observations are consistent with the induction by EVs of accelerated corneal epithelial wound healing and reduced corneal epithelial defects [114, 115]. The therapeutic development of EVs is still at an early stage, and the EV mechanism of action in ocular surface diseases remains to be fully elucidated. Nevertheless, the solid evidence obtained from preclinical studies strongly suggests that, in the near future, isolated MSC-derived EVs could become a new therapeutic strategy for patients suffering from ocular surface diseases.

Take Home Notes

- MSC-based treatments for ocular surface pathology have shown potential therapeutic value.
- Preclinical studies have revealed that MSCs can prolong corneal allograft survival.
- Preclinical evidence supporting the use of MSCs for treating LSCD and DED has already been translated into clinical practice.
- Although the results obtained so far on the use of MSCs for ocular surface pathology are very encouraging, more preclinical and clinical studies are needed to confirm them.
- The clinical future of MSC-based therapy, and potentially MSC-derived EV therapy, in the ocular surface, is undoubtedly very promising.

Acknowledgements We thank B. Bromberg (Certified Editor in Life Sciences, Xenofile Editing) for his assistance in the final editing and preparation of this manuscript. This work was funded by the Ministry of Science and Innovation (grant PID2019-105525RB-100/AEI/10.13039/501100011033 MICINN/FEDER, EU), Spain; the Carlos III National Institute of Health, CIBER-BBN (CB06/01/003 MICINN/FEDER, EU), Spain; and the Regional Center for Regenerative Medicine and Cell Therapy of Castilla y León, Spain.

References

1. Flaxman SR, Bourne RRA, Resnikoff S, Ackland P, Braithwaite T, Cicinelli MV, Das A, Jonas JB, Keeffe J, Kempen J, Leasher J, Limburg H, Naidoo K, Pesudovs K, Silvester A, Stevens GA, Tahhan N, Wong T, Taylor H, Arditi A, Barkana Y, Bozkurt B, Bron A, Budenz D, Cai F, Casson R, Chakravarthy U, Choi J, Congdon N, Dana R, Dandona R, Dandona L, Dekaris I, Del Monte M, Deva J, Dreer L, Ellwein L, Frazier M, Frick K, Friedman D, Furtado J, Gao H, Gazzard G, George R, Gichuhi S, Gonzalez V, Hammond B, Hartnett ME, He M, Hejtmancik J, Hirai F, Huang J, Ingram A, Javitt J, Joslin C, Khairallah M, Khanna R, Kim J, Lambrou G, Lansingh VC, Lanzetta P, Lim J, Mansouri K, Mathew A, Morse A, Munoz B, Musch D, Nangia V, Palaiou M, Parodi MB, Pena FY, Peto T, Quigley H, Raju M, Ramulu P, Reza D, Robin A, Rossetti L, Saaddine J, Sandar M, Serle J, Shen T, Shetty R, Sieving P, Silva JC, Sitorus RS, Stambolian D, Tejedor J, Tielsch J, Tsilimbaris M, van Meurs J, Varma R, Virgili G, Wang YX, Wang NL, West S, Wiedemann P, Wormald R, Zheng Y. Global causes of blindness and distance vision impairment 1990–2020: a systematic review and meta-analysis. Lancet Glob Health. 2017;5:e1221–34. https://doi.org/10.1016/S2214-109X(17)30393-5.
2. Cotsarelis G, Cheng SZ, Dong G, Sun TT, Lavker RM. Existence of slow-cycling limbal epithelial basal cells that can be preferentially stimulated to proliferate: implications on epithelial stem cells. Cell. 1989;57:201–9. https://doi.org/10.1016/0092-8674(89)90958-6.
3. Li W, Hayashida Y, Chen Y-T, Tseng SC. Niche regulation of corneal epithelial stem cells at the limbus. Cell Res. 2007;17:26–36. https://doi.org/10.1038/sj.cr.7310137.
4. Schermer A, Galvin S, Sun TT. Differentiation-related expression of a major 64K corneal keratin in vivo and in culture suggests limbal location of corneal epithelial stem cells. J Cell Biol. 1986;103:49–62. https://doi.org/10.1083/jcb.103.1.49.
5. Dua HS, Saini JS, Azuara-Blanco A, Gupta P. Limbal stem cell deficiency: concept, aetiology, clinical presentation, diagnosis and management. Indian J Ophthalmol. 2000;48:83–92.
6. Rama P, Matuska S, Paganoni G, Spinelli A, De Luca M, Pellegrini G. Limbal stem-cell therapy and long-term corneal regeneration. N Engl J Med. 2010;363:147–55. https://doi.org/10.1056/NEJMoa0905955.
7. Ramírez BE, Sánchez A, Herreras JM, Fernández I, García-Sancho J, Nieto-Miguel T, Calonge M. Stem cell therapy for corneal epithelium regeneration following good manufacturing and clinical procedures. Biomed Res Int. 2015;2015:1–19. https://doi.org/10.1155/2015/408495.
8. Calonge M, Pérez I, Galindo S, Nieto-Miguel T, López-Paniagua M, Fernández I, Alberca M, García-Sancho J, Sánchez A, Herreras JM. A proof-of-concept clinical trial using mesenchymal stem cells for the treatment of corneal epithelial stem cell deficiency. Transl Res. 2019;206:18–40. https://doi.org/10.1016/J.TRSL.2018.11.003.
9. Behaegel J, Zakaria N, Tassignon M-J, Leysen I, Bock F, Koppen C, Ní Dhubhghaill S. Short- and long-term results of xenogeneic-free cultivated autologous and allogeneic limbal epithelial stem cell transplantations. Cornea. 2019;38:1543–9. https://doi.org/10.1097/ICO.0000000000002153.
10. Shimazaki J, Satake Y, Higa K, Yamaguchi T, Noma H, Tsubota K. Long-term outcomes of cultivated cell sheet transplantation for treating total limbal stem cell deficiency. Ocul Surf. 2020;18:663–71. https://doi.org/10.1016/j.jtos.2020.06.005.
11. Calonge M, Nieto-Miguel T, de la Mata A, Galindo S, Herreras JM, López-Paniagua M. Goals and challenges of stem cell-based therapy for corneal blindness due to limbal deficiency. Pharmaceutics. 2021;13:1483. https://doi.org/10.3390/pharmaceutics13091483.
12. Rohban R, Pieber TR. Mesenchymal stem and progenitor cells in regeneration: tissue specificity and regenerative potential. Stem Cells Int. 2017;2017:1–16. https://doi.org/10.1155/2017/5173732.
13. Dominici M, Le Blanc K, Mueller I, Slaper-Cortenbach I, Marini F, Krause DS, Deans RJ, Keating A, Prockop DJ, Horwitz EM. Minimal criteria for defining multipotent mesenchymal stromal cells. The International Society for Cellular Therapy position statement. Cytotherapy. 2006;8:315–7. https://doi.org/10.1080/14653240600855905.
14. Zhang L, Coulson-Thomas VJ, Ferreira TG, Kao WWY. Mesenchymal stem cells for treating ocular surface diseases. BMC Ophthalmol. 2015;15:155. https://doi.org/10.1186/s12886-015-0138-4.
15. O'Callaghan AR, Daniels JT. Concise Review: Limbal epithelial stem cell therapy: controversies and challenges. Stem Cells. 2011;29:1923–32. https://doi.org/10.1002/stem.756.
16. Luetzkendorf J, Nerger K, Hering J, Moegel A, Hoffmann K, Hoefers C, Mueller-Tidow C, Mueller LP. Cryopreservation does not alter main characteristics of good manufacturing process–grade human multipotent mesenchymal stromal cells including immunomodulating potential and lack of malignant transformation. Cytotherapy. 2015;17:186–98. https://doi.org/10.1016/j.jcyt.2014.10.018.

17. Ho MSH, Mei SHJ, Stewart DJ. The immunomodulatory and therapeutic effects of mesenchymal stromal cells for acute lung injury and sepsis. J Cell Physiol. 2015;230:2606–17. https://doi.org/10.1002/jcp.25028.

18. Griffin MD, Ritter T, Mahon BP. Immunological aspects of allogeneic mesenchymal stem cell therapies. Hum Gene Ther. 2010;21:1641–55. https://doi.org/10.1089/hum.2010.156.

19. Zuk PA, Zhu M, Mizuno H, Huang J, Futrell JW, Katz AJ, Benhaim P, Lorenz HP, Hedrick MH. Multilineage cells from human adipose tissue: implications for cell-based therapies. Tissue Eng. 2001;7:211–28. https://doi.org/10.1089/107632701300062859.

20. Phinney DG, Prockop DJ. concise review: mesenchymal stem/multipotent stromal cells: the state of transdifferentiation and modes of tissue repair—current views. Stem Cells. 2007;25:2896–902. https://doi.org/10.1634/stemcells.2007-0637.

21. Kuo TK, Ho JH, Lee OK. Mesenchymal stem cell therapy for nonmusculoskeletal diseases: emerging applications. Cell Transplant. 2009;18:1013–28. https://doi.org/10.3727/096368909X471206.

22. Joe AW, Gregory-Evans K. Mesenchymal stem cells and potential applications in treating ocular disease. Curr Eye Res. 2010;35:941–52. https://doi.org/10.3109/02713683.2010.516466.

23. Chamberlain G, Fox J, Ashton B, Middleton J. Concise Review: Mesenchymal stem cells: their phenotype, differentiation capacity, immunological features, and potential for homing. Stem Cells. 2007;25:2739–49. https://doi.org/10.1634/stemcells.2007-0197.

24. Ren G, Chen X, Dong F, Li W, Ren X, Zhang Y, Shi Y. Concise Review: Mesenchymal stem cells and translational medicine: emerging issues. Stem Cells Transl Med. 2012;1:51–8. https://doi.org/10.5966/sctm.2011-0019.

25. Nieto-Miguel T, Galindo S, López-Paniagua M, Pérez I, Herreras JM, Calonge M. Cell therapy using extraocular mesenchymal stem cells. In: Alió J, Alió del Barrio J, Arnalich-Montiel F, editors. Corneal regeneration. Essentials in ophthalmology. Cham: Springer; 2019. p. 231–62.

26. Beeken LJ, Ting DSJ, Sidney LE. Potential of mesenchymal stem cells as topical immunomodulatory cell therapies for ocular surface inflammatory disorders. Stem Cells Transl Med. 2021;10:39–49. https://doi.org/10.1002/sctm.20-0118.

27. Galindo S, de la Mata A, López-Paniagua M, Herreras JM, Pérez I, Calonge M, Nieto-Miguel T. Subconjunctival injection of mesenchymal stem cells for corneal failure due to limbal stem cell deficiency: state of the art. Stem Cell Res Ther. 2021;12:60. https://doi.org/10.1186/s13287-020-02129-0.

28. Galindo S, Herreras JM, López-Paniagua M, Rey E, de la Mata A, Plata-Cordero M, Calonge M, Nieto-Miguel T. Therapeutic effect of human adipose tissue-derived mesenchymal stem cells in experimental corneal failure due to limbal stem cell niche damage. Stem Cells. 2017;35:2160–74. https://doi.org/10.1002/stem.2672.

29. Di G, Du X, Qi X, Zhao X, Duan H, Li S, Xie L, Zhou Q. Mesenchymal stem cells promote diabetic corneal epithelial wound healing through TSG-6–dependent stem cell activation and macrophage switch. Invest Opthalmol Vis Sci. 2017;58:4344. https://doi.org/10.1167/iovs.17-21506.

30. Yao L, Li Z, Su W, Li Y, Lin M, Zhang W, Liu Y, Wan Q, Liang D. Role of mesenchymal stem cells on cornea wound healing induced by acute alkali burn. PLoS ONE. 2012;7:e30842. https://doi.org/10.1371/journal.pone.0030842.

31. Ke Y, Wu Y, Cui X, Liu X, Yu M, Yang C, Li X. Polysaccharide hydrogel combined with mesenchymal stem cells promotes the healing of corneal alkali burn in rats. PLoS ONE. 2015;10:e0119725. https://doi.org/10.1371/journal.pone.0119725.

32. Lin H-F, Lai Y-C, Tai C-F, Tsai J-L, Hsu H-C, Hsu R-F, Lu S-N, Feng N-H, Chai C-Y, Lee C-H. Effects of cultured human adipose-derived stem cells transplantation on rabbit cornea regeneration after alkaline chemical burn. Kaohsiung J Med Sci. 2013;29:14–8. https://doi.org/10.1016/j.kjms.2012.08.002.

33. Ghazaryan E, Zhang Y, He Y, Liu X, Li Y, Xie J, Su G. Mesenchymal stem cells in corneal neovascularization: comparison of different application routes. Mol Med Rep. 2016;14:3104–12. https://doi.org/10.3892/mmr.2016.5621.

34. Shukla S, Mittal SK, Foulsham W, Elbasiony E, Singhania D, Sahu SK, Chauhan SK. Therapeutic efficacy of different routes of mesenchymal stem cell administration in corneal injury. Ocul Surf. 2019;17:729–36. https://doi.org/10.1016/j.jtos.2019.07.005.

35. Li G, Zhang Y, Cai S, Sun M, Wang J, Li S, Li X, Tighe S, Chen S, Xie H, Zhu Y. Human limbal niche cells are a powerful regenerative source for the prevention of limbal stem cell deficiency in a rabbit model. Sci Rep. 2018;8:6566. https://doi.org/10.1038/s41598-018-24862-6.

36. Pan J, Wang X, Li D, Li J, Jiang Z. MSCs inhibits the angiogenesis of HUVECs through the miR-211/Prox1 pathway. J Biochem. 2019;166:107–13. https://doi.org/10.1093/jb/mvz038.

37. Zhang N, Luo X, Zhang S, Liu R, Liang L, Su W, Liang D. Subconjunctival injection of tumor necrosis factor-α pre-stimulated bone marrow-derived mesenchymal stem cells enhances anti-inflammation and anti-fibrosis in ocular alkali burns. Graefes Arch Clin Exp Ophthalmol. 2021;259:929–40. https://doi.org/10.1007/s00417-020-05017-8.

38. Zeppieri M, Salvetat ML, Beltrami AP, Cesselli D, Bergamin N, Russo R, Cavaliere F, Varano GP, Alcalde I, Merayo J, Brusini P, Beltrami CA, Parodi PC. Human adipose-derived stem cells for the treatment of chemically burned rat cornea: preliminary

results. Curr Eye Res. 2013;38:451–63. https://doi.org/10.3109/02713683.2012.763100.

39. Oh JY, Kim MK, Shin MS, Lee HJ, Ko JH, Wee WR, Lee JH. The anti-inflammatory and anti-angiogenic role of mesenchymal stem cells in corneal wound healing following chemical injury. Stem Cells. 2008;26:1047–55. https://doi.org/10.1634/stemcells.2007-0737.

40. Ma Y, Xu Y, Xiao Z, Yang W, Zhang C, Song E, Du Y, Li L. Reconstruction of chemically burned rat corneal surface by bone marrow-derived human mesenchymal stem cells. Stem Cells. 2006;24:315–21. https://doi.org/10.1634/stemcells.2005-0046.

41. Rohaina CM, Then KY, Ng AMH, Wan Abdul Halim WH, Zahidin AZM, Saim A, Idrus RBH. Reconstruction of limbal stem cell deficient corneal surface with induced human bone marrow mesenchymal stem cells on amniotic membrane. Transl Res. 2014;163:200–10. https://doi.org/10.1016/j.trsl.2013.11.004.

42. Pınarlı FA, Okten G, Beden U, Fışgın T, Kefeli M, Kara N, Duru F, Tomak L. Keratinocyte growth factor-2 and autologous serum potentiate the regenerative effect of mesenchymal stem cells in cornea damage in rats. Int J Ophthalmol. 2014;7:211–9. https://doi.org/10.3980/j.issn.2222-3959.2014.02.05.

43. Jiang T-S, Cai L, Ji W-Y, Hui Y-N, Wang Y-S, Hu D, Zhu J. Reconstruction of the corneal epithelium with induced marrow mesenchymal stem cells in rats. Mol Vis. 2010;16:1304–16.

44. Cejkova J, Trosan P, Cejka C, Lencova A, Zajicova A, Javorkova E, Kubinova S, Sykova E, Holan V. Suppression of alkali-induced oxidative injury in the cornea by mesenchymal stem cells growing on nanofiber scaffolds and transferred onto the damaged corneal surface. Exp Eye Res. 2013;116:312–23. https://doi.org/10.1016/j.exer.2013.10.002.

45. Cejka C, Cejkova J, Trosan P, Zajicova A, Sykova E, Holan V. Transfer of mesenchymal stem cells and cyclosporine A on alkali-injured rabbit cornea using nanofiber scaffolds strongly reduces corneal neovascularization and scar formation. Histol Histopathol. 2016;31:969–80. https://doi.org/10.14670/HH-11-724.

46. Cejka C, Holan V, Trosan P, Zajicova A, Javorkova E, Cejkova J. The favorable effect of mesenchymal stem cell treatment on the antioxidant protective mechanism in the corneal epithelium and renewal of corneal optical properties changed after alkali burns. Oxidative Med Cell Longev. 2016;2016:1–12. https://doi.org/10.1155/2016/5843809.

47. Holan V, Trosan P, Cejka C, Javorkova E, Zajicova A, Hermankova B, Chudickova M, Cejkova J. A comparative study of the therapeutic potential of mesenchymal stem cells and limbal epithelial stem cells for ocular surface reconstruction. Stem Cells Transl Med. 2015;4:1052–63. https://doi.org/10.5966/sctm.2015-0039.

48. Mittal SK, Omoto M, Amouzegar A, Sahu A, Rezazadeh A, Katikireddy KR, Shah DI, Sahu SK, Chauhan SK. Restoration of corneal transparency by mesenchymal stem cells. Stem Cell Rep. 2016;7:583–90. https://doi.org/10.1016/j.stemcr.2016.09.001.

49. Lee RH, Yu JM, Foskett AM, Peltier G, Reneau JC, Bazhanov N, Oh JY, Prockop DJ. TSG-6 as a biomarker to predict efficacy of human mesenchymal stem/progenitor cells (hMSCs) in modulating sterile inflammation in vivo. Proc Natl Acad Sci. 2014;111:16766–71. https://doi.org/10.1073/pnas.1416121111.

50. Lan Y, Kodati S, Lee HS, Omoto M, Jin Y, Chauhan SK. Kinetics and function of mesenchymal stem cells in corneal injury. Invest Opthalmol Vis Sci. 2012;53:3638. https://doi.org/10.1167/iovs.11-9311.

51. Roddy GW, Oh JY, Lee RH, Bartosh TJ, Ylostalo J, Coble K, Rosa RH, Prockop DJ. Action at a distance: systemically administered adult stem/progenitor cells (mscs) reduce inflammatory damage to the cornea without engraftment and primarily by secretion of TNF-α stimulated gene/protein 6. Stem Cells. 2011;29:1572–9. https://doi.org/10.1002/stem.708.

52. Ye J, Yao K, Kim JC. Mesenchymal stem cell transplantation in a rabbit corneal alkali burn model: engraftment and involvement in wound healing. Eye. 2006;20:482–90. https://doi.org/10.1038/sj.eye.6701913.

53. Yun YI, Park SY, Lee HJ, Ko JH, Kim MK, Wee WR, Reger RL, Gregory CA, Choi H, Fulcher SF, Prockop DJ, Oh JY. Comparison of the anti-inflammatory effects of induced pluripotent stem cell–derived and bone marrow–derived mesenchymal stromal cells in a murine model of corneal injury. Cytotherapy. 2017;19:28–35. https://doi.org/10.1016/j.jcyt.2016.10.007.

54. Acar U, Pinarli FA, Acar DE, Beyazyildiz E, Sobaci G, Ozgermen BB, Sonmez AA, Delibasi T. Effect of allogeneic limbal mesenchymal stem cell therapy in corneal healing: role of administration route. Ophthalmic Res. 2015;53:82–9. https://doi.org/10.1159/000368659.

55. Nili E, Li FJ, Dawson RA, Lau C, McEwan B, Barnett NL, Weier S, Walshe J, Richardson NA, Harkin DG. The impact of limbal mesenchymal stromal cells on healing of acute ocular surface wounds is improved by pre-cultivation and implantation in the presence of limbal epithelial cells. Cell Transplant. 2019;28:1257–70. https://doi.org/10.1177/0963689719858577.

56. Gomes JÁP, Geraldes Monteiro B, Melo GB, Smith RL, Pereira C, da Silva M, Lizier NF, Kerkis A, Cerruti H, Kerkis I. Corneal reconstruction with tissue-engineered cell sheets composed of human immature dental pulp stem cells. Invest Opthalmol Vis Sci. 2010;51:1408. https://doi.org/10.1167/iovs.09-4029.

57. Espandar L, Caldwell D, Watson R, Blanco-Mezquita T, Zhang S, Bunnell B. Application of adipose-derived stem cells on scleral contact lens carrier in an animal model of severe acute alkaline burn. Eye

Contact Lens Sci Clin Pract. 2014;40:243–7. https://doi.org/10.1097/ICL.0000000000000045.

58. Ahmed SK, Soliman AA, Omar SMM, Mohammed WR. Bone marrow mesenchymal stem cell transplantation in a rabbit corneal alkali burn model (a histological and immune histo-chemical study). Int J Stem Cells. 2015;8:69–78. https://doi.org/10.15283/ijsc.2015.8.1.69.

59. Almaliotis D, Koliakos G, Papakonstantinou E, Komnenou A, Thomas A, Petrakis S, Nakos I, Gounari E, Karampatakis V. Mesenchymal stem cells improve healing of the cornea after alkali injury. Graefes Arch Clin Exp Ophthalmol. 2015;253:1121–35. https://doi.org/10.1007/s00417-015-3042-y.

60. Gu S, Xing C, Han J, Tso MOM, Hong J. Differentiation of rabbit bone marrow mesenchymal stem cells into corneal epithelial cells in vivo and ex vivo. Mol Vis. 2009;15:99–107.

61. Reinshagen H, Auw-Haedrich C, Sorg RV, Boehringer D, Eberwein P, Schwartzkopff J, Sundmacher R, Reinhard T. Corneal surface reconstruction using adult mesenchymal stem cells in experimental limbal stem cell deficiency in rabbits. Acta Ophthalmol. 2011;89:741–8. https://doi.org/10.1111/j.1755-3768.2009.01812.x.

62. Craig JP, Nichols KK, Akpek EK, Caffery B, Dua HS, Joo C-K, Liu Z, Nelson JD, Nichols JJ, Tsubota K, Stapleton F. TFOS DEWS II definition and classification report. Ocul Surf. 2017;15:276–83. https://doi.org/10.1016/j.jtos.2017.05.008.

63. Gayton J. Etiology, prevalence, and treatment of dry eye disease. Clin Ophthalmol. 2009;3:405. https://doi.org/10.2147/OPTH.S5555.

64. Calonge M, Enríquez-de-Salamanca A, Diebold Y, González-García MJ, Reinoso R, Herreras JM, Corell A. Dry eye disease as an inflammatory disorder. Ocul Immunol Inflamm. 2010;18:244–53. https://doi.org/10.3109/09273941003721926.

65. Wei Y, Asbell PA. The core mechanism of dry eye disease is inflammation. Eye Contact Lens Sci Clin Pract. 2014;40:248–56. https://doi.org/10.1097/ICL.0000000000000042.

66. Hagan S, Martin E, Enríquez-de-Salamanca A. Tear fluid biomarkers in ocular and systemic disease: potential use for predictive, preventive and personalised medicine. EPMA J. 2016;7:15. https://doi.org/10.1186/s13167-016-0065-3.

67. Choi SW, Cha BG, Kim J. Therapeutic contact lens for scavenging excessive reactive oxygen species on the ocular surface. ACS Nano. 2020;14:2483–96. https://doi.org/10.1021/acsnano.9b10145.

68. Xu J, Wang D, Liu D, Fan Z, Zhang H, Liu O, Ding G, Gao R, Zhang C, Ding Y, Bromberg JS, Chen W, Sun L, Wang S. Allogeneic mesenchymal stem cell treatment alleviates experimental and clinical Sjögren syndrome. Blood. 2012;120:3142–51. https://doi.org/10.1182/blood-2011-11-391144.

69. Beyazyıldız E, Pınarlı FA, Beyazyıldız Ö, Hekimoğlu ER, Acar U, Demir MN, Albayrak A, Kaymaz F, Sobacı G, Delibaşı T. Efficacy of topical mesenchymal stem cell therapy in the treatment of experimental dry eye syndrome model. Stem Cells Int. 2014;2014:1–9. https://doi.org/10.1155/2014/250230.

70. Lee MJ, Ko AY, Ko JH, Lee HJ, Kim MK, Wee WR, Khwarg SI, Oh JY. Mesenchymal stem/stromal cells protect the ocular surface by suppressing inflammation in an experimental dry eye. Mol Ther. 2015;23:139–46. https://doi.org/10.1038/mt.2014.159.

71. Aluri HS, Samizadeh M, Edman MC, Hawley DR, Armaos HL, Janga SR, Meng Z, Sendra VG, Hamrah P, Kublin CL, Hamm-Alvarez SF, Zoukhri D. Delivery of bone marrow-derived mesenchymal stem cells improves tear production in a mouse model of Sjögren's syndrome. Stem Cells Int. 2017;2017:1–10. https://doi.org/10.1155/2017/3134543.

72. Abughanam G, Elkashty OA, Liu Y, Bakkar MO, Tran SD. Mesenchymal stem cells extract (MSCsE)-based therapy alleviates xerostomia and keratoconjunctivitis sicca in Sjogren's syndrome-like disease. Int J Mol Sci. 2019;20:4750. https://doi.org/10.3390/ijms20194750.

73. Park SA, Reilly CM, Wood JA, Chung DJ, Carrade DD, Deremer SL, Seraphin RL, Clark KC, Zwingenberger AL, Borjesson DL, Hayashi K, Russell P, Murphy CJ. Safety and immunomodulatory effects of allogeneic canine adipose-derived mesenchymal stromal cells transplanted into the region of the lacrimal gland, the gland of the third eyelid and the knee joint. Cytotherapy. 2013;15:1498–510. https://doi.org/10.1016/j.jcyt.2013.06.009.

74. Villatoro AJ, Fernández V, Claros S, Rico-Llanos GA, Becerra J, Andrades JA. Use of adipose-derived mesenchymal stem cells in keratoconjunctivitis sicca in a canine model. Biomed Res Int. 2015;2015:1–10. https://doi.org/10.1155/2015/527926.

75. Bittencourt MKW, Barros MA, Martins JFP, Vasconcellos JPC, Morais BP, Pompeia C, Bittencourt MD, Evangelho KDS, Kerkis I, Wenceslau CV. Allogeneic mesenchymal stem cell transplantation in dogs with keratoconjunctivitis sicca. Cell Med. 2016;8:63–77. https://doi.org/10.3727/215517916X693366.

76. Lu X, Li N, Zhao L, Guo D, Yi H, Yang L, Liu X, Sun D, Nian H, Wei R. Human umbilical cord mesenchymal stem cells alleviate ongoing autoimmune dacryoadenitis in rabbits via polarizing macrophages into an anti-inflammatory phenotype. Exp Eye Res. 2020;191:107905. https://doi.org/10.1016/j.exer.2019.107905.

77. Dietrich J, Ott L, Roth M, Witt J, Geerling G, Mertsch S, Schrader S. MSC transplantation improves lacrimal gland regeneration after surgically induced dry eye disease in mice. Sci Rep. 2019;9:18299. https://doi.org/10.1038/s41598-019-54840-5.

78. Li F, Zhao S. Control of cross talk between angiogenesis and inflammation by mesenchymal stem cells for the treatment of ocular surface dis-

eases. Stem Cells Int. 2016;2016:1–8. https://doi.org/10.1155/2016/7961816.

79. Ogawa Y, Shimmura S, Dogru M, Tsubota K. Immune processes and pathogenic fibrosis in ocular chronic graft-versus-host disease and clinical manifestations after allogeneic hematopoietic stem cell transplantation. Cornea. 2010;29:S68–77. https://doi.org/10.1097/ICO.0b013e3181ea9a6b.

80. Ogawa Y, Okamoto S, Wakui M, Watanabe R, Yamada M, Yoshino M, Ono M, Yang H-Y, Mashima Y, Oguchi Y, Ikeda Y, Tsubota K. Dry eye after haematopoietic stem cell transplantation. Br J Ophthalmol. 1999;83:1125–30. https://doi.org/10.1136/bjo.83.10.1125.

81. Shikari H, Antin JH, Dana R. Ocular graft-versus-host disease: a review. Surv Ophthalmol. 2013;58:233–51. https://doi.org/10.1016/j.survophthal.2012.08.004.

82. Ogawa Y, Kawakami Y, Tsubota K. Cascade of inflammatory, fibrotic processes, and stress-induced senescence in chronic GVHD-related dry eye disease. Int J Mol Sci. 2021;22:6114. https://doi.org/10.3390/ijms22116114.

83. Shimizu S, Sato S, Taniguchi H, Shimizu E, He J, Hayashi S, Negishi K, Ogawa Y, Shimmura S. Observation of chronic graft-versus-host disease mouse model cornea with in vivo confocal microscopy. Diagnostics. 2021;11:1515. https://doi.org/10.3390/diagnostics11081515.

84. Sanchez-Abarca LI, Hernandez-Galilea E, Lorenzo R, Herrero C, Velasco A, Carrancio S, Caballero-Velazquez T, Rodriguez-Barbosa JI, Parrilla M, Del Canizo C, San Miguel J, Aijon J, Perez-Simon JA. Human bone marrow stromal cells differentiate into corneal tissue and prevent ocular graft-versus-host disease in mice. Cell Transplant. 2015;24:2423–33. https://doi.org/10.3727/096368915x687480.

85. Martínez-Carrasco R, Sánchez-Abarca LI, Nieto-Gómez C, Martín García E, Sánchez-Guijo F, Argüeso P, Aijón J, Hernández-Galilea E, Velasco A. Subconjunctival injection of mesenchymal stromal cells protects the cornea in an experimental model of GVHD. Ocul Surf. 2019;17:285–94. https://doi.org/10.1016/j.jtos.2019.01.001.

86. Rusch RM, Ogawa Y, Sato S, Morikawa S, Inagaki E, Shimizu E, Tsubota K, Shimmura S. MSCs become collagen-type I producing cells with different phenotype in allogeneic and syngeneic bone marrow transplantation. Int J Mol Sci. 2021;22:4895. https://doi.org/10.3390/ijms22094895.

87. Al-Jaibaji O, Swioklo S, Connon CJ. Mesenchymal stromal cells for ocular surface repair. Expert Opin Biol Ther. 2019;19:643–53. https://doi.org/10.1080/14712598.2019.1607836.

88. Dietrich J, Schrader S. Towards lacrimal gland regeneration: current concepts and experimental approaches. Curr Eye Res. 2020;45:230–40. https://doi.org/10.1080/02713683.2019.1637438.

89. Baiula M, Spampinato S. Experimental pharmacotherapy for dry eye disease: a review. J Exp Pharmacol. 2021;13:345–58. https://doi.org/10.2147/JEP.S237487.

90. Gain P, Jullienne R, He Z, Aldossary M, Acquart S, Cognasse F, Thuret G. Global survey of corneal transplantation and eye banking. JAMA Ophthalmol. 2016;134:167–73. https://doi.org/10.1001/jamaophthalmol.2015.4776.

91. Williams KA, Esterman AJ, Bartlett C, Holland H, Hornsby NB, Coster DJ. How effective is penetrating corneal transplantation? Factors influencing long-term outcome in multivariate analysis. Transplantation. 2006;81:896–901. https://doi.org/10.1097/01.tp.0000185197.37824.35.

92. Alio JL, Montesel A, El Sayyad F, Barraquer RI, Arnalich-Montiel F, Alio Del Barrio JL. Corneal graft failure: an update. Br J Ophthalmol. 2021;105:1049–58. https://doi.org/10.1136/bjophthalmol-2020-316705.

93. Tahvildari M, Amouzegar A, Foulsham W, Dana R. Therapeutic approaches for induction of tolerance and immune quiescence in corneal allotransplantation. Cell Mol Life Sci. 2018;75:1509–20. https://doi.org/10.1007/s00018-017-2739-y.

94. Renfro L, Snow JS. Ocular effects of topical and systemic steroids. Dermatol Clin. 1992;10:505–12.

95. Murphy N, Lynch K, Lohan P, Treacy O, Ritter T. Mesenchymal stem cell therapy to promote corneal allograft survival. Curr Opin Organ Transplant. 2016;21:559–67. https://doi.org/10.1097/MOT.0000000000000360.

96. Oh JY, Kim E, Yun YI, Lee RH. Mesenchymal stromal cells for corneal transplantation: literature review and suggestions for successful clinical trials. Ocul Surf. 2021;20:185–94. https://doi.org/10.1016/j.jtos.2021.02.002.

97. Treacy O, Lynch K, Murphy N, Chen X, Donohoe E, Canning A, Lohan P, Shaw G, Fahy G, Ryan AE, Ritter T. Subconjunctival administration of low-dose murine allogeneic mesenchymal stromal cells promotes corneal allograft survival in mice. Stem Cell Res Ther. 2021;12:227. https://doi.org/10.1186/s13287-021-02293-x.

98. Lynch K, Treacy O, Chen X, Murphy N, Lohan P, Islam MN, Donohoe E, Griffin MD, Watson L, McLoughlin S, O'Malley G, Ryan AE, Ritter T. TGF-β1-licensed murine MSCs show superior therapeutic efficacy in modulating corneal allograft immune rejection in vivo. Mol Ther. 2020;28:2023–43. https://doi.org/10.1016/j.ymthe.2020.05.023.

99. Murphy N, Treacy O, Lynch K, Morcos M, Lohan P, Howard L, Fahy G, Griffin MD, Ryan AE, Ritter T. TNF-α/IL-1β—licensed mesenchymal stromal cells promote corneal allograft survival via myeloid cell-mediated induction of Foxp3 + regulatory T cells in the lung. FASEB J. 2019;33:9404–21. https://doi.org/10.1096/fj.201900047R.

100. Oh JY, Lee RH, Yu JM, Ko JH, Lee HJ, Ko AY, Roddy GW, Prockop DJ. Intravenous mesenchymal stem cells prevented rejection of allogeneic corneal transplants by aborting the early inflammatory

response. Mol Ther. 2012;20:2143–52. https://doi.org/10.1038/mt.2012.165.

101. Mittal SK, Foulsham W, Shukla S, Elbasiony E, Omoto M, Chauhan SK. Mesenchymal stromal cells modulate corneal alloimmunity via secretion of hepatocyte growth factor. Stem Cells Transl Med. 2019;8:1030–40. https://doi.org/10.1002/sctm.19-0004.

102. Ramos T, Scott D, Ahmad S. An update on ocular surface epithelial stem cells: cornea and conjunctiva. Stem Cells Int. 2015;2015:1–7. https://doi.org/10.1155/2015/601731.

103. Elhusseiny AM, Soleimani M, Eleiwa TK, ElSheikh RH, Frank CR, Naderan M, Yazdanpanah G, Rosenblatt MI, Djalilian AR. Current and emerging therapies for limbal stem cell deficiency. Stem Cells Transl Med. 2022;11:259–68. https://doi.org/10.1093/stcltm/szab028.

104. Keivyon KR, Tseng SCG. Limbal autograft transplantation for ocular surface disorders. Ophthalmology. 1989;96:709–23. https://doi.org/10.1016/S0161-6420(89)32833-8.

105. Pellegrini G, Traverso CE, Franzi AT, Zingirian M, Cancedda R, De Luca M. Long-term restoration of damaged corneal surfaces with autologous cultivated corneal epithelium. Lancet. 1997;349:990–3. https://doi.org/10.1016/S0140-6736(96)11188-0.

106. Sangwan VS, Basu S, MacNeil S, Balasubramanian D. Simple limbal epithelial transplantation (SLET): a novel surgical technique for the treatment of unilateral limbal stem cell deficiency. Br J Ophthalmol. 2012;96:931–4. https://doi.org/10.1136/bjophthalmol-2011-301164.

107. López-Paniagua M, De La Mata A, Galindo S, Blázquez F, Calonge M, Nieto-Miguel T. Advanced therapy medicinal products for the eye: definitions and regulatory framework. Pharmaceutics. 2021;13:347. https://doi.org/10.3390/pharmaceutics13030347.

108. Jacobs R, Tran U, Chen H, Kassim A, Engelhardt BG, Greer JP, Goodman SG, Clifton C, Lucid C, Vaughan LA, Savani BN, Jagasia M. Prevalence and risk factors associated with development of ocular GVHD defined by NIH consensus criteria. Bone Marrow Transplant. 2012;47:1470–3. https://doi.org/10.1038/bmt.2012.56.

109. Weng J, He C, Lai P, Luo C, Guo R, Wu S, Geng S, Xiangpeng A, Liu X, Du X. Mesenchymal stromal cells treatment attenuates dry eye in patients with chronic graft-versus-host disease. Mol Ther. 2012;20:2347–54. https://doi.org/10.1038/mt.2012.208.

110. Møller-Hansen M, Larsen A-C, Toft PB, Lynggaard CD, Schwartz C, Bruunsgaard H, Haack-Sørensen M, Ekblond A, Kastrup J, Heegaard S. Safety and feasibility of mesenchymal stem cell therapy in patients with aqueous deficient dry eye disease. Ocul Surf. 2021;19:43–52. https://doi.org/10.1016/j.jtos.2020.11.013.

111. Zhou T, He C, Lai P, Yang Z, Liu Y, Xu H, Lin X, Ni B, Ju R, Yi W, Liang L, Pei D, Egwuagu CE, Liu X. miR-204–containing exosomes ameliorate GVHD-associated dry eye disease. Sci Adv. 2022;8:eabj9617. https://doi.org/10.1126/sciadv.abj9617.

112. Rani S, Ryan AE, Griffin MD, Ritter T. Mesenchymal stem cell-derived extracellular vesicles: toward cell-free therapeutic applications. Mol Ther. 2015;23:812–23. https://doi.org/10.1038/mt.2015.44.

113. Fuloria S, Subramaniyan V, Dahiya R, Dahiya S, Sudhakar K, Kumari U, Sathasivam K, Meenakshi DU, Wu YS, Sekar M, Malviya R, Singh A, Fuloria NK. Mesenchymal stem cell-derived extracellular vesicles: regenerative potential and challenges. Biology. 2021;10:172. https://doi.org/10.3390/biology10030172.

114. Deng SX, Dos Santos A, Gee S. Therapeutic potential of extracellular vesicles for the treatment of corneal injuries and scars. Transl Vis Sci Technol. 2020;9:1. https://doi.org/10.1167/tvst.9.12.1.

115. McKay TB, Yeung V, Hutcheon AEK, Guo X, Zieske JD, Ciolino JB. Extracellular vesicles in the cornea: insights from other tissues. Anal Cell Pathol. 2021;2021:1–12. https://doi.org/10.1155/2021/9983900.

Induced Pluripotent Stem Cells in Epithelial Lamellar Keratoplasty

16

Sanja Bojic, Francisco Figueiredo, and Majlinda Lako

Abbreviations

ATMP	Advanced therapeutic medicinal products
CLET	Cultivated limbal epithelial transplantation
ECM	Extracellular matrix
EGF	Epithelial growth factor
ESC	Embryonic stem cells
FACS	Fluorescence-activated cell sorting
FBS	Fetal bovine serum
FGF	Fibroblast growth factor
GMP	Good manufacturing practice
HAM	Human amniotic membrane
iPSC	Induced pluripotent stem cells
KGF	Keratinocyte growth factor
KRT	Cytokeratin
LSC	Limbal stem cells
LSCD	Limbal stem cell deficiency
MSC	Mesenchymal stem cells
MZOC	Multizone ocular cells
PMC	Post-mitotic cells
RA	Trans-retinoic acid
RPE	Retinal pigmented epithelium
SDIA	Stromal cell-derived inducing activity
SEAM	Self-formed ectodermal autonomous multizone
SLET	Simple limbal epithelial transplantation
SMILE	Small incision lenticule extraction
TAC	Transient amplifying ell
TDC	Terminally differentiated cells
TGF	Transforming growth factor

Key Points

- Limbal stem cell biology and limbal stem cell deficiency;
- Limbal stem cell transplantation—advantages and limitations;
- History and biology of induced pluripotent stem cells;
- Differentiation of induced pluripotent stem cells to corneal epithelial lineages—advantages and limitations;
- Main strategies for inducing corneal epithelial differentiation in induced pluripotent stem cells.

S. Bojic (✉) · M. Lako
Faculty of Medical Sciences, Biosciences Institute, Newcastle University, Newcastle upon Tyne, UK
e-mail: sanja.bojic@newcastle.ac.uk; majlinda.lako@newcastle.ac.uk

F. Figueiredo
Faculty of Medical Sciences, Biosciences Institute, Newcastle University, Newcastle upon Tyne, UK

Department of Ophthalmology, Royal Victoria Infirmary, Newcastle upon Tyne Hospitals NHS Foundation Trust, Newcastle upon Tyne, UK
e-mail: francisco.figueiredo@newcastle.ac.uk

"""

Introduction

As the outermost part and a major protective shield of the eye, the cornea is directly exposed to the environment. Corneal scarring and opacity are the fourth most common cause of blindness globally, according to the World Health Organization [1]. Corneal diseases represent a major cause of blindness with the affected population estimated to be more than 10 million people worldwide [2, 3]. Physical injuries such as abrasions, thermal or chemical burns, infections, refractive surgeries, contact lens wearing, or insufficient tear production are common reasons for corneal damage [4]. Besides its barrier function, the cornea is also responsible for three-fourths of the total refractive power of the human eye, and preserving its transparency is vital for normal sight.

The cornea is composed of three cellular layers of different developmental origins: the outer epithelial layer (of ectodermal origin), the stroma, and the inner endothelial layer (both of neural crest origin) [5]. The epithelium as the outermost layer serves as a principal barrier to foreign materials, including pathogens, due to the presence of tight junctions between the epithelial cells and continuous cell turnover. The integrity of the corneal surface is vital for its transparency. The epithelial layer of the cornea renews continuously throughout life. A pool of epithelial stem cells located in the limbal region of the cornea serves as a lifetime reservoir of undifferentiated cells which enables constant regeneration of the cornea. Due to their location, corneal epithelial stem cells are known as limbal stem cells (LSCs). LSCs were reported for the first time in 1989 by Cotsarelis and colleagues, as slow cycling, label retaining cells [6].

The constant corneal renewal and homeostasis are achieved by three different processes that happen simultaneously in the corneal epithelium: proliferation, migration, and differentiation. Crucial for maintaining corneal integrity is the balance between proliferation and differentiation [7]. Preserving the constant pool of stem cells in the limbus throughout the lifetime is achieved by their sparse asymmetric cell divisions. During asymmetric division, stem cells give rise to one daughter cell that remains in the niche as a stem cell, while the other daughter cell enters differentiation and becomes a transient amplifying cell (TAC). Unlike stem cells that divide sparsely, TACs show very high mitotic activity. By going through multiple divisions to increase the number of cells resulting from each stem cell, they protect stem cells from going through the cell cycle too often, which could result in DNA damage accumulation in the stem cell pool over time. Eventually, after a certain number of divisions, TACs differentiate into post-mitotic cells (PMCs), incapable of further division. PMCs are fully committed to differentiation and mature into terminally differentiated cells (TDCs). Similar to the other squamous epithelia, the corneal TDCs are continuously shed from the corneal surface, while new TACs are continuously produced from LSCs residing in the basal layers of the limbus. TACs migrate from the corneal periphery toward the central region of the cornea, and simultaneously ascend from basal to superficial layers of the cornea, to differentiate and replace cells continuously lost from the corneal surface [8]. In homeostasis, the rate of cell proliferation is equal to the rate of cell desquamation, maintaining the corneal epithelial mass constant. The lifespan of human corneal epithelial cells is approximately 7–14 days [5].

Limbal Stem Cells (LSCs)

Stem cells are undifferentiated cells, with unlimited potential for self-renewal and the potential to differentiate into different cell types [9].

Tissue-specific stem cells, also known as adult stem cells, are present in almost every adult tissue, serving as a constant reservoir of new cells for tissue regeneration. LSCs as adult stem cells are responsible for lifetime-long corneal epithelial maintenance and regeneration. Most of the time stem cells are quiescent (in a growth-arrested state), but they can enter the cell cycle on demand (e.g., when tissue is injured) and give rise to their highly proliferative progenies—TACs. Although dividing less frequently, LSCs show a high clonogenic potential [10].

A critical role in preventing differentiation and maintaining a balance between quiescence, proliferation, and regeneration is played by the stem cell microenvironment, known as the stem cell niche [11]. The concept of stem cell niche as a unique microenvironment that supports an undifferentiated state ("stemness") and self-renewal of stem cells was proposed by Schofield in the late 70s [12]. Some of the key LSC niche factors are limbal extracellular matrix (ECM), the basement membrane, in particular, as well as soluble growth factors and survival molecules released by different niche cells, cell–matrix interactions, and cell–cell contacts of limbal stem cells with surrounding niche cells [13–15]. Anatomically, the LSC niche is located deep in the Palisades of Vogt, radially oriented fibrovascular ridges of the limbal stroma [16]. Interpalisade ridges are occupied by the epithelial pegs that contain limbal stem cells [17].

Mature corneal epithelial cells express differentiation markers such as cytokeratin 3 (KRT3) and 12 (KRT12). Limbal epithelial cells, on the contrary, express putative stem cell markers and lack the expression of differentiation markers such as KRT3 and KRT12 [18]. The unique, exclusive marker of LSCs, has not yet been discovered. There is, however, an extensive set of putative LSC markers proposed so far [4, 19, 20]. The correct identification of LSCs relies on a combination of the expression of putative LSC markers together with a lack of expression of corneal differentiation markers. The most widely used putative LSC marker is the epithelial transcription factor p63 and its isoform p63α (particularly ΔNp63α, which is an N-terminally truncated transcript of the alpha isoform of p63) [21, 22]. Another form of p63 commonly used is p40 (ΔNp63) [23]. Other transcription factors characteristic of LSCs are C/EBPδ and Bmi1 [24]. Different cytoplasmatic proteins (certain cytokeratins such as KRT14, KRT15, and KRT19) and cell membrane or transmembrane proteins (e.g., ABCG2, ABCB5, Notch-1, and CD200) are also proposed as potential positive LSC markers [25–29]. Recently, novel LSC markers were discovered using single-cell tran-

Table 16.1 Commonly used molecular markers of iPSC, limbal stem cells, and corneal epithelial cells

	iPSC	Limbal stem cells	Corneal epithelial cells
Intracellular markers	Nanog	p63, ΔNp63 (p40), ΔNp63α	KRT3
	Oct4	KRT14	KRT12
	Sox2	KRT15	
	c-Myc	KRT19	
	Lin28	Sox17	
Surface markers	SSEA4	ABCG2	Connexin 43
	TRA-1-60	ABCB5	Integrin α2 and α6
	TRA-1-81	Integrin β1 and α9	
		GPHA2	
		TSPAN7	

scriptomics including GPHA2, CCL20, SOX17, and TSPAN7 [19, 20, 30, 31].

The full list of positive and negative LSC markers is provided in Table 16.1.

Limbal Stem Cell Deficiency (LSCD)

LSCs could be depleted or destroyed by numerous factors, such as burns, infections, and autoimmune diseases, causing disturbance of the corneal regeneration process, which results in an ocular surface disorder called limbal stem cell deficiency (LSCD). LSCD is a chronic, painful, progressive disorder that leads to conjunctival ingrowth (conjunctivalization) and neovascularization of the corneal surface, inflammation, corneal scarring, consequential loss of transparency, and eventually loss of vision.

The common causes of LSCD are chemical and thermal burns, chronic inflammation, microbial infections, and extended contact lens wear, among others. Inherited conditions such as congenital aniridia, ectodermal dysplasia, and xeroderma pigmentosum, but also autoimmune diseases such as Stevens-Johnson syndrome and ocular cicatricial pemphigoid, could also lead to LSCD [32].

LSCD can affect only one eye (unilateral) or both eyes (bilateral) while depending on the extent of the damage could be classified as either partial or total [33]. The ablation of the LSC pool for continuous regeneration of the corneal surface results in recurrent corneal erosions or persistent epithelial defects accompanied by inflammation, and consequential, pain, irritation, tearing, redness, photophobia, epiphora, and blepharospasm [34, 35]. This may further lead to corneal scarring, thinning, and even perforation. In LSCD, not only does the regenerative stem cell function of the limbus fail but also its barrier function. As a result, conjunctival epithelium along with blood vessels invades the surface of the cornea leading to conjunctivalization of the cornea, a hallmark of LSCD. Other signs of LSCD are corneal epithelial haze, loss of limbal architecture, persistent epithelial defects, corneal neovascularization, corneal scarring, and possibly keratinization [4, 36].

Early diagnosis is very important as it can prevent further damage to the ocular surface. Although the diagnosis is largely made on clinical grounds based on slit-lamp examination, further diagnostic methods, such as corneal impression cytology and *in vivo* confocal microscopy, are very useful to confirm LSCD [4, 37].

The main aims of LSCD treatment are to support the disturbed or absent corneal regeneration by restoring the number of LSCs by transplantation and to re-establish the normal LSC niche microenvironment. However, an optimization of the corneal surface is a very important initial step as part of the LSCD management. The choice of treatment depends on the severity and the extent of the disease. For patients with severe LSCD, ocular surface reconstruction is required. In those cases, cell replacement therapy using autologous or allogeneic limbal grafts is the treatment of choice [4, 36].

Transplantation of LSCs can be achieved by taking a large biopsy for direct transplantation of whole limbal grafts from the contralateral healthy eye in unilateral LSCD or a living-related donor in bilateral LSCD (which might result in iatrogenic LSCD). A safer option is taking a smaller biopsy for either simple limbal epithelial transplantation (SLET), which includes direct transplantation of limbal epithelial tissue pieces, or *ex vivo* cultivated limbal epithelial transplantation (CLET), which requires expansion of LSCs *in vitro* before transplantation [4].

The choice of LSC source for transplantation depends on whether the disease is unilateral or bilateral. Acquired forms of LSCD could be unilateral or bilateral, while autoimmune diseases such as Steven Johnson syndrome usually have bilateral manifestations. In the case of unilateral LSCD, a limbal biopsy is taken from the healthy contralateral eye (autologous transplantation). In bilateral cases, donor tissue is obtained from a living related or unrelated donor, or a cadaver (allogeneic transplantation). In the case of allogeneic transplantation, long-term systemic immunosuppression is necessary to try to prevent the risk of allograft rejection [4]. Although LSC transplantation can improve vision in LSCD, evaluation of the 3-year outcomes of allogeneic CLET showed a decrease in LSCD severity and an increase in visual acuity up to 12 months posttreatment, but thereafter LSCD severity score and visual acuity progressively deteriorated [38]. Moreover, the 5-year graft survival defined by the absence of recurrence of the clinical signs of LSCD was 71% for autologous CLET and 0% for allogeneic LSC transplantation [39].

Long-term immunosuppressive therapy, potential risk of allograft rejection and disease transfection, shortage of donors, a limited number of LSC passages, and risk of cell/gene contamination by 3T3 feeder cells are some of the drawbacks of LSC transplantation [40, 41]. To overcome the limiting factors of LSC transplantation, alternative sources of cells for cell replacement therapy have been investigated. Other autologous epithelial stem cells such as conjunctival, epidermal, oral mucosal, and hair follicle cells, or allogeneic amniotic epithelial cells have been proposed, but none of these cell types represents a better solution than transplantation of LSCs so far.

Most of the cells were used only in preclinical models, with exemptions of oral mucosal epithelial stem cells and mesenchymal stem cells that have been used in clinical trials [42, 43].

Mesenchymal stem cells (MSCs) are easily accessible and nonimmunogenic, thereby their clinical use would not require immunosuppression. However, the potential for trans-differentiation of MSCs of neural crest and mesoderm origin into corneal epithelial cells of ectodermal origin is still questionable, particularly *in vivo* [44, 45].

Other possible sources for the generation of LSCs and corneal epithelial cells are pluripotent stem cells such as embryonic stem cells (ESCs) and induced pluripotent stem cells (iPSCs). Pluripotent stem cells represent a renewable source of autologous cells and are easily expandable and bankable [46, 47]. Besides representing an unlimited source of autologous cells, the other advantage of pluripotent stem cells compared to tissue-specific, adult stem cells, is their wider differentiation potential—they can differentiate into virtually any cell type. To date, multiple protocols have been developed for directed differentiation of both ESCs and iPSCs toward LSCs and corneal epithelium but were only tested in pre-clinical studies.

The discovery of iPSCs unlocked an abundance of possibilities in multiple areas of regenerative medicine including corneal regeneration. Although with a similar capacity to iPSCs, ESCs are the subject of serious ethical debates and therefore less interesting for wider application than iPSCs. The possibility to use cells derived from an individual patient's own iPSCs could represent a cornerstone of personalized and precision medicine. The important advantage of using a patient's own iPSCs to derive cells for cell replacement therapy is the lack of immune response (rejection) toward the body's own cells. Consequently, autologous cell transplantation with a patient's own cells would not require a long-term immunosuppression [48]. However, there is still a long way to go to achieve a safe clinical application of cells derived from iPSCs. The negative side of iPSC clinical use including potential mutagenesis and tumorigenesis, high costs of both iPSCs and iPSC-derived cell production, as well as the reproducibility of differentiation in different clones are yet to be resolved [49].

Induced Pluripotent Stem Cells (iPSCs)

In 2006, Yamanaka and his team created mouse iPSCs using retroviral transduction into mouse somatic cells, by triggering the ectopic expression of four specific genes—POU domain class 5 transcription factor 1 (*OCT3/4*), the sex-determining region Y-box2 (*SOX2*), Kruppel-like factor 4 (*KLF4*), and myelocytomatosis oncogene (*c-MYC*), under ESC culture conditions [50]. Just a year later, they created the human iPSCs [51]. Human iPSCs were generated by retroviral transduction of the same four transcription factors *OCT3/4, SOX2, KLF4,* and *c-MYC*, also known as "OSKM factors" or "Yamanaka's cocktail" [51]. OSKM factors were selected after testing many genes potentially involved in the first stages of ESC development [50]. Since then, iPSCs have been produced from a wide variety of cell types across different species, suggesting a universal molecular mechanism behind the somatic cell reprogramming [52]. This revolutionary discovery led Yamanaka to be awarded a Nobel Prize in Physiology and Medicine in 2012.

Human iPSCs are remarkably similar to human ESCs in terms of morphology, gene expression, surface antigens, proliferative potential, pluripotency, and telomerase activity. They can differentiate into cell types of all three primary germ layers (ectoderm, endoderm, and mesoderm), both *in vitro* and *in vivo* (teratoma formation). The formation of teratomas after iPSC transplantation into immunosuppressed mice is one of their hallmark characteristics [53]. Their pluripotent potential and capability to differentiate into cells of all three germ layers make iPSCs very valuable for regenerative medicine, but at the same time, limit their potential clinical use, as undifferentiated cells can give rise to teratoma upon transplantation [53].

The use of proto-oncogenes *c-MYC* and *KLF4* should be avoided in reprogramming events before the clinical use of iPSC-derived cells. Reactivation of transgene(s) could lead to tumor formation after transplantation [53]. Replacement of *c-MYC* and *KLF4* by *NANOG* and *LIN28* was also used for the successful reprogramming of human somatic cells

[54, 55]. Converting cells from one cell type to another without prior dedifferentiation into iPSCs could eliminate the risk of teratoma formation [53], in a process known as direct trans-differentiation which will be explained later.

Since iPSCs' discovery, different cellular reprogramming strategies have been introduced, which could be classified into two major groups—integrating and non-integrating. The integrating strategies rely on viral transduction of retrovirus or lentivirus, or transposons [56, 57]. The nonintegrating approach includes the use of adenovirus, Sendai virus, episomal vectors, synthetic mRNAs, recombinant proteins, or small molecules [58–60].

Initially, human skin fibroblasts were used as a starting material for iPSC generation. However, skin fibroblasts are not suitable for large-scale production, which creates a need for repeated invasive skin biopsies [61]. Peripheral blood represents a particularly desirable source, as it can be routinely obtained without the need for invasive procedures. So far, it seems that any somatic cell can be reprogrammed to become iPSCs but with variable efficiencies [62]. The origin of cells used for the generation of iPSCs might play a very important role in the iPSC phenotype and transplantation outcome [63]. Residual epigenetic memory might be responsible for the propensity of iPSC cell lines to preferentially differentiate toward cell types of their origin, especially in the initial passages.

Another important point to consider is the rather common use of feeder cells and animal-derived products in the iPSC generation process. Murine-derived feeder cells are widely used for iPSC production. Conventional iPSC culture systems also use serum-containing media, while fetal bovine serum (FBS)-containing medium is routinely used for the culture of feeder cells. However, the reduction or complete removal of serum and animal-derived products and implementation of feeder-free culture systems is a mandatory step for the generation of clinical-grade iPSCs [64].

Importantly, since iPSCs are not derived from human embryos, their use circumvents moral and ethical considerations related to the use of ESCs. Another great advantage of iPSCs is immuno-logical compatibility, as possible complications related to immune rejection would be eliminated by the generation and application of autologous iPSCs from individual patients.

Directed differentiation protocols were developed for the generation of various cell types. Sequential addition of small molecules, growth factors, vitamins, survival factors, and exposure to different substrates that are part of the natural stem cell niche induce and direct iPSC differentiation toward desired cell types. In the absence of inductive cues, spontaneous differentiation of iPSCs occurs, and they spontaneously shift toward the neuroectodermal fate [65, 66].

Takahashi and Yamanaka's breakthrough discovery of the underlying molecular mechanism of somatic cell reprogramming opened a virtually unlimited number of possibilities for their use in human models of disease and development, regenerative medicine, drug screening and discovery, and toxicological research [18, 67, 68].

The possibility of deriving human iPSCs from almost any somatic cell has created an invaluable opportunity for studying specific hereditary diseases. Patient-specific disease models can help in identifying new disease biomarkers, which can support earlier diagnosis, or serve as a ground for developing novel screening procedures. iPSC disease models can also help to identify new compounds capable of alleviating disease pathology *in vitro*, thereby supporting drug discovery and screening. Directed differentiation of iPSCs toward different tissues creates a ground for the generation of future advanced therapeutic medicinal products (ATMPs) for tissue and organ repair, offering ground-breaking new opportunities in the field of regenerative medicine. Normal developmental processes, such as ocular morphogenesis, can also be studied using iPSC differentiation models [2, 69, 70].

iPSC Differentiation to Corneal Epithelial Cells

Since 2012 when the first two studies on methods for directed differentiation of iPSCs toward corneal epithelial cells were reported, multiple research groups published protocols for the generation of corneal and limbal epithelial cells from iPSCs. We will summarize those studies with a focus on the directed differentiation of human iPSCs toward corneal epithelium. The relevance of studies related to murine iPSC-derived corneal epithelium from the clinical point of view is much lower due to the differences between mouse and human physiology.

The microenvironment of a stem cell niche, including various ECM proteins and secreted growth factors, as well as physical characteristics of the surrounding tissue, plays a vital role in the determination of stem cell fate [71]. Culture substrates (surfaces on which cells live and grow) such as feeder cells, human amniotic membrane, or various ECM proteins, together with soluble components in the culture medium (e.g., vitamins, growth factors, survival molecules, among others), provide cues for iPSC fate decision and specification. Collagen IV and laminin in the limbal basement membrane, as well as limbal fibroblasts in the stroma, are some of the important components of the LSC niche [14]. Therefore, collagen IV, a key component of limbal stroma, and laminin, a basement membrane protein, are widely used as substrates for cell cultivation [72].

Many of the studies tried to mimic the LSC niche environment in order to induce and direct differentiation toward corneal epithelium by using collagen IV or laminin coating as a substrate for cell cultivation, in combination with conditioned medium produced by corneal or limbal fibroblasts. Other studies, on the other hand, tried to mimic natural ocular surface development by inducing a cascade of signals that are known to direct the development of the corneal epithelium.

iPSCs Differentiation Toward Corneal Epithelial Cells Using Limbal Niche Cues

The first study reporting the successful differentiation of human pluripotent stem cells into corneal epithelial cells was published in 2007, by Ahmad and colleagues [73]. Their concept of replicating the corneal stem cell niche by exposing human ESCs seeded on collagen IV to a medium conditioned by limbal fibroblast to induce corneal epithelial differentiation led to a successful generation of corneal epithelial-like cells. The method published by Ahmad *et al.* inspired multiple future studies on iPSCs and served as a baseline for the development of many iPSC differentiation protocols toward corneal epithelial-like cells.

In vitro mimicking of LSC niche cues could be achieved using a conditioned medium (conditioned by either limbal or corneal fibroblasts), feeder cells (such as 3T3-J2 mouse embryonic fibroblasts or PA6 mouse stromal cell line), or natural scaffolds (such as denuded human amniotic membrane—HAM, decellularized human organ-cultured corneas, or corneal stromal lenticules).

iPSCs Differentiation Toward Corneal Epithelial Cells Using Conditioned Medium

In 2012, using an improved protocol for ESC differentiation toward corneal epithelium published by Ahmad *et al.* [73], Shalom-Feuerstein and colleagues successfully induced corneal differentiation in iPSCs and developed a cellular model of iPSC-derived corneal epithelial cells in a follow-up study. They reported using BMP4 coupled with collagen IV and corneal fibroblasts-derived conditioned medium, in a protocol that recapitulates corneal epithelial linage development, for induction of corneal epithelial differentiation of iPSCs [68]. They introduced two major modifications to the method designed for ESC differentiation toward corneal epithelium by Ahmad *et al.* [73]. Instead of limbal fibroblasts, they used corneal fibroblasts, isolated from the entire cornea. Moreover, they added BMP4, a major regulator of embryonic epithelial commitment and found that this enhanced the efficiency of corneal epithelial differentiation. Most of the cells generated using this protocol expressed mature corneal epithelial cell marker KRT3 (>90%), while 20–25% of cells were limbal epithelial progenitor cells as evidenced by the expression of KRT14 [68].

iPSCs Differentiation Toward Corneal Epithelial Cells Using Feeder Cells

In 2012, Hayashi *et al.* used dermal fibroblasts and, for the first time, limbal epithelial cells, to derive iPSCs which were then directed toward corneal epithelial differentiation using the so-called "stromal cell-derived inducing activity (SDIA) method" [74]. SDIA method was initially used for the induction of neuroectodermal differentiation of iPSCs toward dopaminergic neurons and retinal pigmented epithelium (RPE) [75]. In this study, Hayashi and colleagues showed that the long-term SDIA differentiation method could induce the generation of corneal epithelial cells, but only after the induction of differentiation of neural, RPE, and lens cells. This finding is consistent with the ocular development timeline, as corneal epithelial cells develop after RPE and lens, supporting the authors' theory that the "SDIA differentiation method *in vitro* mimics the process of ocular development *in vivo*" [74]. Importantly, limbal epithelial cell-derived iPSCs exhibited higher corneal epithelial marker expression and larger corneal epithelial cell colony numbers than dermal fibroblast-derived iPSCs. This difference may be caused by the retention of the epigenomic signature of their original parent cells after reprogramming.

In 2017, Aberdam *et al.* published an improved protocol based on their previous work [68]. In their previous study, most of the cells produced were mature corneal epithelial cells [68]. In this study, they thoroughly modified their previous culture conditions in an attempt to produce a pure population of iPSC-derived limbal epithelial cells, able to further differentiate [18]. In the first phase, they introduced feeders made of irradiated fibroblasts isolated from the peripheral cornea which were seeded on collagen IV-coated dishes. In phase two, cells were seeded on collagen IV coated dishes containing irradiated mouse 3T3-J2 feeder layer. Furthermore, the addition of TGFβ inhibitor, the cell survival rock inhibitor (Y-27632), EGF (epidermal growth factor) or KGF (keratinocyte growth factor) was added at different time points of the newly developed protocol. This modified protocol improved the lim-

bal commitment of iPSCs. Moreover, generated cells were capable of further maturation toward corneal epithelial cells [18].

iPSCs Differentiation Toward Corneal Epithelial Cells Using Natural Scaffolds (Denuded HAM, Decellularized Human Organ-Cultured Corneas, or Corneal Stromal Lenticules)

Sareen *et al.* published a study that maintained the iPSCs on a natural niche replacement represented by de-epithelialized human organ-cultured corneas and denuded HAM, both closely resembling limbal basement membrane in composition. In this study again limbal-derived iPSCs cultured on de-epithelialized human corneas, showed more advanced differentiation, evidenced by the expression of the mature corneal epithelial markers, and compared to fibroblast-derived iPSCs cultured on HAM. A certain level of retention of methylation-related epigenetic signatures in limbal-derived iPSCs could support the limbal epithelial differentiation [46].

Qin *et al.* proposed the utilization of decellularized corneal stromal lenticules, by-products of small incision lenticule extraction (SMILE), as potential scaffolds that could support the survival and proliferation of corneal epithelial-like cells derived from iPSCs [76]. Lenticules were decellularized to remove any cellular or nuclear material that could potentially cause allograft rejection. The growth of corneal epithelial stem cells on lenticules was previously investigated, and it was demonstrated that they were capable of proliferating for at least three passages in culture, suggesting that lenticules might not interfere with the stemness and proliferative potential of corneal epithelial stem cells [77].

iPSCs Differentiation Toward Corneal Epithelial Cells Using Defined Factors

While previous studies on pluripotent stem cells induction of corneal differentiation relied on various undefined or animal-derived components (such as feeder cells, amniotic membrane or use of the conditioned medium, alone or in combinations), in 2014, Mikhailova *et al.* proposed for the first time the use of defined factors for directed differentiation of iPSCs toward corneal epithelial progenitors. They used two small molecular inhibitors (i.e., SB-505124 and IWP-2) in combination with basic fibroblast growth factor (bFGF) to mimic "signalling cues active during ocular surface ectoderm development" [78].

They showed that inhibition of the TGFβ pathway using SB-505124 and the Wnt signalling pathway using IWP-2 together with activation of the FGF signaling pathway directed iPSC differentiation toward a relatively pure population of corneal epithelial-like progenitor cells, capable of terminal differentiation into mature corneal epithelial-like cells [78]. In their next study, the same group of authors evaluated the protein expression of both ESC- and iPSC-derived limbal epithelial stem cells and compared it to native human corneal epithelial cells [79]. They identified 860 unique proteins present in all three samples and showed that protein expression profiles were nearly identical in limbal epithelial cells derived from ESCs and iPSCs, proving that their differentiation protocol is reproducible and leads to the production of homogeneous cell populations [79]. Mikhailova *et al.* further investigated the use of the cells generated by their protocol on bioengineered collagen matrices in serum-free conditions for potential clinical application showing that the proliferation of cells on bioengineered matrices was significantly higher than on collagen-coated control wells [80].

iPSCs Differentiation Toward Corneal Epithelial Cells Using a Combination of Limbal Niche Cues with Defined Factors

Many studies use a combined approach, a combination of limbal niche cues (different ECM components such as collagen IV, laminin, or Matrigel) with defined chemical factors.

iPSCs Differentiation Toward Corneal Epithelial Cells Using a Combination of Limbal Niche Cues with Defined Factors Containing Animal-Derived Components

In their attempt to better reflect the complexity of the whole eye development, Hayashi *et al.* generated a so-called "self-formed ectodermal autonomous multi-zone (SEAM)" of ocular cells derived from iPSCs [69]. A proportion of iPSCs exposed to this protocol spontaneously formed circular 2D colonies composed of four concentric zones: the innermost zone 1 containing neuronal cells, zone 2 containing neural crest cell-like cells and retina-like cells (neuro-retina and RPE), zone 3 containing ocular surface epithelial-like cells (corneal, limbal, and conjunctival-like cells), and the outermost zone 4 with nonocular surface epithelial-like cells. Lens-like cells could be found at the margin of zones 2 and 3. Each zone had distinctive cell morphology, with the visible delineation with adjacent zones. The innermost zone was formed first, followed by the emergence of three more radial concentric cell zones. To some extent, the concentric SEAM seems to mimic the whole eye development, which might be useful for studies of ocular morphogenesis [69]. In this study, a laminin 511 E8 fragment (LN511E8) was used as a substrate in combination with defined factors for the full length of the protocol. Corneal epithelium-like cells generated using this protocol can be purified and sorted by fluorescence-activated cell sorting (FACS), expanded, and differentiated to form a transplantable corneal epithelial sheet that was able to recover corneal function in an animal model of LSCD [69, 70].

Shibata *et al.* continued work previously done by Hayashi *et al.* (the same research group) and reported that laminin isoforms differentially regulate the ocular cell differentiation from iPSCs, and that SEAM contains four concentric zones only when iPSCs are cultivated on LN511E8 form of laminin [71]. To investigate the capability of various laminin isoforms to facilitate the generation of iPSC-derived corneal epithelial cells, iPSCs were differentiated on five different laminin isoforms (i.e., LN111E8, LN211E8, LN332E8, LN411E8, and LN511E8). iPSCs differentiated on LN332E8 isoform generated the highest proportion of corneal epithelial-like cells. Their results suggest that iPSCs differentiation on LN332E8 enhances the yield of iPSC-derived corneal epithelial cells, and it shortens the culture period needed for corneal epithelial-like cell sheet preparation compared to iPSC differentiation on LN511E8 [71]. Although successful in corneal epithelial-like cell sheet preparation, the SEAM method is very time-consuming, complex, and requires a certain level of expertise, therefore, the outcome is not easily reproducible. Better yield, shorter differentiation time, and simpler methodology make this protocol easier to follow and reproduce compared to the one on LN511E8. Moreover, Shibata *et al.* further simplified the protocol excluding the need for FACS sorting, by introducing magnetic-activated cell sorting as an alternative to further facilitate the efficient production of transplantable corneal epithelial-like cell sheets [71].

In 2018, Kamarudin *et al.* published their defined feeder-free monolayer differentiation method [8]. Induction of corneal differentiation was achieved in pluripotent stem cells (two iPSC lines and one ESC line) by supplementation of growth factors and small molecules during the two-stage differentiation protocol. For the first seven days (the first stage of differentiation) ESCs and iPSCs seeded on Matrigel-coated plates were exposed to BMP4, all-trans-retinoic acid (RA) and EGF, alone or in combination. BMP4 and RA were selected according to their capability to promote non-neural ectodermal commitment. EGF, on the other hand, stimulates the proliferation of corneal epithelial progenitors. Importantly, this study revealed certain intra-line differences in the capability of iPSCs to differentiate into corneal epithelial-like cells which were dependent on the level of endogenous BMP signaling and could be restored via the activation of this pathway by a specific TGFβ inhibitor SB431542. The nonresponsive iPSC line had a lower level of BMP signaling activity due to lower expression of receptors and effectors, which led to low expression of BMP target genes. The addition of SB431542, influenced the balance of co-SMADS in favor of BMP signaling, leading to successful differentiation of the nonresponsive iPSC line toward corneal epithelial progenitor-like cells [8].

In 2019, Li *et al.* published a stepwise, chemically defined method to induce the differentiation of "multizone ocular cells (MZOC)" from iPSCs, which contained differentiated cell types including the neural retina, retinal pigment epithelium, surface ectoderm, neural crest, and lens cells. Resembling the SEAM method, the surface ectoderm zone of MZOC could be mechanically isolated and further induced into corneal epithelial-like cells [2]. The differentiating cells "spontaneously and progressively formed five identifiable zones" (zones 1 and 2 formed first, followed by zones 3 and 4, with zone 5 formed last). Zone 1 expressed the neural retina markers, zone 2 RPE markers, and zone 3 the surface ectodermal markers together with the LSC marker, in the peripheral region. Zone 4 cells primarily expressed neural crest markers and zone 5 lens markers. The ocular surface ectoderm (zone 3) was mechanically isolated from MZOCs and directed into corneal epithelial cells. Comparable with LSC reaching replicative senescence *in vitro* after a certain number of passages, the iPSC-derived corneal epithelial-like cells also exhibited limited proliferative capacity in a continuous passage. Therefore, further optimization of this method is necessary for the long-term expansion of these cells [2].

Xeno-Free iPSCs Differentiation Toward Corneal Epithelial Cells Using a Combination of Limbal Niche Cues with Defined Factors

To fulfil the need for more standardized, xeno-free methods for the generation of iPSC-derived ocular cells for transplantation purposes, Hongisto *et al.* developed a protocol for the generation of a relatively pure population of limbal epithelial-like cells and RPE-like cells from pluripotent stem cells (both ESCs and iPSCs), to help with efficient and large-scale production of autologous cells for cell therapies. They proposed a relatively simple, short, and easily reproducible protocol that relies on the utilization of defined molecular cues and circumvents the use of undefined animal components, such as serum and feeders. iPSCs differentiation toward limbal epithelial cells included two phases: the first one, corneal induction, conducted in suspension culture (without any plate coating) and the second one, corneal differentiation, in adherent culture (using a combination of collagen IV and laminin-521 used for coating). iPSCs-derived limbal epithelial-like cells derived by this protocol were capable of further maturation and differentiation after exposure to appropriate conditions [65]. Besides proposing the xeno-free differentiation protocol, they also implemented a monolayer culture of undifferentiated iPSCs on recombinant laminin-521 in a defined, commercially available xeno-free medium before the start of induction, ensuring the xeno-free generation of starting cell material for further differentiation. Moreover, they also developed a xeno-free cryopreservation method to provide a readily available stock of iPSC-derived limbal epithelial stem cells for potential cell therapy, as well as for quality and safety testing. Importantly, the purity of derived cells improved after cryopreservation, and even further after passaging and prolonged culture, which was documented by the increased expression of the putative stem cell marker ΔNp63 [65]. In 2018, the same protocol was published as a detailed video article, showing step-by-step instructions for robust, xeno-and feeder-free production of limbal epithelial stem cells from pluripotent stem cells [81].

Although the feeder-free culture might be more scalable and less laborious than feeder-based systems, the major drawback of this protocol, and most likely feeder-free iPSC culture in general, is that prolonged feeder-free culture using single cell passaging led to an accumulation of karyotype changes. Therefore, frequent karyotyping is necessary, and the use of low passage iPSCs for differentiation is required [65].

Direct Trans-differentiation

The risk of teratoma formation hinders the clinical use of iPSC-derived corneal epithelial cells. If rigorous purification of corneal epithelial-like cells is not performed adequately, and some undifferentiated iPSCs remained, their remaining pluripotent capacity has the potential to form teratomas after transplantation [53].

An alternative to the directed differentiation of iPSCs into corneal epithelial-like cells is a direct reprogramming method (also known as direct trans-differentiation), which is a process wherein mature, fully differentiated somatic cells are induced to become the other cell type without going through the intermediate state of pluripotency (iPSC stage) [82]. Following that approach, rat hair follicle stem cells were transdifferentiated into corneal epithelial-like cells by induced overexpression of *PAX6* together with the use of soluble factors [83], as well as murine vibrissa hair follicle stem cells [84]. Moreover, human skin-derived precursor cells were directly trans-differentiated into corneal epithelial-like cells by culturing them with a set of three growth factors (EGF, KGF, and HGF) [85]. Trans-differentiation of stem cells from human-exfoliated deciduous teeth toward a phenotype of corneal epithelium was also reported [86]. More recently, Kitazawa *et al.* reported direct reprogramming of human fibroblasts into corneal epithelial cells by overexpression of *PAX6*, *OVOL2*, and *KLF4* [87]. Some of the advantages of direct reprogramming are the circumvention of the pluripotent state, which is potentially tumorigenic, and carcinogenic, but also avoiding expensive and lengthy production and characterization of iPSC lines [88].

To examine the trans-differentiation approach, Cieslar-Pobuda and colleagues tried different combinations of transcription factors—a combination of three transcription factors important for limbal epithelial development ΔNp63, *TCF4,* and *C/EBPδ*, plus either *OCT4* or *KLF4* or both. Cells infected with any combination of transcription factors showed the same strong expression of mature corneal epithelial cell markers KRT3 and KRT12, but cells infected with ΔNp63, *TCF4,* and *C/EBPδ* proliferated and differentiated much faster than cells transduced with four or five factors. Although KRT3 and KRT12 expression suggests a change toward the corneal epithelial state, no further markers were examined, nor clonogenicity of generated cells [53].

Conclusions

Recently, in the first clinical trial based on iPSC-derived cells, iPSC-derived RPE cells were transplanted into a patient with neovascular age-related macular degeneration [89]. iPSC-derived corneal epithelial cells might be the next candidate for transplantation as LSCD is a promising target for future transplantation trials [65, 90].

Only a few thousand p63-bright limbal epithelial cells are required for cell transplantation onto the human eye. A minimum of approximately p63-bright 3000 cells is required for successful transplantation as reported by Rama *et al.* [22].

One of the limiting factors in LSC transplantation is the fact that primary *ex vivo* expanded LSCs undergo rapid replicative senescence *in vitro*. iPSCs as a potentially unlimited source of corneal epithelial cells opened the possibility to overcome replicative senescence of LSCs and enable the production of sufficient cell numbers for transplantation and cell banking. Moreover, iPSCs can be obtained from the patient's own cells, and then directed toward differentiation into the desired cell type, making them suitable for autologous cell transplantation. However, undefined culture conditions and the use of animal-derived components impede the clinical translation of iPSC-derived cells into therapeutics. GMP-compliant generation, culture, and differentiation protocols are mandatory for cell-based medicinal products. There is certainly a need for more standardized, xenogeneic-free protocols for iPSC generation, culture, and differentiation together with reasonable financial costs. Strictly defined conditions would prevent batch-to-batch variations, which is an important advantage of serum-free, xeno-free, and feeder-free protocols. Several defined xeno-free protocols for a prolonged culture of iPSCs are already

commercially available, but it was documented that long-term feeder-free culture of iPSCs leads to accumulation of karyotypic abnormalities which could influence growth and differentiation but also the safety profile of the final cell product [65, 81]. Therefore, further optimization of protocols for iPSC generation and differentiation toward corneal epithelial cells is necessary.

Multiple groups published methods for preferential differentiation of iPSCs into corneal and limbal epithelial cells. It has been documented that different iPSC clones show a different propensity for corneal differentiation, likely caused by differences in levels of endogenous signaling pathways involved in corneal epithelial development (such as BMP4) or their epigenetic status. This issue might be resolved by further optimization of the protocol specifically for each iPSC line, which unfortunately is a time-consuming, expensive, and nonsustainable process.

Most of the protocols include two steps: the induction phase and the differentiation phase.

In the induction phase direction of iPSC differentiation toward surface ectoderm is essential. TGFβ and Wnt antagonists as well as the FGF pathway activators are used to induce ectodermal differentiation, while BMP4 is used to propel differentiation toward surface ectoderm. Components of basement membrane such as collagen IV and different isoforms of laminin are used to mimic the natural niche microenvironment. Monolayer culture might be a more easily reproducible, quicker method compared to 3D corneal organoids, or 2D SEAM which are longer, more complex and difficult to standardize across different laboratories and different iPSC lines [81].

A rigorous purification to get a highly homogenous cell population, safe for transplantation purposes, is necessary before clinical utilization as sufficient purity is mandatory for cell therapies. The final product must be devoid of any undifferentiated cells, noncorneal iPSC-derived cells or cellular impurities that might originate from feeder cells. For that reason, improved protocols for highly homogenous production of corneal epithelial cells from iPSCs are necessary to consider their potential future use in cell therapy. Hayashi *et al.* included the FACS purification step to gain a homogenous population of corneal epithelial cells, including corneal stem cells, before transplantation of *ex vivo* expanded corneal epithelial cell sheets in an experimentally induced rabbit model of LSCD. Shibata *et al.* further simplified the purification process, by introducing magnetic-activated cell sorting as an alternative to FACS, intending to facilitate efficient production of the transplantable corneal epithelial-like cell sheets. So far, iPSC-derived corneal epithelial cell sheets are transplanted successfully in an experimentally induced animal model of LSCD. For the next step, in human transplantation of iPSC-derived corneal and limbal epithelial cells, the development of safe, robust, and GMP-compliant differentiation protocols is necessary. Although Hongisto *et al.* developed a xeno-free protocol, no GMP-compliant protocols for iPSC differentiation toward corneal epithelium have been published yet. Adaptation of research protocols relying on research-grade ingredients to clinical-grade protocols using GMP-grade reagents is a crucial step in the clinical translation of iPSC-derived corneal and limbal epithelial cells.

Besides their therapeutical use in regenerative medicine, iPSC-derived corneal and limbal epithelial cells can be potentially used for research purposes, including investigation of ocular morphogenesis, disease modeling, drug screening, toxicity testing, or genetic engineering.

Take Home Notes

- Induced pluripotent stem cells represent an unlimited source of autologous cells and a powerful resource for cell-based replacement corneal therapies;
- Two main strategies are used for the induction of corneal epithelial differentiation of induced pluripotent stem cells (alone or in combination)—mimicking the LSC niche environment and mimicking natural ocular surface development;
- Mimicking the limbal stem cell niche environment is achieved by using feeder cells or various extracellular protein matrix coatings in combination with a conditioned medium produced by corneal or limbal fibroblasts;
- Mimicking the ocular surface development is achieved by inducing a cascade of defined signals known to direct the development of corneal epithelium;
- Improved protocols for highly homogenous production of corneal epithelial cells from induced pluripotent stem cells as well as GMP-compliant generation, culture, and differentiation protocols are necessary to consider their use in cell therapy.

References

1. Resnikoff S, Pascolini D, Mariotti SP, Pokharel GP. Global magnitude of visual impairment caused by uncorrected refractive errors in 2004. Bull World Health Organ. 2008;86(1):63–70. https://doi.org/10.2471/blt.07.041210.
2. Li Z, Duan H, Li W, Hu X, Jia Y, Zhao C, et al. Rapid differentiation of multi-zone ocular cells from human induced pluripotent stem cells and generation of corneal epithelial and endothelial cells. Stem Cells Dev. 2019;28(7):454–63. https://doi.org/10.1089/scd.2018.0176.
3. Whitcher JP, Srinivasan M, Upadhyay MP. Corneal blindness: a global perspective. Bull World Health Organ. 2001;79(3):214–21.
4. Bojic S. Optimisation of protocols for ex vivo expansion of limbal stem cells and their enrichment. Doctoral dissertation, Institute of Genetic Medicine: Newcastle University, Newcastle upon Tyne, United Kingdom; 2020.
5. Eghrari AO, Riazuddin SA, Gottsch JD. Overview of the cornea: structure, function, and development. Prog Mol Biol Transl Sci. 2015;134:7–23. https://doi.org/10.1016/bs.pmbts.2015.04.001.
6. Cotsarelis G, Cheng S-Z, Dong G, Sun T-T, Lavker RM. Existence of slow-cycling limbal epithelial basal cells that can be preferentially stimulated to proliferate: implications on epithelial stem cells. Cell. 1989;57(2):201–9. https://doi.org/10.1016/0092-8674(89)90958-6.
7. Thoft RA, Friend J. The X, Y, Z hypothesis of corneal epithelial maintenance. Invest Ophthalmol Vis Sci. 1983;24(10):1442–3.
8. Kamarudin TA, Bojic S, Collin J, Yu M, Alharthi S, Buck H, et al. Differences in the activity of endogenous bone morphogenetic protein signaling impact on the ability of induced pluripotent stem cells to differentiate to corneal epithelial-like cells. Stem Cells. 2018;36(3):337–48. https://doi.org/10.1002/stem.2750.

9. Weissman IL. Stem cells: units of development, units of regeneration, and units in evolution. Cell. 2000;100(1):157–68. https://doi.org/10.1016/s0092-8674(00)81692-x.

10. Takács L, Tóth E, Berta A, Vereb G. Stem cells of the adult cornea: from cytometric markers to therapeutic applications. Cytometry A. 2009;75(1):54–66. https://doi.org/10.1002/cyto.a.20671.

11. Mushtaq M, Kovalevska L, Darekar S, Abramsson A, Zetterberg H, Kashuba V, et al. Cell stemness is maintained upon concurrent expression of RB and the mitochondrial ribosomal protein S18-2. Proc Natl Acad Sci. 2020;117(27):15673–83. https://doi.org/10.1073/pnas.1922535117.

12. Schofield R. The relationship between the spleen colony-forming cell and the haemopoietic stem cell. Blood Cells. 1978;4(1-2):7–25.

13. Dziasko MA, Daniels JT. Anatomical features and cell-cell interactions in the human limbal epithelial stem cell niche. Ocul Surf. 2016;14(3):322–30. https://doi.org/10.1016/j.jtos.2016.04.002.

14. Mei H, Gonzalez S, Deng SX. Extracellular matrix is an important component of limbal stem cell niche. J Funct Biomater. 2012;3(4):879–94. https://doi.org/10.3390/jfb3040879.

15. Redondo PA, Pavlou M, Loizidou M, Cheema U. Elements of the niche for adult stem cell expansion. J Tissue Eng. 2017;8:2041731417725464. https://doi.org/10.1177/2041731417725464.

16. Davanger M, Evensen A. Role of the pericorneal papillary structure in renewal of corneal epithelium. Nature. 1971;229(5286):560–1. https://doi.org/10.1038/229560a0.

17. Townsend WM. The limbal palisades of Vogt. Trans Am Ophthalmol Soc. 1991;89:721–56.

18. Aberdam E, Petit I, Sangari L, Aberdam D. Induced pluripotent stem cell-derived limbal epithelial cells (LiPSC) as a cellular alternative for in vitro ocular toxicity testing. PLoS One. 2017;12(6):e0179913. https://doi.org/10.1371/journal.pone.0179913.

19. Collin J, Queen R, Zerti D, Bojic S, Dorgau B, Moyse N, et al. A single cell atlas of human cornea that defines its development, limbal progenitor cells and their interactions with the immune cells. Ocul Surf. 2021;21:279–98. https://doi.org/10.1016/j.jtos.2021.03.010.

20. Altshuler A, Amitai-Lange A, Tarazi N, Dey S, Strinkovsky L, Hadad-Porat S, et al. Discrete limbal epithelial stem cell populations mediate corneal homeostasis and wound healing. Cell Stem Cell. 2021;28(7):1248–61. https://doi.org/10.1016/j.stem.2021.04.003.

21. Di Iorio E, Barbaro V, Ruzza A, Ponzin D, Pellegrini G, De Luca M. Isoforms of DeltaNp63 and the migration of ocular limbal cells in human corneal regeneration. Proc Natl Acad Sci U S A. 2005;102(27):9523–8. https://doi.org/10.1073/pnas.0503437102.

22. Rama P, Matuska S, Paganoni G, Spinelli A, De Luca M, Pellegrini G. Limbal stem-cell therapy and long-term corneal regeneration. N Engl J Med. 2010;363(2):147–55. https://doi.org/10.1056/NEJMoa0905955.

23. Yu M, Bojic S, Figueiredo GS, Rooney P, de Havilland J, Dickinson A, et al. An important role for adenine, cholera toxin, hydrocortisone and tri-iodothyronine in the proliferation, self-renewal and differentiation of limbal stem cells in vitro. Exp Eye Res. 2016;152:113–22. https://doi.org/10.1016/j.exer.2016.09.008.

24. Barbaro V, Testa A, Di Iorio E, Mavilio F, Pellegrini G, De Luca M. C/EBPdelta regulates cell cycle and self-renewal of human limbal stem cells. J Cell Biol. 2007;177(6):1037–49. https://doi.org/10.1083/jcb.200703003.

25. Bojic S, Hallam D, Alcada N, Ghareeb A, Queen R, Pervinder S, et al. CD200 expression marks a population of quiescent limbal epithelial stem cells with holoclone forming ability. Stem Cells. 2018;36(11):1723–35. https://doi.org/10.1002/stem.2903.

26. Umemoto T, Yamato M, Nishida K, Yang J, Tano Y, Okano T. Limbal epithelial side-population cells have stem cell-like properties, including quiescent state. Stem Cells. 2006;24(1):86–94. https://doi.org/10.1634/stemcells.2005-0064.

27. Ksander BR, Kolovou PE, Wilson BJ, Saab KR, Guo Q, Ma J, et al. ABCB5 is a limbal stem cell gene required for corneal development and repair. Nature. 2014;511(7509):353–7. https://doi.org/10.1038/nature13426.

28. Thomas PB, Liu YH, Zhuang FF, Selvam S, Song SW, Smith RE, et al. Identification of notch-1 expression in the limbal basal epithelium. Mol Vis. 2007;13:337–44.

29. Merjava S, Neuwirth A, Tanzerova M, Jirsova K. The spectrum of cytokeratins expressed in the adult human cornea, limbus and perilimbal conjunctiva. Histol Histopathol. 2011;26(3):323–31. https://doi.org/10.14670/hh-26.323.

30. Li DQ, Kim S, Li JM, Gao Q, Choi J, Bian F, et al. Single-cell transcriptomics identifies limbal stem cell population and cell types mapping its differentiation trajectory in limbal basal epithelium of human cornea. Ocul Surf. 2021;20:20–32. https://doi.org/10.1016/j.jtos.2020.12.004.

31. Dou S, Wang Q, Qi X, Zhang B, Jiang H, Chen S, et al. Molecular identity of human limbal heterogeneity involved in corneal homeostasis and privilege. Ocul Surf. 2021;21:206–20. https://doi.org/10.1016/j.jtos.2021.04.010.

32. Ahmad S. Concise review: limbal stem cell deficiency, dysfunction, and distress. Stem Cells Transl Med. 2012;1(2):110–5. https://doi.org/10.5966/sctm.2011-0037.

33. Kolli S, Ahmad S, Lako M, Figueiredo F. Successful clinical implementation of corneal epithelial stem cell therapy for treatment of unilateral limbal stem cell deficiency. Stem Cells. 2010;28(3):597–610. https://doi.org/10.1002/stem.276.

34. Espana EM, Grueterich M, Romano AC, Touhami A, Tseng SC. Idiopathic limbal stem cell deficiency. Ophthalmology. 2002;109(11):2004–10. https://doi.org/10.1016/s0161-6420(02)01250-2.

35. Utheim TP, Aass Utheim Ø, Salvanos P, Jackson CJ, Schrader S, Geerling G, et al. Concise Review: Altered versus unaltered amniotic membrane as a substrate for limbal epithelial cells. Stem Cells Transl Med. 2018;7(5):415–27. https://doi.org/10.1002/sctm.17-0257.

36. Ghareeb AE, Lako M, Figueiredo FC. Recent advances in stem cell therapy for limbal stem cell deficiency: a narrative review. Ophthalmol Therapy. 2020;9(4):809–31. https://doi.org/10.1007/s40123-020-00305-2.

37. Osei-Bempong C, Figueiredo FC, Lako M. The limbal epithelium of the eye–a review of limbal stem cell biology, disease and treatment. Bioessays. 2013;35(3):211–9. https://doi.org/10.1002/bies.201200086.

38. Shortt AJ, Bunce C, Levis HJ, Blows P, Doré CJ, Vernon A, et al. Three-year outcomes of cultured limbal epithelial allografts in aniridia and Stevens-Johnson syndrome evaluated using the clinical outcome assessment in surgical trials assessment tool. Stem Cells Transl Med. 2014;3(2):265–75. https://doi.org/10.5966/sctm.2013-0025.

39. Borderie VM, Ghoubay D, Georgeon C, Borderie M, de Sousa C, Legendre A, et al. Long-term results of cultured limbal stem cell versus limbal tissue transplantation in stage III limbal deficiency. Stem Cells Transl Med. 2019;8(12):1230–41. https://doi.org/10.1002/sctm.19-0021.

40. Tseng SC, Chen SY, Shen YC, Chen WL, Hu FR. Critical appraisal of ex vivo expansion of human limbal epithelial stem cells. Curr Mol Med. 2010;10(9):841–50. https://doi.org/10.2174/156652410793937796.

41. Baylis O, Figueiredo F, Henein C, Lako M, Ahmad S. 13 years of cultured limbal epithelial cell therapy: a review of the outcomes. J Cell Biochem. 2011;112(4):993–1002. https://doi.org/10.1002/jcb.23028.

42. Kolli S, Ahmad S, Mudhar HS, Meeny A, Lako M, Figueiredo FC. Successful application of ex vivo expanded human autologous oral mucosal epithelium for the treatment of total bilateral limbal stem cell deficiency. Stem Cells. 2014;32(8):2135–46. https://doi.org/10.1002/stem.1694.

43. Calonge M, Pérez I, Galindo S, Nieto-Miguel T, López-Paniagua M, Fernández I, et al. A proof-of-concept clinical trial using mesenchymal stem cells for the treatment of corneal epithelial stem cell deficiency. Transl Res. 2019;206:18–40. https://doi.org/10.1016/j.trsl.2018.11.003.

44. Zhang L, Coulson-Thomas VJ, Ferreira TG, Kao WW. Mesenchymal stem cells for treating ocular surface diseases. BMC Ophthalmol. 2015;15(Suppl 1):155. https://doi.org/10.1186/s12886-015-0138-4.

45. Nieto-Nicolau N, Martín-Antonio B, Müller-Sánchez C, Casaroli-Marano RP. In vitro potential of human mesenchymal stem cells for corneal epithelial regeneration. Regen Med. 2020;15(3):1409–26. https://doi.org/10.2217/rme-2019-0067.

46. Sareen D, Saghizadeh M, Ornelas L, Winkler MA, Narwani K, Sahabian A, et al. Differentiation of human limbal-derived induced pluripotent stem cells into limbal-like epithelium. Stem Cells Transl Med. 2014;3(9):1002–12. https://doi.org/10.5966/sctm.2014-0076.

47. Huang CY, Liu CL, Ting CY, Chiu YT, Cheng YC, Nicholson MW, et al. Human iPSC banking: barriers and opportunities. J Biomed Sci. 2019;26(1):87. https://doi.org/10.1186/s12929-019-0578-x.

48. Shi Y, Inoue H, Wu JC, Yamanaka S. Induced pluripotent stem cell technology: a decade of progress. Nat Rev Drug Discov. 2017;16(2):115–30. https://doi.org/10.1038/nrd.2016.245.

49. Erbani J, Aberdam D, Larghero J, Vanneaux V. Pluripotent stem cells and other innovative strategies for the treatment of ocular surface diseases. Stem Cell Rev Rep. 2016;12(2):171–8. https://doi.org/10.1007/s12015-016-9643-y.

50. Takahashi K, Yamanaka S. Induction of pluripotent stem cells from mouse embryonic and adult fibroblast cultures by defined factors. Cell. 2006;126(4):663–76. https://doi.org/10.1016/j.cell.2006.07.024.

51. Takahashi K, Tanabe K, Ohnuki M, Narita M, Ichisaka T, Tomoda K, et al. Induction of pluripotent stem cells from adult human fibroblasts by defined factors. Cell. 2007;131(5):861–72. https://doi.org/10.1016/j.cell.2007.11.019.

52. Karagiannis P, Takahashi K, Saito M, Yoshida Y, Okita K, Watanabe A, et al. Induced pluripotent stem cells and their use in human models of disease and development. Physiol Rev. 2019;99(1):79–114. https://doi.org/10.1152/physrev.00039.2017.

53. Cieślar-Pobuda A, Rafat M, Knoflach V, Skonieczna M, Hudecki A, Małecki A, et al. Human induced pluripotent stem cell differentiation and direct transdifferentiation into corneal epithelial-like cells. Oncotarget. 2016;7(27):42314–29. https://doi.org/10.18632/oncotarget.9791.

54. Yu J, Vodyanik MA, Smuga-Otto K, Antosiewicz-Bourget J, Frane JL, Tian S, et al. Induced pluripotent stem cell lines derived from human somatic cells. Science. 2007;318(5858):1917–20. https://doi.org/10.1126/science.1151526.

55. Okita K, Ichisaka T, Yamanaka S. Generation of germline-competent induced pluripotent stem cells. Nature. 2007;448(7151):313–7. https://doi.org/10.1038/nature05934.

56. Kang X, Yu Q, Huang Y, Song B, Chen Y, Gao X, et al. Effects of integrating and non-integrating reprogramming methods on copy number variation and genomic stability of human induced pluripotent stem cells. PLoS One. 2015;10(7):e0131128. https://doi.org/10.1371/journal.pone.0131128.

57. Kumar D, Talluri TR, Anand T, Kues WA. Transposon-based reprogramming to induced pluripotency. Histol Histopathol. 2015;30(12):1397–409. https://doi.org/10.14670/hh-11-656.

58. Ma X, Kong L, Zhu S. Reprogramming cell fates by small molecules. Protein Cell. 2017;8(5):328–48. https://doi.org/10.1007/s13238-016-0362-6.

59. Gurumoorthy N, Nordin F, Tye GJ, Wan Kamarul Zaman WS, Ng MH. Non-integrating lentiviral vectors in clinical applications: a glance through. Biomedicine. 2022;10(1):107. https://doi.org/10.3390/biomedicines10010107.

60. Haridhasapavalan KK, Borgohain MP, Dey C, Saha B, Narayan G, Kumar S, et al. An insight into non-integrative gene delivery approaches to generate transgene-free induced pluripotent stem cells. Gene. 2019;686:146–59. https://doi.org/10.1016/j.gene.2018.11.069.

61. Raab S, Klingenstein M, Liebau S, Linta L. A comparative view on human somatic cell sources for iPSC generation. Stem Cells Int. 2014;2014:768391. https://doi.org/10.1155/2014/768391.

62. Yamanaka S. Induced pluripotent stem cells: past, present, and future. Cell Stem Cell. 2012;10(6):678–84. https://doi.org/10.1016/j.stem.2012.05.005.

63. Scesa G, Adami R, Bottai D. iPSC preparation and epigenetic memory: does the tissue origin matter? Cell. 2021;10(6):1470. https://doi.org/10.3390/cells10061470.

64. Nakagawa M, Taniguchi Y, Senda S, Takizawa N, Ichisaka T, Asano K, et al. A novel efficient feeder-free culture system for the derivation of human induced pluripotent stem cells. Sci Rep. 2014;4:3594. https://doi.org/10.1038/srep03594.

65. Hongisto H, Ilmarinen T, Vattulainen M, Mikhailova A, Skottman H. Xeno- and feeder-free differentiation of human pluripotent stem cells to two distinct ocular epithelial cell types using simple modifications of one method. Stem Cell Res Ther. 2017;8(1):291. https://doi.org/10.1186/s13287-017-0738-4.

66. Klimanskaya I, Hipp J, Rezai KA, West M, Atala A, Lanza R. Derivation and comparative assessment of retinal pigment epithelium from human embryonic stem cells using transcriptomics. Cloning Stem Cells. 2004;6(3):217–45. https://doi.org/10.1089/clo.2004.6.217.

67. Eintracht J, Toms M, Moosajee M. The use of induced pluripotent stem cells as a model for developmental eye disorders. Front Cell Neurosci. 2020;14:265. https://doi.org/10.3389/fncel.2020.00265.

68. Shalom-Feuerstein R, Serror L, De La Forest DS, Petit I, Aberdam E, Camargo L, et al. Pluripotent stem cell model reveals essential roles for miR-450b-5p and miR-184 in embryonic corneal lineage specification. Stem Cells. 2012;30(5):898–909. https://doi.org/10.1002/stem.1068.

69. Hayashi R, Ishikawa Y, Sasamoto Y, Katori R, Nomura N, Ichikawa T, et al. Co-ordinated ocular development from human iPS cells and recovery of corneal function. Nature. 2016;531(7594):376–80. https://doi.org/10.1038/nature17000.

70. Hayashi R, Ishikawa Y, Katori R, Sasamoto Y, Taniwaki Y, Takayanagi H, et al. Coordinated generation of multiple ocular-like cell lineages and fabrication of functional corneal epithelial cell sheets from human iPS cells. Nat Protoc. 2017;12(4):683–96. https://doi.org/10.1038/nprot.2017.007.

71. Shibata S, Hayashi R, Okubo T, Kudo Y, Katayama T, Ishikawa Y, et al. Selective laminin-directed differentiation of human induced pluripotent stem cells into distinct ocular lineages. Cell Rep. 2018;25(6):1668–79.e5. https://doi.org/10.1016/j.celrep.2018.10.032.

72. Schlötzer-Schrehardt U, Dietrich T, Saito K, Sorokin L, Sasaki T, Paulsson M, et al. Characterization of extracellular matrix components in the limbal epithelial stem cell compartment. Exp Eye Res. 2007;85(6):845–60. https://doi.org/10.1016/j.exer.2007.08.020.

73. Ahmad S, Stewart R, Yung S, Kolli S, Armstrong L, Stojkovic M, et al. Differentiation of human embryonic stem cells into corneal epithelial-like cells by in vitro replication of the corneal epithelial stem cell niche. Stem Cells. 2007;25(5):1145–55. https://doi.org/10.1634/stemcells.2006-0516.

74. Hayashi R, Ishikawa Y, Ito M, Kageyama T, Takashiba K, Fujioka T, et al. Generation of corneal epithelial cells from induced pluripotent stem cells derived from human dermal fibroblast and corneal limbal epithelium. PLoS One. 2012;7(9):e45435. https://doi.org/10.1371/journal.pone.0045435.

75. Kawasaki H, Suemori H, Mizuseki K, Watanabe K, Urano F, Ichinose H, et al. Generation of dopaminergic neurons and pigmented epithelia from primate ES cells by stromal cell-derived inducing activity. Proc Natl Acad Sci U S A. 2002;99(3):1580–5. https://doi.org/10.1073/pnas.032662199.

76. Qin S, Zheng S, Qi B, Guo R, Hou G. Decellularized human stromal lenticules combine with corneal epithelial-like cells: a new resource for corneal tissue engineering. Stem Cells Int. 2019;2019:4252514. https://doi.org/10.1155/2019/4252514.

77. Barbaro V, Ferrari S, Fasolo A, Ponzin D, Di Iorio E. Reconstruction of a human hemicornea through natural scaffolds compatible with the growth of corneal epithelial stem cells and stromal keratocytes. Mol Vis. 2009;15:2084–93.

78. Mikhailova A, Ilmarinen T, Uusitalo H, Skottman H. Small-molecule induction promotes corneal epithelial cell differentiation from human induced pluripotent stem cells. Stem Cell Rep. 2014;2(2):219–31. https://doi.org/10.1016/j.stemcr.2013.12.014.

79. Mikhailova A, Jylhä A, Rieck J, Nättinen J, Ilmarinen T, Veréb Z, et al. Comparative proteomics reveals human pluripotent stem cell-derived limbal epithelial stem cells are similar to native ocular surface epithelial cells. Sci Rep. 2015;5:14684. https://doi.org/10.1038/srep14684.

80. Mikhailova A, Ilmarinen T, Ratnayake A, Petrovski G, Uusitalo H, Skottman H, et al. Human pluripotent

stem cell-derived limbal epithelial stem cells on bio-engineered matrices for corneal reconstruction. Exp Eye Res. 2016;146:26–34. https://doi.org/10.1016/j.exer.2015.11.021.

81. Hongisto H, Vattulainen M, Ilmarinen T, Mikhailova A, Skottman H. Efficient and scalable directed differentiation of clinically compatible corneal limbal epithelial stem cells from human pluripotent stem cells. JoVE. 2018;140:58279. https://doi.org/10.3791/58279.

82. Kelaini S, Cochrane A, Margariti A. Direct reprogramming of adult cells: avoiding the pluripotent state. Stem Cells Cloning. 2014;7:19–29. https://doi.org/10.2147/sccaa.S38006.

83. Yang K, Jiang Z, Wang D, Lian X, Yang T. Corneal epithelial-like transdifferentiation of hair follicle stem cells is mediated by pax6 and beta-catenin/Lef-1. Cell Biol Int. 2009;33(8):861–6. https://doi.org/10.1016/j.cellbi.2009.04.009.

84. Blazejewska EA, Schlötzer-Schrehardt U, Zenkel M, Bachmann B, Chankiewitz E, Jacobi C, et al. Corneal limbal microenvironment can induce transdifferentiation of hair follicle stem cells into corneal epithelial-like cells. Stem Cells. 2009;27(3):642–52. https://doi.org/10.1634/stemcells.2008-0721.

85. Saichanma S, Bunyaratvej A, Sila-Asna M. In vitro transdifferentiation of corneal epithelial-like cells from human skin-derived precursor cells. Int J Ophthalmol. 2012;5(2):158–63. https://doi.org/10.3980/j.issn.2222-3959.2012.02.08.

86. Tsai CL, Chuang PC, Kuo HK, Chen YH, Su WH, Wu PC. Differentiation of stem cells from human exfoliated deciduous teeth toward a phenotype of corneal epithelium in vitro. Cornea. 2015;34(11):1471–7. https://doi.org/10.1097/ico.0000000000000532.

87. Kitazawa K, Hikichi T, Nakamura T, Nakamura M, Sotozono C, Masui S, et al. Direct reprogramming into corneal epithelial cells using a transcriptional network comprising PAX6, OVOL2, and KLF4. Cornea. 2019;38(Suppl 1):S34–41. https://doi.org/10.1097/ico.0000000000002074.

88. Casaroli-Marano RP, Nieto-Nicolau N, Martínez-Conesa EM, Edel M. Potential role of induced pluripotent stem cells (IPSCs) for cell-based therapy of the ocular surface. J Clin Med. 2015;4(2):318–42. https://doi.org/10.3390/jcm4020318.

89. Mandai M, Watanabe A, Kurimoto Y, Hirami Y, Morinaga C, Daimon T, et al. Autologous induced stem-cell-derived retinal cells for macular degeneration. N Engl J Med. 2017;376(11):1038–46. https://doi.org/10.1056/NEJMoa1608368.

90. Susaimanickam PJ, Maddileti S, Pulimamidi VK, Boyinpally SR, Naik RR, Naik MN, et al. Generating minicorneal organoids from human induced pluripotent stem cells. Development. 2017;144(13):2338–51. https://doi.org/10.1242/dev.143040.

Part IV

Stromal Lamellar Keratoplasty

Bowman Layer Transplantation

Achraf Laouani, Lydia van der Star, Silke Oellerich, Korine van Dijk, Gerrit R. J. Melles, and Viridiana Kocaba

Key Points

- The standard treatment options for eyes with advanced progressive keratoconus that are not eligible for UV-cross-linking or intracorneal ring segments are DALK and PK.
- Eyes with advanced progressive keratoconus and subjectively good vision would benefit from less invasive treatment options.
- In this chapter, we present Bowman layer transplantation as a new treatment option for eyes with advanced progressive keratoconus.

Introduction

The Bowman layer (BL) is an acellular and non-regenerating layer located between the corneal epithelial basement membrane and the anterior corneal stroma. The collagen fibrils are randomly interwoven, forming a dense, felt-like sheet, in contrast to the underlying stroma, where collagen fibers run in alignment across the diameter of the cornea to form characteristic lamellae [1]. The disruption of this anatomical barrier can be congenital, or more commonly secondary to fragmentation seen in keratoconus (KC) [2, 3]. It has also been suggested that disruption of this layer may result in an abnormal wound-healing

A. Laouani · L. van der Star · K. van Dijk
Netherlands Institute for Innovative Ocular Surgery, Rotterdam, The Netherlands

Melles Cornea Clinic, Rotterdam, The Netherlands
e-mail: laouani@niios.com; vanderstar@niios.com

S. Oellerich
Netherlands Institute for Innovative Ocular Surgery, Rotterdam, The Netherlands
e-mail: Oellerich@niios.com

G. R. J. Melles (✉)
Netherlands Institute for Innovative Ocular Surgery, Rotterdam, The Netherlands

Melles Cornea Clinic, Rotterdam, The Netherlands

Amnitrans Eye Bank, Rotterdam, The Netherlands
e-mail: melles@niioc.nl

V. Kocaba
Netherlands Institute for Innovative Ocular Surgery, Rotterdam, The Netherlands

Melles Cornea Clinic, Rotterdam, The Netherlands

Amnitrans Eye Bank, Rotterdam, The Netherlands

Tissue and Cell Therapy Group, Singapore Eye Research Institute, Singapore, Singapore
e-mail: vandijk@niios.com

© The Author(s), under exclusive license to Springer Nature Switzerland AG 2023
J. L. Alió, J. L. A. del Barrio (eds.), *Modern Keratoplasty*, Essentials in Ophthalmology,
https://doi.org/10.1007/978-3-031-32408-6_17

a

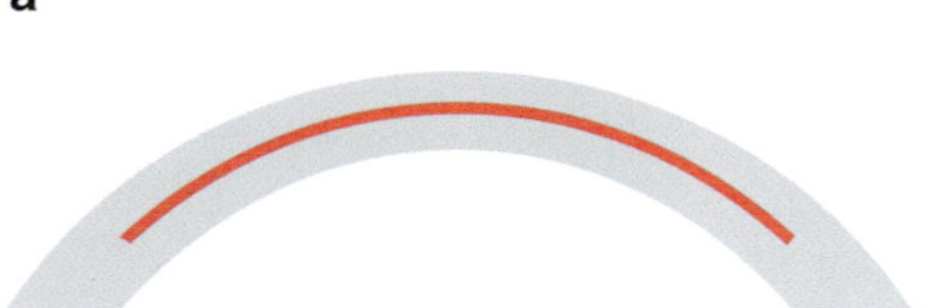

b

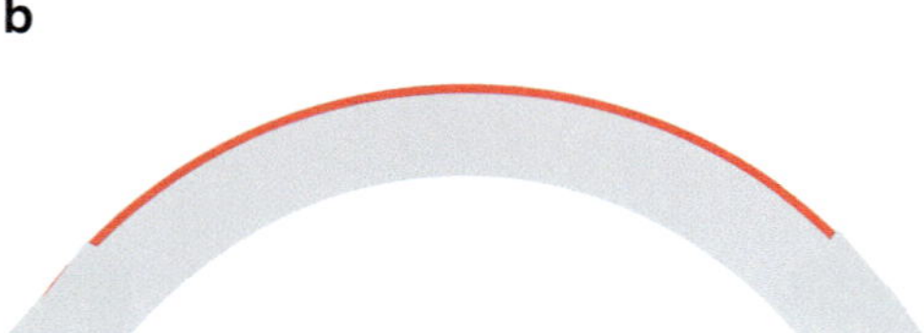

Fig. 17.1 Schematic representation of Bowman layer (BL) inlay and onlay transplantation techniques. (**a**) Bowman layer inlay. An isolated BL graft (red) is implanted intrastromally in a manually dissected pocket. (**b**) Bowman layer onlay. BL graft (red) is positioned onto the patient's anterior stroma

response, manifesting clinically as subepithelial stromal scarring [4, 5]. In view of these observations, it has been suggested that restoring this anatomical barrier, by transplanting a healthy donor BL graft, may help to stabilize the cornea against further ectasia and maintain a better epithelial–stromal interaction [6].

BL transplantation was first developed as an "inlay" graft, by inserting the BL graft in a manually created intrastromal pocket [6, 7]. In eyes with advanced, progressive KC (preoperative maximum keratometry (Kmax) >69 Diopter), this technique resulted in a flattening of 5–7 Diopter and stabilization of the corneas against further ectasia [6–8]. This technique, however, may be technically challenging, since performing a midstromal dissection in eyes with advanced KC and very thin corneas bears an increased risk for Descemet membrane perforation as also seen with deep anterior lamellar keratoplasty (DALK) [9]. To avoid the stromal dissection and the associated risk of perforation, BL transplantation was further developed into an onlay procedure in which the isolated BL graft is placed directly onto the anterior stroma resulting in a safer and technically easier procedure (Fig. 17.1) [10, 11].

Indications

Bowman layer inlay transplantation was developed to treat patients with advanced, progressive keratoconus that were not considered to be eligible anymore for ultraviolet corneal cross-linking or intracorneal ring segments treatments [6–8, 12, 13]. Based on recent clinical outcomes, the BL inlay procedure is most effective in eyes with a preoperative maximum keratometry (Kmax) of more than 69 Diopter [14]. For those advanced, progressive KC eyes with a subjectively acceptable contact lens-corrected visual acuity before BL transplantation, even with poor contact lens tolerance, BL transplantation can be indicated to postpone or even avoid the more invasive penetrating keratoplasty (PK) or DALK procedures, which were previously the only available treatment options for this group of patients [6–8, 12–14].

Advanced, progressive KC is also an indication for the recently introduced BL onlay transplantation [10]. In addition, the BL onlay procedure can help in managing subepithelial haze after excimer laser surface ablation and has the potential of reducing superficial corneal scaring and anterior corneal irregularities after herpetic infection [15, 16]. BL onlay grafting was additionally applied to reduce fluctuation in visual acuity and refractive error after previous radial keratotomy (RK) surgery and to treat a case with recurrent corneal erosions [17, 18].

Surgical Technique

Bowman Layer Graft Preparation

Isolated BL grafts can either be prepared from whole donor globes that were obtained less than 24 h postmortem and whose corneas are considered ineligible for PK or from an anterior corneal button after stripping a Descemet membrane endothelial keratoplasty (DMEK) graft [15, 19–21].

For the preparation, donor globes or anterior corneal buttons are mounted with the epithelial side up on a globe holder or artificial anterior chamber, respectively, and the epithelium is removed using surgical spears. To incise the BL, a 30-gauge needle is used just within the limbal area, 360° around. In a next step, the peripheral BL can be lifted and grasped with a McPherson forceps. With careful peeling to avoid tearing of the graft, the entire BL can be removed from the underlying stroma. The resulting BL graft usually has a diameter of 9 to 11 mm (Fig. 17.2). After removal of remnant epithelial cells, the grafts can be stored in organ-culture medium until the time of transplantation.

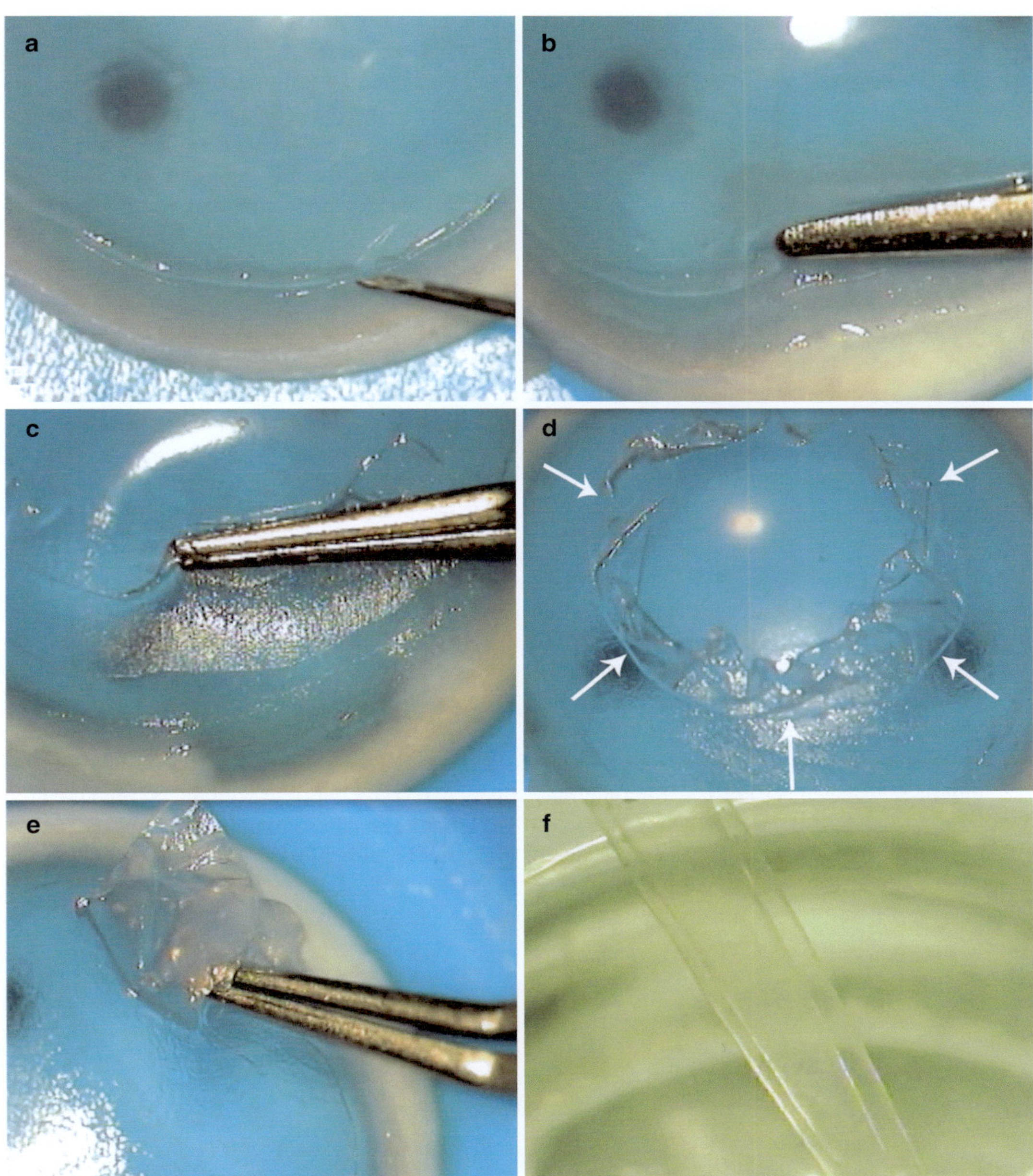

Fig. 17.2 Bowman layer (BL) graft preparation. (**a**) The donor tissue is fixed with its epithelial side up. After epithelial removal, a 30-gauge needle is used just within the limbal area, 360° around, to incise the BL. (**b**) The peripheral BL can be lifted and grasped with a McPherson forceps. (**c–e**) By careful and circular peeling, the entire BL can be removed from the underlying stroma. (**f**) The resulting BL graft usually has a diameter of 9 to 11 mm and forms a single or a double roll. (Figure reprinted from Dragnea DC, Birbal RS, Ham L, Dapena I, Oellerich S, van Dijk K, Melles GRJ. Bowman layer transplantation in the treatment of keratoconus. Eye Vis (Lond). 2018;5:24)

As the manual preparation of BL grafts may require a high technical ability and is rather time consuming, the use of a femtosecond laser to facilitate the preparation has also been explored [22, 23]. Bowman layer grafts prepared with the femtosecond laser seemed to be significantly thicker, containing anterior stroma, but were relatively smoother than manually prepared tissue [19, 22]. The potential optical impact of these differences between manually and femtosecond laser-prepared graft has not been evaluated yet.

Bowman Layer Inlay Grafting

Under retrobulbar anesthesia, a localized, superior conjunctival peritomy is performed. Then, 1–2 mm behind the limbus, a 5 mm partial thickness scleral groove is created and dissected up to the cornea using a crescent knife. A paracentesis is then fashioned, through which the anterior chamber is completely filled with air. Next, a dedicated set of curved spatulas (Melles spatula set; DORC International, Zuidland, The Netherlands) is used to dissect a mid-stromal pocket. Utilizing the air–endothelial reflex, the dissection plane aims to be at 50% stromal depth, from limbus-to-limbus, 360° around, within the recipient cornea. After the lamellar pocket has been created and most air is removed from the anterior chamber, a surgical glide [BD Visitec (Fichman); Beaver-Visitec International, Waltham, MA, USA] is inserted into the created pocket. The BL graft, which is once again immersed in 70% alcohol to remove any residual epithelial cells, and rinsed with balanced salt solution, is stained with trypan blue (VisionBlue; DORC International BV) and inserted along the surgical glide into the lamellar pocket. The BL graft is then unfolded and centered, using a cannula and jets of balanced salt solution (Fig. 17.3) [6–8]. Once the BL graft is fully unfolded, the anterior chamber is inflated up to physiological pressure with balanced salt solution, and the conjunctiva is re-approximated to the superior limbus. No sutures are required. Postoperative medications include antibiotics for the first postoperative week and corticosteroids for the first month after which the steroids are tapered.

As manual dissection in very advanced keratoectatic, thin corneas may be challenging and can result in a Descemet membrane perforation as also described for DALK [9, 12], the use of an operating microscopy with intraoperative anterior segment optical coherence tomography (AS-OCT) has been described to facilitate visualization of the dissection plane especially when blood, edema, or scarring obscures the surgeon's view of the air–endothelial reflex during the manual dissection [24, 25].

The use of a femtosecond laser to facilitate the dissection of the stromal pocket has also been explored [20, 23]. As the presence of anterior corneal scarring and/or an uneven thickness profile (which are often seen in advanced keratoconus patients) could interfere with the optimal creation of the femtosecond stromal pocket, this technique may not be suited for all KC patients [11].

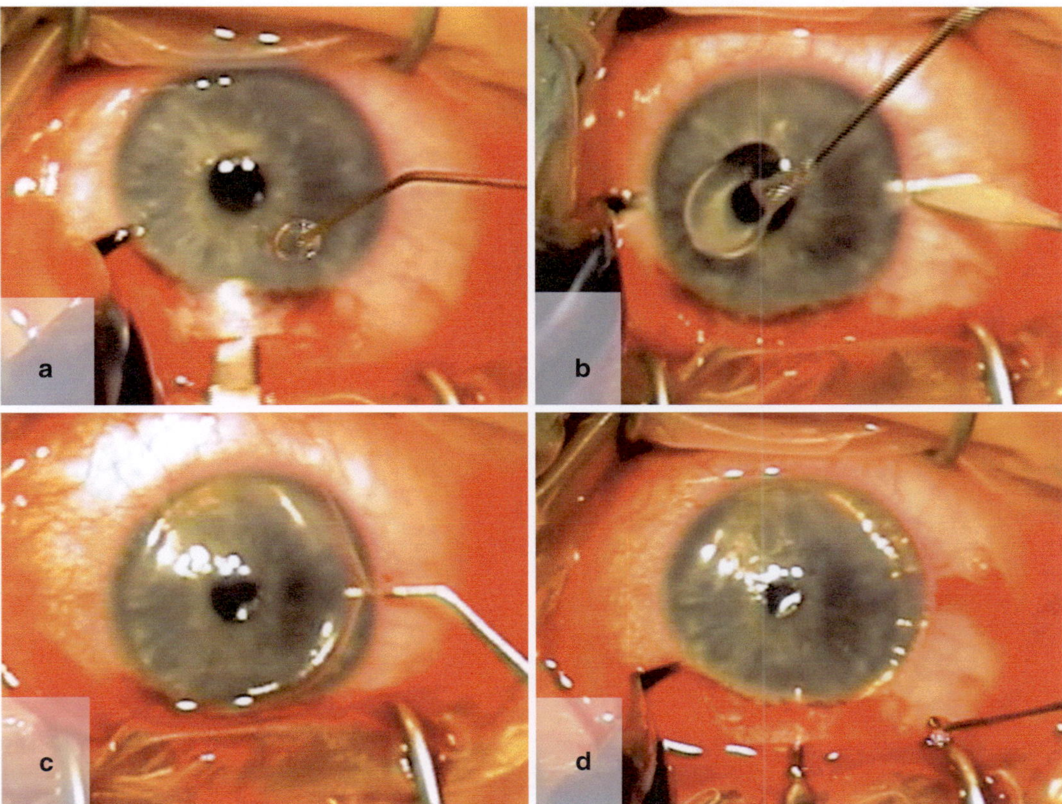

Fig. 17.3 Bowman layer (BL) inlay surgical technique. (**a**) A scleral groove is created and dissected up to the cornea and (**b**) paracentesis is then fashioned, (**c**) through which air is injected filling the anterior chamber. (**d–f**) With curved spatulas, a mid-stromal pocked is made. After air removal, (**g**, **h**) the BL graft is inserted using a glide. (**i**, **j**) The graft is then unfolded and centered using a cannula. (Figure reprinted from Dragnea DC, Birbal RS, Ham L, Dapena I, Oellerich S, van Dijk K, Melles GRJ. Bowman layer transplantation in the treatment of keratoconus. Eye Vis (Lond). 2018;5:24)

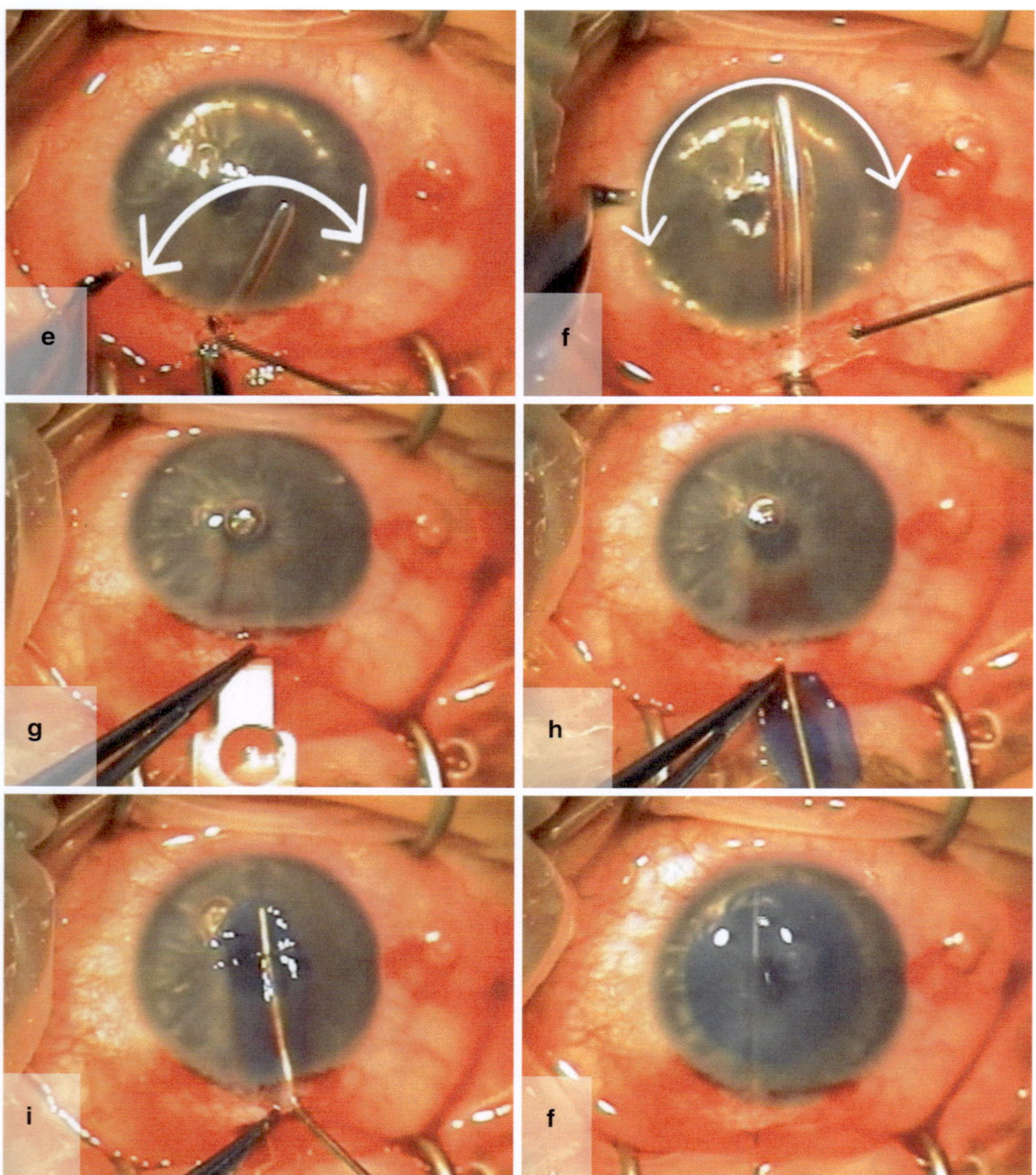

Fig. 17.3 (continued)

Bowman Layer Onlay Grafting

In very advanced KC eyes, the stromal dissection can be challenging since the apex of the cone may be very thin and fragile, with an increasing risk of perforation into the anterior chamber during surgery. Unlike the inlay technique, no corneal dissection is performed in the recently introduced BL onlay grafting technique, reducing the intraoperative risk of this procedure [10, 11].

During the procedure [10], first the recipient epithelium is removed from the corneal surface with a hockey stick knife. In case of anterior stromal scar-ring, a manual keratotomy is carefully performed. Epithelial remnants are removed by thoroughly rinsing the stromal bed with BSS. The BL graft (8.5–9.5 mm in diameter) is stained with 0.06% trypan blue (VisionBlue; DORC International) and positioned onto the recipient cornea. The graft is then stretched at the periphery 360° by using thin forceps and flattened with a bent 30-gauge cannula to squeeze out any interface fluid and to ensure the adhesion of the BL graft onto the anterior stromal bed without folds (Fig. 17.4). The BL transplant is subsequently allowed to dry-in for 45 min and a soft bandage lens is placed on the eye [10].

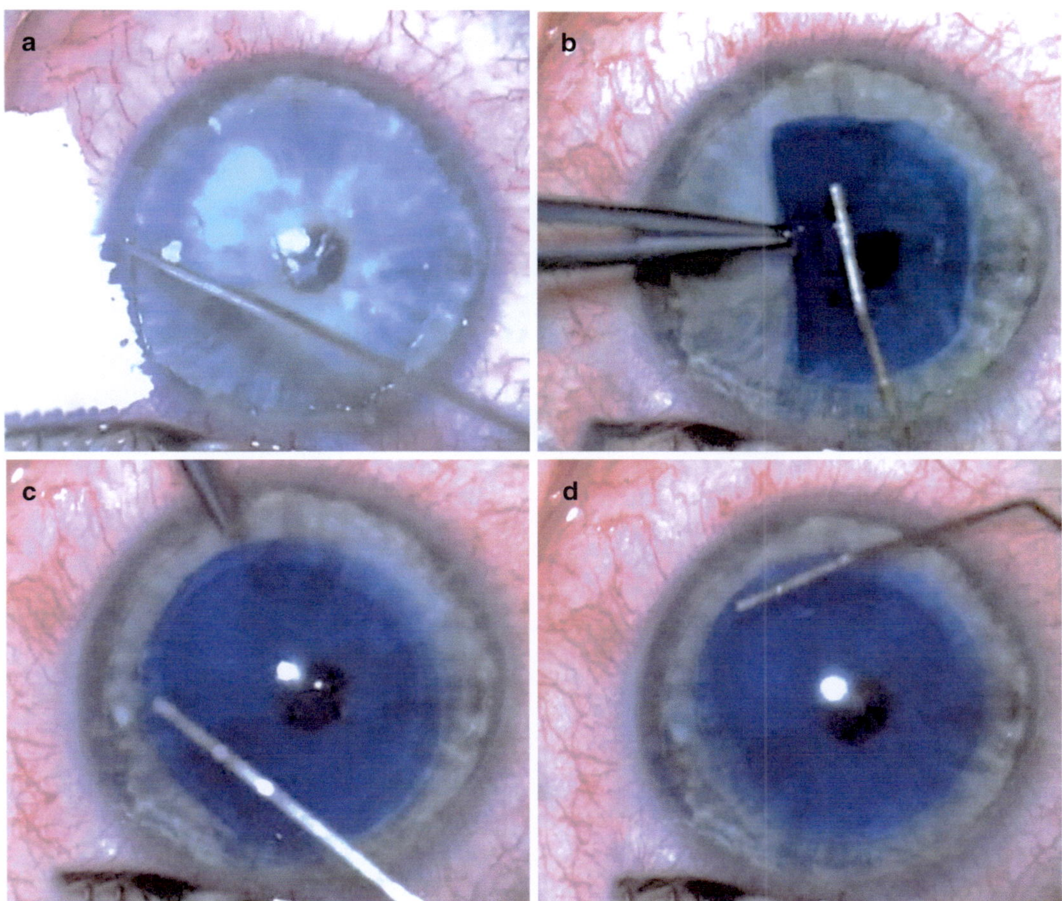

Fig. 17.4 Bowman layer onlay surgical technique. (**a**) The epithelium is first removed using a hockey stick knife. (**b**) The stained graft is positioned onto the recipient stroma. (**c**) The graft is stretched using thin forceps. (**d**) The graft is flattened with a 30-gauge cannula

Clinical Outcomes

Bowman Layer Inlay Grafting

BL inlay transplantation resulted in a stabilization of progressive KC in 88% of the eyes up to 8 years postoperatively, which is comparable to the success rate of both UV cross-linking and intracorneal ring segments [14]. Furthermore, a flattening effect with an average Kmax reduction of 7 Diopter was observed within the first postoperative month for eyes with preoperative Kmax of more than 69 Diopters with no significant further changes up to 8 years postoperatively. For eyes with preoperative Kmax of less than 69 Diopters, on the other hand, no significant change in Kmax was observed after the procedure [14]. For eyes with a preoperative Kmax of more than 69 Diopters, van Dijk et al. also showed that the posterior corneal curvature flattens postoperatively and stabilizes thereafter [7]. A similar flattening effect was also described in other reports [21, 26], while no consistent conclusion can yet be drawn on the effect of BL inlay transplantation on the posterior surface [7, 27].

While most patients achieved a subjectively acceptable vision with contact lenses and full daily wear after BL inlay transplantation, average best contact lens corrected visual acuity did not change significantly from pre- to postoperatively [13, 14, 28]. Possibly as a result of the corneal flattening for some eyes an improvement in spectacle-corrected visual acuity and a decrease in corneal higher order aberrations (especially spherical aberration) in the first postoperative year were observed [8, 29]. The mid-stromal positioning of the BL graft resulted, however, in an increase in corneal backscatter, which was found to occur up to 5 years postoperatively, and may be caused by interface irregularities [8, 13]. However, these changes did not correlate with a decrease of best-corrected visual acuity [8, 13].

Bowman Layer Onlay Graft

The clinical outcomes of BL onlay transplantation have been reported for a pilot study including five patients with advanced KC [10]. The grafts are usually re-epithelialized and appeared to be well integrated in the corneal surface within 2–3 weeks. The average Kmax decreased in this group from 75 Diopters to 70 Diopters up to 1 year after surgery [10]. No changes were observed in the posterior corneal parameters. Anterior- and posterior-order aberrations, especially the corneal front lower order aberrations, also seemed to improve throughout the postoperative follow-up period. The best contact lens corrected visual acuity remained stable [10, 11].

BL onlay transplantation was also performed to reduce fluctuations in visual acuity and refractive error in an eye after RK and the authors reported a reduction in the subjective complaints of visual fluctuation after the procedure [17]. In two cases with superficial corneal scarring secondary to herpes simplex and varicella zoster virus (HSV and VZV, respectively), BL onlay transplantation led to an improvement in corneal clarity, and no viral reactivation occurred throughout the follow-up period [16]. Finally, a case report on a patient with a history of recurrent painful corneal erosions, BL onlay grafting was performed to restore the corneal surface. Until 1.5 years postoperatively, the epithelium was smooth over the graft, and the patients had no complaints and no recurrence of the epithelial corneal erosion [18].

Complications

Since no sutures are required for both the BL inlay and onlay procedure, suture-related complications can be avoided with these procedures. Due to the acellularity of the BL graft, allograft rejection may be unlikely for both procedures and topical steroids may be rapidly discontinued, minimizing the risk of glaucoma development or cataract formation [8, 11].

Bowman Layer Inlay Graft

In the case of the inlay graft technique, the main intraoperative complication (7.9–12.5%) [14, 21] may be a Descemet membrane perforation while

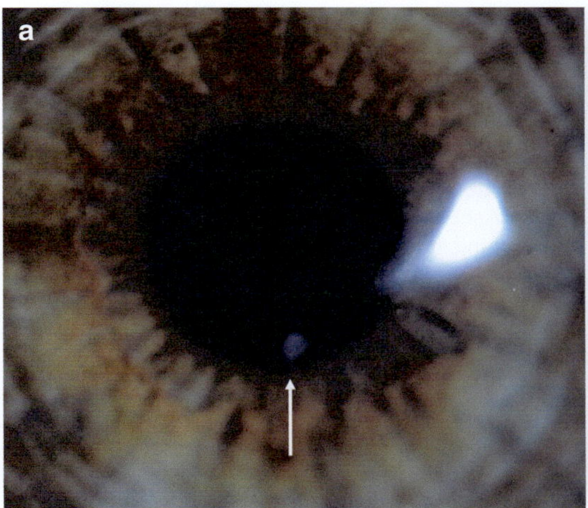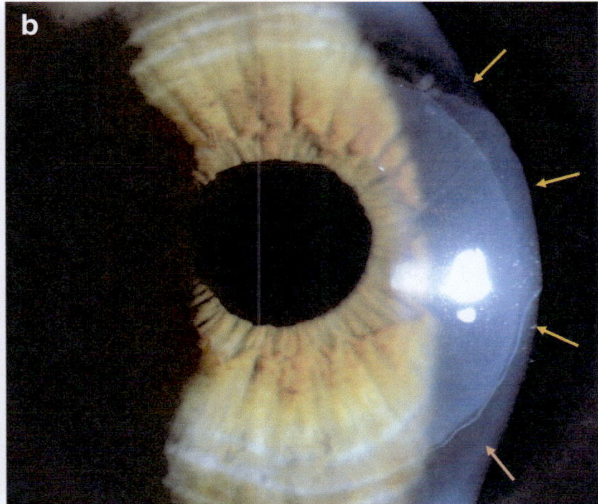

Fig. 17.5 Pre- and postoperative images of an eye that underwent Bowman layer onlay transplantation for advanced keratoconus. (**a**) Preoperative and (**b**) 2 years after Bowman layer onlay transplantation. Note that the scar (white arrow in **a**) is no longer present in **b**. Orange arrows point to notches in the BL-onlay graft

dissecting the mid-stromal pocket [7, 14, 21]. As with DALK, these perforations can be managed expectantly by aborting the operation, which allows healing, and reattempting again at a later date [9, 11, 12]. Alternatively, the surgeon may proceed with PK, depending on the size and position of the perforation.

In a group of 35 eyes undergoing BL inlay transplantation, 4 eyes (11.4%) showed continued corneal steepening and one patient underwent successful BL inlay retransplantation for unsatisfactory visual performance at 22 months after the initial BL inlay transplantation [14]. Five eyes (four patients) developed an acute corneal hydrops within 8 years after surgery (at 43–82 months postoperatively). These patients had a history of severe eye rubbing and atopy and had continued with eye rubbing after BL inlay transplantation. The eyes were treated with topical dexamethasone and NaCl, which resulted in corneal clearing with some residual scarring and visual restoration to pre-hydrops levels [14].

Bowman Layer Onlay Graft

For the five eyes included in the proof-of-concept study of the BL onlay technique, it was reported that one eye with a partial dislocation of the graft on the first postoperative day due to inadvertent removal of the bandage lens [10]. The graft was then repositioned and covered with amniotic membrane and a new bandage lens. It was also observed that most BL onlay grafts showed some notches located at the peripheral edges progressing over time (Fig. 17.5), but without any detectable effect on the corneal curvature [10]. These notches could be secondary to a difference in thickness of the graft or a variable wound-healing response.

For the BL onlay procedures performed for indications other than advanced, progressive KC, no postoperative complications have been reported [16–18].

Conclusion

BL graft transplantation is a promising new surgical technique for the treatment of advanced, progressive keratoconus in order to postpone or prevent a more invasive corneal surgery.

In eyes with advanced, progressive keratoconus, both BL inlay and onlay grafting seem to show comparable clinical outcomes in the first postoperative months, resulting in corneal flattening, stabilization against further ectasia, and enabling continued contact lens wear with high tolerance. In addition, the BL onlay procedure was successfully applied to reduce superficial corneal scarring and/or anterior corneal irregularities and as a treatment of last resort in patients with recurrent corneal erosions.

Overall, the BL onlay approach is technically less challenging and shows promising results, which need to be confirmed in a larger cohort of patient. Less invasive and completely extraocular, the BL onlay procedure has the potential to become the preferred surgical option for advanced KC.

Take Home Notes

- Bowman layer inlay or onlay transplantation may become an alternative treatment option for eyes with advanced progressive keratoconus in order to postpone or prevent a more invasive corneal surgery.
- Bowman layer transplantation can be performed intrastromally or as an onlay graft and induces a corneal flattening and stabilization of the keratoconus, maintaining the visual acuity and the comfort of the contact lens wear.
- Bowman layer onlay grafting is technically less challenging, less invasive and completely extraocular.
- Bowman layer onlay grafts may also be applied to reduce superficial corneal scarring and/or anterior corneal irregularities and as a treatment of last resort in patients with recurrent corneal erosions.

References

1. Wilson SE, Hong JW. Bowman's layer structure and function: critical or dispensable to corneal function? A hypothesis. Cornea. 2000;19(4):417–20.
2. Romero-Jiménez M, Santodomingo-Rubido J, Wolffsohn JS. Keratoconus: a review. Cont Lens Anter Eye. 2010;33(4):157–66.
3. Ambekar R, Toussaint KC Jr, Wagoner Johnson A. The effect of keratoconus on the structural, mechanical, and optical properties of the cornea. J Mech Behav Biomed Mater. 2011;4(3):223–36.
4. Melles GRJ, Binder PS. A comparison of wound healing in sutured and unsutured corneal wounds. Arch Ophthalmol. 1990;108(10):1460–9.
5. Melles GRJ, Binder PS, Anderson JA. Variation in healing throughout the depth of long-term, unsutured, corneal wounds in human autopsy specimens and monkeys. Arch Ophthalmol. 1994;112(1):100–9.
6. Van Dijk K, Parker J, Tong CM, Ham L, Lie JT, Groeneveld-van Beek EA, Melles GRJ. Midstromal isolated Bowman layer graft for reduction of advanced keratoconus – a technique to postpone penetrating or deep anterior lamellar keratoplasty. JAMA Ophthalmol. 2014;132(4):495–501.
7. Van Dijk K, Liarakos VS, Parker J, Ham L, Lie JT, Groeneveld-van Beek EA, Melles GRJ. Bowman layer transplantation to reduce and stabilize progressive, advanced keratoconus. Ophthalmology. 2015;122(5):909–17.
8. Dragnea DC, Birbal RS, Ham L, Dapena I, Oellerich S, van Dijk K, Melles GRJ. Bowman layer transplantation in the treatment of keratoconus. Eye Vis. 2018;5:24.
9. Karimian F, Feizi S. Deep anterior lamellar keratoplasty: indications, surgical techniques and complications. Mid E Afr J Ophthalmol. 2010;17(1):28–37.
10. Dapena I, van der Star L, Groeneveld-van Beek EA, Quilendrino R, van Dijk K, Parker JS, Oellerich S, Melles GRJ. Bowman layer onlay grafting: proof-of-concept of a new technique to flatten corneal curvature and reduce progression in keratoconus. Cornea. 2021;40(12):1561–6.
11. Dapena I, Parker JS, Melles GRJ. Potential benefits of modified corneal tissue grafts for keratoconus: Bowman layer 'inlay' and 'onlay' transplantation, and allogenic tissue ring segments. Curr Opin Ophthalmol. 2020;31(4):276–83.
12. Parker JS, van Dijk K, Melles GR. Treatment options for advanced keratoconus: a review. Surv Ophthalmol. 2015;60(5):459–80.
13. Van Dijk K, Parker JS, Baydoun L, Ilyas A, Dapena I, Groeneveld-van Beek EA, Melles GRJ. Bowman layer transplantation: 5-year results. Graefes Arch Clin Exp Ophthalmol. 2018;256(6):1151–8.
14. Van der Star L, van Dijk K, Vasiliauskaitė I, Dapena I, Oellerich S, Melles GRJ. Long-term outcomes of Bowman layer inlay transplantation for the treatment of progressive keratoconus. Cornea. 2021;41:1150.
15. Lie J, Droutsas K, Ham L, Dapena I, Ververs B, Otten H, van der Wees J, Melles GRJ. Isolated Bowman layer transplantation to manage persistent subepithelial haze after excimer laser surface ablation. J Cataract Refract Surg. 2010;36(6):1036–41.
16. Dapena I, Musayeva A, Dragnea DC, Groeneveld-van Beek EA, Ní Dhubhghaill S, Parker JS, van Dijk K, Melles GRJ. Bowman layer onlay transplantation to manage herpes corneal scar. Cornea. 2020;39(9):1164–6.
17. Parker JS, Dockery PW, Parker JS, Dapena I, van Dijk K, Melles GRJ. Bowman layer onlay graft for reducing fluctuation in visual acuity after previous radial keratotomy. Cornea. 2020;39(10):1303–6.
18. Mulders-Al-Saady R, van der Star L, van Dijk K, Parker JS, Dapena I, Melles GRJ. Bowman layer

onlay graft for recurrent corneal erosions in map–dot–fingerprint dystrophy. Cornea. 2022;41:1062.

19. Groeneveld-van Beek EA, Parker J, Lie JT, et al. Donor tissue preparation for Bowman layer transplantation. Cornea. 2016;35(12):1499–502.

20. García de Oteyza G, González Dibildox LA, Vázquez-Romo KA, Tapia-Vazquez A, Davila-Alquisiras JH, Martínez-Báez BE, Garcia-Albisua AM, Ramirez M, Hernández-Quintela E. Bowman layer transplantation using a femtosecond laser. J Cataract Refract Surg. 2019;45(3):261–6.

21. Tourkmani AK, Mohammad T, McCance E, Potts J, Ford R, Anderson DF. One-year front versus central and paracentral corneal changes after Bowman layer transplantation for keratoconus. Cornea. 2021;41(2):165–70.

22. Parker JS, Huls F, Cooper E, Graves P, Groeneveld-van Beek EA, Lie J, Melles GRJ. Technical feasibility of isolated Bowman layer graft preparation by femtosecond laser: a pilot study. Eur J Ophthalmol. 2017;27(6):675–7.

23. Mittal V, Rathod D, Sehdev N. Bowman-stromal inlay using an intraocular lens injector for management of keratoconus. J Cataract Refract Surg. 2021;47(12):e49–55.

24. Tong CM, van Dijk K, Melles GRJ. Update on Bowman layer transplantation. Curr Opin Ophthalmol. 2019;30(4):249–55.

25. Tong CM, Parker JS, Dockery PW, Birbal RS, Melles GRJ. Use of intraoperative anterior segment optical coherence tomography for Bowman layer transplantation. Acta Ophthalmol. 2019;97(7):e1031–2.

26. Shah Z, Hussain I, Borroni D, Khan BS, Wahab S, Mahar PS. Bowman's layer transplantation in advanced keratoconus; 18-months outcome. Int Ophthalmol. 2021;42:1161.

27. Tourkmani AK, Lyons C, Hossain PN, Konstantopoulos A, Anderson DF, Alio JL. 1 year posterior corneal changes after Bowman layer transplantation for keratoconus. Eur J Ophthalmol. 2021;32:1370.

28. Zygoura V, Birbal RS, van Dijk K, Parker JS, Baydoun L, Dapena I, Melles GRJ. Validity of Bowman layer transplantation for keratoconus: visual performance at 5–7 years. Acta Ophthalmol. 2018;96(7):e901–2.

29. Luceri S, Parker J, Dapena I, Baydoun L, Oellerich S, van Dijk K, et al. Corneal densitometry and higher order aberrations after Bowman layer transplantation: 1-year results. Cornea. 2016;35(7):959–66.

Anterior Lamellar Keratoplasty: Current State of the Art

Enrica Sarnicola, Caterina Sarnicola, and Vincenzo Sarnicola

Key Points

- Anterior lamellar keratoplasty (ALK) includes techniques whereby the diseased corneal stroma is partially or totally replaced by donor tissue, provided that the endothelium is still functioning.
- Among ALK major advantages there is the avoidance of endothelial rejection, which is one the most common cause of graft failure with penetrating keratoplasty (PK).
- Unsatisfactory visual outcomes related to the thick residual host bed and interface issue are a main downside in ALK. These techniques never gain popularity and have progressively been dismissed.
- Only procedures that accomplish a very deep stromal dissection, deep anterior lamellar keratoplasty (DALK), can achieve good visual results, comparable with PK.

- In order to achieve good visual outcome and be classified as DALK, the stromal dissection has to create a residual bed that is thin (≤80 μm), smooth, and uniform in its thickness.
- Surgical techniques used to be divided into two classes: predescemetic DALK (pdDALK) to indicate manual dissections techniques, which may be considered challenging and time consuming; and descemetic DALK (dDALK) to refer to techniques that were thought to expose the Descemet's membrane (DM) making the surgery faster and more reliable, like with big bubble (BB) and viscodissection.
- It has been recently demonstrated that BB type 1 does not separate DM from stroma but is in fact an intrastromal bubble, whereas only BB type 2 truly exposes the DM. This newer knowledge has made the term dDALK and pdDALK confusing, creating the need for a new classification.
- A new classification has been proposed: Deep anterior lamellar keratoplasty (DALK) for all the manual dissection techniques that are sufficiently deep; subtotal anterior lamellar keratoplasty (STALK) for all the previous dDALK techniques where a very thin layer of stroma is left behind together with the DM and the endothelium indeed, and total anterior lamellar keratoplasty (TALK) for the cases were the DM is truly exposed.

Supplementary Information The online version contains supplementary material available at https://doi.org/10.1007/978-3-031-32408-6_18.

E. Sarnicola · V. Sarnicola (✉)
Ambulatorio di Chirurgia Oculare Santa Lucia, Grosseto, Italy

Clinica degli Occhi Sarnicola, Grosseto, Italy

C. Sarnicola
Clinica degli Occhi Sarnicola, Grosseto, Italy

Ospedale San Donato, U.O.C. Oculistica, Arezzo, Italy

Introduction

Corneal transplantation has been evolved rapidly in the past 20 years. Penetrating keratoplasty (PK) has been the dominant procedure for more than half century, but it has now been substituted by lamellar keratoplasties (LKs), less invasive procedures that selectively replace only the diseased corneal layer [1–5]. These include deep anterior lamellar keratoplasty (DALK) to address stromal diseases; a variety of endothelial keratoplasty (EK) procedures for endothelial diseases, including Descemet stripping endothelial keratoplasty (DSEK), Descemet stripping automated endothelial keratoplasty (DSAEK), and Descemet membrane endothelial keratoplasty (DMEK); as well as ocular surface stem cell transplantation for epithelial diseases due to limbal stem cell deficiency (LSCD) [1, 2, 6–8]. This chapter will discuss LK for stromal diseases with a healthy endothelium.

Initially, the expression LK was used to refer only to anterior lamellar keratoplasty and only to manual dissection techniques, regardless of the depth of the stromal removal [9]. Somewhat less than the entire thickness of cornea was removed, preserving the recipient endothelium, Descemet's membrane (DM), and a portion of deep stroma. An intrastromal interface was thereby produced where donor and host collagen lamellae meet in apposition; hence the term "lamellar keratoplasty" [3]. With the development of endothelial keratoplasty, LK necessarily became anterior lamellar keratoplasty (ALK) [9].

Despite its undeniable advantages, including the avoidance of endothelial rejection and longer graft survival, ALK did not gain popularity, mainly due to unsatisfactory visual results related to the thick residual host bed and interface issues [9–15]. Advances in technology and techniques, as well as a greater understanding of corneal physiology and optics, facilitated the resumption of lamellar surgery, showing that the key to obtain a good visual outcome, and to reduce the donor–host interface, is to perform the deepest possible stromectomy, reaching a smooth and uniform in thickness recipient surface [9, 16–19]. In fact, it was only with the introduction of newer *deep* anterior lamellar keratoplasty (DALK) techniques that surgeons were able to achieve visual outcomes similar to PK and shift the paradigm of corneal transplantation [2, 10]. It was Archila, in 1984, who first wrote the term " deep lamellar keratoplasty (DLK)" to differentiate his technique from all others ALKs that were too superficial, emphasizing the need of a deep dissection. Due to the lack of a proper categorization, however, misclassification between DALK and ALK has been unfortunately common, and the two terms have been often inappropriately used as synonymous [9, 14, 20].

A clear distinction between ALK and DALK is pivotal, especially when comparing visual outcomes with PK. Today, we know that the achieved residual host bed has to be equal or thinner than 80 μm, smooth, and uniform in thickness to be classified as a DALK, weather techniques that leave a significant thicker/uneven residual bed should not be included in this category, and they should be indicated as ALK (that are not deep or deep enough indeed) [9, 14, 15, 21, 22].

Anterior Lamellar Keratoplasty (ALK)

ALK techniques have always had a poor diffusion and are progressively being dismissed; today they are mostly the unintended result of a manual DALK that does not reach the appropriate depth. There are some exceptions, however, that deserve at list a brief mention.

Epikeratoplasty (EPK)

Epikeratoplasty (EPK), also known as "epikeratophakia" or "onlay lamellar keratoplasty," is an older surgical procedure initially conceived to correct aphakia, first described by Werblin and Kaufman in 1981 [23]. Other indications later included high myopia, hyperopia, and keratoconus [24]. The technique consists in placing a lamellar donor graft on top of a de-epithelialized host cornea and suturing it into a prepared groove. The advantages of this procedure are similar to those of other ALK procedure, plus its potential reversibility. The procedure, however, has been forsaken due to poorly predictable visual outcomes, long visual recovery, risk of postoperative irregular astigmatism, progressive myopia, reduced contrast sensitivity, and interface opacity [25]. Today, this technique may still have some very limited indications like the management of extremely advanced keratoglobus, or thinning/perforation in brittle corneal syndrome cases [26–29].

Lamellar Patch Grafts

This group of ALKs includes different techniques in which the graft is harvested in various shapes and depths, in accordance with the shape and the depth of the affected cornea (i.e. lamellar crescentic keratoplasty, "banana" graft, partial ring lamellar keratoplasty, D-shaped lamellar keratoplasty, C-shaped lamellar keratoplasty, "donut" lamellar keratoplasty, annular lamellar keratoplasty, ring lamellar keratoplasty, etc.). These techniques have been used mainly for tectonic purposes and are best suitable in cases with peripheral corneal perforations/descemetoceles, providing acceptables visual rehabilitation because of the graft eccentric location.

Although the technique of eccentric lamellar patch grafting is technically challenging and lacks of standardized procedure, current indications include the management of a variety of corneal disorders characterized by peripheral thinning and/or ectasia, with the aim of providing tectonic stability and/or improvement in corneal surface regularity: pellucid marginal degeneration (PMD), peripheral ulcerative keratitis (PUK), Mooren's ulcer, Fuchs marginal keratitis, advanced Terrien's marginal degeneration, and also infectious disorders with peripheral melting [15, 30–34].

Superficial Anterior Lamellar Keratoplasty (SALK)

Superficial anterior lamellar keratoplasty (SALK) is an intended superficial ALK technique, first described by Kaufman et al. in 2003, usually reserved for the treatment of corneal opacities confined to the anterior third of the corneal stroma (within the first 160 µm) [35, 36].

The procedure includes both superficial keratectomy, as well as the preparation of an anterior lamella from the donor tissue of the same thickness to be placed onto the recipient bed, with or without overlay sutures. Results obtained with manual dissection are suboptimal due to the irregular interface and thus poor visual outcome, while better results are reported with the use of microkeratome or femtosecond laser. Compared to the microkeratome, the femtosecond laser might be more accurate and precise; however, it is more expensive and, in the presence of significant corneal opacities, the quality of the stromal bed could be inferior compared with that created using a microkeratome [35, 37–39].

The indications for SALK are very limited, including only superficial irregular opacities, such as anterior corneal dystrophies and superficial scars, which are conditions where phototherapeutic keratectomy (PTK) is largely considered the treatment of choice. Recurrence of corneal dystrophy after PTK or DALK is common and often eventually requires repeated interventions. SALK has the theoretical advantage that it could be repeated with no increased risk of hyperopic shift or corneal thinning, as it could instead occur with repeated PTK. Only few small case series are published on this matter [35, 38, 40, 41].

Contraindications of these techniques are superficial scars that are depressed because the microkeratome cut follows the surface profile and would lead to the same defect on the stromal bed; thin and/or irregular corneas; and deep-set eyes with small palpebral aperture that can pose difficulty in the fitting of the microkeratome [15] (Fig. 18.1).

Possible complications include dystrophy recurrence, stromal melting, graft dislocation, epithelial ingrowth, infectious keratitis, and astigmatism [37, 42].

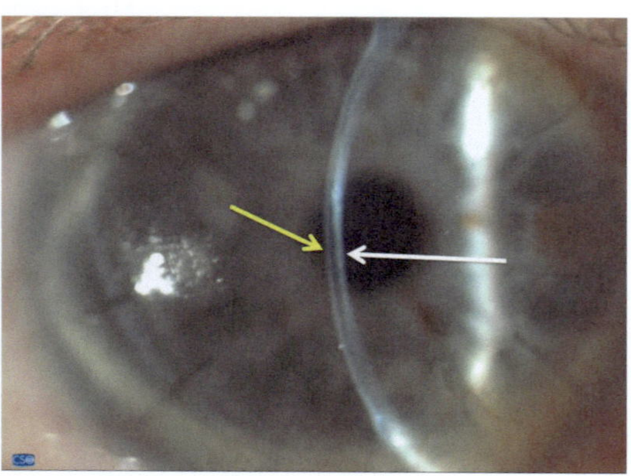

Fig. 18.1 Postoperative clinical photograph of a patient who underwent microkeratome assisted SALK for postinfective scar. The slit lamp illumination shows the interface between the donor (yellow arrow) and the recipient (white arrow). The recipient bed has an uneven pachymetry, being thinner in the center and thicker in the periphery, and some residual scarring, which both affect the visual outcome

Deep Anterior Lamellar Keratoplasty

Classifications of Surgical Techniques

Several DALK techniques have been described in the past 25 years, each aiming to expose the Descemet membrane (DM)-endothelium complex or to leave behind as little residual stroma as possible, aiming to create a good optical graft–host interface and optimize visual recovery [16, 22, 35].

These techniques have been broadly classified in the literature as **descemetic DALK (dDALK)** and **predescemetic DALK (pdDALK)** [17]. In dDALK cases, the dissection is achieved up to the DM (or at least what it was thought to be up to the DM) thanks to a forceful deep stromal injection of air (big bubble) or viscoelastic (viscodissection) which creates bubble formation that detaches the DM-endothelium from the posterior stromal. This type of stromal dissection makes the surgery become faster and more reliable, allowing the surgeon to be confident to have performed an optimal procedure with a good visual prognosis [9, 17, 43, 44]. In pdDALK cases, a small amount of posterior stroma is left in place along with the DM-endothelium, which is usually the result of manual dissection techniques [17]. How much stroma can be left in place to provide good visual outcome? Josè Barraquer, who outlined the requirements to achieve good visual results with LK, addressed this matter in 1972 already. These requisites were later on better refined with measured values, but they essentially remain the same: obtain the deepest possible interface to reduce scarring, attain a posterior layer of uniform thickness, and create a smooth surface of both the graft and the recipient bed [9, 18].

Although there is no unanimous agreement yet, the vast majority of articles in the literature show that visual recovery after pdDALK is slower (2–5 years of follow-up) but comparable with dDALK and PK, as long as the residual recipient bed thickness does not measures more than 80 μm and is homogenous in its thickness. However, it is not always easy to judge the depth of the manual dissection intraoperatively; therefore, dDALK techniques are usually preferred, as they make the surgeon confident to have performed optimal stromal removal with a good visual prognosis [9, 10, 19].

The more recent description of **Dua's layer (DL)**, also called **pre-descemetic Layer (PDL)**, has demonstrated that the recipient bed created in dDALK cases, which was thought to be a DM–endothelium surgical exposure, in fact also includes a very thin layer of stroma in most cases [45]. Although the existence of the sixth new layer of cornea remains a contested subject, the presence of some very thin stroma that remains on top of was thought to be just DM–endothelium is unquestionable [46]. This knowledge generated confusion about what is intended with the terms "dDALK" and " pdDALK," supporting the need for a more appropriate nomenclature.

A new nomenclature has been proposed in 2019, trying to respect both the previous classification and the new findings in microscopic anatomy. The new proposed classification goes as follow [9]:

- **DALK—Deep Anterior Lamellar Keratoplasty**: it includes all the previously called pdDALK techniques. This group basically includes manual techniques that leave along with the DM a small amount of posterior stroma, which is macroscopically evident during surgery, but that does not measure more than 80 μm of thickness (i.e. peeling off, layer by layer manual dissection, hydrodissection, etc.).
- **STALK—Sub-Total Anterior Lamellar Keratoplasty**: this group encompasses what was called dDALK (except for the type 2 big bubble), in which the DM seems to be intraoperatively exposed, but where a microscopic layer of stroma is in fact left in place too (i.e. big bubble type 1, viscodissection, air-viscobubble).
- **TALK—Total Anterior Lamellar Keratoplasty**: it includes the type 2 big bubble, the only technique previously classified as dDALK, which actually exposes the DM.

Surgical Techniques

Several techniques have been employed to achieve deep stromal dissection [16, 35, 47] however, in the authors' opinion, the most common are big bubble [43], viscodissection [44, 48, 49], and some manual techniques [22, 50, 51].

Big Bubble (BB)

The big bubble (BB) technique was originally described by Anwar and Teichmann in 2002, and it is probably the most commonly used technique [9, 43, 52]. It was one of the first STALK/TALK techniques (previously dDALK) described, and it helped the world transitioning from PK to DALK. This technique involves a forceful injection of air into the corneal stroma to produce a sudden separation of the stroma from the DM–endothelium, resulting in rapid formation of a circular air pocket that is seen as a big bubble [45] (Fig. 18.2).

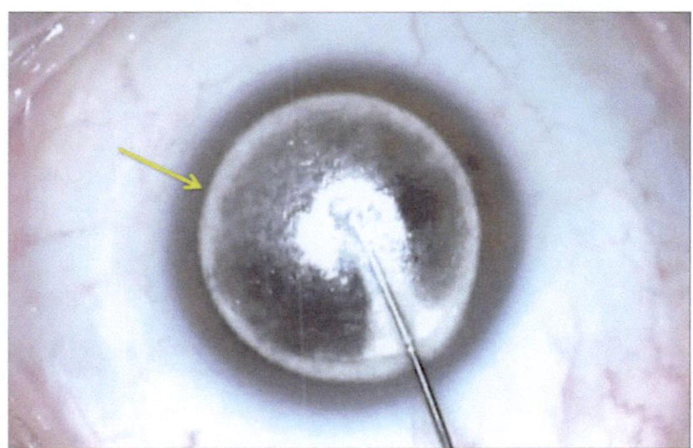

Fig. 18.2 Big bubble (BB) type 1. This type of BB is well circumscribed, it has white margins (yellow arrow), its diameter measures up to 8.5 mm, and it starts in the center and enlarges circumferentially toward the periphery

Types of Big Bubble

There are three types of bubbles. **BB Type 1** is the most common type and exposes a residual bed that intraoperatively looks like DM–endothelium, but that is in fact intrastromal. The recipient bed obtained histologically also contains some residual stroma, the alleged PDL. This type of bubble has some distinctive features: it is well-circumscribed, it has white margins, its diameter measures up to 8.5 mm, it starts in the center and enlarges circumferentially toward the periphery, and it is quite resistant [45] (Fig. 18.2). BB type 1 was erroneously considered a dDALK for many years, but it has now been re-classified as STALK.

BB type 2 is larger (up to 10.5 mm), typically eccentric, it usually starts in the periphery and enlarges centrally, and it has clear margins, almost looking like a bubble of air in the anterior chamber that does not move when the eye is rotated (Fig. 18.3). This type of bubble is pretty rare and it is the only type of bubble that really cleaves off the DM–endothelium from the stroma (TALK) and therefore it is very fragile [45, 53]. One should be extremely careful when opening this type of bubble; given the high risk of DM rupture, some surgeons even suggest no to open the bubble and to perform a manual dissection on top of it instead [54]. The bubble usually resolves itself in the early postoperative time [55].

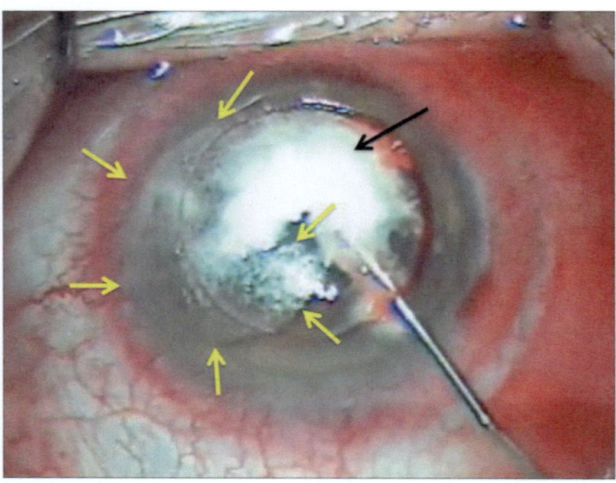

Fig. 18.3 Big bubble (BB) type 2. BB type 2 (yellow arrows) is typically eccentric, it usually starts in the periphery and enlarges centrally, and it has clear margins, almost looking like a bubble of air in the anterior chamber that does not move when the eye is rotated. The black arrow shows some central stromal emphysema (no bubble)

BB type 3 consists in mixed type of bubbles: BB type 1 and one or more smaller type 2 bubbles [45].

Needle Big Bubble Technique

With the original BB technique, a trephine is used to perform a partial thickness corneal trephination at about a 60–80% depth. A 27- or 30-gauge **needle**, attached to an air-filled syringe, is then inserted deep into the paracentral stroma through the bottom of the trephination groove, and advanced with the bevel parallel to the DM, facing downward. Air is injected, and a big bubble is formed between DM–endothelium and the corneal stroma (BB type 2) or, more frequently, between the posterior stroma and the PDL layer (BB type 1). Subsequently, anterior keratectomy is performed and a small opening at the center of the anterior wall of the bubble is created. This opening should be performed using the sharp tip of a pointed blade, held almost parallel to the surface. As the collapse of the air bubble occurs, the knife has to be quickly withdrawn to avoid inadvertent perforations. The remaining corneal stromal layers are lifted with an iris spatula, severed with a blade, and excised with scissors, before suturing the donor [43].

The deeper the air is injected, the higher are the chances to create a big bubble [56]; therefore, several modifications of the original technique have been described trying to increase the bubble success rate [22].

Cannula Big Bubble Technique

Aiming to inject the air as close as possible to DM, the use of blunt instrument has been proposed instead of a needle, by Sarnicola and Toro in 2011, to let surgeons go as deeply as possible into the corneal stroma, without being afraid of perforating: the **"cannula big bubble"** technique. The surgical steps are similar to the BB technique described by Anwar, but with two important modifications. (1) After a partial corneal trephination, a smooth spatula is inserted at the deepest point in the peripheral trephination groove, and it is moved toward central/paracentral cornea using a wiggling motion, creating a very deep track. When a very deep plane is reached, two signs may be observed: reduced resistance of the advancement of the spatula and the appearance of DM folds. (2) The spatula can then be withdrawn, leaving a corneal track where to insert a 27-gauge, blunt tipped, bottom port, air injection cannula, attached to a 5 cc air filled syringe. After advancing the cannula, a little more forward to the center of the cornea, the air is then injected using a firm continuous pressure till the formation of big bubble is noted [57]. A comparative study over 507 eyes affected by keratoconus showed a significantly higher percentage of successful BB using a cannula (82%) compared to using a needle (61%) ($p < 0.01$) [58]. The advantages of using a blunt tipped bottom port cannula have been confirmed by several studies [59–61].

Pachy Bubble and Newer Devices

Intraoperative corneal thickness measurement to create a pachymetry-guided intrastromal air injection to increase the rate of BB formation has been proposed by Ghanem in 2012; the **"pachybubble"** technique. After an initial partial trephination (about 60–70%), intraoperative corneal thickness measurements using ultrasound pachymetry are taken 0.8 mm internally from the trephination groove in the 11–1 o' clock position.

In this area, a 2-mm incision is made, parallel to the groove, with a micrometer diamond knife, calibrated to 90% depth of the thinnest measurement. The incision is then opened with toothed forceps and widened superficially with a 15-degree blade and used to start the stromal track for the cannula BB technique [57, 62]. **Intraoperative anterior segment optical coherence tomography** (AS-OCT) and **femtosecond lasers** have been suggested to guide or create the deep stromal track to allow proper placement of needle/cannula; these tool seems to be helpful and promising; however, they are very expensive, and there are limited data in literature [63–67]. The use of femtosecond lasers in DALK has also been employed to substitute manual trephination and create precise shaped wound. The shaped wound configuration may offer the advantage of better donor host apposition, with increased surface area contact, resulting in faster wound healing, greater tectonic stability, allowing earlier suture removal, and possibly reducing astigmatism as well. However, there is no consensus on a standardized approach for wound design or postoperative management, and most of the reports on the matter are laboratory studies or small case series with short-term outcomes [65]. The use of femtosecond laser to prepare the residual stromal bed, on the other hand, has generated a lot of concern about its efficacy and safeness when used [35, 68, 69]. Studies have showed that deep femtosecond laser ablation, using high energy, creates irregularities and bridges that give poor optical quality. This is due to different biomechanics between the posterior corneal lamellae and the anterior stroma [70]. Newer femtosecond laser settings are the object of current studies to create a cut that resembles the optimum cut achieved in the anterior cornea during refractive surgery. However, there are also limitations in creating a residual host bed thinner than 100 µm without damaging the endothelial cells and in producing a pachymetrically homogeneous host bed given the different curvature between anterior and posterior surface, especially in advanced keratoconus patients [71].

Bubble Test

While injecting air into the stroma, trying to obtain a BB, corneal emphysema can occur and it may hinder visualization of the BB, making the surgeon uncertain about how to proceed. Parthasarathy et al. described a technique in which a small air bubble is injected into the anterior chamber (AC) via a limbal paracentesis. If the small air bubble is seen at the periphery of the AC, it will confirm that separation of the DM induced by BB has been successfully accomplished. This is noted also while rotating the eye trying to make the air bubble move centrally; the air bubble moves circumferentially and remains in the periphery of the AC, usually with a sausage configuration. If the small bubble is not seen at the periphery of the AC and is instead located centrally beneath the opaque corneal stroma, this would suggest that the big bubble has not been obtained [72] (Fig. 18.4).

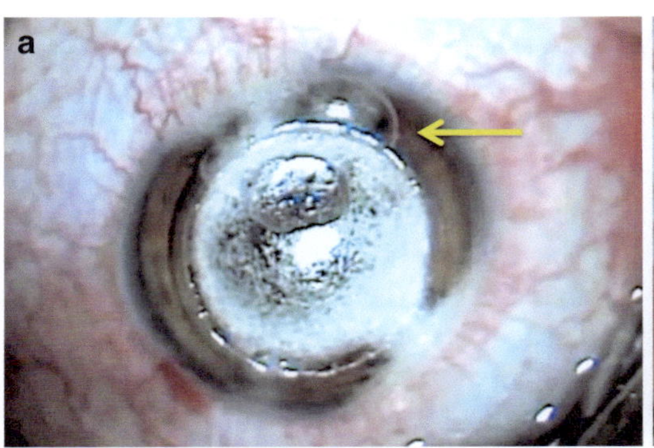
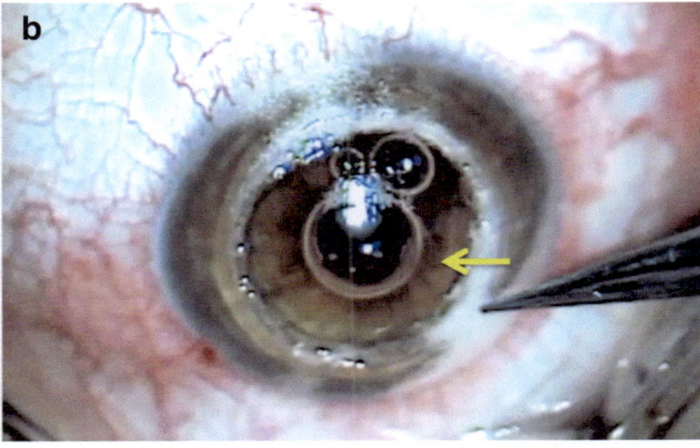

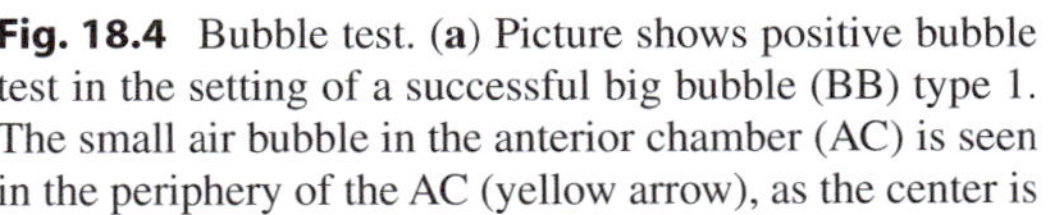

Fig. 18.4 Bubble test. (**a**) Picture shows positive bubble test in the setting of a successful big bubble (BB) type 1. The small air bubble in the anterior chamber (AC) is seen in the periphery of the AC (yellow arrow), as the center is occupied by the BB. (**b**) When the BB is opened, the bubble test becomes negative, as the air bubble into the AC is free to move into the center of the AC (yellow arrow)

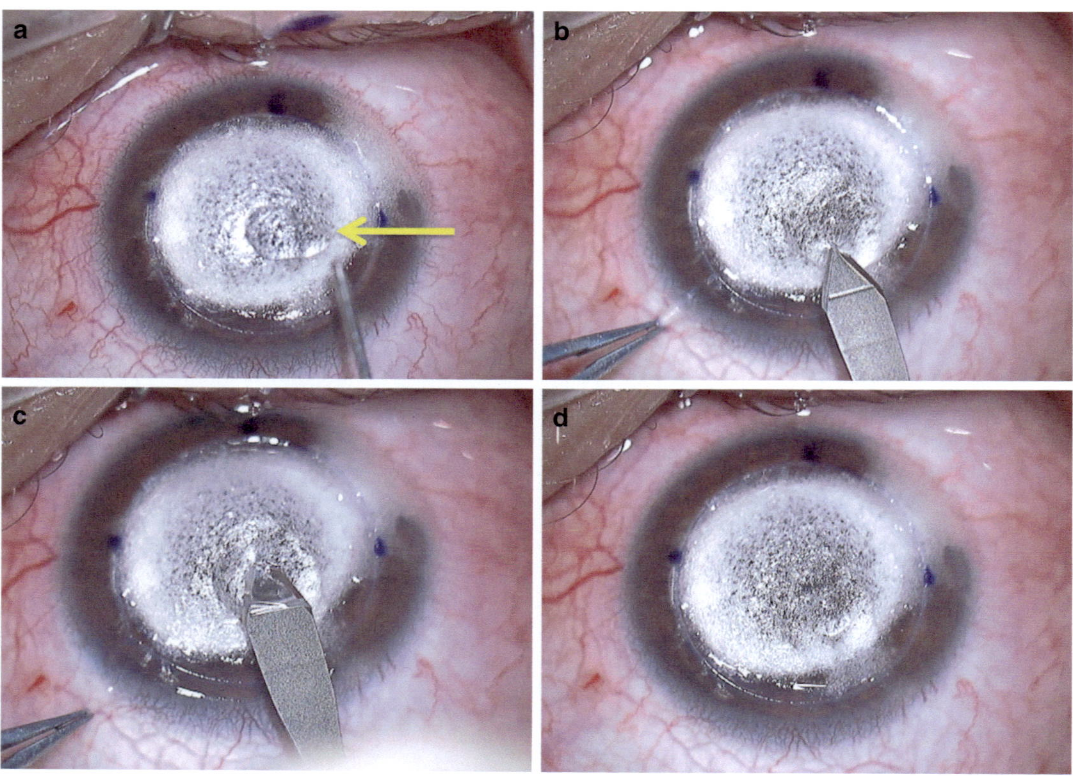

Fig. 18.5 New big bubble (BB) opening. (**a**) Once the BB has been achieved, an anterior keratectomy should be performed and the stroma overlying the BB should be coated with a cohesive viscoelastic (yellow arrow); (**b**, **c**) a 2.2 keratome is used to incise the bubble, with a bottom upwards incision; (**d**) no collapse of the BB after the withdraw of the keratome

New Technique to Open the Big Bubble

The technique to open the big bubble, as originally described by Anwar (see section "Needle Big Bubble Technique"), is associated with a known risk of DM perforation; the maneuver is in fact called "the brave slash" by many corneal surgeons [43]. The BB opening technique has been refined by Goshe et al. to avoid perforation. They suggested to coat the stroma overlying the BB with a cohesive viscoelastic prior to entering the big bubble, and to incise the bubble using only the tip of the blade in a "lifting" motion. These measures limit the escape of air from the bubble, preventing a sudden collapse of the BB while entering in it with the blade. Furthermore, they suggested an air–viscoelastic exchange to maintain space in the bubble, to facilitate the removal of the anterior wall of the bubble [73]. To further limit the escape of air from the BB during its

opening, a bottom upward incision cut using a 2.2 mm keratotome can be considered instead of the lifting motion cut and to perform a paracentesis to reduce the eye pressure before opening the bubble [16, 22] (Fig. 18.5).

Viscodissection

Intrastromal injection of ophthalmic viscoelastic can be used too to create a bubble and achieve a quick and deep stromal dissection [44, 48, 74]. This technique, also known as "**visco-bubble**," has been described by Melles et al. in 1999. This bubble mimics the behavior of the air BB type 1 and it usually results in a STALK [9]. In this technique, a 30-gauge needle (or a blunt tipped bottom port cannula) attached to a viscoelastic-filled syringe, is inserted into the corneal stroma as close to the DM as possible [48]. To visualize the depth of the corneal track dissection during surgery, Melles et al. proposed the creation of an air-to-endothelium interface, which behaves as a convex mirror, exchanging anterior chamber aqueous fluid with air [49]. A dark, nonreflective band can be seen between the tip of the needle/cannula and the light reflex, representing the residual corneal tissue. Because the dark band becomes thinner when advancing the needle/cannula into the deeper stromal layers, the corneal depth of the needle/cannula can be judged from the thickness of the dark band, helping to decide when to inject the viscoelastic. A typical reflex, that we like to call "golden ring", outlines the formation of a visco-bubble. Once the bubble has formed, it can be opened, the stroma over the bubble is excised, and the recipient bed is thoroughly irrigated to remove all residual viscoelastic before suturing the donor [44, 48, 49].

Although this procedure provides good results, it is not always easy to identify the reflex. Some surgeons prefer to de-bulk the cornea before attempting the viscobubble to enhance the chances to inject the viscoelastic as close as possible to the DM. In the authors' opinion, the use of cohesive viscoelastic should to be preferred because it is easier to remove, reducing the risk of postoperative double anterior chamber [22].

Intrastromal viscoelastic injection has also been suggested, by Sarnicola et al. in 2010, as a rescue bubble technique, thus as a second approach after a failed air bubble: **air-viscobubble (AVB)** [17, 57, 75]. With this technique, when air BB fails, a superficial keratectomy is performed with a crescent blade and a new deeper corneal track is created into the stroma by using a blunt spatula. A visco-bubble is then attempted as a second strategy to obtain a STALK, by using the same blunt tipped bottom port cannula used for the cannula BB technique [17, 57, 75]. In a case series of 507 eyes affected by keratoconus, this combined technique (AVB) incremented of 12% the percentage of bubble formation, bringing the total cases of successful bubble formation (STALK) to 94% [58]. When the BB fails, the cornea is generally pneumatized and offers many pathways of less resistance to air compared to the pre-Descemet space (i.e. leakage of air through the stroma, the trabecular meshwork, or the

trephination groove). Because of its high viscosity, the viscoelastic device does not escape as easily, creating a much higher intrastromal pressure and increasing the chances of bubble formation, probably also increasing the pressure inside the small stromal air bubbles (from the failed BB attempt) that spontaneously merge to form a large DM detachment [75].

Manual DALK Techniques

Despite technically more challenging, manual dissection techniques are still a valid option; they are mainly adopted in cases where air- and/or visco-dissection fail or when they are not indicated (i.e. keratoconus with history of previous hydrops, deep dense stromal scars, opaque cornea with poor visibility, penetrating corneal wounds, etc.). These techniques used to be classified as pdDALK, today just DALK (see section "Classifications of Surgical Techniques").

Peeling Off (Video 18.1)

Malbran described this easy and rapid technique in 1966, which still represents a useful option, especially in eyes with keratoconus. In the original technique, a partial corneal trephination is deepened 360° with a blade and the edges are then raised with a Paufique knife until there is enough tissue to grasp; two forceps are then used to pull the stroma away from the deeper layers [51, 76, 77].

This surgical technique basically separates the anterior corneal stroma by pulling the deep stromal lamellae following the plane of their lowest adhesion, which is usually very deep, allowing an optimal visual recovery (formerly classified as pdDALK). The pulling does not require great force, and it is very easy especially in the area of the cone of the keratoconus cases [9, 22, 78].

Recently, the peeling off technique has been re-proposed by some surgeons (Sarnicola, Fogla, etc.) with some modifications, namely performing a partial debulking before the pulling and the use of dedicated blunt instruments to deepen the trephination grove and find the appropriate very deep plane that allows for the stroma to be peeled away (blunt tipped pocket stromal forceps or a blunt tipped 27 G DALK spatula) [22, 79] (Fig. 18.6).

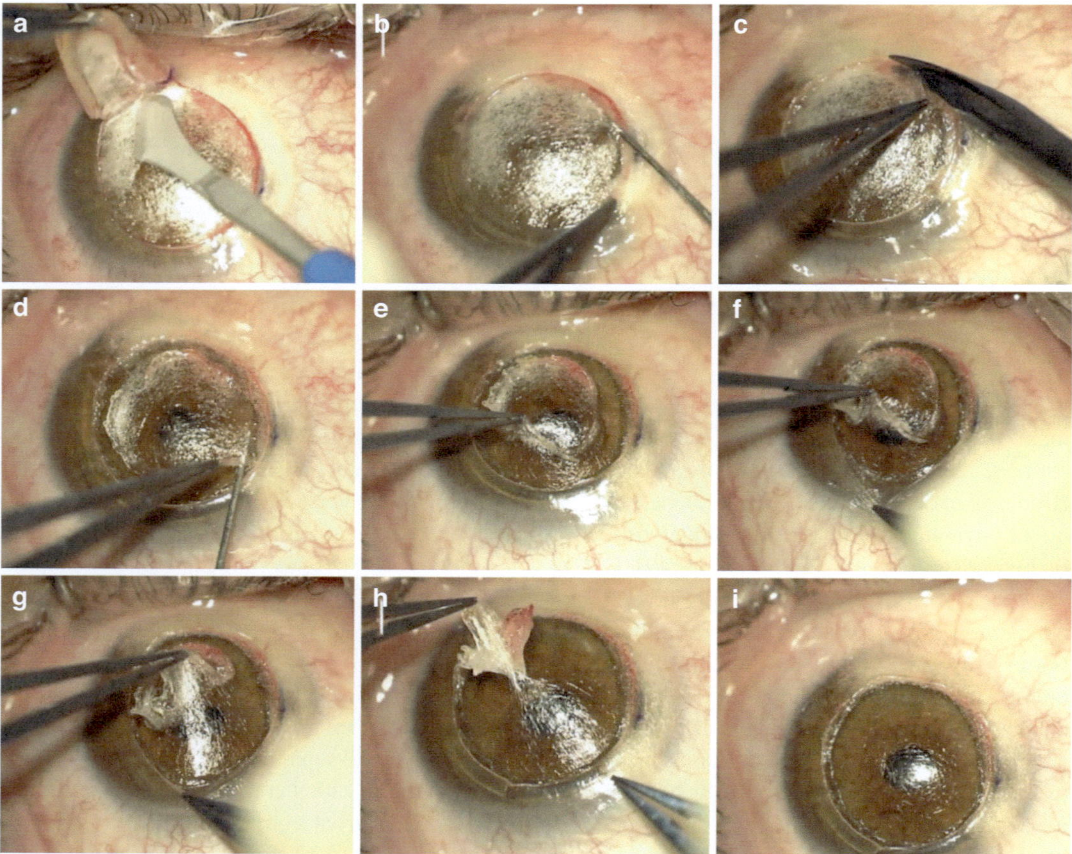

Fig. 18.6 Peeling off DALK technique. In this specific case, the peeling off technique has to be used after a failed attempt of big bubble. (**a**) Anterior keratectomy using a crescent blade. The white emphysema is the result of failed big bubble; (**b–d**) The trephination groove is deepened by creating a deep stromal track along the groove, using a 27 G DALK blunt spatula. Once the track has reached the length of the spatula, it is opened using corneal scissors. This maneuver is repeated until a very deep plane is exposed 360°; (**e**) the appropriate depth of the plane can be identified by its shiny and smooth appearance, and by the absence of any area of air emphysema; (**f–h**) once the stromal periphery is freed, the inner stromal edges of the central stroma are grasped securely with forceps, which are used to pull the stromal tissue and to peel it from underlying deeper layers; (**i**) deep and smooth residual recipient bed

Layer-by-Layer Manual Dissection

Dry manual dissection is probably the oldest described technique of LK, which reclaimed attention when Tsubota et al. applied the cataract surgery principle of "divide-and-conquer" to corneal transplantation. After the initial trephination, the recipient cornea is divided into four quadrants in order to facilitate lamellar dissection at approximately 70% of corneal depth. This division is then continued until a proper deep plane is exposed [50].

Although Tsubota et al. reported just one case of DM rupture over 17 eyes (repaired by injecting air into the anterior chamber), this technique has a high risk of intraoperative perforations [50, 80]. In order to reduce the risk of DM rupture, it might be helpful to reduce the intraocular pressure, by evacuating some aqueous through a peripheral paracentesis, and to wet the stroma with some balanced salt solution (BSS) during the procedure [22].

Injecting air into the stroma to create emphysema can be helpful to understand the depth of the stromal dissection, as described by Archila in 1984 [20, 81]. Some newest technological tools such as intraoperative AS-OCT or a hand holder pachymeter might be helpful as well [22, 66].

This technique is still a valid option, although it is rarely the first technique of choice giving that it is more challenging and time consuming than the others, and it requires a certain surgical experience to understand intraoperatively the depth of the obtained dissection.

Donor Preparation

Donor cornea preparation can be performed using punch of the surgeon's choice (with/without suction). It is usually prepared from the endothelial side and centration is crucial to avoid creating an oval donor button with higher postoperative astigmatism [82]. The DM–endothelium complex has to be gently stripped off the donor by using a dry weck surgical sponge, or with fine non tooth forceps, taking care not to damage the stroma. Trypan blue dye can be used to stain DM and aid peeling; gently damaging the donor endothelium with a swab before coloring with the Trypan blue makes the staining stronger [16].

Most of the studies published in literature show that the diameter of the donor cornea generally oversized the recipient by 0.25 mm [52]. Nonetheless, we suggest the use of equivalent diameters in order to reduce postoperative myopic shift due to an oversized donor [82, 83]. The use of a smaller sized graft is still a matter of discussion; it could help to reduce postoperative myopia, but it has also been associated with a higher risk of DM wrinkles and glaucoma. We suggest the use of a smaller sized graft in cases with anisometropia greater than 3 D myopic spherical equivalent is present in the eye to operate, or when both eyes require a DALK and have a myopic spherical equivalent greater than 5 D. In case of DM wrinkles appearance while suturing the donor, these should be managed by applying the suture, so that the wrinkles form in the periphery and therefore limit possible negative effect on the VA. DM wrinkles become usually less visible and may completely disappear over time.

However, it is important to underline that a smaller donor cannot be used in the presence of an intraoperative DM rupture because the disparity of curvature between the donor and the recipient prevents the management of DM rupture [16, 22, 84, 85].

DALK Long-Term Outcomes

A major advantage of DALK is the **avoidance of endothelial rejection**, one of the leading causes of graft failure in PK [10–12]. When considering the endothelial cell count (ECC) as a proxy for graft survival, it is reasonable to think that DALK surgery may provide a major advantage in patients with long life expectancy [10].

A study by Sarnicola et al. presented data on 660 eyes, with various diagnoses, that underwent to DALK surgery with a mean follow-up of 4.5 years (range 0.5–10 years). **Graft survival** average was **99.3%** (range 98.5–100%) [11]. Interestingly, patients were divided into five subgroups by different follow-ups (10–9 year, 8–7 year, 6–5 year, 4–3 year, 2–1 year), and no significant difference was found in terms of graft survival. These findings may indicate that, with DALK, patients can expect having a clear graft for a long period, as opposed to the progressive decline of graft survival over time that occurs with PK. Similarly, the ECC with DALK shows an average 11–12% loss only in the first 6 months after surgery, and then it remains stable over time. The endothelial cell loss might be higher in cases that experienced an intraoperative DM rupture (19%); however, this does not seem to significantly impact the graft survival [11, 80, 86, 87]. **Graft failure** rate was 0.6% and occurred only within the first year postoperatively, due to infection or ocular surface complications. After the initial postoperative period, thanks to the recovery of the ocular surface defenses and to a good stable ECC, DALK graft survival becomes not "time dependent" and is likely to last lifetime, whereas with PK, the cumulative rate of graft failure increases significantly over time [2, 11]. These findings have been recently confirmed by a 10-year graft survival comparative study from Arundhati et al. of 362 primary DALK procedures and 306 primary PK procedures. The survival rate for PK was 94.4%, 80.4%, and 72.0% at 1 year, 5 years, and 10 years, respectively, and 95.8%, 93.9%, and 93.9% at 1 year, 5 years, and 10 years respectively for DALK ($p = 0.001$). Arundhati et al. also found that DALK resulted in fewer post-operative complications and lower rates of graft rejection and failure; patients who underwent PK developed more complications of glaucoma (29.3% vs. 11.6%, respectively; $p < 0.001$), allograft rejection (16.6% vs. 1.7%, respectively; $p < 0.001$), epithelial problems (10.4% vs. 5.5%, respectively; $p = 0.018$), and nonimmunological failure (7.8% vs. 1.9%, respectively; $p < 0.001$), compared to DALK [88].

DALK failures are not related to endothelial rejection and DALK **re-graft** does not seems to increase the risk of rejection [21, 89–92]. On the contrary, a registry study over 4834 PKs by Kelly et al. reports Kaplan–Meier survival rates of first grafts for keratoconus to be 89%, 49%, and 17% at 10 years, 20 years, and 23 years, respectively [93]. Interestingly, a longitudinal review of 3992 PKs for various diagnosis by Thompson et al. showed that primary grafts had a twofold higher 10-year survival rate (82%) compared with initial re-grafts (41%) [86]. Second and third re-grafts have even a worse survival prognosis. Maguire et al. reported that the risk of failure 3 years after PK increases from 17% with no previous grafts to 53% with two or more previous PKs [94]. With re-grafts, the recipient's immune system might become sensitized to foreign corneal tissue, developing an increased risk for immunologic rejection.

Despite endothelial rejection is avoided with DALK, **epithelial,** and **stromal rejection** can still occur; however, these are usually easily managed with topical steroids [10]. The followings have been identified as main risks factor for rejection after DALK: shorter time of postoperative local steroids (7-week median duration versus 1–4 years), younger age, African American ethnicity, atopy, corneal neo-vascularization, and large limbus-to-limbus graft [95, 96].

Visual outcomes of DALK are comparable to PK [9, 10, 17]. To be thorough, the reported results about DALK visual outcome actually vary among the published studies. Although few studies have found the outcomes of DALK to be inferior to PK, many other studies have found comparable outcomes between PK and DALK. The reason for this incongruity may be imputed to a misclassification between DALK and ALK. In fact, no significant difference in postoperative best spectacle-corrected visual acuity (BSCVA) between STALK/TALK (previously dDALK) and PK has been found, whereas conflicting opinions have arisen only regarding PK versus manual DALK (previously pdDALK). Although there is not unanimous agreement yet, the vast majority of papers in the literature show that visual recovery after manual DALK (previously pdDALK) is slower but comparable with STALK/TALK (previously dDALK) at a longer follow-up (usually 2–5 years), as long as the residual recipient bed thickness is equal or less than 80 μm, regular in its thickness, and with a smooth surface [9, 10].

Among the main advantages of DALK over PK, we also find that DALK is a "**closed sky**" procedure, carrying a lower risk of endophthalmitis and expulsive hemorrhage [10]. DALK also offers a stronger wound integrity, lower risk of glaucoma, and it allows for a safer staged cataract surgery, with all the related advantages [10, 97].

Current Indications and New Prospectives

DALK should be offered to patients suffering from stromal diseases that have a presumably functioning endothelium, for optical, therapeutic, or tectonic purposes. Cases with history of preoperative DM rupture (i.e. penetrating corneal wound, acute hydrops, etc.), or presumed previous DM ruptures (i.e. radial keratotomy (RK), deep scars, etc.), can still be addressed with DALK; however, careful manual dissection should be the preferred technique, as the DM can break at the site of previous scarring/rupture when air, fluid, or viscoelastic is injected [15]. Let us review some of the most common indications.

Keratoconus and Other Ectatic Disorders

Keratoconus is probably the most common indication for DALK; the disease affects young patients with a long life expectancy; therefore, it is easy to understand how they can definitely benefit from the long-term graft survival of DALK [98–100]. Patients affected by keratoconus are typically young, therefore with a healthy endothelium; concomitant endothelial dystrophy is rare and usually does not compromise the endothelium function at the age requiring stromal surgery [101]. In a series of 158 eyes affected by keratoconus, DALK showed a long-term graft survival of 98% (6 years of average follow-up, range 4–19 years) [102].

DALK can and should be performed even in keratoconus cases with a positive history for **previous acute hydrops**. Manual dissection techniques should be the procedure of choice, given the presumable presence of a DM break in the site of the previous hydrops. The key of performing a successful surgery is to start the stromectomy from the opposite site of the presumed DM break spot, dissecting the area of the hydrops as last, and managing it as any other intraoperative DM rupture [15, 80, 103–105].

Recurrence of keratoconus after keratoplasty is largely related to placement of a small graft that did not remove the entire cone. A repeated larger DALK, or even DALK in a previous PK, can successfully manage this condition. In the specific case of a DALK over a PK, manual dissection techniques should be considered as preferred choice, to avoid the risk of a big bubble burst when enlarging outside the full thickness penetrating trephination grove [15, 106].

The surgical management of **keratoglobus** is particularly challenging due to diffuse limbus-to-limbus corneal thinning. There is not a unanimous agreement about the best surgical treatment for this disease; however, in order to avoid the placement of the graft–host junction at the thinned mid-periphery and to create better stability, these cases require very large limbus-to-limbus grafts [107]. The graft proximity to the limbus is well known as risk factor for graft rejection. Registry data have shown us that PK outcomes are dependent on the indication for surgery and are best for keratoconus and worse in cases with active vascularization or when a large graft has to be performed [108]. It is intuitive that DALK would have a better prognosis in these patients. The preferred DALK surgical technique for keratoglobus should be manual dissection [15, 85]. Vajpayee et al. have described a very interesting DALK modification called the "tuck in" technique, with the aim of providing additional tectonic support to the peripheral cornea and facilitate the donor suturing. The technique involves the creation of a peripheral, partial-thickness flange of about 2.5–3 mm of posterior stromal tissue of the donor lenticule. The flange of the donor button is integrated into a 360° inferior stromal pocket in the host cornea, followed by graft suturing. This procedure is indicated not only for keratoglobus but also for any case with advanced peripheral corneal thinning, like PMD (PMD) [109, 110].

PMD is a rare ectatic disorder, which typically affects the inferior-peripheral cornea in a crescentic fashion. Surgery is indicated when spectacles and contact lenses are unsuccessful in providing satisfactory vision. Although a number of surgical techniques are available for patients with PMD, there is currently no consensus on which method provides the most effective treatment. Considering the peripheral location of the diseases, the advantages in term of rejections of lamellar techniques are evident [111, 112]. Among these options, good outcomes have been reported with very large DALK for highly ectatic cases, even in eyes with previous perforations [113, 114].

Leukoma

Although superficial corneal opacities may be treated with PTK, deeper leukoma that are visually significant are candidates for DALK. Causes of leukoma can vary and some of them deserve few specifications.

Among the post infective stromal scars, **herpes simplex virus (HSV) related scars** are the ones that may benefit the most from the low immunological insult of DALK. In HSV infections, especially for immune stromal keratitis, the relationship between rejection and recurrence of the infection is particularly significant. Rejection can trigger an HSV recurrence and vice versa. In a large cases series of 52 eyes, the combination of DALK, long-term oral antiviral therapy, and long-term local steroids has shown good efficacy in in both rehabilitating vision and preventing recurrence of infection [115] (Fig. 18.7). Several other studies, despite confirming DALK as a good surgical treatment for post-herpetic stromal scar, reported a certain percentage of HSV recurrence, probably due to a shorter postoperative prophylactic antiviral treatment. On the contrary, PK outcomes are poor in cases with active vascularization and should be avoided, as the survival rate in these cases is only 60% with the first graft [116]. Interestingly, a case report about the management of a stromal scar secondary to a HSV recurrence on a PK graft shows that DALK is technically possible even in such cases, as long as the endothelium is functional [117].

Severe thermal/chemical injuries often result in corneal opacity and LSCD. Eyes with significant LSCD are not candidates for conventional keratoplasty as the outcome of a corneal transplant alone is poor in these patients because of the LSCD will recur in the graft as soon as the donor epithelium fails; it is mandatory to perform ocular surface stem cell grafting first. Once the ocular surface has been restored, residual corneal scarring can be addressed with keratoplasty. These eyes often present some degree of inflammation and corneal neovascularization, hence performing a DALK improves the graft survival prognosis [2, 6, 108, 118–120].

Stromal scarring in optical zone, resulting from **penetrating or perforating corneal wounds**, is usually considered an indication to PK. The frequent associated traumatic cataract is very often addressed together with the keratoplasty performing a triple procedure. Although providing satisfactory anatomical results, this approach does not allow an easy choice of the refractive power of the IOL, with risk of poor visual results [97, 121, 122]. Recently, DALK has been proposed to address this condition too, as long as there has been no significant loss of corneal tissue. In addition to the known advantages over PK, DALK allows the surgeon to perform a staged procedure safely. Postponing cataract surgery for a year after DALK provides the surgeon with stable and more reliable parameters to choose the appropriate IOL power and even to reduce the residual post keratoplasty astigmatism. Performing DALK in eyes with a history of full-thickness perforating wound, and therefore with a DM break, might be challenging; however, it is not impossible. Given the presence of a break in the DM, the technique of choice is manual dissection. It is advisable to perform

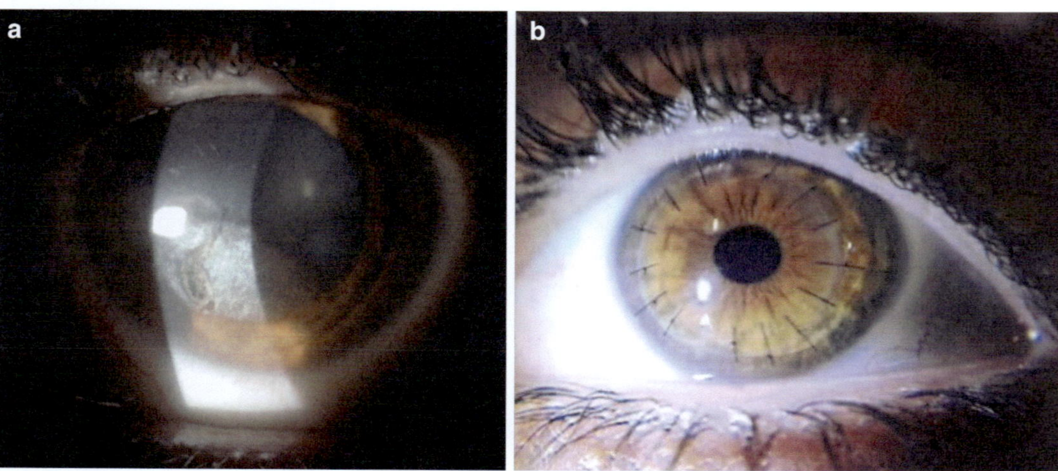

Fig. 18.7 DALK performed in herpes simplex scar. (**a**) Preoperative; (**b**) 1-year postoperative

DALK at list 1 year after the injury, to give enough time to the cornea to cicatrize. In these cases, it is important to perform peripheral paracentesis immediately after the trephination and before starting the stromal dissection, as the creation of the paracentesis would be difficult in the case of AC collapse. Stromal dissection should be started from the opposite side of the corneal injury and continued in a manner that encircles the corneal injury. Therefore, the perforated area is deliberately treated last. During the manual dissection, once the deep plane is found, stromal removal may be carried on with a crescent blade to avoid any stromal traction that could open the existing DM break, or potentially enlarge it. When dissecting the area of the previous injury, aqueous leakage and collapse of the AC are usually seen, making the surgery more challenging. The leaking of the aqueous can be managed, alternating fluid drainage with a sponge and careful stromal dissection maneuvers. A second operator can keep gently drying the stroma to enhance the visibility of the stroma, while the first surgeon completes the stromectomy. In cases without high posterior pressure, a gentle injection of air into the AC may reform the AC and stop the leakage of the fluid, making the completion of the stromectomy easier. At the end of the surgery, once the donor is sutured, an air bubble should be left into the AC to promote the adherence between the donor and recipient and reduce the risk of postoperative double AC [123].

Stromal Dystrophies

PTK is usually the preferred initial therapeutic modality to treat stromal dystrophies that primarily affect the anterior corneal stroma. However, patients that show pan-stromal or posterior stromal involvement are best managed by DALK [124]. Good visual outcomes have been reported for different types of stromal dystrophies with both DALK and PK [125–129]. However, recurrence of the dystrophy may occur in the donor cornea, regardless of the type of keratoplasty performed, and clinically significant recurrence may require multiple re-grafts. Performing DALK represents a better choice, since re-grafting in DALK is relatively easy and is not burdened by

progressive increase in the risk of rejection as with PK [130, 131].

To be thorough, it has to be said that macular corneal dystrophy may also have an associated endothelial dysfunction. However, in advanced cases, it might not be easy to properly evaluate the endothelial function, since corneal pachymetry is usually also abnormal. Given its remarkable advantages, DALK should nonetheless be performed where there is no clear evidence of endothelial dysfunction [126, 132].

Active Infections Unresponsive to Medical Treatment

Misdiagnosis, lack of effective medical therapy, and delay of treatment often compromise the success of treating fungal or amoebic infections. Conventional therapeutic PK (TPK) is the most commonly employed surgical procedure; however, it is burdened with the risk of intraocular spread of infectious organisms during the procedure resulting in secondary endophthalmitis. Furthermore, given the frequent presence of severe inflammation, TPK is also considered at high risk of endothelial rejection [133]. Graft clarity at 1 year postoperatively and the recurrence of infection have been found as high as 51.3% and 30% respectively in TPK for fungal keratitis [134]. The graft survival after TPK performed in cases of *Acanthamoeba* keratitis (AK) is also known to be poor and has been reported to be ranging from 55% to 78% at 1 year postoperatively, with a recurrence rate ranging from 38% to 13% [134, 135]. For these reasons, TPK is usually delayed and is performed in desperate cases in order to prevent impending corneal perforation or scleral extension [136, 137].

Thanks to the sparing of the host endothelium, therapeutic DALK (TDALK) may represent a better surgical option in these inflamed eyes, avoiding the risk of endothelial rejection. Additionally, TDALK prevents the intraocular spread of the infection, because the entry of the anterior chamber can be largely avoided. However, TDALK could be less effective than PK in eradicating the infection in very advanced cases; therefore, an early surgical timing is crucial to increase the chances of DALK to be radi-

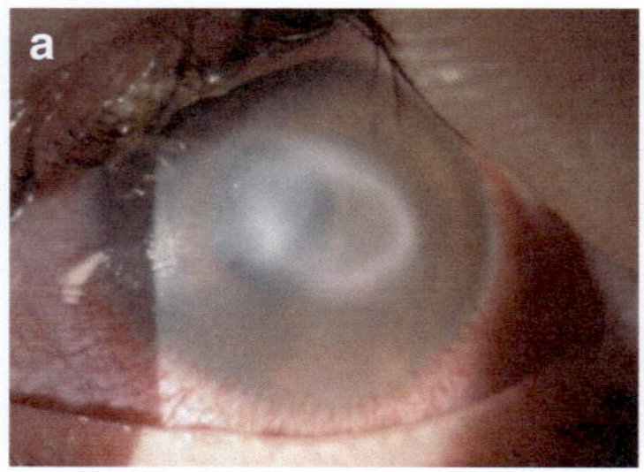
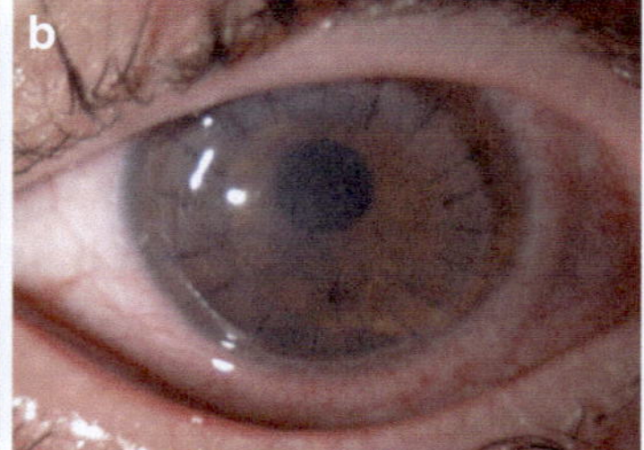
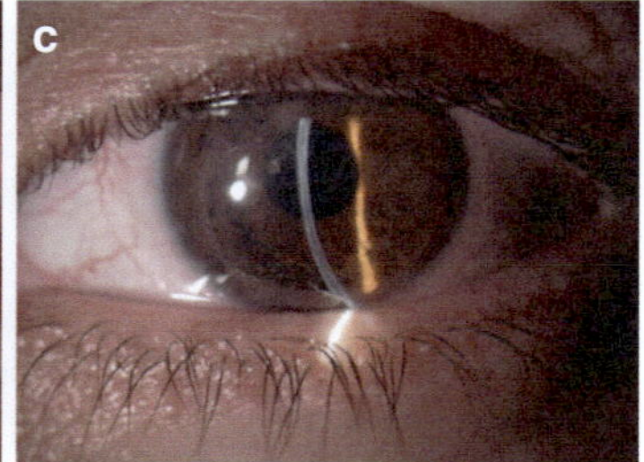

Fig. 18.8 Early therapeutic DALK performed in a case of active *Acanthamoeba* keratitis, poorly responsive to medical treatment. (**a**) Preoperative; (**b**) 1-week postoperative, (**c**) 18-months postoperative

cal [138–141]. Earlier surgical timing seems to be also the key to avoid complications due to prolonged inflammation and protracted toxic topical medical treatment [142–144].

In a comparative study between TDALK versus TPK for advanced microbial keratitis, Anshu et al. reported an infection recurrence rate of 15.3% (4 cases over 26 eyes) after TDALK and a recurrence rate of 12% (12 cases over 100 eyes) after TPK [141]. However, all the recurrent cases in the TDALK group were seen in manual DALK cases. Three of them were successively treated with a second deeper/larger manual DALK, without further recurrence. The remaining patient opted to be treated medically with resolution of infection but developed graft failure. On the contrary, the recurrent cases belonging to the TPK group were characterized by poor final outcome and 9 out of 12 eyes ultimately required evisceration. Considering that patients of the TPK group had actually more extensive and advanced lesions, and that the TDALK group had more favorable outcomes, Anshu et al. concluded that earlier intervention with lamellar surgery might have been a reasonable option [141].

Sarnicola et al. have more recently published two studies demonstrating very good results of early TDALK in dangerous corneal infections, precisely in 11 eyes affected by active *Acanthamoeba* keratitis and 23 eyes affected by active fungal keratitis. In both series, no episodes of rejection, recurrence, or graft failure were observed at 1 year of follow-up. Indications for an early TDALK were: poor response to targeted medical therapy, a significant ulcer in optical zone that had not yet involved the entire stroma (deeper than 150 µm but less than 300 µm), severity and dangerousness of the infection (*Acanthamoeba* and fungal keratitis), and, in some cases, patient compliance. Despite these very good results, it is critical that only surgeons with a low PK conversion rate should perform these procedures [138, 140] (Fig. 18.8; Video 18.1).

Descemetocele

Descemetocele is a severe complication of corneal ulceration. A small descemetocele can be successfully repaired with multilayer amniotic membrane grafting; however, surgical management of larger, or recurring, or infected descemetocele may require a keratoplasty. DALK can be technically performed even in these cases. Manual dissection should be the DALK technique of choice, and we recommend dissecting the area of the descemetocele as last, using the same precautions/approach suggested when performing DALK for corneal penetrating injury, because the descemetocele might break during the surgery [15, 145, 146] (Fig. 18.9).

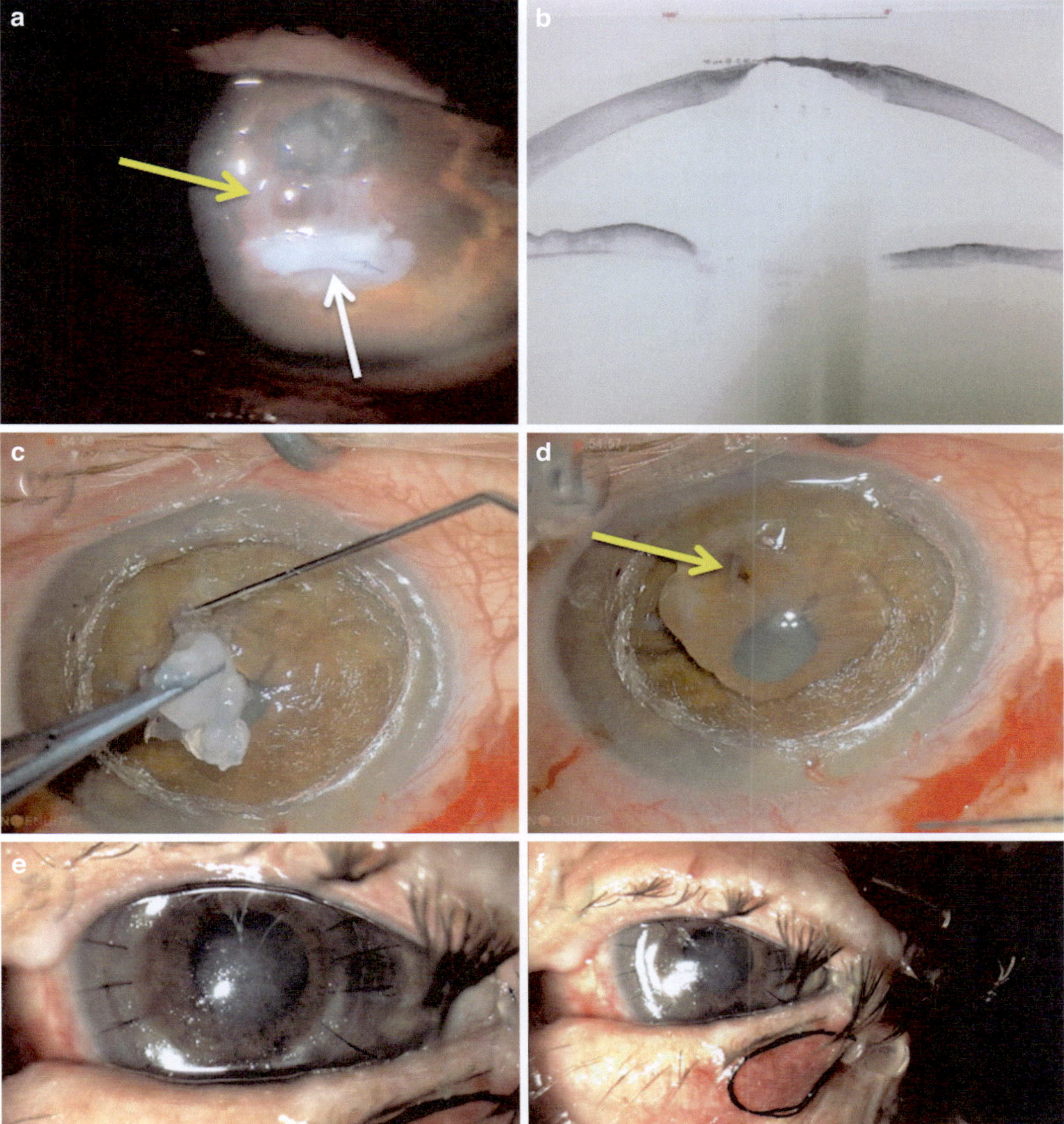

Fig. 18.9 DALK performed in descemetocele, in the setting of HSV-related neurotrophic keratopathy. (**a**) Preoperative: the picture shows the recurrence of a descemetocele (yellow arrow) after the reabsorbing of amniotic membrane (white arrow); (**b**) Preoperative anterior segment OCT; (**c**) manual DALK dissecting the area of descemetocele intentionally as last; (**d**) recipient bed rupture in the area of the descemetocele (yellow arrow) with aqueous leakage; (**e**) 1-week postoperative; (**f**) 1-week postoperative showing the presence of temporary tarsorrhaphy to promote epithelial healing

Post Radial Keratotomy Corneal Shape Disorders

RK was a popular refractive procedure used to correct myopia before the era of excimer ablative procedures. Despite initial satisfactory results, long-term follow-up of patients has shown corneal instability with frequent fluctuations of visual acuity and hyperopic shifts, leading to poor visual acuity [147]. According to a recent study on DALK performed in patients with RK, the indications for corneal transplant were significant irregular astigmatism (50%), central scarring or haze (40%), and progressive hyperopia with visual fluctuation (10%) [148]. Although big bubble technique has been shown to be feasible, manual dissection DALK techniques may be safer, considering the significant risk that the RK incisions may have reached the DM [15, 148].

Complications Unique to DALK Surgery

Intraoperative unintentional **rupture of recipient bed** is a complication unique to DALK surgery, which can occur even in expert hands. The need of subsequent PK conversion cannot be eliminated, but it can be largely avoided by learning how to manage recipient bed ruptures and their consequences [80, 149, 150].

The rate of DM perforation varies in literature from 4.5% to 45% of cases, leading to a PK conversion in 0–86% of cases, depending of surgeon's skill [79]. In fact, the rate of DM rupture and PK conversion gradually decreases as surgeons become more experienced [149]. In a case series of 1443 DALK procedures, Sarnicola et al. reported 119 (8%) intraoperative recipient bed ruptures, which were all successfully repaired with no need for PK conversion. One hundred (84%) of the cases with ruptures resolved by the first postoperative day, whereas 19 cases (16%) developed double AC, which were all fixed by using different strategies. Graft survival of the eyes that experienced an intraoperative rupture was 99% at last follow up, showing that it is worth trying to repair all DM ruptures in DALK, whereas immediate PK conversion should be avoided [80].

Only a few other studies in the literature have reported on outcomes of intraoperative DM ruptures. Two large comparative studies about DALK with and without DM ruptures (Senoo et al. [150] and Huang et al. [151]) also found that intraoperative recipient bed perforation did not affect the graft survival or the visual acuity [150, 151].

Understanding the physiomechanical mechanisms in DALK allows to correctly choose a proper rescue strategy to successfully repair DM ruptures. Sarnicola et al. have described in detail different approaches to adopt based on specific scenarios of rupture. However, there are some general rules that can be valid in most cases [16, 80, 85, 152, 153]. Once a recipient bed rupture is encountered, the stromal removal should to be continued and completed as deep and as smooth as possible, trying to minimize any stromal irregularities between the donor and recipient layers that could keep the recipient bed rupture patent. When completing the stromectomy in the area of DM rupture, it is not uncommon for the rupture to enlarge, especially in STALK (through BB type 1 or AVB) and TALK (through BB type 2) cases, making subsequent stromectomy elsewhere more difficult to perform. Therefore, when completing the stromectomy, the area of DM rupture should always intentionally dissected last. Once the stromectomy is completed, the donor graft, denuded of its endothelium, can be sutured to the recipient. After suturing the donor, an air bubble can be injected into the AC (about 70% of the AC) to tamponade the rupture. Same size diameter for donor and recipient should be used in cases of DM ruptures to avoid curvature disparity between the graft donor and recipient cornea, which could create a refractory double AC. At the end of surgery, rotating the eye in different positions may facilitate the drainage of interface fluid, promoting adherence between the recipient bed and donor graft. The postoperative head's position of the patient plays a very important role; it has to be set so that the air bubble in the AC would tamponade the rupture (i.e. sitting position for superior ruptures, lying on the opposite site of a DM break for lateral ruptures, and supine position with chin hyperextension for inferior ruptures). Pharmacological pupil dilation and close patient monitoring (for at list the first 6 h after surgery) are pivotal to prevent/manage pupillary block. At the patient's discharge, the air in the AC should not be more than 50–60% and with good pupil dilation [80].

Double AC is the most frequent postoperative complication, and it usually occurs in cases that experienced intraoperative recipient bed rupture. The reasons why such complication may occur are multiples. In some cases, the air bubble left in the AC at the end of surgery can shrink, becoming insufficient to tamponade the rupture. These cases can be fixed with simple re-bubbling. Another reason for double AC can be the patient's noncompliance with the head positioning; this is more common for cases with inferior rupture because the required head position can be quite uncomfortable. Re-bubbling emphasizing the importance of head positioning to the patient can be resolutive. In case of persistent double AC, the regularity of the sutures should carefully be assessed. Sometimes, certain sutures can be considerably tighter than others, pushing the donor on the recipient bed not homogeneously and causing a persistent double chamber. In these cases, the tight sutures should be replaced right after the re-bubbling. The shape of the air bubble in the AC during the re-bubbling can help evaluating the tension of the sutures; a circular shape of the bubble indicates a uniform distribution of the tension generated by the sutures, whereas an oval or irregular shape of the air bubble suggests otherwise. Finally, significant donor–recipient disparity of curvature, in the presence of a recipient's bed rupture during manual DALK, may cause a persistent double chamber. In these cases, re-bubbling may not work, requiring surgical correction [80, 85, 153].

Take Home Notes

- DALK has become the gold standard technique to treat stromal diseases, when the endothelium is functioning.
- DALK avoidance of endothelial rejection makes a very meaningful impact not only in the prognosis of patients with keratoconus but also for high-risk corneal transplants (i.e. disorders that need large grafts, presence of neovascularization, inflammation, active infections, etc.).
- The big bubble (BB) technique is the most common procedure; however, the mastership

of other effective techniques is useful in cases were BB fails or is not indicated.

- When properly executed, DALK manual dissection techniques can be as effective as subtotal anterior lamellar keratoplasty (STALK) techniques.
- Despite technically more challenging, DALK can be performed even in cases with a history of hydrops, RK, perforating wounds and descemetocele. Manual dissection techniques should be preferred in such cases.
- With appropriate rescue techniques to repair the recipient bed rupture and to manage postoperative double AC, conversion to PK can be avoided in the majority of cases.

References

1. Colby K. Update on corneal transplant in 2021. JAMA. 2021;325(18):1886–7. https://doi.org/10.1001/jama.2020.17382.
2. Tan DT, Dart JK, Holland EJ, Kinoshita S. Corneal transplantation. Lancet. 2012;379(9827):1749–61. https://doi.org/10.1016/S0140-6736(12)60437-1.
3. Rich LF. Expanding the scope of lamellar keratoplasty. Trans Am Ophthalmol Soc. 1999;97:771–814. PMCID: PMC1298281.
4. America EBAo. Eye banking statistical report. Washington, DC: Eye Bank Association of America; 1997.
5. Sarnicola C, Sarnicola E, Perri P, Sarnicola V. Recent developments in cornea and corneal transplants. In: Grzybowski A, editor. Current concepts in ophthalmology. Cham: Springer International Publishing; 2020. p. 35–53. https://doi.org/10.1007/978-3-030-25389-9.
6. Cheung AY, Sarnicola E, Denny MR, Sepsakos L, Auteri NJ, Holland EJ. Limbal stem cell deficiency: demographics and clinical characteristics of a large retrospective series at a single tertiary referral center. Cornea. 2021;40(12):1525–31. https://doi.org/10.1097/ICO.0000000000002770.
7. Cheung AY, Sarnicola E, Kurji KH, Govil A, Mogilishetty G, Eslani M, et al. Cincinnati protocol for preoperative screening and donor selection for ocular surface stem cell transplantation. Cornea. 2018;37(9):1192–7. https://doi.org/10.1097/ICO.0000000000001662.
8. Cheung AY, Sarnicola E, Govil A, Holland EJ. Combined conjunctival limbal autografts and living-related conjunctival limbal allografts for severe unilateral ocular surface failure. Cornea.

2017;36(12):1570–5. https://doi.org/10.1097/ICO.0000000000001376.

9. Sarnicola E, Sarnicola C, Cheung AY, Holland EJ, Sarnicola V. Surgical corneal anatomy in deep anterior lamellar keratoplasty: suggestion of new acronyms. Cornea. 2019;38(4):515–22. https://doi.org/10.1097/ICO.0000000000001845.

10. Reinhart WJ, Musch DC, Jacobs DS, Lee WB, Kaufman SC, Shtein RM. Deep anterior lamellar keratoplasty as an alternative to penetrating keratoplasty a report by the American Academy of Ophthalmology. Ophthalmology. 2011;118(1):209–18. https://doi.org/10.1016/j.ophtha.2010.11.002.

11. Sarnicola V, Toro P, Sarnicola C, Sarnicola E, Ruggiero A. Long-term graft survival in deep anterior lamellar keratoplasty. Cornea. 2012;31(6):621–6. https://doi.org/10.1097/ICO.0b013e31823d0412.

12. Borderie VM, Sandali O, Bullet J, Gaujoux T, Touzeau O, Laroche L. Long-term results of deep anterior lamellar versus penetrating keratoplasty. Ophthalmology. 2012;119(2):249–55. https://doi.org/10.1016/j.ophtha.2011.07.057.

13. Fontana L, Parente G, Sincich A, Tassinari G. Influence of graft-host interface on the quality of vision after deep anterior lamellar keratoplasty in patients with keratoconus. Cornea. 2011;30(5):497–502. https://doi.org/10.1097/ico.0b013e3181d25e4d.

14. Sarnicola E, Sarnicola C, Cheung AY, Holland EJ, Sarnicola V. Reply. Cornea. 2019;38(10):e45–e6. https://doi.org/10.1097/ICO.0000000000002077.

15. Sarnicola C, Sarnicola E, Sarnicola V, Anwar M. Indications for anterior lamellar keratoplasty. In: Mannis MJ, Holland EJ, editors. Cornea, vol. 2. 5th ed. Amsterdam: Elsevier; 2021.

16. Sarnicola E, Sarnicola C, Sarnicola V. Deep anterior lamellar keratoplasty: surgical technique, indications, clinical results and complications. In: Guell JL, editor. Cornea. ESASO Course series, vol. 6. Basel: Karger; 2015. https://doi.org/10.1159/000381495.

17. Sarnicola V, Toro P, Gentile D, Hannush SB. Descemetic DALK and predescemetic DALK: outcomes in 236 cases of keratoconus. Cornea. 2010;29(1):53–9. https://doi.org/10.1097/ICO.0b013e3181a31aea.

18. Barraquer JI. Lamellar keratoplasty. (Special techniques). Ann Ophthalmol. 1972;4(6):437–69.

19. Ardjomand N, Hau S, McAlister JC, Bunce C, Galaretta D, Tuft SJ, et al. Quality of vision and graft thickness in deep anterior lamellar and penetrating corneal allografts. Am J Ophthalmol. 2007;143(2):228–35. https://doi.org/10.1016/j.ajo.2006.10.043.

20. Archila EA. Deep lamellar keratoplasty dissection of host tissue with intrastromal air injection. Cornea. 1984;3(3):217–8.

21. Sarnicola C, Sarnicola E, Cheung AY, Panico E, Panico C, Sarnicola V. Deep anterior lamellar keratoplasty after previous anterior lamellar keratoplasty to improve the visual outcomes.

22. Enrica S, Caterina S, Vincenzo S. Techniques of anterior lamellar keratoplasty. In: Mannis MJ, Holland EJ, editors. Cornea, vol. 2. 5th ed. Amsterdam: Elsevier; 2021.

23. Werblin TP, Kaufman HE, Friedlander MH, Granet N. Epikeratophakia: the surgical correction of aphakia. III. Preliminary results of a prospective clinical trial. Arch Ophthalmol. 1981;99(11):1957–60. https://doi.org/10.1001/archopht.1981.03930020833002.

24. Kang J, Cabot F, Yoo SH. Long-term follow-up of epikeratophakia. J Cataract Refract Surg. 2015;41(3):670–3. https://doi.org/10.1016/j.jcrs.2014.11.035.

25. Uusitalo RJ, Uusitalo HM. Long-term follow-up of pediatric epikeratophakia. J Refract Surg. 1997;13(1):45–54. https://doi.org/10.3928/1081-597X-19970101-12.

26. Cameron JA, Cotter JB, Risco JM, Alvarez H. Epikeratoplasty for keratoglobus associated with blue sclera. Ophthalmology. 1991;98(4):446–52. https://doi.org/10.1016/s0161-6420(91)32271-1.

27. Javadi MA, Kanavi MR, Ahmadi M, Yazdani S. Outcomes of epikeratoplasty for advanced keratoglobus. Cornea. 2007;26(2):154–7. https://doi.org/10.1097/01.ico.0000244878.38621.fc.

28. Macsai MS, Lemley HL, Schwartz T. Management of oculus fragilis in Ehlers-Danlos type VI. Cornea. 2000;19(1):104–7. https://doi.org/10.1097/00003226-200001000-00020.

29. Walkden A, Burkitt-Wright E, Au L. Brittle cornea syndrome: current perspectives. Clin Ophthalmol. 2019;13:1511–6. https://doi.org/10.2147/OPTH.S185287.

30. Jhanji V, Young AL, Mehta JS, Sharma N, Agarwal T, Vajpayee RB. Management of corneal perforation. Surv Ophthalmol. 2011;56(6):522–38. https://doi.org/10.1016/j.survophthal.2011.06.003.

31. Huang D, Qiu WY, Zhang B, Wang BH, Yao YF. Peripheral deep anterior lamellar keratoplasty using a cryopreserved donor cornea for Terrien's marginal degeneration. J Zhejiang Univ Sci B. 2014;15(12):1055–63. https://doi.org/10.1631/jzus.B1400083.

32. Cheng CL, Theng JT, Tan DT. Compressive C-shaped lamellar keratoplasty: a surgical alternative for the management of severe astigmatism from peripheral corneal degeneration. Ophthalmology. 2005;112(3):425–30. https://doi.org/10.1016/j.ophtha.2004.10.033.

33. Cheung AY, Sarnicola E, Kurji KH, Genereux BM, Holland EJ. Three hundred sixty-degree fuchs superficial marginal keratitis managed with annular lamellar keratoplasty. Cornea. 2018;37(2):260–2. https://doi.org/10.1097/ICO.0000000000001433.

34. Lohchab M, Prakash G, Arora T, Maharana P, Jhanji V, Sharma N, et al. Surgical management of peripheral corneal thinning disorders. Surv Ophthalmol.

2019;64(1):67–78. https://doi.org/10.1016/j.survophthal.2018.06.002.

35. Arenas E, Esquenazi S, Anwar M, Terry M. Lamellar corneal transplantation. Surv Ophthalmol. 2012;57(6):510–29. https://doi.org/10.1016/j.survophthal.2012.01.009.

36. Kaufman HE, Insler MS, Ibrahim-Elzembely HA, Kaufman SC. Human fibrin tissue adhesive for sutureless lamellar keratoplasty and scleral patch adhesion: a pilot study. Ophthalmology. 2003;110(11):2168–72. https://doi.org/10.1016/S0161-6420(03)00832-7.

37. Patel AK, Scorcia V, Kadyan A, Lapenna L, Ponzin D, Busin M. Microkeratome-assisted superficial anterior lamellar keratoplasty for anterior stromal corneal opacities after penetrating keratoplasty. Cornea. 2012;31(1):101–5. https://doi.org/10.1097/ICO.0b013e31820c9fd1.

38. Fogla R, Knyazer B. Microkeratome-assisted two-stage technique of superficial anterior lamellar keratoplasty for Reis-Bücklers corneal dystrophy. Cornea. 2014;33(10):1118–22. https://doi.org/10.1097/ICO.0000000000000189.

39. Shousha MA, Yoo SH, Kymionis GD, Ide T, Feuer W, Karp CL, et al. Long-term results of femtosecond laser-assisted sutureless anterior lamellar keratoplasty. Ophthalmology. 2011;118(2):315–23. https://doi.org/10.1016/j.ophtha.2010.06.037.

40. Seitz B, Lisch W. Stage-related therapy of corneal dystrophies. Dev Ophthalmol. 2011;48:116–53. https://doi.org/10.1159/000324081.

41. Deshmukh R, Reddy JC, Rapuano CJ, Vaddavalli PK. Phototherapeutic keratectomy: indications, methods and decision making. Indian J Ophthalmol. 2020;68(12):2856–66. https://doi.org/10.4103/ijo.IJO_1524_20.

42. Beltz J, Madi S, Santorum P. Superficial anterior lamellar keratoplasty: description of technique and presentation of results. Min Oftalmol. 2018;60:156–61. https://doi.org/10.23736/S0026-4903.18.01811-1. Madi S, editor.

43. Anwar M, Teichmann KD. Big-bubble technique to bare Descemet's membrane in anterior lamellar keratoplasty. J Cataract Refract Surg. 2002;28(3):398–403. https://doi.org/10.1016/s0886-3350(01)01181-6.

44. Melles GR, Lander F, Rietveld FJ, Remeijer L, Beekhuis WH, Binder PS. A new surgical technique for deep stromal, anterior lamellar keratoplasty. Br J Ophthalmol. 1999;83(3):327–33. https://doi.org/10.1136/bjo.83.3.327.

45. Dua HS, Faraj LA, Said DG, Gray T, Lowe J. Human corneal anatomy redefined: a novel pre-Descemet's layer (Dua's layer). Ophthalmology. 2013;120(9):1778–85. https://doi.org/10.1016/j.ophtha.2013.01.018.

46. Jafarinasab MR, Rahmati-Kamel M, Kanavi MR, Feizi S. Dissection plane in deep anterior lamellar keratoplasty using the big-bubble technique. Cornea. 2010;29(4):388–91. https://doi.org/10.1097/ICO.0b013e3181ba7016.

47. Luengo-Gimeno F, Tan DT, Mehta JS. Evolution of deep anterior lamellar keratoplasty (DALK). Ocul Surf. 2011;9(2):98–110. https://doi.org/10.1016/s1542-0124(11)70017-9.

48. Melles GR, Remeijer L, Geerards AJ, Beekhuis WH. A quick surgical technique for deep, anterior lamellar keratoplasty using visco-dissection. Cornea. 2000;19(4):427–32. https://doi.org/10.1097/00003226-200007000-00004.

49. Melles GR, Rietveld FJ, Beekhuis WH, Binder PS. A technique to visualize corneal incision and lamellar dissection depth during surgery. Cornea. 1999;18(1):80–6.

50. Tsubota K, Kaido M, Monden Y, Satake Y, Bissen-Miyajima H, Shimazaki J. A new surgical technique for deep lamellar keratoplasty with single running suture adjustment. Am J Ophthalmol. 1998;126(1):1–8. https://doi.org/10.1016/s0002-9394(98)00067-1.

51. Polack FM. Lamellar keratoplasty. Malbran's "peeling off" technique. Arch Ophthalmol. 1971;86(3):293–5. https://doi.org/10.1001/archopht.1971.01000010295010.

52. Fogla R, Sahay P, Sharma N. Preferred practice pattern and observed outcome of deep anterior lamellar keratoplasty - a survey of Indian corneal surgeons. Indian J Ophthalmol. 2021;69(6):1553–8. https://doi.org/10.4103/ijo.IJO_3067_20.

53. McKee HD, Irion LC, Carley FM, Jhanji V, Brahma AK. Dissection plane of the clear margin big-bubble in deep anterior lamellar keratoplasty. Cornea. 2013;32(4):e51–2. https://doi.org/10.1097/ICO.0b013e318262e8ce.

54. Goweida MB, Ragab AM, Liu C. Management of type 2 bubble formed during big bubble deep anterior lamellar keratoplasty. Cornea. 2019;38(2):189–93. https://doi.org/10.1097/ICO.0000000000001815.

55. Gujar P. Type 2 big bubble deep anterior lamellar keratoplasty-serial anterior segment optical coherence tomography documentation showing resolution of bubble in the postoperative period. Indian J Ophthalmol. 2017;65(10):1017–8. https://doi.org/10.4103/ijo.IJO_343_17.

56. Pasricha ND, Shieh C, Carrasco-Zevallos OM, Keller B, Cunefare D, Mehta JS, et al. Needle depth and big-bubble success in deep anterior lamellar keratoplasty: an ex vivo microscope-integrated OCT study. Cornea. 2016;35(11):1471–7. https://doi.org/10.1097/ICO.0000000000000948.

57. Sarnicola V, Toro P. Blunt cannula for descemetic deep anterior lamellar keratoplasty. Cornea. 2011;30(8):895–8. https://doi.org/10.1097/ICO.0b013e3181e848c3.

58. Sarnicola E, Sarnicola C, Sabatino F, Tosi GM, Perri P, Sarnicola V. Cannula DALK versus needle DALK for keratoconus. Cornea. 2016;35(12):1508–11. https://doi.org/10.1097/ICO.0000000000001032.

59. Fogla R, Padmanabhan P. Results of deep lamellar keratoplasty using the big-bubble technique in patients with keratoconus. Am J Ophthalmol. 2006;141(2):254–9. https://doi.org/10.1016/j.ajo.2005.08.064.

60. Fogla R. Deep anterior lamellar keratoplasty in the management of keratoconus. Indian J Ophthalmol. 2013;61(8):465–8. https://doi.org/10.4103/0301-4738.116061.

61. Fournié P, Malecaze F, Coullet J, Arné JL. Variant of the big bubble technique in deep anterior lamellar keratoplasty. J Cataract Refract Surg. 2007;33(3):371–5. https://doi.org/10.1016/j.jcrs.2006.10.053.

62. Ghanem RC, Ghanem MA. Pachymetry-guided intrastromal air injection ("pachy-bubble") for deep anterior lamellar keratoplasty. Cornea. 2012;31(9):1087–91. https://doi.org/10.1097/ICO.0b013e31823f8f2d.

63. Scorcia V, Busin M, Lucisano A, Beltz J, Carta A, Scorcia G. Anterior segment optical coherence tomography-guided big-bubble technique. Ophthalmology. 2013;120(3):471–6. https://doi.org/10.1016/j.ophtha.2012.08.041.

64. Buzzonetti L, Laborante A, Petrocelli G. Standardized big-bubble technique in deep anterior lamellar keratoplasty assisted by the femtosecond laser. J Cataract Refract Surg. 2010;36(10):1631–6. https://doi.org/10.1016/j.jcrs.2010.08.013.

65. Chamberlain WD. Femtosecond laser-assisted deep anterior lamellar keratoplasty. Curr Opin Ophthalmol. 2019;30(4):256–63. https://doi.org/10.1097/ICU.0000000000000574.

66. Price FW. Intraoperative optical coherence tomography: game-changing technology. Cornea. 2021;40(6):675–8. https://doi.org/10.1097/ICO.0000000000002629.

67. De Benito-Llopis L, Mehta JS, Angunawela RI, Ang M, Tan DT. Intraoperative anterior segment optical coherence tomography: a novel assessment tool during deep anterior lamellar keratoplasty. Am J Ophthalmol. 2014;157(2):334–41.e3. https://doi.org/10.1016/j.ajo.2013.10.001.

68. de Macedo JP, de Oliveira LA, Hirai F, de Sousa LB. Femtosecond laser-assisted deep anterior lamellar keratoplasty in phototherapeutic keratectomy versus the big-bubble technique in keratoconus. Int J Ophthalmol. 2018;11(5):807–12. https://doi.org/10.18240/ijo.2018.05.15.

69. Farid M, Steinert RF. Femtosecond laser-assisted corneal surgery. Curr Opin Ophthalmol. 2010;21(4):288–92. https://doi.org/10.1097/ICU.0b013e32833a8dbc.

70. Ziebarth NM, Dias J, Hürmeriç V, Shousha MA, Yau CB, Moy VT, et al. Quality of corneal lamellar cuts quantified using atomic force microscopy. J Cataract Refract Surg. 2013;39(1):110–7. https://doi.org/10.1016/j.jcrs.2012.07.040.

71. Lu Y, Shi YH, Yang LP, Ge YR, Chen XF, Wu Y, et al. Femtosecond laser-assisted deep anterior lamellar keratoplasty for keratoconus and keratecta-sia. Int J Ophthalmol. 2014;7(4):638–43. https://doi.org/10.3980/j.issn.2222-3959.2014.04.09.

72. Parthasarathy A, Por YM, Tan DT. Using a "small bubble technique" to aid in success in Anwar's "big bubble technique" of deep lamellar keratoplasty with complete baring of Descemet's membrane. Br J Ophthalmol. 2008;92(3):422. https://doi.org/10.1136/bjo.2006.113357.

73. Goshe J, Terry MA, Shamie N, Li J. Ophthalmic viscosurgical device-assisted incision modification for the big-bubble technique in deep anterior lamellar keratoplasty. J Cataract Refract Surg. 2011;37(11):1923–7. https://doi.org/10.1016/j.jcrs.2011.09.014.

74. Manche EE, Holland GN, Maloney RK. Deep lamellar keratoplasty using viscoelastic dissection. Arch Ophthalmol. 1999;117(11):1561–5. https://doi.org/10.1001/archopht.117.11.1561.

75. Muftuoglu O, Toro P, Hogan RN, Bowman RW, Cavanagh HD, McCulley JP, et al. Sarnicola air-visco bubble technique in deep anterior lamellar keratoplasty. Cornea. 2013;32(4):527–32. https://doi.org/10.1097/ICO.0b013e31826cbe99.

76. Malbran E, Stefani C. Lamellar keratoplasty in corneal ectasias. Ophthalmologica. 1972;164(1):50–8. https://doi.org/10.1159/000306704.

77. Malbran E. Lamellar keratoplasty in keratoconus. Int Ophthalmol Clin. 1966;6(1):99–109.

78. Smolek MK, McCarey BE. Interlamellar adhesive strength in human eyebank corneas. Invest Ophthalmol Vis Sci. 1990;31(6):1087–95.

79. Sarnicola C, Sarnicola V, Romani A, Sarnicola E. Rediscovering a valuable manual Deep Anterior Lamellar Keratoplasty (DALK) technique: outcomes of 42 "Peeling-off" DALK. Eur J Ophthalmol. 2022;33:900. https://doi.org/10.1177/11206721221132622.

80. Sarnicola C, Sarnicola E, Cheung AY, Sarnicola V. Deep anterior lamellar keratoplasty: can all ruptures be fixed? Cornea. 2023;42:80–8. https://doi.org/10.1097/ICO.0000000000003054.

81. Price FW. Air lamellar keratoplasty. Refract Corneal Surg. 1989;5(4):240–3.

82. Nanavaty MA, Vijjan KS, Yvon C. Deep anterior lamellar keratoplasty: a surgeon's guide. J Curr Ophthalmol. 2018;30(4):297–310. https://doi.org/10.1016/j.joco.2018.06.004.

83. Huang T, Ouyang C, Hou C, Wu Q, Hu Y. Outcomes of same-size host and donor trephine in deep anterior lamellar keratoplasty for keratoconus. Am J Ophthalmol. 2016;166:8–13. https://doi.org/10.1016/j.ajo.2016.03.018.

84. Shi W, Li S, Gao H, Wang T, Xie L. Modified deep lamellar keratoplasty for the treatment of advanced-stage keratoconus with steep curvature. Ophthalmology. 2010;117(2):226–31. https://doi.org/10.1016/j.ophtha.2009.07.005.

85. Sarnicola E, Sarnicola C, Cheung AY, Panico E, Panico C, Sarnicola V. Total or subtotal full thickness recipient bed cut to repair donor-recipient cur-

vature disparity in cases of DM rupture with manual DALK. Eur J Ophthalmol. 2020;30:1172. https://doi.org/10.1177/1120672120932833.

86. Thompson RW, Price MO, Bowers PJ, Price FW. Long-term graft survival after penetrating keratoplasty. Ophthalmology. 2003;110(7):1396–402. https://doi.org/10.1016/S0161-6420(03)00463-9.

87. Zadok D, Schwarts S, Marcovich A, Barkana Y, Morad Y, Eting E, et al. Penetrating keratoplasty for keratoconus: long-term results. Cornea. 2005;24(8):959–61. https://doi.org/10.1097/01.ico.0000159729.51015.b4.

88. Arundhati A, Chew MC, Lim L, Mehta JS, Lang SS, Htoon HM, et al. Comparative study of long-term graft survival between penetrating keratoplasty and deep anterior lamellar keratoplasty. Am J Ophthalmol. 2021;224:207–16. https://doi.org/10.1016/j.ajo.2020.11.006.

89. Woo JH, Tan YL, Htoon HM, Tan DTH, Mehta JS. Outcomes of repeat anterior lamellar keratoplasty. Cornea. 2020;39(2):200–6. https://doi.org/10.1097/ICO.0000000000002167.

90. Alió Del Barrio JL, Bhogal M, Ang M, Ziaei M, Robbie S, Montesel A, et al. Corneal transplantation after failed grafts: options and outcomes. Surv Ophthalmol. 2021;66(1):20–40. https://doi.org/10.1016/j.survophthal.2020.10.003.

91. Montesel A, Alió Del Barrio JL, Yébana Rubio P, Alió JL. Corneal graft surgery: a monocentric long-term analysis. Eur J Ophthalmol. 2021;31(4):1700–8. https://doi.org/10.1177/1120672120947592.

92. Gómez-Benlloch A, Montesel A, Pareja-Aricò L, Mingo-Botín D, Michael R, Barraquer RI, et al. Causes of corneal transplant failure: a multicentric study. Acta Ophthalmol. 2021;99(6):e922–e8. https://doi.org/10.1111/aos.14708.

93. Kelly TL, Williams KA, Coster DJ, Registry ACG. Corneal transplantation for keratoconus: a registry study. Arch Ophthalmol. 2011;129(6):691–7. https://doi.org/10.1001/archophthalmol.2011.7.

94. Maguire MG, Stark WJ, Gottsch JD, Stulting RD, Sugar A, Fink NE, et al. Risk factors for corneal graft failure and rejection in the collaborative corneal transplantation studies. Collaborative Corneal Transplantation Studies Research Group. Ophthalmology. 1994;101(9):1536–47. https://doi.org/10.1016/s0161-6420(94)31138-9.

95. Gonzalez A, Price MO, Feng MT, Lee C, Arbelaez JG, Price FW. Immunologic rejection episodes after deep anterior lamellar keratoplasty: incidence and risk factors. Cornea. 2017;36(9):1076–82. https://doi.org/10.1097/ICO.0000000000001223.

96. Watson SL, Tuft SJ, Dart JK. Patterns of rejection after deep lamellar keratoplasty. Ophthalmology. 2006;113(4):556–60. https://doi.org/10.1016/j.ophtha.2006.01.006.

97. Sarnicola C, Sarnicola E, Panico E, Panico C, Sarnicola V. Cataract surgery in corneal transplantation. Curr Opin Ophthalmol. 2020;31(1):23–7. https://doi.org/10.1097/ICU.0000000000000635.

98. Williams KA, Keane MC. Outcomes of corneal transplantation in Australia, in an era of lamellar keratoplasty. Clin Exp Ophthalmol. 2022;50(4):374–85. https://doi.org/10.1111/ceo.14089.

99. Eye Bank Association of America (EBAA). Eye banking statistical report 2017. Washington, DC: EBAA; 2018.

100. Arnalich-Montiel F, Alió Del Barrio JL, Alió JL. Corneal surgery in keratoconus: which type, which technique, which outcomes? Eye Vis. 2016;3:2. https://doi.org/10.1186/s40662-016-0033-y.

101. Cremona FA, Ghosheh FR, Rapuano CJ, Eagle RC, Hammersmith KM, Laibson PR, et al. Keratoconus associated with other corneal dystrophies. Cornea. 2009;28(2):127–35. https://doi.org/10.1097/ICO.0b013e3181859935.

102. Romano V, Iovieno A, Parente G, Soldani AM, Fontana L. Long-term clinical outcomes of deep anterior lamellar keratoplasty in patients with keratoconus. Am J Ophthalmol. 2015;159(3):505–11. https://doi.org/10.1016/j.ajo.2014.11.033.

103. Chew AC, Mehta JS, Tan DT. Deep lamellar keratoplasty after resolution of hydrops in keratoconus. Cornea. 2011;30(4):454–9. https://doi.org/10.1097/ICO.0b013e3181f0b1f3.

104. Fuest M, Mehta JS. Strategies for deep anterior lamellar keratoplasty after hydrops in keratoconus. Eye Contact Lens. 2018;44(2):69–76. https://doi.org/10.1097/ICL.0000000000000383.

105. Jacob S, Narasimhan S, Agarwal A, Sambath J, Umamaheshwari G, Saijimol AI. Primary modified predescemetic deep anterior lamellar keratoplasty in acute corneal hydrops. Cornea. 2018;37(10):1328–33. https://doi.org/10.1097/ICO.0000000000001693.

106. Lake D, Hamada S, Khan S, Daya SM. Deep anterior lamellar keratoplasty over penetrating keratoplasty for host rim thinning and ectasia. Cornea. 2009;28(5):489–92. https://doi.org/10.1097/ICO.0b013e31818d3b3c.

107. Wallang BS, Das S. Keratoglobus. Eye. 2013;27(9):1004–12. https://doi.org/10.1038/eye.2013.130.

108. Williams KA, Lowe M, Bartlett C, Kelly TL, Coster DJ, Contributors A. Risk factors for human corneal graft failure within the Australian corneal graft registry. Transplantation. 2008;86(12):1720–4. https://doi.org/10.1097/TP.0b013e3181903b0a.

109. Vajpayee RB, Bhartiya P, Sharma N. Central lamellar keratoplasty with peripheral intralamellar tuck: a new surgical technique for keratoglobus. Cornea. 2002;21(7):657–60. https://doi.org/10.1097/00003226-200210000-00005.

110. Kaushal S, Jhanji V, Sharma N, Tandon R, Titiyal JS, Vajpayee RB. "Tuck In" Lamellar Keratoplasty (TILK) for corneal ectasias involving corneal periphery. Br J Ophthalmol. 2008;92(2):286–90. https://doi.org/10.1136/bjo.2007.12462.

111. Jinabhai A, Radhakrishnan H, O'Donnell C. Pellucid corneal marginal degeneration: a review. Cont

Lens Anter Eye. 2011;34(2):56–63. https://doi.org/10.1016/j.clae.2010.11.007.

112. Moshirfar M, Edmonds JN, Behunin NL, Christiansen SM. Current options in the management of pellucid marginal degeneration. J Refract Surg. 2014;30(7):474–85. https://doi.org/10.3928/1081597X-20140429-02.

113. Millar MJ, Maloof A. Deep lamellar keratoplasty for pellucid marginal degeneration: review of management options for corneal perforation. Cornea. 2008;27(8):953–6. https://doi.org/10.1097/ICO.0b013e31816ed516.

114. Al-Torbak AA. Deep anterior lamellar keratoplasty for pellucid marginal degeneration. Saudi J Ophthalmol. 2013;27(1):11–4. https://doi.org/10.1016/j.sjopt.2012.04.001.

115. Sarnicola V, Toro P. Deep anterior lamellar keratoplasty in herpes simplex corneal opacities. Cornea. 2010;29(1):60–4. https://doi.org/10.1097/ICO.0b013e3181a317d3.

116. Skarentzos K, Chatzimichael E, Panagiotopoulou EK, Taliantzis S, Konstantinidis A, Labiris G. Corneal graft success rates in HSV keratitis: a systematic review. Acta Med (Hradec Kralove). 2020;63(4):150–8. https://doi.org/10.14712/18059694.2020.57.

117. Ramamurthi S, Cornish KS, Steeples L, Ramaesh K. Deep anterior lamellar keratoplasty on a previously failed full-thickness graft. Cornea. 2009;28(4):456–7. https://doi.org/10.1097/ICO.0b013e31818c2af7.

118. Sepsakos L, Cheung AY, Holland EJ. Outcomes of keratoplasty after ocular surface stem cell transplantation. Cornea. 2017;36(9):1025–30. https://doi.org/10.1097/ICO.0000000000001267.

119. Yao YF, Zhang B, Zhou P, Jiang JK. Autologous limbal grafting combined with deep lamellar keratoplasty in unilateral eye with severe chemical or thermal burn at late stage. Ophthalmology. 2002;109(11):2011–7. https://doi.org/10.1016/s0161-6420(02)01258-7.

120. Fogla R, Padmanabhan P. Deep anterior lamellar keratoplasty combined with autologous limbal stem cell transplantation in unilateral severe chemical injury. Cornea. 2005;24(4):421–5. https://doi.org/10.1097/01.ico.0000151550.51556.2d.

121. Inoue Y. Corneal triple procedure. Semin Ophthalmol. 2001;16(3):113–8. https://doi.org/10.1076/soph.16.3.113.4202.

122. Oie Y, Nishida K. Triple procedure: cataract extraction, intraocular lens implantation, and corneal graft. Curr Opin Ophthalmol. 2017;28(1):63–6. https://doi.org/10.1097/ICU.0000000000000337.

123. Sarnicola E, Sarnicola C, Cheung AY, Sarnicola V. Deep anterior lamellar keratoplasty for corneal penetrating wounds. Eur J Ophthalmol. 2021;17:28. https://doi.org/10.1177/11206721211014385.

124. Moshirfar M, Bennett P, Ronquillo Y. Corneal dystrophy. Treasure Island, FL: StatPearls Publishing; 2021.

125. Mohamed A, Chaurasia S, Ramappa M, Murthy SI, Garg P. Outcomes of keratoplasty in lattice corneal dystrophy in a large cohort of Indian eyes. Indian J Ophthalmol. 2018;66(5):666–72. https://doi.org/10.4103/ijo.IJO_1150_17.

126. Sogutlu Sari E, Kubaloglu A, Unal M, Pinero D, Bulut N, Erol MK, et al. Deep anterior lamellar keratoplasty versus penetrating keratoplasty for macular corneal dystrophy: a randomized trial. Am J Ophthalmol. 2013;156(2):267–74.e1. https://doi.org/10.1016/j.ajo.2013.03.007.

127. Unal M, Arslan OS, Atalay E, Mangan MS, Bilgin AB. Deep anterior lamellar keratoplasty for the treatment of stromal corneal dystrophies. Cornea. 2013;32(3):301–5. https://doi.org/10.1097/ICO.0b013e31825718ca.

128. Vajpayee RB, Tyagi J, Sharma N, Kumar N, Jhanji V, Titiyal JS. Deep anterior lamellar keratoplasty by big-bubble technique for treatment corneal stromal opacities. Am J Ophthalmol. 2007;143(6):954–7. https://doi.org/10.1016/j.ajo.2007.02.036.

129. Shimazaki J, Shimmura S, Ishioka M, Tsubota K. Randomized clinical trial of deep lamellar keratoplasty vs penetrating keratoplasty. Am J Ophthalmol. 2002;134(2):159–65. https://doi.org/10.1016/s0002-9394(02)01523-4.

130. Lewis DR, Price MO, Feng MT, Price FW. Recurrence of granular corneal dystrophy type 1 after phototherapeutic keratectomy, lamellar keratoplasty, and penetrating keratoplasty in a single population. Cornea. 2017;36(10):1227–32. https://doi.org/10.1097/ICO.0000000000001303.

131. Marcon AS, Cohen EJ, Rapuano CJ, Laibson PR. Recurrence of corneal stromal dystrophies after penetrating keratoplasty. Cornea. 2003;22(1):19–21. https://doi.org/10.1097/00003226-200301000-00005.

132. Reddy JC, Murthy SI, Vaddavalli PK, Garg P, Ramappa M, Chaurasia S, et al. Clinical outcomes and risk factors for graft failure after deep anterior lamellar keratoplasty and penetrating keratoplasty for macular corneal dystrophy. Cornea. 2015;34(2):171–6. https://doi.org/10.1097/ICO.0000000000000327.

133. Sharma N, Jain M, Sehra SV, Maharana P, Agarwal T, Satpathy G, et al. Outcomes of therapeutic penetrating keratoplasty from a tertiary eye care centre in northern India. Cornea. 2014;33(2):114–8. https://doi.org/10.1097/ICO.0000000000000025.

134. Chen WL, Wu CY, Hu FR, Wang IJ. Therapeutic penetrating keratoplasty for microbial keratitis in Taiwan from 1987 to 2001. Am J Ophthalmol. 2004;137(4):736–43. https://doi.org/10.1016/j.ajo.2003.11.010.

135. Kashiwabuchi RT, de Freitas D, Alvarenga LS, Vieira L, Contarini P, Sato E, et al. Corneal graft survival after therapeutic keratoplasty for Acanthamoeba keratitis. Acta Ophthalmol. 2008;86(6):666–9. https://doi.org/10.1111/j.1600-0420.2007.01086.x.

136. Dart JK, Saw VP, Kilvington S. Acanthamoeba keratitis: diagnosis and treatment update 2009. Am J Ophthalmol. 2009;148(4):487–99.e2. https://doi.org/10.1016/j.ajo.2009.06.009.

137. Kaufman AR, Tu EY. Advances in the management of Acanthamoeba keratitis: a review of the literature and synthesized algorithmic approach. Ocul Surf. 2022;25:26–36. https://doi.org/10.1016/j.jtos.2022.04.003.

138. Sarnicola E, Sarnicola C, Sabatino F, Tosi GM, Perri P, Sarnicola V. Early Deep Anterior Lamellar Keratoplasty (DALK) for acanthamoeba keratitis poorly responsive to medical treatment. Cornea. 2016;35(1):1–5. https://doi.org/10.1097/ICO.0000000000000681.

139. Sarnicola V, Sarnicola E, Sarnicola C, Sabatino F, Tosi GM, Perri P. Reply. Cornea. 2016;35(6):e14–5. https://doi.org/10.1097/ICO.0000000000000832.

140. Sabatino F, Sarnicola E, Sarnicola C, Tosi GM, Perri P, Sarnicola V, et al. Early deep anterior lamellar keratoplasty for fungal keratitis poorly responsive to medical treatment. Eye. 2017;31(12):1639–46. https://doi.org/10.1038/eye.2017.228.

141. Anshu A, Parthasarathy A, Mehta JS, Htoon HM, Tan DT. Outcomes of therapeutic deep lamellar keratoplasty and penetrating keratoplasty for advanced infectious keratitis: a comparative study. Ophthalmology. 2009;116(4):615–23. https://doi.org/10.1016/j.ophtha.2008.12.043.

142. Bagga B, Garg P, Joseph J, Mohamed A, Kalra P. Outcome of therapeutic deep anterior lamellar keratoplasty in advanced. Indian J Ophthalmol. 2020;68(3):442–6. https://doi.org/10.4103/ijo.IJO_307_19.

143. Laurik KL, Szentmáry N, Daas L, Langenbucher A, Seitz B. Early penetrating keratoplasty à chaud may improve outcome in therapy-resistant acanthamoeba keratitis. Adv Ther. 2019;36(9):2528–40. https://doi.org/10.1007/s12325-019-01031-3.

144. Ehlers N, Hjortdal J. Are cataract and iris atrophy toxic complications of medical treatment of acanthamoeba keratitis? Acta Ophthalmol Scand. 2004;82(2):228–31. https://doi.org/10.1111/j.1600-0420.2004.00237.x.

145. Sharma N, Kumar C, Mannan R, Titiyal JS, Vajpayee RB. Surgical technique of deep anterior lamellar keratoplasty in descemetoceles. Cornea. 2010;29(12):1448–51. https://doi.org/10.1097/ICO.0b013e3181e2ef9c.

146. Gabison EE, Doan S, Catanese M, Chastang P, Ben M'hamed M, Cochereau I. Modified deep anterior lamellar keratoplasty in the management of small and large epithelialized descemetoceles. Cornea. 2011;30(10):1179–82. https://doi.org/10.1097/ICO.0b013e3182031c81.

147. Waring GO, Lynn MJ, McDonnell PJ. Results of the prospective evaluation of radial keratotomy (PERK) study 10 years after surgery. Arch Ophthalmol. 1994;112(10):1298–308. https://doi.org/10.1001/archopht.1994.01090220048022.

148. Einan-Lifshitz A, Belkin A, Sorkin N, Mednick Z, Boutin T, Kreimei M, et al. Evaluation of big bubble technique for deep anterior lamellar keratoplasty in patients with radial keratotomy. Cornea. 2019;38(2):194–7. https://doi.org/10.1097/ICO.0000000000001811.

149. Smadja D, Colin J, Krueger RR, Mello GR, Gallois A, Mortemousque B, et al. Outcomes of deep anterior lamellar keratoplasty for keratoconus: learning curve and advantages of the big bubble technique. Cornea. 2012;31(8):859–63. https://doi.org/10.1097/ICO.0b013e318242fdae.

150. Senoo T, Chiba K, Terada O, Hasegawa K, Obara Y. Visual acuity prognosis after anterior chamber air replacement to prevent pseudo-anterior chamber formation after deep lamellar keratoplasty. Jpn J Ophthalmol. 2007;51(3):181–4. https://doi.org/10.1007/s10384-006-0421-2.

151. Huang OS, Htoon HM, Chan AM, Tan D, Mehta JS. Incidence and outcomes of intraoperative descemet membrane perforations during deep anterior lamellar keratoplasty. Am J Ophthalmol. 2019;199:9–18. https://doi.org/10.1016/j.ajo.2018.10.026.

152. Sarnicola E, Sarnicola C, Cheung AY, Panico E, Panico C, Sarnicola V. Manual deep anterior lamellar keratoplasty after partial unintentional full-thickness trephination. Eur J Ophthalmol. 2020;31:774. https://doi.org/10.1177/1120672120932108.

153. Sarnicola V, Sarnicola E, Sarnicola C. Recovery techniques in DALK. In: Mannis MJ, Holland EJ, editors. Cornea, vol. 2. 4th ed. Amsterdam: Elsevier; 2016.

Stromal Lenticule Addition Keratoplasty (SLAK)

19

Leonardo Mastropasqua, Niccolò Salgari, Manuela Lanzini, and Mario Nubile

Key Points

- The concept of "remodeling" the keratoconic cornea, by intrapocket implantation of human stromal lenticules, is presented in this chapter. The main difference resides in the fact that diseased stroma is not replaced by the keratoplasty technique but "augmented" in order to reshape the transparent ectatic cornea.

- The use of femtosecond lasers system for the preparation of both the recipient intracorneal dissection and the "shaped" lenticule from donor corneas is clearly presented in the chapter. The main clinical advantages reside in the quick and simple surgical procedure that can be performed suture-less under topical anesthesia.

- The results as well as the pros and cons of the technique are presented, with updated literature review and description of the tomographic, refractive, and microscopic tissue changes occurring after SLAK. Finally, future perspectives and field of improvement are described.

Supplementary Information The online version contains supplementary material available at https://doi.org/10.1007/978-3-031-32408-6_19.

L. Mastropasqua · M. Lanzini · M. Nubile
National High-Tech Eye Center, University of Chieti and Pescara, Chieti, Italy
e-mail: mastropa@unich.it; m.lanzini@unich.it

N. Salgari (✉)
Department of Translational Medicine, University of Ferrara, Ferrara, Italy

Introduction

Keratoconus is a non-inflammatory degenerative ectatic disorder of the cornea in which progressive stromal thinning and apex protrusion produce corneal optical function impairment [1]. Up to the advanced stage, the corneal stromal is transparent, and visual function is mainly impeded by irregular astigmatism [2].

Visual rehabilitation in keratoconus relies on spectacle lenses when ectasia is in its early stages but, when protrusion evolves, contact lens is the only option to achieve acceptable vision quality. When gas-permeable lenses fail on multiple attempts, surgery has to be considered [3]. At present, keratoconus is the second indication for keratoplasty worldwide. The first indication for keratoplasty became graft replacement in the 2019 USA Eye-Bank report, which demonstrates the increasing demand of tissues for keratoplasty repetition. Keratoconus usually develops in the second decade of life [4] and this, combined with limited graft survival and disease recurrence, could be one of the reasons for the increasing incidence of re-grafting in recent years [5].

Deep anterior lamellar keratoplasty (DALK) is considered the gold standard procedure for the surgical treatment of keratoconus thanks to the lower risk of rejection, increased postoperative biomechanical corneal strength and longer graft survival compared to penetrating keratoplasty (PK) [6, 7]. DALK is a challenging procedure that may require conversion to PK if descemet-endothelial rupture occurs [6, 8]. Unfortunately, visual outcomes can be threatened by severe intraoperative (e.g. endophthalmitis, choroidal hemorrhage) along with postoperative (e.g. rejection, cataract, glaucoma, wound dehiscence, and stromal melting) complications that could also require lifelong medical treatment or further surgeries [9]. Despite successful surgery, over a third of patients should continue the use of contact lenses due to astigmatism or anisometropia after keratoplasty [10].

Attempts to modify corneal shape in order to avoid keratoplasty have been made in recent years with variable results. Photorefractive keratectomy (PTK) and intracorneal ring segments (ICRS) implantation combined with corneal collagen cross-linking (CXL) is available procedures but not widely adopted due to the difficult prediction of visual results and application limited to moderate cases [11, 12].

History of Stromal Keratophakia

The optical function of the cornea relies on the high regularity of its central area and small changes of this portion produce great modification of its dioptric power [13, 14]. Attempts to modify corneal shape by incision have been made since the 1800s but it was in the 1950s when a novel concept introduced by José Ignacio Barraquer led to the beginning of the refractive surgery era [15–17]. Amid the first experiments in this exciting surgery field, Barraquer proposed two approaches to reshape corneal curvature by means of tissue addition or subtraction [16, 18]. The latter is now the cornerstone of all refractive surgery procedures, while the first has been rapidly abandoned due to poor visual results mainly due to technological limitations [19, 20].

The original idea of keratophakia (from Greek words "kerato" for cornea and "phakia" for "lens") was to produce corneal curvature changes by the addition of stromal tissue into the recipient stromal bed. The Barraquer's "thickness law" states that corneal flattening can be obtained by tissue subtraction from the center or tissue addition in the periphery and vice-versa [16]. The

procedure was complex at first and after lenticule preparation with cryolathe, it involved lamellar cap dissection of the recipient cornea, donor lenticule implantation on keratectomy bed, and then repositioning and suturing of the recipient cap [21, 22]. Parallel to this work, a similar approach was proposed by Kaufman based on suturing the donor lenticule to the anterior corneal surface after epithelium removal in a procedure called "epikeratophakia" [23, 24].

Dissection depth of early microkeratomes was quite variable and inadvertent perforation was even possible. Lenticule customization was based on mechanical carving and cutting. Wound dehiscence of the lamellar cap was possible with risk of infections, epithelial ingrowth, and irregular astigmatism development. Visual recovery was generally poor due to structural cryodamages to the lenticules during grinding procedure. In a group of 32 patients, Troutman reported CDVA >20/40 in 84% of patients and a target refraction within 1.00 D in only 38.5% [19]. Similarly, Swinger and Barraquer achieved CDVA >20/40 in only 46.4% of their 46 patients [16]. Refractive results were far away from the desired target with a mean postoperative astigmatism of 2.45 ± 0.37 D [25]. Given the increasing accuracy and reproducibility of the laser subtractive techniques in the following years, keratophakia and epikeratophakia were soon abandoned.

Recent Advancements in Corneal Surgery

A renewed interest in stromal keratophakia began in 2011 when, following the introduction of femtosecond laser technology in the refractive surgery field, a novel group of techniques capable of producing precise and optically functioning stromal lenticules was presented: the Refractive Lenticule Extraction (ReLEx) techniques [26]. The small incision refractive lenticule extraction (SMILE) became a valid alternative to the excimer laser-based techniques available since the 1980s [27].

In 2011, Mohamed-Noriega et al. proved that fresh extracted tissues after ReLEx are vital and their vitality and optical efficiency were maintained after cryopreservation [28]. Angunawela et al. showed that lenticules could be safely reimplanted to reverse the refractive procedure in a rabbit model [29], and Riau et al. showed that this procedure was feasible also in nonhuman primate model [30].

Following these early insights, many authors showed interest in this field and numerous experiments took place. Liu et al. [31] investigated autologous lenticule implantation in rabbit cornea the same year of Angunawela and later, in 2015, Zhang et al. and Liu et al. showed the results of allogenic lenticule implantation in rabbit and monkey animal models [32, 33]. The first human case of FSL-derived allogenic lenticule implantation was reported by Pradhan et al. in 2013 who implanted a convex lenticule produced by myopic SMILE of -10.50 D (127 μm central thickness) with 5.75 mm diameter in a lamellar pocket at 110 μm depth to treat a high positive refractive error due to aphakia [34]. In fact, thanks to the capability of increasing corneal curvature with convex positive meniscus-shaped lenticule implantation, the first attempted applications of this concept were in hyperopia and presbyopia treatment [35–37].

Treatment of Keratoconus by Stromal Lenticule Addition

Therapeutic use of SMILE-derived lenticules is another possible application of this innovative concept of keratoplasty. Ganesh et al. proposed in 2015 the implantation of modified lenticules combined with corneal collagen cross-linking to treat keratoconus in a modification of the original technique he proposed in 2014 named femtosecond intrastromal lenticular implantation (FILI) [38, 39].

Inclusion criteria were grade 1–3 keratoconus with or without documented evidence of progression. The lenticule diameter was 6.0–7.0 mm with side-cut angle of 90°. The authors tried to calculate based on corneal topography the best match with available donor lenticules, but calculations were too complex and not reliable, so they

decided to rely on a spherical equivalent as matching parameter. Cryopreserved lenticules were thawed and washed, soaked with riboflavin, and then underwent a central 3-mm trephination to obtain a donut-like shape. Intrastromal pocket was created into the recipient cornea at 100-μm depth with 7.0- to 8.0-mm diameter (1 mm larger than the donor lenticule) and a 4-mm superior incision. The procedure was combined with accelerated collagen cross-linking. Improvement was reported for uncorrected distance visual acuity (1.06 ± 0.48 to 0.38 ± 0.27 logMAR) and corrected distance visual acuity (0.51 ± 0.20 to 0.20 ± 0.24 logMAR), and manifest spherical equivalent (23.47 ± 1.15 D to 21.77 ± 1.7 D). Mean keratometry in 3-mm and 5-mm zones reduced by 3.42 ± 2.09 D and 1.70 ± 1.31 D, respectively. Mean pachymetry in the central and mid peripheral zones increased by 18.3 ± 7.3 mm and 33.0 ± 8.8 mm, respectively. All eyes had reduction in higher order aberrations, specifically coma with no loss of lines of corrected distance visual acuity. No adverse events were reported [39].

Nearly contemporary to the first lenticule implantation experiments performed by many authors for refractive error correction, Mastropasqua et al. hypothesized the possibility of treating corneal ectasia making advantage of the tissue addition concept [40].

Stromal Lenticule Addition Keratoplasty (SLAK)

Taking cues from the results of early experiments with positive meniscus-shaped lenticule, Matropasqua et al. hypothesized that a lenticule with a negative profile can induce opposite changes to corneal curvature. This concept is part of the knowledge we learned from intracorneal ring segment implantation (ICRS), despite the working principle of ICRS is not fully understood yet. According to this hypothesis and the ongoing development of a novel negative meniscus-shaped lenticule model for application of SMILE in hyperopia treatment [41], we proposed the use of that lenticule geometry to obtain the desired effect in a novel procedure of keratoplasty [40]. The negative meniscus lenticule presents a concave profile with a maximum thickness in the peripheral region of the optical zone that gradually reduces toward the thinnest point located in the center.

The first ex vivo preliminary SLAK study on normal cornea was designed in 2015 to understand the effect of negative meniscus lenticule addition [40]. Following the promising results experienced ex vivo, a human in vivo noncomparative interventional case series was performed in a group of subjects affected by advanced central keratoconus who were already candidates for keratoplasty in 2018 [42]. Treatment was reserved to central keratoconus because only symmetrical lenticule geometry was available.

Surgical Technique

The first phase of the surgical procedure consists of lenticule preparation in donor cornea by means of a femtosecond laser (FSL). Corneo-scleral buttons are mounted on an artificial anterior chamber and pressure is standardized with a BSS bottle at 180 cm of height to inflate the anterior chamber.

All the surgical procedure is performed under topical anesthesia. Corneal epithelium is removed using a blunt spatula, and a modified femtosecond laser flap-cut procedure (flocket) [43] is performed to fashion an intrastromal pocket with a 500-kHz VisuMax femtosecond laser (Carl Zeiss Meditec, Jena, Germany) centered on the corneal central zone (Figs. 19.1a and 19.2a). A hinge length of 21.7 mm is set in order to produce a circular planar plane of dissection with a single 4-mm superior opening, a diameter of 8.2 mm, and depth from surface of 120 µm. After the laser phase, the patient is moved to the surgical microscope and flocket dissected by means of a blunt dissector (Figs. 19.1b and 19.2b) [40, 42].

Donor lenticule is produced by means of femtosecond lenticule extraction procedure (FLEx) with VisuMax femtosecond laser platform. The lenticule parameters are set as follows: flap thickness 110 µm, flap diameter 8 mm, hyperopic correction 8.00 D, optical zone 6 mm. The maximum lenticule thickness obtained is 148 µm with a central lenticule minimal thickness of 30 µm. The overall transition zone in the periphery of the lenticules is 0.70 mm in diameter [40, 42].

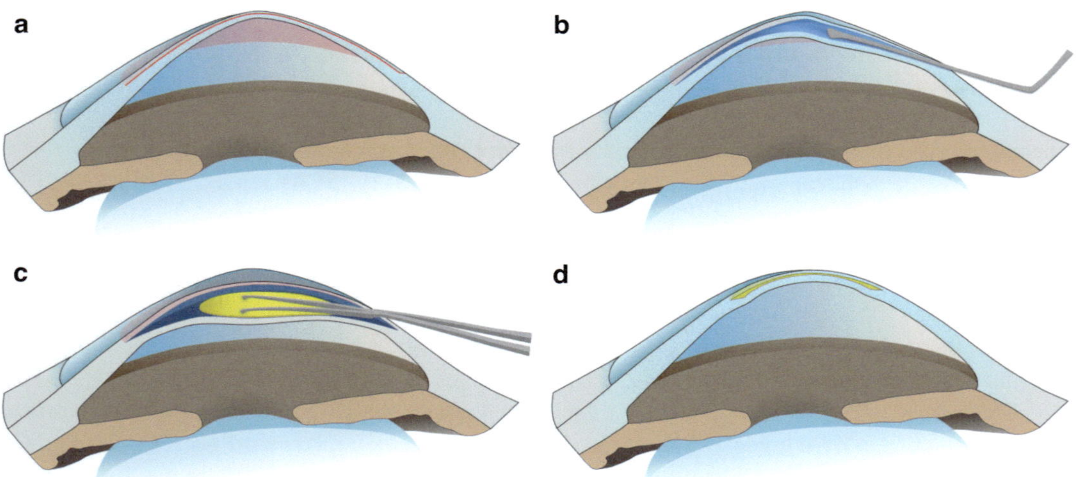

Fig. 19.1 Illustration of the surgical technique. Intrastromal pocket is created in the recipient cornea by means of femtosecond laser (**a**). Stromal dissection is performed with a blunt spatula (**b**) and then the lenticule is inserted through the incision and spread out with a dedicated forceps (**c**). Lenticule in its final position produces peripheral thickening and central flattening (**d**)

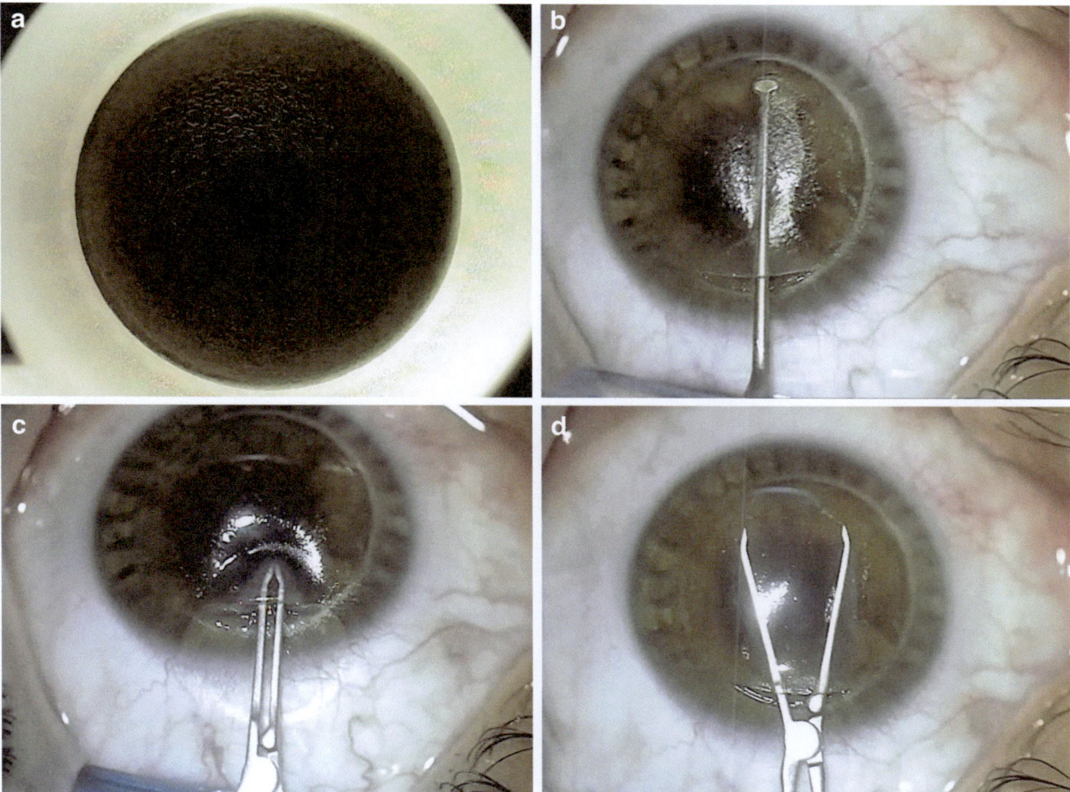

Fig. 19.2 Surgical phases of stromal lenticule addition keratoplasty. Stromal pocket is created by means of a femtosecond laser in the recipient cornea (**a**) and plane dissection is manually performed with a blunt spatula (**b**). Stromal lenticule is implanted through the small incision (**c**) and spread out in a single maneuver with a dedicated forceps (**d**)

After completion of the FSL dissection phase, the flap is lifted by means of a blunt spatula under the surgical microscope and then the lenticule is separated and transferred to the patient's eye maintaining its original orientation. The incision of the recipient pocket is opened with a Seibel spatula and the plane dissected with a blunt dissection spatula (Mastropasqua SMILE kit, Janach, Como, Italy). The lenticule is placed on the patient's cornea close to the incision opening and while grasping its distal edge, the lenticule is dragged into the pocket through the incision and spread out (Figs. 19.1c, d and 19.2c, d). Final distention is achieved from the surface using the spatula (Video 19.1). The lenticule is carefully centered onto the apex of the cone and correct distension and centration should be assessed by the operator using an intraoperative microscope, AS-OCT, and topography [40, 42].

Results

The results of the first human in vivo noncomparative interventional case series of SLAK proved that corneal flattening is possible by selective tissue addition (Fig. 19.3). Despite lack of customization, the addition of a standardized negative meniscus lenticule centered on the cone apex produced a significant improvement of corneal topography along with best corrected visual acuity in our first case series in 2015 [42]. Uncorrected distance visual acuity (UDVA) at 6 months improved in 8 of 10 eyes ($p < 0.01$; Fisher's exact test), whereas all but one eye had improvement of corrected distance visual acuity

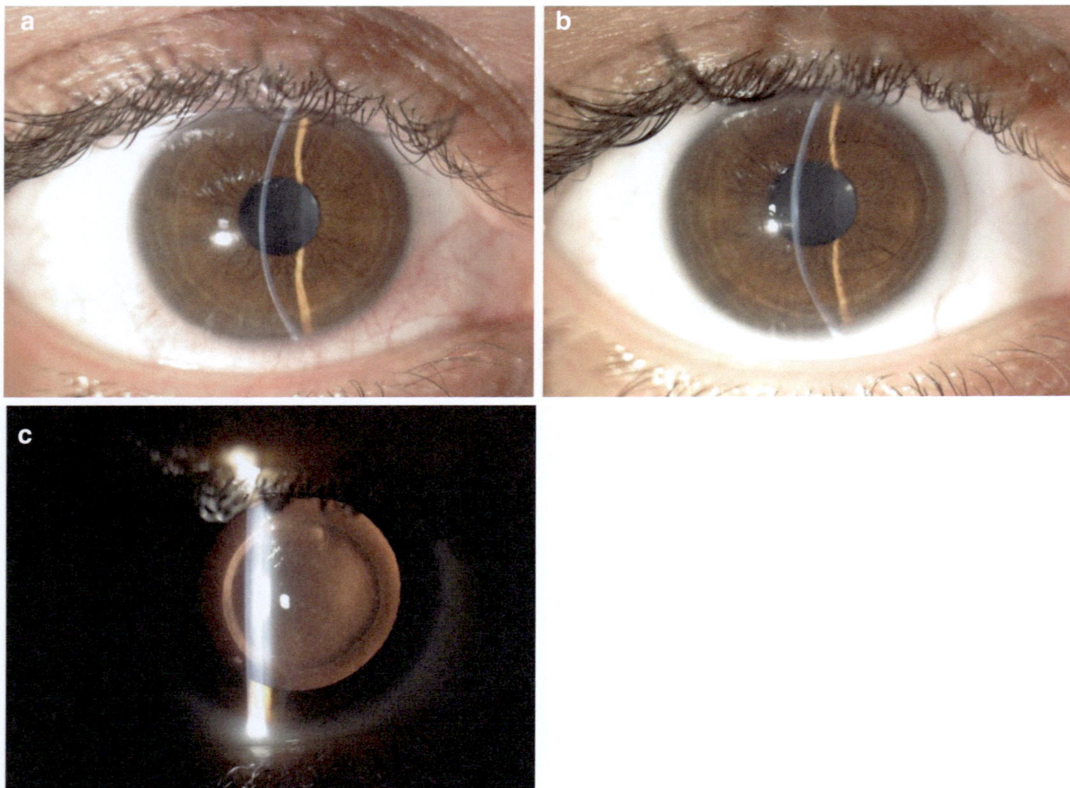

Fig. 19.3 Recipient cornea before (**a**) and 1 month after SLAK (**b**). Lenticule inside the stroma was barely noticeable on slit light direct illumination but clearly visible on retro-illumination (**c**)

(CDVA). UDVA improved from 1.58 ± 0.36 to 1.22 ± 0.37 logMAR (p = 0.024; Wilcoxon signed-rank test), whereas CDVA improved from 1.07 ± 0.17 to 0.70 ± 0.23 logMAR (p = 0.007). One eye gained three lines, three eyes gained two lines, five eyes gained one line, and one eye had no change in lines of CDVA. Spherical equivalent significantly reduced from −7.46 ± 2.49 D to −3.61 D ± 1.99 D at 6 months (p = 0.021).

Corneal Topography

On corneal topography, a generalized flattening of the cone can be observed after SLAK (Fig. 19.4). We reported a mean anterior keratometry value reduction from 58.69 ± 3.59 to 53.59 ± 3.50 diopters at 6 months after surgery in the first in vivo study (p < 0.05; Wilcoxon signed-rank test) along with negligible variation of the posterior corneal mean keratometry. Anterior

corneal asphericity (Q value) was reduced indicating a reduction of corneal irregular high prolacity (p < 0.05; Wilcoxon signed-rank test) [42].

Corneal topography after SLAK shows an area of central curvature reduction surrounded by a red ring of increased curvature corresponding to the transition zone from the addition area to the peripheral recipient cornea. Anterior topographic flattening appears similar on color-graded map to corneal flattening pattern experienced after conventional myopic refractive laser treatment [42].

In Vivo Confocal Microscopy

Intrastromal FSL-based refractive surgery procedures proved to induce a lower level of inflammation and apoptosis combined with a better preservation of anterior stromal lamellae structure and nerve plexus compared to traditional

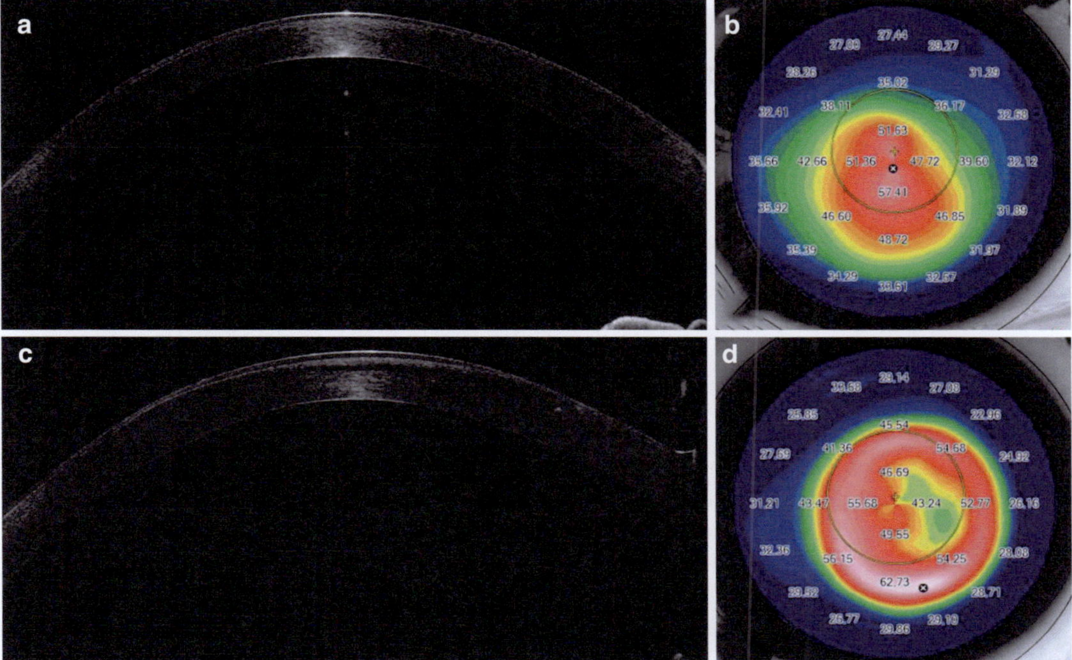

Fig. 19.4 Anterior segment OCT and tangential corneal curvature map before (**a** and **b**, respectively) and 6 months (**c** and **d**, respectively) after SLAK. Lenticule profile is clearly visible inside the recipient cornea (**c**), while the cone flattening effect is appreciable on the anterior corneal curvature map (**d**) surrounded by a red ring of curvature transition zone

ablative techniques [44–49]. Interfaces produced by FSL-cut appear optically clear and highly regular [50]. Thanks to the low energy delivered into the recipient stroma, a low incidence of corneal haze was reported after ReLEx treatments. Preservation of anterior lamellar structure proved to be relevant to corneal biomechanics, while subepithelial nerve sparing induces faster recovery of corneal sensitivity and epithelial integrity [46, 49, 51, 52].

On IVCM, corneal epithelium appeared regularly stratified after SLAK all over the follow-up [53]. Mean subbasal nerve density was restored to preoperative values at 3 months after surgery, and no significant variations of dendritic immune cell density were reported. Mild anterior stromal edema was present in all cases but rapidly subsided during the first month. At 6 months postoperatively, no sign of stromal reaction or keratocyte activation was visible. Interface reflectivity significantly reduced at 3 months with persistence of some cellular debris consisting of roundish appearing elements with small diameter. Interfaces remained visible up to the end of the follow-up of 12 months on IVCM but with decreasing reflectivity. Interface appearance was similar to what was previously documented after refractive lenticule extraction procedure.

No significant endothelial or keratocyte cell density changes nor signs of rejection were reported following SLAK. Lenticule microfolds were variably visible in some cases on IVCM but never documented on slit lamp examination [53].

Epithelial and Stromal Remodeling

Remodeling of corneal structure is a progressive phenomenon that requires time after surgery [54–58]. Epithelial compensation is a documented process that can affect final corneal curvature and induce refractive changes after corneal surgery and laser treatments [59, 60]. Epithelial thickness map 1 month after SLAK showed a central thickness increase and a mid-peripheral thickness reduction corresponding to the zone of increased curvature [61]. Epithelial thickness outside the addition area experienced a progressive increase up to 6 months after surgery. No significant changes were reported on optical coherence tomographic analysis regarding lenticule thickness profile and anterior or posterior recipient stromal thicknesses throughout the follow-up [61].

Discussion

Technical limitations of early stromal keratophakia procedures (e.g. coarse mechanical dissection of stromal bed, freezing-chiseling and subsequent thawing of tissues, and flap suturing) were linked to poor visual results [21, 22].

The introduction of femtosecond laser refractive lenticule extraction not only brought advantages in the refractive surgery field but also allowed novel surgical approaches to corneal pathologies. Stromal lenticules produced by FSL have accurate geometry, smooth surfaces, preserved vitality, and undamaged collagen structure [28, 50]. Moreover, FSL can be used to fashion intra-stromal dissection planes in the recipient cornea minimally affecting biomechanics of anterior stromal layers [49]. The possibility of transplanting refractive lenticules was validated in studies conducted with animal models at first [29, 30, 32, 33], then stromal transplantation of refractive lenticules derived from myopic SMILE has been proposed as a possible tissue addition approach to successfully steepen the cornea for treating hyperopia and aphakia [34, 35, 62, 63].

Nearly contemporary to Ganesh and Brar in 2014 [39], we hypothesized the possibility of making use of this principle to treat keratoconus in 2015.

Ganesh and Brar proposed the implantation of donut-shaped stromal lenticules, obtained by a 3-mm central punching of cryopreserved myopic lenticules combined with collagen cross-linking, in keratoconus [39]. The result of the addition of stromal tissue in the mid-periphery and around the cone caused a relative flattening in the center and a reduction of hyper-prolate shape [39]. The theoretical mechanism of action of this technique is thought to be partially similar to the intracorneal ring segments (ICRS) implantation because both techniques involve addition of volume and local elevation in the mid-periphery [64].

Topographical analysis after SLAK showed that all eyes had a detectable reduction of central anterior corneal curvature, indicating a significant relative flattening of the cone, with negligible effects on the posterior corneal curvature (Fig. 19.5). Vision rehabilitation with current technique is limited by the lack of a customized lenticule profile. Lenticule dioptric power is technically limited to maximum +8.00 D with a maximum peripheral thickness of +148 μm. Despite the enrolled cases in the first series were advanced keratoconus with curvature of 58.69 ± 3.59 D, mean UDVA and CDVA significantly increased: 9 of 10 eyes showed an increase in CDVA that ranged from one to three Snellen lines [42].

Interestingly, lenticule dimensions analyzed by means of AS-OCT showed minimal but consistent differences in the central lenticule thickness; on average the central lenticule thickness

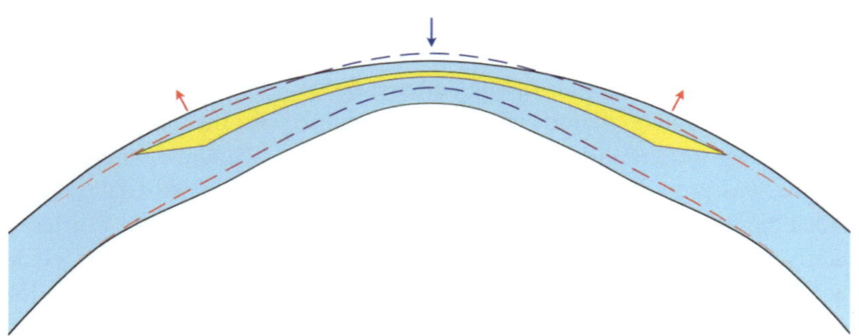

Fig. 19.5 Illustration of corneal curvature and thickness changes following SLAK. The red arrows indicate forward displacement of the anterior surface, while the blue arrow indicates central flattening. Dashed lines represent the original keratoconus profile

was measured to be 47 μm compared to a programmed thickness of 30 μm [42, 61]. Despite stromal edema rapidly regressed over the first month, this increase was documented up to the 6 months. Ganesh and Brar reported an increase in CCT after implantation of donut-shaped myopic lenticules, although there was no addition of stroma in the central area in their procedure [39]. They proposed that this might be related to a mild lifting of the anterior corneal layers and creation of a potential space in the center after peripheral tissue addition. They also observed a trend toward a decrease in CCT at 6 months after surgery [39]. Stromal wound-healing process can be accounted as a possible explanation of this phenomena in our opinion. New extracellular matrix (ECM) may be produced in response to keratocyte activation and less volume addition in central cornea concomitantly to a mechanical stress displacement in mid-periphery, where the lamellae become compacted by volume addition, may be the cause of increased ECM apposition in central area. Further histological study must be performed to clear this hypothesis.

Biomechanical redistribution of tensile strength on collagen lamellae and viscosity of ECM could be responsible for the slow changes of anterior and posterior surfaces observed during the first month, as already reported in other refractive surgery procedures [65].

Epithelial remodeling participates in the overall corneal thickness increase after SLAK. Epithelial map produced by ultrahigh-resolution OCT documented that cone flattening was associated with significantly increased epithelial thickness increase at 1 month after surgery, stabilizing at 3-months. Observed epithelial thickness values were close to normality after 1 month with an increase of about 15%. Epithelial remodeling occurred also in the mid peripheral and peripheral regions, with a slight decrease in the first and increase in the second consistent with anterior corneal profile variations [61]. This phenomenon should be taken into account in future study of predictability. On the other side, corneal epithelial restoration can also improve contact lens tolerance and reduce the risk for epithelial breakdown or keratoconic "pips" observed in patients with thin epithelium [66].

Stress redistribution and biomechanical changes in lenticule addition procedures are processes that should be evaluated in future study. We can hypothesize that Bowman Membrane (BM) could affect predictability of curvature changes after SLAK, while on the other hand the procedure could affect disease progression changing shear stress distribution on BM. In SLAK, a significant amount of tissue is added to the conus apex thus improving the corneal thinning of keratoconus. Increasing thickness may be not enough to halt disease progression on itself since donor tissue integration with recipient stroma remains to be demonstrated. The contact alongside the interfaces between host and donor, probably create at least a minimum improvement to shear stress resistance but, as already proved in LASIK, tissues mechanically separated never integrate completely and can be easily separated even after years. The improved wound healing produced by FSL lamellar cut may positively affect this integration, as proved in corneal trephination [67]. ICRS implantation does not stop the disease progression and central distention of collagen fibers, despite inducing flattening, theoretically may produce more stress on conus apex [68, 69]. On the contrary, the addition of tissue around the cone base produced by SLAK may reduce the apex fiber stress displacing tensile stress to the peripheral intact Bowman membrane, thus affecting the progression process and apical scarring in some way. These considerations need to be evaluated in further long-term in vivo studies also including progressive keratoconus and less advanced stages.

The in vivo confocal microscopy (IVCM) examination did not show a significant modification of dendritic cell population after SLAK, and patients did not experience any type of corneal rejection during the follow-up [53]. The presence of subbasal dendritic cells has been documented after traditional keratoplasty regardless of the presence of a clinically evident rejection. These cells are involved in antigen presentation and are largely recruited in corneal inflammation [70]. This process can have a role in stimulating the immune reaction and onset of a later graft failure [71–73]. DALK is the current gold standard treatment for advanced keratoconus because one of the main advantages of this lamellar technique over penetrating keratoplasty is the reduced rejection rate with longer graft survival [74]. Although the observation period of our IVCM study was limited, we suppose that, given the reduced amount of transplanted tissue and the isolation of the donor tissue inside the stromal pocket, the immunological stimulation in SLAK might be at least similar if not lower with respect to the DALK one.

Corneal reinnervation after keratoplasty is mainly due to subepithelial fiber proliferation rather than stromal reinnervation [75]. In vivo confocal microscopy studies revealed that lamellar cuts produced by SMILE surgery only partially affect subbasal nerve density and nerve fibers are almost recovered by 6 months after surgery. Subbasal fibers are resected only at the level of the incision, and the stromal fibers are resected only at the trespassing of the cap cut [46, 47, 76]. In SLAK, we observed a similar reduction of density shortly after surgery with fiber degeneration within the first few months and a recovery of the original plexus at 3–6 months after surgery [53].

The regularity of the interface between donor and recipient stroma is the main factor affecting visual recovery in lamellar procedures [77–80]. The femtosecond laser produces highly regular stromal cuts that appear as hyperreflective planes in the corneal stroma [50]. Despite the interface reflectivity, SMILE grants excellent visual outcomes but the degree of interface roughness can affect the quality of vision [81]. Similarly to SMILE [82], in SLAK, we documented moderately reflective interfaces with the presence of particles in the first month that gradually reduced over time. Cellular and matrix debris on both the anterior and posterior interfaces significantly reduced over time but persisted until 12 months. The presence of a double interface may affect visual rehabilitation after SLAK but, even though the anterior and posterior interfaces were close to each other in the central area, we did not observe any opacification of the corneal stroma.

Future Perspectives: Lenticule Shape Customization

The main current limit of SLAK is that only eyes affected by central keratoconus are eligible for the treatment because only symmetrical lenticule geometry is available.

Ongoing studies are trying to figure out the proper way to obtain lenticules suitable for implantation in corneas with eccentric keratoconus, which represent more than 70% of cases.

We recently conducted an ex vivo study to assess the effects of different types of lenticule customizations. Human eye bank donor corneas not suitable for transplantation for low endothelial cell density were used to realize keratoconus models (recipients) and customized lenticules (donors). In addition recent findings showed that lenticule customization is possible by the aid for excimer laser photoablation of the FSL-prepared donor lenticules [83]. This will allow to increase the precision of corneal reshaping in the various forms and stages of keratoconic eyes in treated patients and to expand the indications of intrastromal tissue implantation.

The encouraging results bode well for upcoming advancements in corneal additive surgery.

In conclusion, our investigations demonstrated that stromal lenticule in addition to keratoplasty is a feasible and effective technique for stromal remodeling that improves vision and corneal regularity in central keratoconus. Implanted tissues were accepted by host stroma without rejection nor opacification. Corneal remodeling should be further investigated to develop customization algorithms and expand indications to mild keratoconus cases where this technique might ideally offer better results. Currently, no treatment can outperform the results of DALK that is still the gold standard in keratoconus surgical treatment, in particular for advanced cases, but SLAK opened new perspectives on future developments of customized, minimally invasive, additive treatments for keratoconus. It may become a valuable option for treating those cases that have no indication for traditional keratoplasty but may benefit from a minimally invasive procedure capable of reshaping the corneal geometry.

Take Home Notes

- Femtosecond laser lenticule extraction procedures can be used to produce transparent stromal lenticules in donor cornea suitable for additive corneal transplantation techniques.
- Intrastromal lenticule implantation can effectively and predictably change curvature and thickness of the recipient cornea according to the lenticule design.
- Flattening of a central keratoconus is possible by means of negative meniscus-shaped lenticule addition in SLAK, leading to an improvement of visual acuity, thickness, and corneal curvature.
- The SLAK procedure induces mild and transient inflammation rapidly recovering during the first postoperative days and can be performed under topical anesthesia.

In the future, customization of lenticule shape according to corneal topography could optimize the curvature regularization and make possible to treat decentered keratoconus. Lenticule harvesting from living donors undergoing refractive surgery along with eye-banking customization and storage could help standardizing and ease the procedure for the surgeon.

References

1. Gomes JAP, Tan D, Rapuano CJ, Belin MW, Ambrósio R, Guell JL, et al. Global consensus on keratoconus and ectatic diseases. Cornea. 2015;34(4):359–69.
2. Belin MW, Duncan JK. Keratoconus: the ABCD grading system. Klin Monatsbl Augenheilkd. 2016;233(6):701–7.
3. Parker JS, van Dijk K, Melles GRJ. Treatment options for advanced keratoconus: a review. Surv Ophthalmol. 2015;60(5):459–80.
4. Olivares Jiménez JL, Guerrero Jurado JC, Bermudez Rodriguez FJ, Serrano Laborda D. Keratoconus: age of onset and natural history. Optom Vis Sci. 1997;74(3):147–51.
5. Yoshida J, Murata H, Miyai T, Shirakawa R, Toyono T, Yamagami S, et al. Characteristics and risk factors of recurrent keratoconus over the long term after penetrating keratoplasty. Graefes Arch Clin Exp Ophthalmol. 2018;256(12):2377–83.
6. Han DCY, Mehta JS, Por YM, Htoon HM, Tan DTH. Comparison of outcomes of lamellar keratoplasty and penetrating keratoplasty in keratoconus. Am J Ophthalmol. 2009;148(5):744–751.e1.
7. Yu AC, Franco E, Caruso L, Myerscough J, Spena R, Fusco F, et al. Ten-year outcomes of microkeratome-assisted lamellar keratoplasty for keratoconus. Br J Ophthalmol. 2020;105:1651.
8. Myerscough J, Roberts H, Yu AC, Elkadim M, Bovone C, Busin M. Five-year outcomes of converted mushroom keratoplasty from intended Deep Anterior Lamellar Keratoplasty (DALK) mandate 9-mm diameter DALK as the optimal approach to keratoconus. Am J Ophthalmol. 2020;220:9–18.
9. Liu H, Chen Y, Wang P, Li B, Wang W, Su Y, et al. Efficacy and safety of deep anterior lamellar keratoplasty vs. penetrating keratoplasty for keratoconus: a meta-analysis. PLoS One. 2015;10(1):e0113332.
10. Smiddy WE, Hamburg TR, Kracher GP, Stark WJ. Keratoconus. Contact lens or keratoplasty? Ophthalmology. 1988;95(4):487–92.
11. Arnalich-Montiel F, Alió Del Barrio JL, Alió JL. Corneal surgery in keratoconus: which type, which technique, which outcomes? Eye Vis. 2016;3:2.
12. Mastropasqua L. Collagen cross-linking: when and how? A review of the state of the art of the technique and new perspectives. Eye Vis. 2015;2:19.
13. Doss JD, Hutson RL, Rowsey JJ, Brown DR. Method for calculation of corneal profile and power distribution. Arch Ophthalmol. 1981;99(7):1261–5.
14. Olsen T. On the calculation of power from curvature of the cornea. Br J Ophthalmol. 1986;70(2):152–4.
15. Nordan LT. Barraquer lecture. José Barraquer: father of modern refractive keratoplasty. Refract Corneal Surg. 1989;5(3):177–8.
16. Swinger CA, Barraquer JI. Keratophakia and keratomileusis--clinical results. Ophthalmology. 1981;88(8):709–15.
17. Barraquer JI. Keratomileusis. Int Surg. 1967;48(2):103–17.
18. Ainslie D. The surgical correction of refractive errors by keratomileusis and keratophakia. Ann Ophthalmol. 1976;8(3):349–67.
19. Troutman RC, Swinger C, Goldstein M. Keratophakia update. Ophthalmology. 1981;88(1):36–8.
20. Friedlander MH, Safir A, McDonald MB, Kaufman HE, Granet N. Update on keratophakia. Ophthalmology. 1983;90(4):365–8.
21. Friedlander MH, Rich LF, Werblin TP, Kaufman HE, Granet N. Keratophakia using preserved lenticules. Ophthalmology. 1980;87(7):687–92.
22. Maguen E, Pinhas S, Verity SM, Nesburn AB. Keratophakia with lyophilized cornea lathed at room temperature: new techniques and experimental surgical results. Ophthalmic Surg. 1983;14(9):759–62.
23. Kaufman HE. The correction of aphakia. XXXVI Edward Jackson Memorial Lecture. Am J Ophthalmol. 1980;89(1):1–10.
24. Busin M, Cusumano A, Spitznas M. Epithelial interface cysts after epikeratophakia. Ophthalmology. 1993;100(8):1225–9.

25. Riau AK, Liu Y-C, Yam GHF, Mehta JS. Stromal keratophakia: corneal inlay implantation. Prog Retin Eye Res. 2020;75:100780.
26. Sekundo W, Kunert K, Russmann C, Gille A, Bissmann W, Stobrawa G, et al. First efficacy and safety study of femtosecond lenticule extraction for the correction of myopia: six-month results. J Cataract Refract Surg. 2008;34(9):1513–20.
27. Sekundo W, Kunert KS, Blum M. Small incision corneal refractive surgery using the small incision lenticule extraction (SMILE) procedure for the correction of myopia and myopic astigmatism: results of a 6 month prospective study. Br J Ophthalmol. 2011;95(3):335–9.
28. Mohamed-Noriega K, Toh K-P, Poh R, Balehosur D, Riau A, Htoon HM, et al. Cornea lenticule viability and structural integrity after refractive lenticule extraction (ReLEx) and cryopreservation. Mol Vis. 2011;17:3437–49.
29. Angunawela RI, Riau AK, Chaurasia SS, Tan DT, Mehta JS. Refractive lenticule re-implantation after myopic ReLEx: a feasibility study of stromal restoration after refractive surgery in a rabbit model. Invest Ophthalmol Vis Sci. 2012;53(8):4975–85.
30. Riau AK, Angunawela RI, Chaurasia SS, Lee WS, Tan DT, Mehta JS. Reversible femtosecond laser-assisted myopia correction: a non-human primate study of lenticule re-implantation after refractive lenticule extraction. PLoS One. 2013;8(6):e67058.
31. Liu H, Zhu W, Jiang AC, Sprecher AJ, Zhou X. Femtosecond laser lenticule transplantation in rabbit cornea: experimental study. J Refract Surg. 2012;28(12):907–11.
32. Zhang T, Sun Y, Liu M, Zhou Y, Wang D, Chen Y, et al. Femtosecond laser-assisted endokeratophakia using allogeneic corneal lenticule in a rabbit model. J Refract Surg. 2015;31(11):775–82.
33. Liu R, Zhao J, Xu Y, Li M, Niu L, Liu H, et al. Femtosecond laser-assisted corneal small incision allogenic intrastromal lenticule implantation in monkeys: a pilot study. Invest Ophthalmol Vis Sci. 2015;56(6):3715–20.
34. Pradhan KR, Reinstein DZ, Carp GI, Archer TJ, Gobbe M, Gurung R. Femtosecond laser-assisted keyhole endokeratophakia: correction of hyperopia by implantation of an allogeneic lenticule obtained by SMILE from a myopic donor. J Refract Surg. 2013;29(11):777–82.
35. Williams GP, Wu B, Liu YC, Teo E, Nyein CL, Peh G, et al. Hyperopic refractive correction by LASIK, SMILE or lenticule reimplantation in a non-human primate model. PLoS One. 2018;13(3):e0194209.
36. Jacob S, Kumar DA, Agarwal A, Agarwal A, Aravind R, Saijimol AI. Preliminary evidence of successful near vision enhancement with a new technique: presbyopic allogenic refractive lenticule (PEARL) corneal inlay using a SMILE lenticule. J Refract Surg. 2017;33(4):224–9.
37. Liu Y-C, Teo EPW, Ang HP, Seah XY, Lwin NC, Yam GHF, et al. Biological corneal inlay for presbyopia derived from small incision lenticule extraction (SMILE). Sci Rep. 2018;8(1):1831.
38. Ganesh S, Brar S, Rao PA. Cryopreservation of extracted corneal lenticules after small incision lenticule extraction for potential use in human subjects. Cornea. 2014;33(12):1355–62.
39. Ganesh S, Brar S. Femtosecond intrastromal lenticular implantation combined with accelerated collagen cross-linking for the treatment of keratoconus--initial clinical result in 6 eyes. Cornea. 2015;34(10):1331–9.
40. Mastropasqua L, Nubile M. Corneal thickening and central flattening induced by femtosecond laser hyperopic-shaped intrastromal lenticule implantation. Int Ophthalmol. 2017;37(4):893–904.
41. Liu Y-C, Ang HP, Teo EPW, Lwin NC, Yam GHF, Mehta JS. Wound healing profiles of hyperopic-small incision lenticule extraction (SMILE). Sci Rep. 2016;6:29802.
42. Mastropasqua L, Nubile M, Salgari N, Mastropasqua R. Femtosecond laser-assisted stromal lenticule addition keratoplasty for the treatment of advanced keratoconus: a preliminary study. J Refract Surg. 2018;34(1):36–44.
43. Konstantopoulos A, Liu Y-C, Teo EPW, Lwin NC, Yam GHF, Mehta JS. Early wound healing and refractive response of different pocket configurations following presbyopic inlay implantation. PLoS One. 2017;12(2):e0172014.
44. Slade SG. Applications for the femtosecond laser in corneal surgery. Curr Opin Ophthalmol. 2007;18(4):338–41.
45. Reinstein DZ, Archer TJ, Gobbe M. Small incision lenticule extraction (SMILE) history, fundamentals of a new refractive surgery technique and clinical outcomes. Eye Vis. 2014;1:3.
46. Vestergaard AH, Grønbech KT, Grauslund J, Ivarsen AR, Hjortdal JØ. Subbasal nerve morphology, corneal sensation, and tear film evaluation after refractive femtosecond laser lenticule extraction. Graefes Arch Clin Exp Ophthalmol. 2013;251(11):2591–600.
47. Li M, Niu L, Qin B, Zhou Z, Ni K, Le Q, et al. Confocal comparison of corneal reinnervation after small incision lenticule extraction (SMILE) and femtosecond laser in situ keratomileusis (FS-LASIK). PLoS One. 2013;8(12):e81435.
48. Mohamed-Noriega K, Riau AK, Lwin NC, Chaurasia SS, Tan DT, Mehta JS. Early corneal nerve damage and recovery following small incision lenticule extraction (SMILE) and laser in situ keratomileusis (LASIK). Invest Ophthalmol Vis Sci. 2014;55(3):1823–34.
49. Reinstein DZ, Archer TJ, Randleman JB. Mathematical model to compare the relative tensile strength of the cornea after PRK, LASIK, and small incision lenticule extraction. J Refract Surg. 2013;29(7):454–60.
50. Riau AK, Angunawela RI, Chaurasia SS, Tan DT, Mehta JS. Effect of different femtosecond laser-firing patterns on collagen disruption during refractive lenticule extraction. J Cataract Refract Surg. 2012;38(8):1467–75.

51. Ivarsen A, Asp S, Hjortdal J. Safety and complications of more than 1500 small-incision lenticule extraction procedures. Ophthalmology. 2014;121(4):822–8.

52. Yang W, Li M, Fu D, Wei R, Cui C, Zhou X. A comparison of the effects of different cap thicknesses on corneal nerve destruction after small incision lenticule extraction. Int Ophthalmol. 2020;40(8):1905–11.

53. Mastropasqua L, Salgari N, D'Ugo E, Lanzini M, Alió Del Barrio JL, Alió JL, et al. In vivo confocal microscopy of stromal lenticule addition keratoplasty for advanced keratoconus. J Refract Surg. 2020;36(8):544–50.

54. Vega-Estrada A, Mimouni M, Espla E, Alió Del Barrio J, Alio JL. Corneal epithelial thickness intrasubject repeatability and its relation with visual limitation in keratoconus. Am J Ophthalmol. 2019;200:255–62.

55. Franco J, White CA, Kruh JN. Analysis of compensatory corneal epithelial thickness changes in keratoconus using corneal tomography. Cornea. 2020;39(3):298–302.

56. Luft N, Ring MH, Dirisamer M, Mursch-Edlmayr AS, Kreutzer TC, Pretzl J, et al. Corneal epithelial remodeling induced by small incision lenticule extraction (SMILE). Invest Ophthalmol Vis Sci. 2016;57(9):OCT176–83.

57. Hwang ES, Schallhorn JM, Randleman JB. Utility of regional epithelial thickness measurements in corneal evaluations. Surv Ophthalmol. 2020;65(2):187–204.

58. Reinstein DZ, Silverman RH, Rondeau MJ, Coleman DJ. Epithelial and corneal thickness measurements by high-frequency ultrasound digital signal processing. Ophthalmology. 1994;101(1):140–6.

59. Reinstein DZ, Archer TJ, Gobbe M. Refractive and topographic errors in topography-guided ablation produced by epithelial compensation predicted by 3D Artemis VHF digital ultrasound stromal and epithelial thickness mapping. J Refract Surg. 2012;28(9):657–63.

60. Kanellopoulos AJ. Comparison of corneal epithelial remodeling over 2 years in LASIK versus SMILE: a contralateral eye study. Cornea. 2019;38(3):290–6.

61. Nubile M, Salgari N, Mehta JS, Calienno R, Erroi E, Bondì J, et al. Epithelial and stromal remodelling following femtosecond laser-assisted stromal lenticule addition keratoplasty (SLAK) for keratoconus. Sci Rep. 2021;11(1):2293.

62. Damgaard IB, Ivarsen A, Hjortdal J. Biological lenticule implantation for correction of hyperopia: an ex vivo study in human corneas. J Refract Surg. 2018;34(4):245–52.

63. Lazaridis A, Messerschmidt-Roth A, Sekundo W, Schulze S. Refractive lenticule implantation for correction of ametropia: case reports and literature review. Klin Monatsbl Augenheilkd. 2017;234(1):77–89.

64. Vega-Estrada A, Alio JL. The use of intracorneal ring segments in keratoconus. Eye Vis. 2016;3:8.

65. Kamiya K, Shimizu K, Ohmoto F. Time course of corneal biomechanical parameters after laser in situ keratomileusis. Ophthalmic Res. 2009;42(3):167–71.

66. Sorbara L, Lopez JCL, Gorbet M, Bizheva K, Lamarca JM, Pastor J-C, et al. Impact of contact lens wear on epithelial alterations in keratoconus. J Opt. 2021;14(1):37–43.

67. Alio JL, Abdelghany AA, Barraquer R, Hammouda LM, Sabry AM. Femtosecond laser assisted deep anterior lamellar keratoplasty outcomes and healing patterns compared to manual technique. Biomed Res Int. 2015;2015:397891.

68. Warrak EL, Serhan HA, Ayash JG, Wahab CH, Baban TA, Daoud RC, et al. Long-term follow up of intracorneal ring segment implantation in 932 keratoconus eyes. J Fr Ophtalmol. 2020;43(10):1020–4.

69. Abreu AC, Malheiro L, Coelho J, Neves MM, Gomes M, Oliveira L, et al. Implantation of intracorneal ring segments in pediatric patients: long-term follow-up. Int Med Case Rep J. 2018;11:23–7.

70. Mastropasqua L, Nubile M, Lanzini M, Carpineto P, Ciancaglini M, Pannellini T, et al. Epithelial dendritic cell distribution in normal and inflamed human cornea: in vivo confocal microscopy study. Am J Ophthalmol. 2006;142(5):736–44.

71. Wang D, Song P, Wang S, Sun D, Wang Y, Zhang Y, et al. Laser scanning in vivo confocal microscopy of clear grafts after penetrating keratoplasty. Biomed Res Int. 2016;2016:5159746.

72. Chirapapaisan C, Abbouda A, Jamali A, Müller RT, Cavalcanti BM, Colon C, et al. In vivo confocal microscopy demonstrates increased immune cell densities in corneal graft rejection correlating with signs and symptoms. Am J Ophthalmol. 2019;203:26–36.

73. Kocaba V, Colica C, Rabilloud M, Burillon C. Predicting corneal graft rejection by confocal microscopy. Cornea. 2015;34(Suppl 10):S61–4.

74. Giannaccare G, Weiss JS, Sapigni L, Bovone C, Mattioli L, Campos EC, et al. Immunologic stromal rejection after deep anterior lamellar keratoplasty with grafts of a larger size (9 mm) for various stromal diseases. Cornea. 2018;37(8):967–72.

75. Al-Aqaba MA, Otri AM, Fares U, Miri A, Dua HS. Organization of the regenerated nerves in human corneal grafts. Am J Ophthalmol. 2012;153(1):29–37.e4.

76. Pang A, Mohamed-Noriega K, Chan AS, Mehta JS. Confocal microscopy findings in deep anterior lamellar keratoplasty performed after Descemet's stripping automated endothelial keratoplasty. Clin Ophthalmol. 2014;8:243–9.

77. Fontana L, Parente G, Sincich A, Tassinari G. Influence of graft-host interface on the quality of vision after deep anterior lamellar keratoplasty in patients with keratoconus. Cornea. 2011;30(5):497–502.

78. Schiano-Lomoriello D, Colabelli-Gisoldi RA, Nubile M, Oddone F, Ducoli G, Villani CM, et al. Descemetic and predescemetic DALK in keratoconus patients: a clinical and confocal perspective study. Biomed Res Int. 2014;2014:123156.

79. Bhatt UK, Fares U, Rahman I, Said DG, Maharajan SV, Dua HS. Outcomes of deep anterior lamellar keratoplasty following successful and failed "big bubble". Br J Ophthalmol. 2012;96(4):564–9.
80. Abdelkader A, Kaufman HE. Descemetic versus predescemetic lamellar keratoplasty: clinical and confocal study. Cornea. 2011;30(11):1244–52.
81. Ganesh S, Brar S, Pandey R, Pawar A. Interface healing and its correlation with visual recovery and quality of vision following small incision lenticule extraction. Indian J Ophthalmol. 2018;66:212.
82. Riau AK, Angunawela RI, Chaurasia SS, Lee WS, Tan DT, Mehta JS. Early corneal wound healing and inflammatory responses after refractive lenticule extraction (ReLEx). Invest Ophthalmol Vis Sci. 2011;52(9):6213–21.
83. Doroodgar F, Jabbarvand M, Niazi S, Karimian F, Niazi F, Sanginabadi A, Ghoreishi M, Alinia C, Hashemi H, Alió JL. Customized stromal lenticule implantation for keratoconus. J Refract Surg. 2020;36(12):786–94.

Lamellar Surgeries with SMILE Lenticules

20

Sri Ganesh and Sheetal Brar

Key Points

SMILE-derived lenticules can be used successfully for the potential management of hyperopia, keratoconus, SMILE ectasia, and presbyopia.

- Long-term clinical outcomes of tissue addition with SMILE-derived lenticules performed in 42 eyes with moderate to high hyperopia showed a mean regression of +0.66 D, at a mean follow-up of 68 months (5.6 years).
- Addition of thick lenticule (>6 D) resulted in posterior curvature changes in the cornea, leading to significant under correction of hyperopia.
- Bowmans membrane relaxation (BMR) may be an easy, practical, and cost-effective technique to reverse the posterior curvature changes and enhance the effect of tissue addition for high hyperopia.

Introduction

In 1949, José Ignacio Barraquer laid the groundwork for the use of natural corneal tissue to change the refractive properties of the eye [1, 2]. Subsequently, Pradhan et al., in 2013, published a case report showing the feasibility of the use of a myopic SMILE lenticule (Endokeratophakia) for correction of aphakia [3]. Followed by this, many researchers successfully reported the use of allogenic and autologous SMILE lenticules for management of conditions such as high hyperopia, keratoconus, presbyopia, and sealing corneal defects [4–8]. Recently, the technique has been shown to provide satisfactory and stable results for managing ectasia after SMILE [9].

This chapter aims at discussing the feasibility of SMILE-derived lenticules for the potential management of hyperopia, keratoconus, SMILE ectasia, presbyopia and reporting the clinical outcomes, and experience of various researchers in this evolving field so far.

Supplementary Information The online version contains supplementary material available at https://doi.org/10.1007/978-3-031-32408-6_20.

S. Ganesh (✉) · S. Brar
Nethradhama Superspeciality Eye Hospital,
Bangalore, India

Lamellar Surgery with SMILE Lenticules for Hyperopia

In the technique of femtosecond intrastromal lenticule implantation (FILI), published by our group in 2014, the cornea was made steeper by the addition of a SMILE lenticule of known thickness and power, into a pocket created in the recipient's cornea using a femtosecond laser [4]. The concept was subsequently adopted by various authors, who reported their results with certain modifications in the technique [5, 9]. Recently, Liu et al. published their 2-year results with SMILE lenticule implantation and suggested that allogenic lenticule transplantation may be a promising option for correcting moderate to high hyperopia [10].

We recently concluded a retrospective study of eligible patients, who underwent FILI for correction of moderate to high hyperopia from July 2013 till October 2020. Inclusion criteria included: age 18 years or older, hyperopic refractive error ranging between +3.00 to +11.00 D, stable refractive error (change of <0.5 D within the past 12 months), pre-op CDVA of 0.6 LogMAR or better, and a strong motivation for refractive correction. Eyes with previous keratitis, severe dry eye disease, cataract, glaucoma, or vitreoretinal disorders, concomitant autoimmune diseases, pregnancy, and patients with unrealistic expectations are excluded.

Surgical Procedure

For FILI, the donor SMILE lenticules used were either cryopreserved or fresh, i.e., the extracted lenticule was used either in the same sitting or within 48 h, when stored in balanced salt solution. Briefly, the FILI procedure involved the insertion of the donor SMILE lenticule into a femtosecond laser-enabled pocket created using VisuMax FS Laser (Carl Zeiss Meditec, Jena, Germany) at a depth of 160 μm, as described earlier [4]. Video 20.1 shows a surgical video of the procedure.

For the enhancement procedure, i.e., Bowman membrane relaxation (BMR), a Hessburg–Barron trephine (Barron Precision Instruments, Grand blanc, Michigan) was used to trephine the Bowman's membrane and part of the anterior stromal fibers. The technique has been explained in detail in a previously published paper by our group [11]. Video 20.2 shows a surgical video of enhancement with BMR.

For the lenticule exchange procedure, a Sinskey's hook was used to open the old incision and enter the corneal interface. A blunt spatula was then used to dissect the tissue above and below the implanted lenticule and separate the same from the surrounding adhesions. The free lenticule was then grasped with a micro-forceps from its edge and extracted from the corneal pocket. The interface was washed with a balanced salt solution, followed by which, the fresh lenticule was implanted into the interface using the standard technique of FILI, described above. Postoperative regimen was similar to the one published earlier [4].

Results

FILI was performed on 42 eyes of 25 patients. Table 20.1 provides the preoperative demographic and baseline data of all recipient patients, as well as the donors whose lenticules were used for implantation. Mean follow-up was

Table 20.1 Preoperative demographic data of the recipient and donor eyes

Parameter	Mean ± SD
Recipient details	
Age (Years)	27.04 ± 5.33
UDVA (LogMAR)	1.03 ± 0.39
CDVA (LogMAR)	0.22 ± 0.23
Sphere (D)	5.24 ± 1.96
Cylinder (D)	0.51 ± 0.48
SE (D)	5.50 ± 1.96
CCT (μm)	550.02 ± 29.68
Km anterior (D)	43.72 ± 1.55
Km posterior (D)	−6.30 ± 0.26
Q-value	−0.34 ± 0.09
HOA (RMS)	0.398 ± 0.15
Donor details	
Age (years)	28 ± 5.33
S.E treated (D)	−6.03 ± 1.99
Optical zone (μm)	6.50 ± 0.28
Lenticule thickness (μm)	114 ± 25.70
Length of cryopreservation (days)	61 ± 103.61

UDVA, uncorrected distant visual acuity; *CDVA*, corrected distant visual acuity; *SE*, spherical equivalent; *D*, diopters; *RMS*, root mean square; *CCT*, central corneal thickness

Table 20.2 Visual and refractive results post FILI ($n = 42$ eyes) at 2 weeks and 68 months post-op

Parameter	Pre mean ± SD (range)	2 weeks mean ± SD (range)	p-value (pre vs. 2 week)	Last follow-up mean ± SD (range)	p-value (2-week vs. last follow-up)
UDVA (LogMAR)	1.03 ± 0.39 (0.22–1.78)	0.21 ± 0.23 (−0.10 to 0.80)	<0.001	0.25 ± 0.23 (−0.10 to 0.60)	0.36
CDVA (LogMAR)	0.22 ± 0.23 (−0.10 to 0.80)	0.19 ± 0.20 (−0.10 to 0.70)	0.51	0.19 ± 0.21 (−0.20 to 0.60)	0.88
Sphere (D)	5.24 ± 1.96 (+3 to +11)	0.57 ± 0.82 (0 to +2.25)	<0.001	0.56 ± 0.94 (−1.50 to +2.25)	0.95
Cylinder (D)	0.51 ± 0.48 (0 to +1.50)	0.14 ± 0.65 (−1.50 to +1.50)	<0.001	0.19 ± 0.67 (−1.25 to +1.50)	0.71
SE (D)	5.54 ± 1.96 (+3 to +11)	0.64 ± 1.05 (−0.625 to +4.50)	<0.001	0.66 ± 1.18 (−2.00 to +2.375)	0.95

UDVA, uncorrected distant visual acuity; *CDVA,* corrected distant visual acuity; *SE,* spherical equivalent; *D,* diopters

68 ± 17.28 months (12–84 months). Table 20.2 shows the postoperative visual and refractive results at 2 weeks and at the end of the mean follow-up.

Efficacy and Safety

At 68 months, the mean efficacy index was 0.86 ± 0.19 (0.39–1.0). The postoperative mean UDVA was 0.25 ± 0.22 (−0.12 to 0.6) LogMAR. Cumulative UDVA of 20/20 or better and 20/40 or better was seen in 38% ($n = 16$) and 81% ($n = 34$) of eyes, respectively (Fig. 20.1a). The mean safety index was 1.17 ± 0.39 (0.63–2.54). Thirty-six percent ($n = 15$) eyes gained one or more lines, 45% ($n = 19$) had no change, whereas 19% ($n = 8$) eyes lost one line of CDVA. No eye lost more than 2 lines of CDVA (Fig. 20.1b).

Spherical Equivalent (SE), Astigmatism Accuracy, and Stability

The accuracy of SE refraction within ±0.5 D was observed in 50% ($n = 21$) eyes; however, 71% ($n = 30$) of all the treated eyes were within ±1.00 D of SE correction. A coefficient of determination value of 0.71 was obtained on the predictability curve (Fig. 20.1c, d). Sixty-four percent ($n = 29$) eyes were within 0.5 D of astigmatism, while 88% ($n = 37$) eyes were within ±1.00 D of astigmatism (Fig. 20.1e). The mean

residual refraction at 2 weeks post-op was 0.64 ± 1.05 D, which showed a nonsignificant increase to 0.66 ± 1.17 D at 68 months post-op, $p = 0.95$ (Fig. 20.1f).

There was a significant increase in the Kmean anterior, central corneal thickness, Q-value, and corneal HOAs, 2 weeks post-op compared to the preoperative values, $p < 0.05$ (Table 20.3). However, no significant change was observed in these parameters at 68 months, when compared to 2 weeks, $p > 0.05$ (Table 20.3). The Kmean posterior, on the other hand, showed a significant change from −6.30 ± 0.26 to −6.13 ± 0.34 D, $p = 0.02$ (i.e., becoming more positive), 2 weeks post FILI, which did not change significantly thereafter (p value, 2 weeks vs. 68 months = 0.23).

Figures 20.2 and 20.3, respectively, show the 2-weeks versus pre-op difference maps of both eyes of a 29 year old male, who underwent FILI for high hyperopia of +6.5 D and +7.0 D in the right and left eye, respectively. Compared to preoperative, an increase in K1, K2, and thinnest pachymetry by 2.7 D, 3.2 D, and 96 μ was observed at 2 weeks in the RE (Fig. 20.2). Similar changes were observed in the LE of the patient, wherein the KI, K2, and thinnest pachymetry increased by 3.0 D, 4.1 D, and 77 μ, respectively (Fig. 20.3). Figures 20.4 and 20.5, respectively, show the difference maps of both eyes of the same patient at a long follow-up of 5.8 years versus 2 weeks post FILI. Figure 20.6a1, b1 show clinical photographs of both eyes of the same patient at 2 weeks post-op, showing the implanted lenticule in situ. Note that, in a freshly

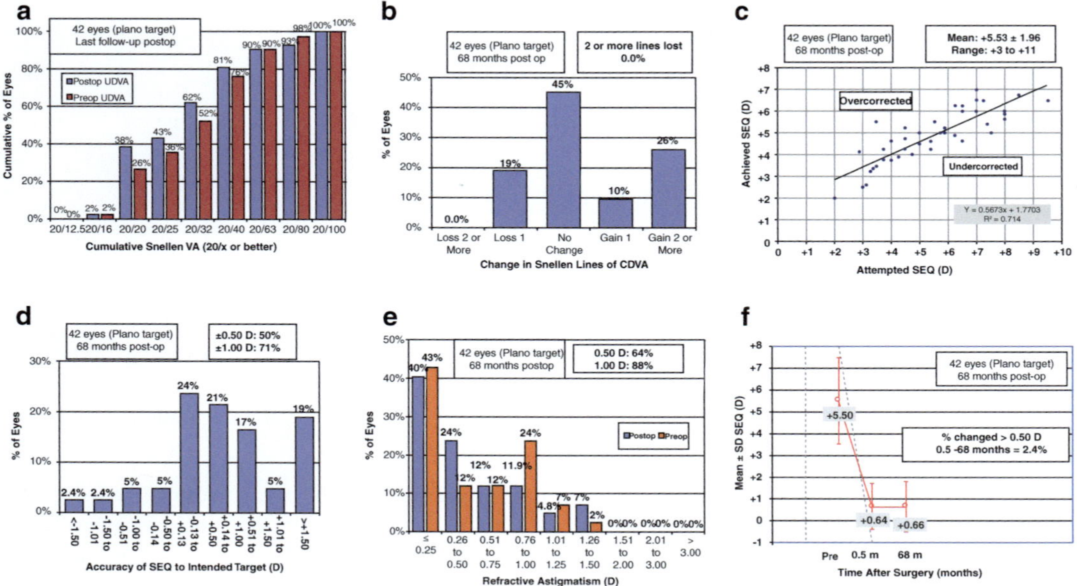

Fig. 20.1 JRS standard graphs for $n = 42$ eyes treated with FILI in the series

Table 20.3 Changes in Kmean anterior, Kmean posterior, central corneal thickness, Q-value, and corneal HOAs at 2 weeks and 68 months post-op

Parameter	Pre mean ± SD (range)	2 weeks mean ± SD (range)	p-value (Pre vs. 2 week)	Last follow-up mean ± SD (Range)	p-value (2-week vs. last follow-up)
Km Anterior (D)	43.72 ± 1.55 (41.50–46.20)	47.45 ± 1.75 (44.20–50.30)	<0.001	47.48 ± 2.02 (44.30–50.90)	0.94
Km Posterior (D)	−6.30 ± 0.26 (−5.70 to −6.80)	−6.13 ± 0.34 (−5.37 to −6.60)	0.02	−6.19 ± 0.31 (−5.50 to −6.70)	0.23
CCT (μm)	550.02 ± 29.68 (494–596)	631.59 ± 37.72 (546–717)	<0.001	625.76 ± 41.69 (530–720)	0.50
Q value	−0.34 ± 0.09 (−0.13 to −0.55)	−0.89 ± 0.23 (−0.43 to −1.69)	<0.001	−0.95 ± 0.28 (−0.40 to 1.94)	0.29
HOA (RMS)	0.39 ± 0.15 (0.07–0.97)	0.83 ± 0.34 (0.13–1.62)	<0.001	0.96 ± 0.34 (0.41–1.94)	0.10

HOA, higher order aberration; *CCT,* central corneal thickness; *RMS,* root mean square

implanted lenticule, the borders are well-defined and mild folds in the tissue can be observed. However, at 5.8 years post-op follow-up (Fig. 20.6a2, b2), the borders of the lenticules are merged with the surrounding host tissue, and a very faint boundary of the lenticule is visible. The lenticule is relatively clear and does not have any folds or interface haze of any kind.

Figure 20.7 demonstrates the corresponding AS-OCT scans with clear and well-centered lenticules in situ.

Four eyes of three patients underwent enhancement with Bowman membrane relaxation (BMR) for a significant residual refractive error. Table 20.4 depicts the visual and refractive outcomes of these eyes following enhancement.

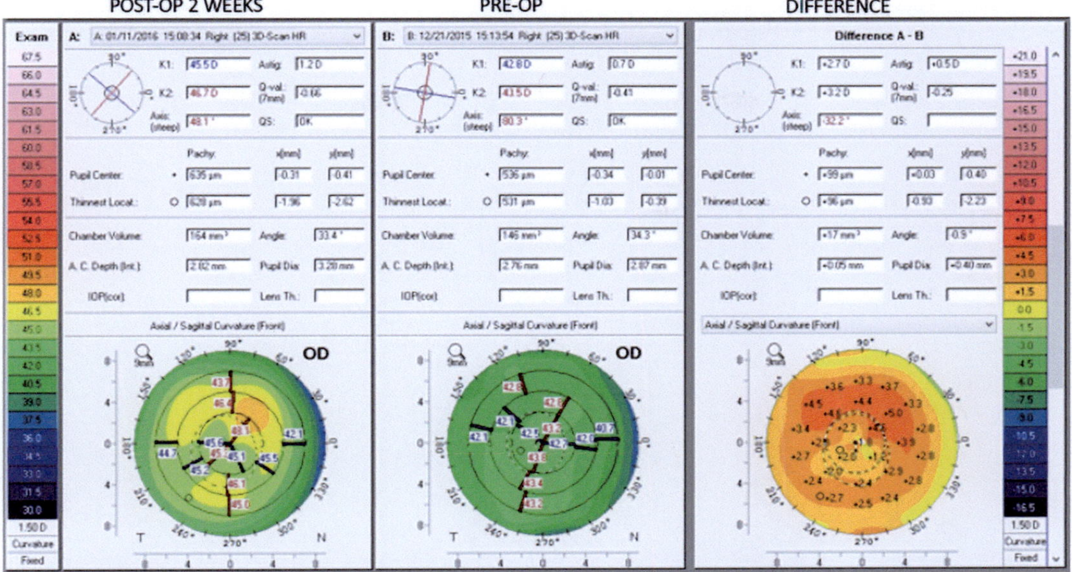

Fig. 20.2 Two weeks versus pre-op difference maps of RE eye of a 29-year-old patient, who underwent FILI for hyperopic refractive error of +6.5 D

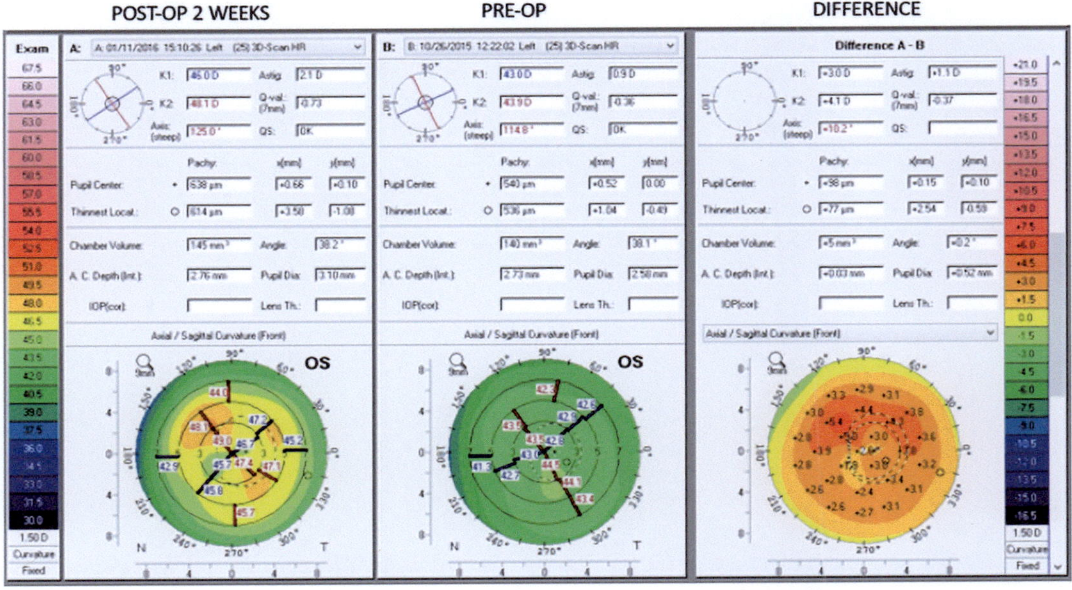

Fig. 20.3 Two weeks versus pre-op difference maps of LE of a 29-year-old patient, who underwent FILI for hyperopic refractive error of +7.0 D

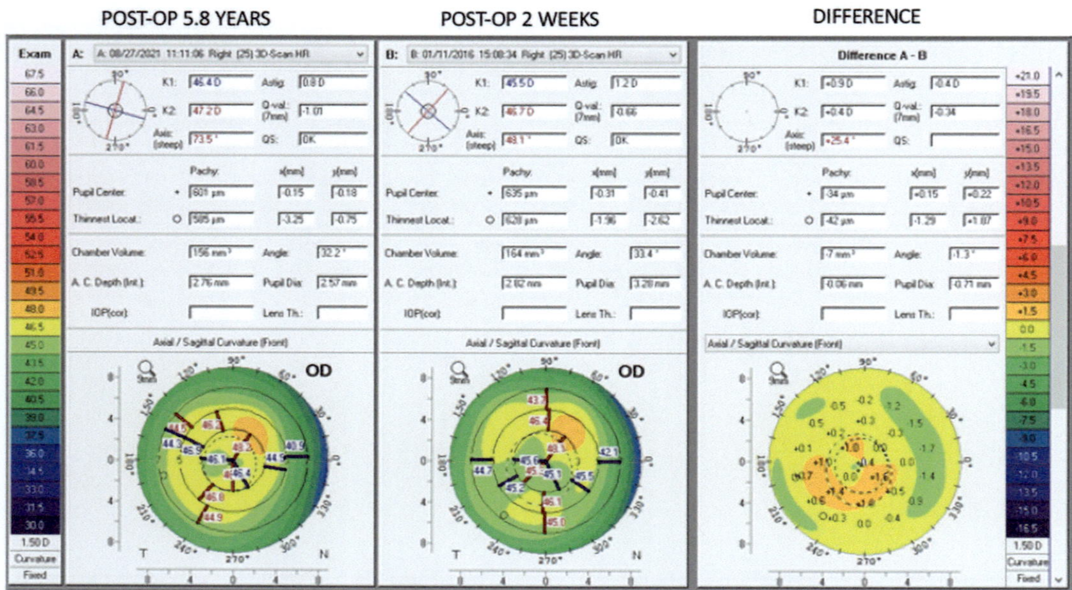

Fig. 20.4 RE difference map of 5.8 years versus 2 weeks post FILI of the same patient

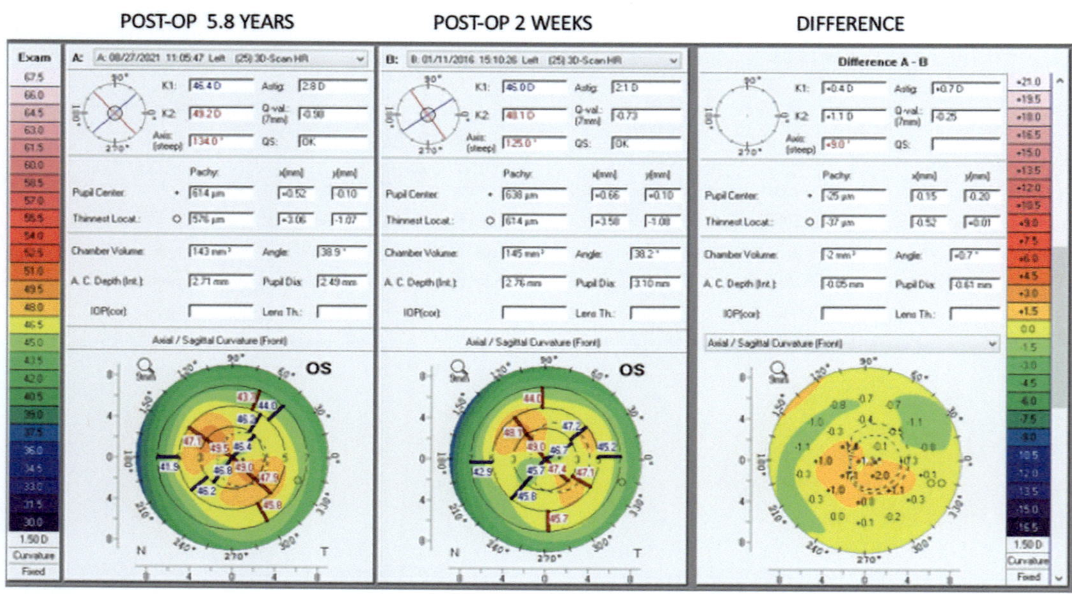

Fig. 20.5 LE difference map of 5.8 years versus 2 weeks post FILI of the same patient

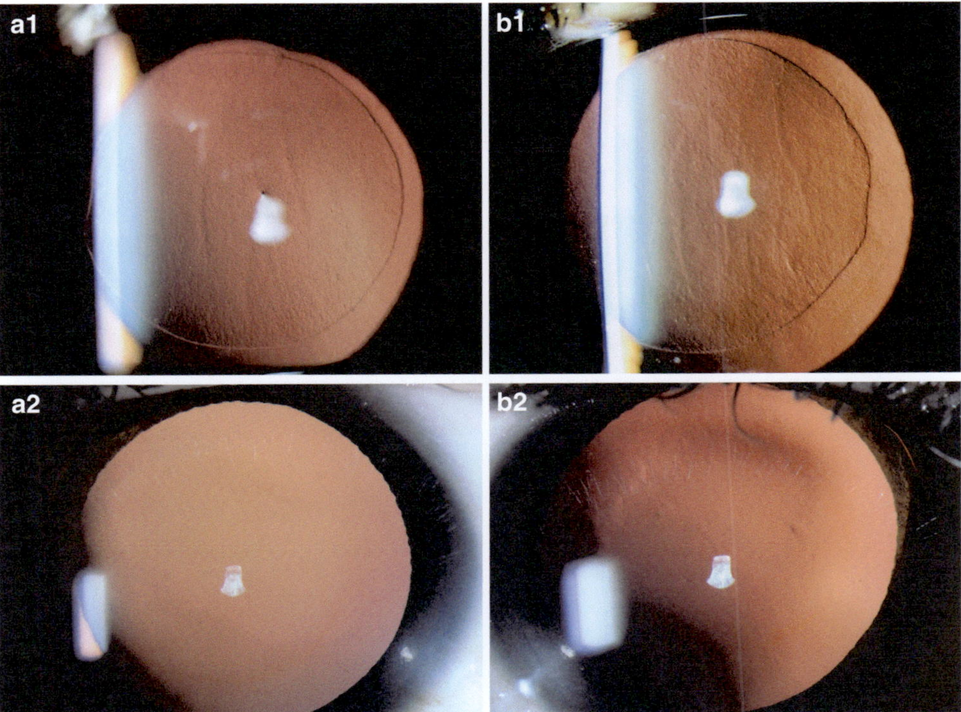

Fig. 20.6 Clinical photographs of the same patient; (**a1**, **b1**) 2 weeks post-op and (**a2**, **b2**) 5.8 years post-op, for the right and left eyes, respectively

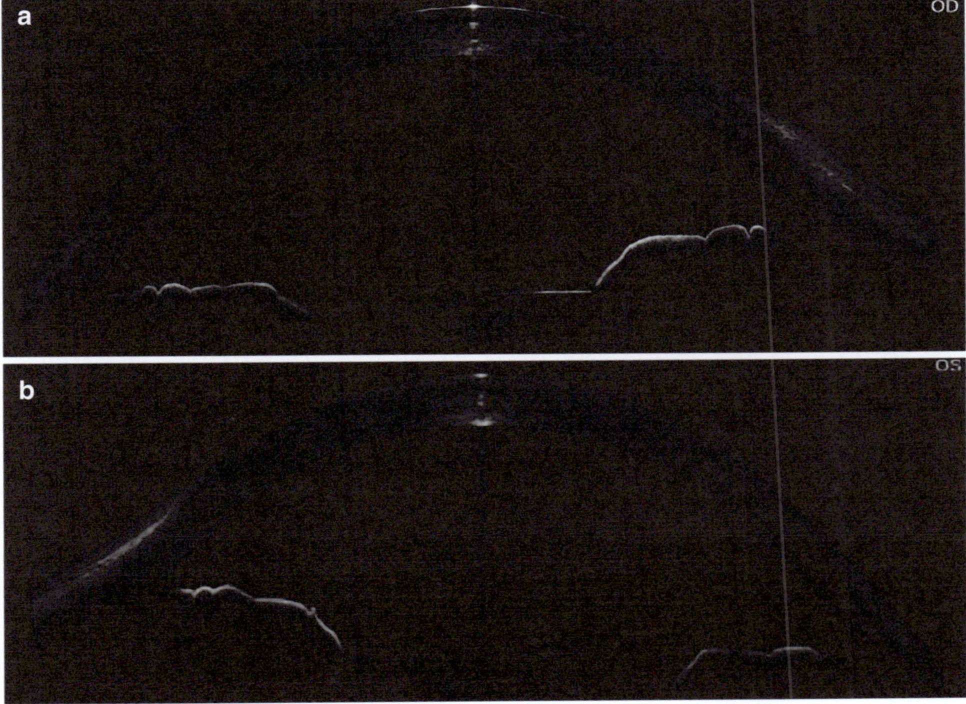

Fig. 20.7 AS-OCT of both eyes of the same patient at 5.8 years follow-up, with clear and well-centered lenticules in situ

Table 20.4 Visual and refractive results of $n = 4$ eyes, enhanced with Bowman membrane relaxation (BMR) in the series

Parameter	Pre-FILI mean (range)	Preenhancement mean (range)	Post-enhancement mean (range)
UDVA (LogMAR)	0.80 (0.50–1.00)	0.55 (0.5–0.6)	0.33 (0.3–0.4)
Sphere (D)	+6.88 (+6.50 to +7.00)	+1.50 (+1.00 to +2.50)	+0.25 (0.00 to +0.50)
Cylinder (D)	+0.69 (+0.50 to +1.00)	+1.50 (+0.50 to +3.00)	+0.12 (−1.50 to +1.25)
SE (D)	+7.22 (+6.75 to +7.50)	+2.25 (+1.75 to +2.50)	+0.31 (−0.50 to +1.125)
CDVA (LogMAR)	0.30 (0.2–0.4)	0.35 (0.3–0.4)	0.30 (0.2–0.4)

UDVA, uncorrected distant visual acuity; *CDVA*, corrected distant visual acuity; *SE*, spherical equivalent; *D*, diopters

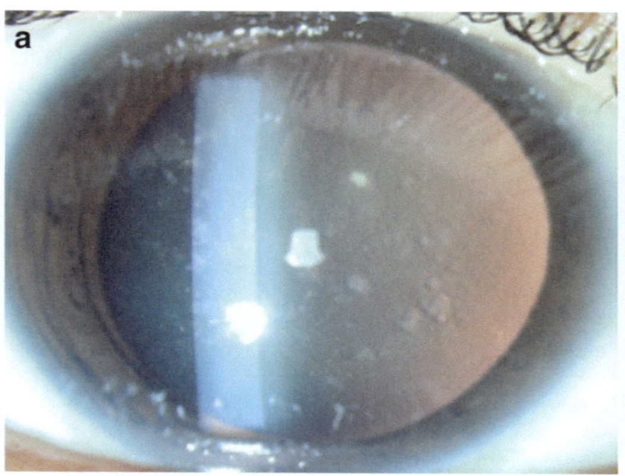
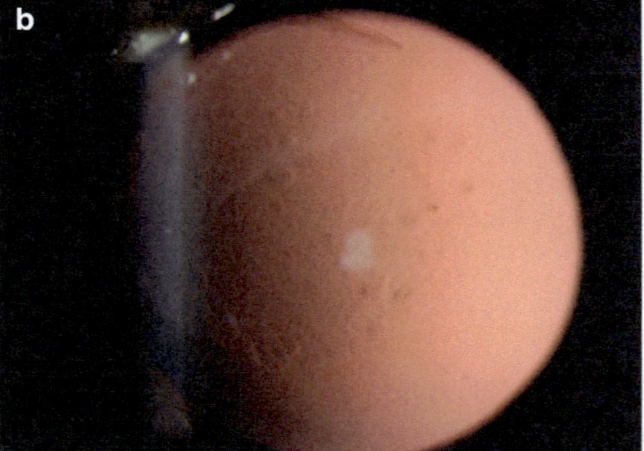

Fig. 20.8 Dilated clinical pictures (**a**) oblique illumination, **b** (retro illumination) of left eye of a patient at 1.5 ±years post-op, showing interface haze due diffuse lenticule scarring. The hazy lenticule was explanted and exchanged with a fresh lenticule 2 weeks later, which remained clear over a follow-up of 6 years

Complications

Four eyes of two patients underwent explantation of the lenticule due to suspected stromal rejection. All the lenticules used in these eyes were cryopreserved. For one patient, the lenticules were exchanged with fresh lenticules. Figure 20.8 shows the dilated clinical pictures of left eye of this patient at 1.5 years post-op, showing interface haze due diffuse lenticule scarring. Post-exchange, the lenticules remained clear with full recovery of patient's visual acuity. For the second patient, lenticules were explanted after 3 years of the FILI procedure, following which hyperopic LASIK was performed, 2 months later.

Discussion

In the present study, we evaluated the long-term clinical outcomes of FILI for the treatment of moderate to high hyperopia in 42 eyes treated with this technique. At a mean follow-up of 68 months (5.6 years), our results were fairly accurate and stable showing reduction of SE from +5.54 D to +0.64 D at 2 weeks, and +0.66 D at 5.6 years. When compared to the long-term results of hyperopic LASIK reported by Dave et al., the mean SE in their study reduced from +3.74 D to +0.84 D at a comparable follow-up of 5 years [12]. Biscevic et al. recently evaluated the safety and efficacy of laser in situ keratomileusis (LASIK) procedure for the correction of high hypermetropia in a retrospective study of 160 patients (266 eyes) who underwent LASIK procedure for the correction of hypermetropia between +3.00 and +7.00 D and cylinder up to 2.00 D, using the Wavelight Allegretto Eye-Q400Hzexcimer laser (Alcon, Forth Worth, TX, USA) with aberration free module and were centered on a corneal vertex. The authors found that 1 week SE was 0.03 ± 0.67 D (−0.50 to +0.63 D), while at 1 year it regressed to 0.58 ± 0.56 D (+0.25 to +0.88 D) [13], which was similar to that observed by Dave et al. at 5 years.

These findings may support the previously proposed mechanisms described in relation with tissue addition, such as lesser epithelial response, induced abberations, and better biomechanical stability, favoring this technique over excimer laser procedures for treating higher degrees of hyperopia [4, 11]. SMILE, as a treatment modality for hyperopia was explored by Pradhan et al., who reported a relative change in SE from +5.61 D to −0.19 D at 12 months follow-up [14]. However, they reported an 11% loss of follow-up at the last visit. The authors suggested SMILE to be a promising modality for high hyperopia; however, a longer follow-up is awaited to assess the long-term stability following this procedure.

Liu et al. recently reported their 2 years clinical experience of treating 14 eyes with implantation of allogenic SMILE lenticule for moderate to high hyperopia [10]. The technique of donor lenticule extraction and implantation in the recipient eye was similar to the one published by our group in 2014 [4]. However, all of their lenticule implantation procedures were scheduled on the same day as the myopic donor eye SMILE. In our series, 24 eyes were implanted with cryopreserved SMILE lenticules, whereas the remaining 18 eyes received fresh lenticules. Contrary to our results, Liu et al. noted a slight overcorrection, as the pre-op SE reduced from +5.53 D to −0.60 D at 2 years post-op. This may be explained by the fact that the depth of the femtolaser pocket at which the donor lenticule was implanted in their study was set at 100 μm as compared to 160 μm in our study, which may have maximized the refractive effect by mainly changing the anterior corneal curvature, without significantly influenc-

ing the posterior curvature. Moshirfar et al. reported a case of high hyperopia of +6.00/−1.00@40 managed with lenticule intrastromal keratoplasty (LIKE) procedure using a thick corneal lenticule of 157 μm (+7.00 D), implanted under a flap at a depth of 100 μm. At 6 months post-op, manifest refraction reduced to 0/−1.25@71, without any noticeable change in the posterior curvature (0.2 D change in steep K) [15]. Damgaard et al. evaluated changes in corneal tomography after stromal lenticule implantation ex vivo, using a combination of two implantation depths (110 and 160 μm) and two lenticule thicknesses (95 μm = 4.00 D, 150 μm = 8.00 D). For the front curvature, a 110 μm implantation depth induced significantly more steepening than a 160 μm depth in all groups [16]. These observations may suggest that a relatively superficial implantation of the lenticule may result in more pronounced anterior curvature changes.

In terms of the changes in front keratometry, corneal thickness, and Q-value, we noted a significant increase in these parameters after FILI at 2 weeks, similar to the results of Liu et al. obtained at 1 month post allogenic lenticule implantation [10]. However, they observed a significant decrease in the anterior keratometry at 2 years when compared to 3 months values (−0.36 D, $p < 0.001$), without a significant corresponding change is the SE refraction. On the contrary, we did not observe any significant change in either anterior keratometry or SE values at 68 months versus 2 weeks post-op. The much anterior placement of the lenticule (at 100 μm) may result in an acute and exaggerated change in the anterior corneal curvature and Q-value, thus, making the cornea prone to regression due to resultant epithelial response. On the other hand, it may be hypothesized that when the lenticule is implanted at a deeper depth of (160 μm), the anterior curvature changes observed for the same amount of tissue may be more gradual, possibly resulting in lesser epithelial response and better refractive stability.

The ideal depth at which the lenticule must be implanted and long-term stability after tissue addition for hyperopia is debatable. Based upon the observations and discussions of the aforementioned studies, it may be proposed that the lenticule be implanted at around 120–130 μm, in order to achieve the desired effect on the anterior curvature, without inducing much posterior changes. Significant over and under corrections may also be avoided by potentially improving the refractive predictability.

Tissue additive procedures for high hyperopia may involve insertion of natural corneal tissue or SMILE lenticule under a LASIK flap (lenticule intrastromal keratoplasty-LIKE) [17] or inside a corneal pocket created using a femtosecond laser (FILI and s-LIKE) [4, 9]. The creation of a flap for tissue addition may pose various challenges such as increased risk of dry eye, DLK, weakening of biomechanics, poor adhesion and dislocation of the flap edge, and epithelial ingrowth that may not be present when the tissue is implanted inside a pocket [9]. Moshirfar et al. reported a case of moderate flap necrosis with epithelial ingrowth following LIKE procedure for high hyperopia, presenting at 1-month post-op [14]. Although, the case was managed with scraping of the epithelial ingrowth, suturing and application of glue at the necrotic flap edge, however, the incidence of such complications may be minimized by implanting the tissue in a stromal pocket, as the incision is small, and amount of surgical manipulation is less.

Liu et al. reported good safety profile with 14.3% eyes gaining one line, 78.6% showing no change, and 7.1% losing one line of CDVA at 2 years post-op [10]. In our study, 45% (19) eyes had no change, 36% (15) eyes gained one line or more, and 19% (8) eyes lost 1 line of CDVA. No eye lost two or more lines of CDVA in either study. However, there were 4 eyes in our series, which required lenticule explantation due to suspected stromal rejection diagnosed at a mean period of 2.25 years. A common factor in these four eyes was the use of a cryopreserved tissue, compared to their study, wherein all the lenticules were harvested and implanted on the same day. Cryopreservation process may alter the physical properties of the stromal collagen and keratocytes, making them susceptible to necrosis, possibly due to a relative lack of cell membrane

protection by cryoprotectants used [18]. However, the cases wherein fresh lenticules were used, may still need to be followed up, due to the potential risk of late stromal rejection, which remains. Pretreatment with gamma radiation has been suggested to deantigenize the donor tissue and prevent future rejection [19, 20]. The feasibility of this option, however, needs to be explored. It may be noteworthy to mention that all the four eyes for which the lenticules were explanted achieved complete visual recovery following reimplantation of fresh lenticules (two eyes) and subsequent excimer treatment (two eyes), suggesting full reversibility of the procedure.

Moshirfar et al. suggested use of CIRCLE [21] software and the side cut only technique to convert the cap into a LASIK flap for the purpose of enhancement after LIKE procedure for high hyperopia [9]. We achieved satisfactory outcomes using the BMR technique for treating residual refractive error after FILI, by potentially reversing the posterior corneal curvature changes [11].

Thus, our tissue addition technique of FILI resulted in satisfactory visual and refractive outcomes with good safety, efficacy, and stability of achieved correction. Truly reversible nature of the procedure could be verified by successful retreatments resulting in complete restoration of visual acuity in eyes requiring explantation of the lenticules. Enhancements with BMR resulted in improved refractive accuracy. However, predictability of refractive results may be further improved by suitable nomograms and modifications in surgical planning and techniques.

Lamellar Surgery with SMILE Lenticules for Keratoconus and SMILE-Ectasia

Recently, the feasibility of use of SMILE tissue to treat corneal ectatic conditions has been successfully shown by our group. The technique has shown promising results when used for potential management of keratoconus [6] and post SMILE ectasia [22]. The surgical technique and guidelines for treatment planning were similar for both the scenarios. Both the donor procedure and the FILI procedure were planned for the same day, after receiving the serology report. The power of the lenticule to be implanted was based on the spherical equivalent of the recipient eye that had signs of ectasia. Exclusion criteria were advanced ectasia with significant decentration, thinnest pachymetry less than 400 mm, maximum keratometry more than 55 dioptre (D), central scarring, or corrected distance visual acuity (CDVA) less than 6/36.

After extraction from the donor eye, the SMILE lenticule was thoroughly rinsed 3 times in a balanced salt solution to remove any debris, tear secretions, or metallic particles that might have attached to the lenticule surface during dissection, extraction, and examination of the lenticule on the corneal surface. The washed lenticule was then placed on a Teflon block and stained with 0.23% riboflavin solution (Peschke L) to enhance its visibility. A 3.0 mm trephine was used to punch the center of the lenticule to create a doughnut-shaped lenticule tissue.

For keratoconus [6], a stromal pocket was created at 100 μm depth using the VisuMax FS laser (Carl Zeiss Meditec, Germany). The pocket was dissected using a blunt spatula followed by injection of 0.25% Vibex Xtra (Avedro) or 0.23% (Peschke-L) dye into the interface for 60 s, after which the interface was washed with normal saline. The corneal vertex was marked with gentian violet using the first Purkinje image as a reference while asking the patient to fixate on the microscope light. The donut-shaped lenticule with the anterior aspect facing upward was held with lenticule forceps and gently inserted into the pocket through the 4-mm superior incision. The lenticule was positioned around the marked center of the cornea and ironed out from the surface using a blunt spatula. Video 20.3 shows the video of surgical procedure of FILI for keratoconus.

For SMILE ectasia [22], the old SMILE incision was opened using the Sinskey side of the Reinstein dissector (Duckworth & Kent Ltd.), followed by dissection of the pocket using the blunt side of the same instrument. This allowed access to the interface, into which 0.23% riboflavin dye (Peschke-L) was then injected. The dye was allowed to soak for 60 s, after which the interface was washed with a balanced salt solution. Following this, the doughnut-shaped lenticule was inserted into the pocket in a similar way as for keratoconus eyes (described earlier).

After the insertion of the tissue, the eye was finally exposed to ultraviolet (UV) A radiation using a power of 18 mW/cm^2 for a period of 5.8 min with an accelerated system (Avedro, Inc.), delivering a total energy of 6.3 J for both keratoconus and SMILE ectasia cases.

Postoperatively, topical steroid in the form of 1% prednisolone (Predforte, Allergan, Inc.) was prescribed for a period of 3 months in tapering dosage, along with 0.5% moxifloxacin antibiotic eyedrops (Vigamox 0.5%, Allergan, Inc.) 4 times a day for 2 weeks. Lubricants were prescribed for 4 times a day for 1 month and as needed thereafter.

Results in Keratoconus

Six eyes from six patients were included in the study. Based on values before and 6 months after the procedure, clinical improvement was noted in uncorrected distance visual acuity (1.06 ± 0.48 logMAR vs. 0.38 ± 0.27 logMAR), corrected distance visual acuity (0.51 ± 0.20 logMAR vs. 0.20 ± 0.24 logMAR), and manifest spherical equivalent (−3.47 ± 1.15 D vs. −1.77 ± 1.7 D). There was flattening of mean keratometry in 3-mm and 5-mm zones by 3.42 ± 2.09 D and 1.70 ± 1.31 D, respectively. Mean pachymetry in the central and midperipheral zones increased by 18.3 ± 7.3 μm and 33.0 ± 8.8 μm, respectively. All eyes had reduction in higher order aberrations, specifically coma. No eye lost lines of corrected distance visual acuity. No adverse events such as haze, infection, or allogeneic graft rejection were observed.

Results in SMILE Ectasia

Four eyes of three patients (mean age 25.7 years) developed features of keraectasia at a mean period of 3 years after myopic SMILE correction.

All cases were managed with insertion of heterologous SMILE lenticules in the previously created pocket, followed by simultaneous accelerated CXL. At a mean follow-up of 7.67 months, there was improvement in corrected distance visual acuity and reduction in keratometry and higher order aberrations in all eyes. The visual, refractive, and topographic parameters remained stable at the last visit compared with the 2-week follow-up visit. No eye developed haze, infection, or rejection requiring tissue explantation.

Early experience showed tissue addition with simultaneous pocket CXL to be a feasible approach for managing ectasia after SMILE. However, further follow-up is required to establish the long-term safety and effects on corneal stabilization.

Lamellar Surgery with SMILE Lenticules for Presbyopia

Jacob et al., recently, described a new technique called PEARL (PrEsbyopic Allogenic Refractive Lenticule) that uses an inlay obtained from a small incision lenticule extraction (SMILE) lenticule [7]. With regard to the methodology, the anterior side of the stored SMILE lenticule was identified, and it was spread out with the anterior side facing up, dried with a surgical sponge, and the center marked with the inked tip of a fine Sinskey hook. A 1-mm trephine was centered on the inked mark to fashion a small donor allogenic presbyopic corneal inlay, which was then centered at co-axially sighted light reflex while it was inserted into a corneal pocket created using a femtosecond laser at 120 μm depth, into the nondominant eye of the presbyopic individuals.

Results

Four emmetropic presbyopic patients underwent PEARL inlay implantation in the nondominant eye. In the operated eye, uncorrected near visual acuity at 33 cm improved from J8 to J2 in one and from J5, J6, and J7, respectively, to J2 in three operated eyes with improvement between three and five lines in

all eyes. Uncorrected intermediate visual acuity ranged between J3 and J5 at 67 cm and uncorrected distance visual acuity remained 20/20 in the operated eye and binocularly. The patients were comfortable and reported independence from glasses for near, intermediate, and distance for all their routine visual tasks for the 6-month follow-up period. There were no complaints of dysphotopsia or troublesome night glare/halos. All lenticules remained well centered during the follow-up, and no lenticule-induced complications were seen.

According to the authors, The PEARL inlay acts as a shape-changing inlay by increasing the central radius of curvature and resulting in a hyperprolate corneal shape. Unlike the synthetic implants, there is unhindered passage of oxygen and nutrients because the PEARL inlay is made of allogenic cornea, thus ensuring stable corneal conditions and decreasing the risk for corneal necrosis and melt. It also has the advantages of reversibility and adjustability. However, larger data and longer follow-ups are needed to establish the long-term safety and efficacy of the procedure in presbyopic individuals.

Other Uses of SMILE-Derived Lenticules

Recently, the initial clinical outcomes of the small incision lenticule extraction (SMILE)-derived glued lenticule patch graft for management of micro-perforations and complicated corneal tears were reported [8, 23]. In our single-center case series, seven eyes that presented with micro-perforations, partial-thickness corneal defect, and traumatic complicated corneal tear were repaired with a lenticule patch graft obtained from the SMILE procedure. The patch was secured to the recipient eye using fibrin glue. Preoperatively, anterior segment optical coherence tomography was used to assess the depth of the defect and to decide the thickness of the lenticule. Patients were followed up on days 1, 7, and 15 and at 1 and 3 months postoperatively. Main outcome parameters measured were best-corrected visual acuity, clarity of the graft, and restoration of optical and tectonic integrity.

Results

Significant improvement in visual acuity was seen from 15 days onward in five of seven eyes. The lenticule graft was well apposed and remained clear until the last follow-up visit in all eyes treated.

Thus, the patch graft from the SMILE-derived lenticule using fibrin glue seems to serve as a safe, feasible, and inexpensive surgical option for the management of micro perforations and complicated corneal tears, especially in centers that perform the SMILE procedure in large numbers.

Take Home Notes

Lamellar corneal surgeries using SMILE lenticules appear to be a feasible and exciting concept with encouraging results for the management of various corneal conditions, which carries a huge potential for further research. Long-term results of hyperopic tissue addition using SMILE lenticules are available; however, further results are awaited for keratoconus and presbyopia. Future research is also suggested in the areas of nomogram refinement, evaluating biomechanical changes, epithelial and stromal remodeling, tissue treatments, and preservation to prevent rejection following this procedure.

References

1. Barraquer JI. Queratomileusis y queratofakia. Bogota: Instituto Barraquer de America; 1980. p. 342.
2. Barraquer JI. Refractive corneal surgery: experience and considerations. An Inst Barraquer. 1993;24:113–8.
3. Pradhan KR, Reinstein DZ, Carp GI, Archer TJ, Gobbe M, Gurung R. Femtosecond laser-assisted keyhole endokeratophakia: correction of hyperopia by implantation of an allogeneic lenticule obtained by SMILE from a myopic donor. J Refract Surg. 2013;29(11):777–82. https://doi.org/10.3928/1081597X-20131021-07. Erratum in: J Refract Surg. 2015;31:60.
4. Ganesh S, Brar S, Rao PA. Cryopreservation of extracted corneal lenticules after small incision lenticule extraction for potential use in human subjects. Cornea. 2014;33(12):1355–62. https://doi.org/10.1097/ICO.0000000000000276.
5. Sun L, Yao P, Li M, Shen Y, Zhao J, Zhou X. The safety and predictability of implanting autologous lenticule obtained by SMILE for hyperopia. J Refract Surg. 2015;31(6):374–9. https://doi.org/10.3928/1081597X-20150521-03.
6. Ganesh S, Brar S. Femtosecond intrastromal lenticular implantation combined with accelerated collagen cross-linking for the treatment of keratoconus—initial clinical result in 6 eyes. Cornea. 2015;34:1331–9.
7. Jacob S, Kumar DA, Agarwal A, Agarwal A, Aravind R, Saijimol AI. Preliminary evidence of successful near vision enhancement with a new technique: PrEsbyopic Allogenic Refractive Lenticule (PEARL) corneal inlay using a SMILE lenticule. J Refract Surg. 2017;33:224–9.
8. Bhandari V, Ganesh S, Brar S, Pandey R. Application of the SMILE-derived glued lenticule patch graft in micro perforations and partial-thickness corneal defects. Cornea. 2016;35(3):408–12. https://doi.org/10.1097/ICO.0000000000000741. PMID: 26764882.
9. Moshirfar M, Shah TJ, Masud M, Fanning T, Linn SH, Ronquillo Y, Hoopes PC Sr. A modified Small-Incision Lenticule Intrastromal Keratoplasty (sLIKE) for the correction of high hyperopia: a description of a new surgical technique and comparison to Lenticule Intrastromal Keratoplasty (LIKE). Med Hypothesis Discov Innov Ophthalmol. 2018;7(2):48–56.
10. Liu S, Wei R, Choi J, Li M, Zhou X. Visual outcomes after implantation of allogenic lenticule in a 100-μm pocket for moderate to high hyperopia: 2-year results. J Refract Surg. 2021;37(11):734–40. https://doi.org/10.3928/1081597X-20210730-02. Epub 2021 Nov 1. PMID: 34756142.
11. Brar S, Ganesh S, Sriganesh SS, Dorennavar L. Long-term outcomes of bowman's membrane relaxation for enhancement of femtosecond intrastromal lenticule implantation performed for the management of high hyperopia. J Refract Surg. 2022;38(2):134–41.
12. Dave R, O'Brart DP, Wagh VK, Lim WS, Patel P, Lee J, Marshall J. Sixteen-year follow-up of hyperopic laser in situ keratomileusis. J Cataract Refract Surg. 2016;42(5):717–24. https://doi.org/10.1016/j.jcrs.2016.03.028. PMID: 27255248.
13. Biscevic A, Pidro A, Pjano MA, Grisevic S, Ziga N, Bohac M. Lasik as a solution for high hypermetropia. Med Arch. 2019;73(3):191–4. https://doi.org/10.5455/medarh.2019.73.191-194. PMID: 31402804; PMCID: PMC6643362.
14. Pradhan KR, Reinstein DZ, Carp GI, Archer TJ, Dhungana P. Small Incision Lenticule Extraction (SMILE) for hyperopia: 12-month refractive and visual outcomes. J Refract Surg. 2019;35(7):442–50. https://doi.org/10.3928/1081597X-20190529-01. PMID: 31298724.
15. Moshirfar M, Hopping GC, Somani AN, et al. Human allograft refractive lenticular implantation for high hyperopic correction. J Cataract Refract Surg. 2020;46(2):305–11. https://doi.org/10.1097/j.jcrs.0000000000000011.
16. Damgaard IB, Ivarsen A, Hjortdal J. Biological lenticule implantation for correction of hyperopia: an ex vivo study in human corneas. J

Refract Surg. 2018;34(4):245–52. https://doi.org/10.3928/1081597X-20180206-01.

17. Jankov M, Mrochen M, Seiler T. Laser intrastromal keratoplasty-case report. J Refract Surg. 2004;20:79–84.

18. Borderie VM, Laroche L. Ultrastructure of cultured and cryopreserved human corneal keratocytes. Cornea. 1999;18(5):589–94. PMID: 10487434.

19. Stevenson W, Cheng SF, Emami-Naeini P, Hua J, Paschalis EI, Dana R, Saban DR. Gamma-irradiation reduces the allogenicity of donor corneas. Invest Ophthalmol Vis Sci. 2012;53:7151–8.

20. Utine CA, Tzu JH, Akpek EK. Lamellar keratoplasty using gamma-irradiated corneal lenticules. Am J Ophthalmol. 2011;151:170–174.e1.

21. Ganesh S, Brar S, Manasa KV. CIRCLE software for the management of retained lenticule tissue following complicated SMILE surgery. J Refract Surg. 2019;35(1):60–5. https://doi.org/10.3928/1081597X-20181120-01. PMID: 30633789.

22. Ganesh S, Brar S, Bowry R. Management of small-incision lenticule extraction ectasia using tissue addition and pocket crosslinking. J Cataract Refract Surg. 2021;47(3):407–12. https://doi.org/10.1097/j.jcrs.0000000000000335. PMID: 32694305.

23. Yang H, Zhou Y, Zhao H, Xue J, Jiang Q. Application of the SMILE-derived lenticule in therapeutic keratoplasty. Int Ophthalmol. 2020;40(3):689–95. https://doi.org/10.1007/s10792-019-01229-y. Epub 2019 Nov 21. PMID: 31754892.

Corneal Allogenic Intrastromal Ring Segments (CAIRS)

21

D. Sravani and Soosan Jacob

Key Points

- CAIRS is a new technique that flattens and regularizes ectatic corneas in patients with keratoconus, post LASIK ectasia, pellucid marginal degeneration, and other ectatic disorders.
- The advantages over synthetic ICRS are many and are discussed further in this chapter.
- CAIRS can be used even in advanced cases where conventional synthetic ICRS would not be implanted. In many cases, DALK can be avoided by combining CAIRS with thin-cornea cross-linking techniques.
- Customized CAIRS: CAIRS can be further customized according to individual refraction and topography to tailor results for each patient.
- Bioptics: CAIRS can be implanted first to create synergy with other procedures such as topography-guided PRK, phakic IOL, refractive lens exchange, etc. by decreasing the amount of residual irregular astigmatism and hence the safety and efficacy of these additional procedures. In many cases, the need for the additional procedures may be done away with by just CAIRS alone.
- CAIRS can be used to treat complications of synthetic ICRS such as corneal melts.

Introduction

Corneal allogenic intrastromal ring segment (CAIRS) is a minimally invasive technique first performed by one of the authors (Soosan Jacob) in 2015 for the treatment of keratoconus and other corneal ectasias with the aim of improving the outcome achieved and decreasing the risks associated with synthetic intrastromal corneal ring segments (ICRS).

Ectatic Corneal Disorders

Ectasia is an abnormal progressive thinning and protrusion of the cornea due to biomechanical failure. Keratoconus, pellucid marginal degeneration, keratoglobus, and post-laser vision correction ectasia are common ectatic disorders seen in clinical practice.

Keratoconus

Keratoconus is an uncommon corneal disorder with progressive thinning and steepening of

Supplementary Information The online version contains supplementary material available at https://doi.org/10.1007/978-3-031-32408-6_21.

D. Sravani · S. Jacob (✉)
Dr. Agarwal's Refractive and Cornea Foundation (DARCF), Chennai, India

Dr. Agarwal's Group of Eye Hospitals, Chennai, India; http://www.dragarwal.com

the central and paracentral cornea. This causes irregular astigmatism affecting the quality of vision [1]. Abnormal curvature maps with abnormal posterior elevation, with or without corneal thinning, are the typical topographic features of keratoconus. The disease is inherited in an autosomal dominant pattern with no gender predilection. With the incidence rate of one in 2000 to upto 5 per hundred, it starts in puberty and progresses over a decade into the mid-30s [2]. Downs syndrome, Marfan's syndrome, Lebers congenital amaurosis, and mitral valve prolapse are some syndromes associated with the disease. Although there are no clear causative factors, postulated risk factors include chronic exposure to ultraviolet light, atopy and constant eye rubbing [3]. The treatment of keratoconus includes medical management such as glasses and various contact lenses. The surgical treatment includes corneal crosslinking, intrastromal corneal ring segments (ICRS), deep anterior lamellar keratoplasty (DALK), and in advanced cases, penetrating keratoplasty (PK).

Intrastromal Corneal Ring Segments (ICRS)

Originally developed for refractive correction of high myopia and astigmatism, ICRS became a key treatment strategy for the treatment of keratoconus. ICRS segments are made from synthetic material polymethylmethacrylate (PMMA). Various types of ICRS are available commercially.

available ICRS include Intacs, Kerarings, Ferrara rings, Myorings, Bisantis segments, etc. Each model of ICRS has its own nomogram. The quality of vision is improved by flattening and regularizing the corneal surface. ICRS is associated with complications such as migration, intrusion, extrusion, and overriding. Melting and stromal necrosis are common with the PMMA segments [4]. Focal edema, deposits in the channels, and neovascularization are the other common complications. Rare trouble encompasses infectious keratitis in a few cases.

Mechanism of Action of ICRS

According to the Barraquers Thickness law, necessary flattening of the central cornea can be achieved either by removing the tissue from the center or placing the tissue in the periphery to achieve an arc shortening effect [5]. The flattening that is achieved with ICRS can be improved by either decreasing the optical zone diameter or by placing a thicker segment. The final cylindrical power correction achieved is proportional to the arc length, and the thickness and diameter of the segment determine the final myopic correction [6]. Combining collagen cross-linking with ICRS improved the corneal biomechanics as well as the quality of the vision achieved.

Cairs or Corneal Allogenic Intrastromal Ring Segments

CAIRS procedure is an alternative to ICRS and replaces synthetic segments with a biocompatible allogenic material thereby reducing the risk of complications [7–9]. Allogenic implants can be prepared from fresh or preserved donor stroma, processed donor stroma, or any other source of allogenic tissue [10]. These segments are then inserted into circular intra-stromal corneal channels created within the keratoconic patient's eye [11, 12]. The mechanism of action is possibly by a combination of different mechanisms—mid-peripheral volume augmentation, arc shortening, and epithelial remodelling. The myopic power decreases secondary to increased posterior corneal curvature and decreased anterior corneal curvature. Regular and irregular astigmatisms decrease because of improvement in topography. The quality of vision is improved secondary to regularization of the anterior corneal surface. CAIRS can be inserted at a more superficial depth than synthetic segments and also in more advanced cases. CAIRS is especially advantageous in progressive keratoconus and in eye rubbers since in these patients, an initially satisfacto-

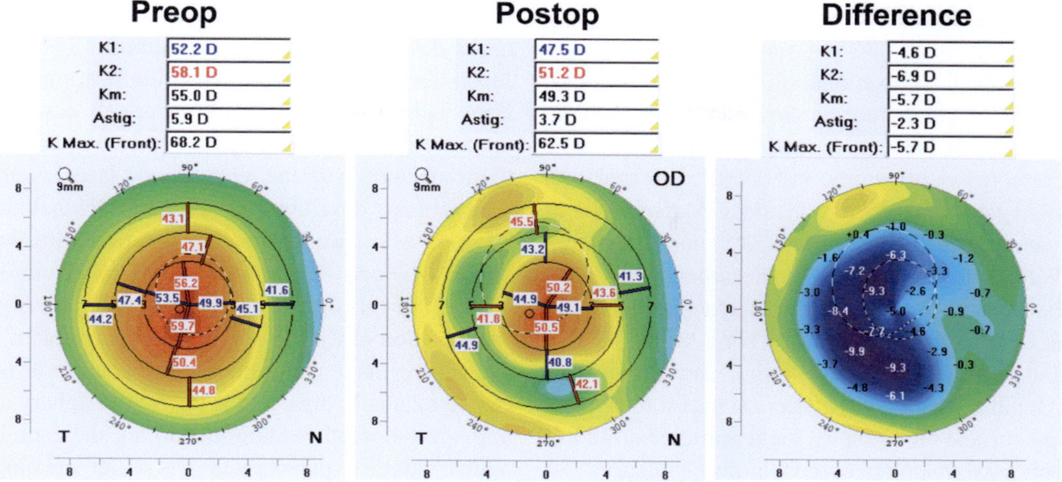

Fig. 21.1 Comparison of the pre-op and post-op topographic map and parameters after CAIRS procedure showing improvement. Difference map shows the flattening achieved together with improvement in all parameters

rily placed synthetic segment may become superficial with time. This fear does not exist with CAIRS [13, 14]. Excellent biocompatibility and biointegration (follow-up range more than 8 years), centralization and regularization of the cone, wide applicability even in patients with a thin cornea, easy learning curve, improved visual quality and quantity, and the ability to exquisitely customize the segments on an individual basis are some of the benefits compared to synthetic ICRS [15, 16].

Though the risk of rejection exists with CAIRS, it is low because of multiple reasons: host keratocytes can quickly repopulate CAIRS tissue due to the low volume of tissue that is transferred and the ensconced position within the host stroma; lack of epithelial and endothelial transfer; distance from the limbus; lack of sutures, etc. The safety and efficacy of CAIRS have been quite good till date with significant improvements noted in refraction, uncorrected and best-corrected visual acuities, topographic parameters, and quality of vision achieved.

The mid-peripheral location and the untouched visual axis mean that even in the rare scenario of a rejection, vision remains unaffected (Figs. 21.1 and 21.2).

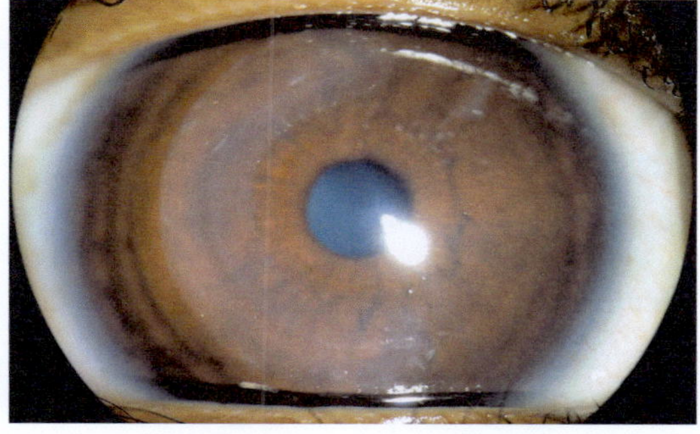

Fig. 21.2 Shows the same case as Fig. 21.1 with single CAIRS segment placed on the temporal side extending superiorly and inferiorly as well

Indications and Contraindications

- Ectatic corneal disorders like keratoconus, pellucid marginal degeneration, post LASIK ectasias, and post-ICRS melts are common indications.
- Systemic contraindications include autoimmune disorders, collagen vascular disorders, immunodeficiency, etc.
- Viral keratitis sequalae, corneal scarring especially in central and paracentral areas and eyes too thin to be cross-linked are ocular contraindications though further studies are required to ascertain these.

Preoperative Workup

A detailed eye examination, automated refractometric reading, retinoscopy, meticulous subjective verification of uncorrected and spectacle corrected visual acuity, and contact lens trial with rigid gas permeable lens are done. Various devices such as Pentacam® (Oculus, Wetzlar, Germany), Wavelight Topolyzer® (Alcon Laboratories, Inc., Fort Worth, Texas), Zywave aberrometer® (Bausch & Lomb Zywave, Rochester, NY), MS39 ASOCT and topography® (CSO Italia), and Corvis® ST (Oculus, Wetzlar, Germany) are useful for assessing corneal tomography, higher order aberrations, epithelial mapping, corneal biomechanics, etc.

Technique

CAIRS segment is prepared from allogenic tissue such as the stroma of an allogenic donor corneoscleral rim. First, the epithelium and endothelium are removed. A 360-degree segment of stromal tissue is trephined using the Jacob double-bladed trephine™ (Madhu Instruments, New Delhi).

Finally, the segments with desired thickness, width, and arc length are prepared. CAIRS may be customized further if required using the technique described by one of the authors (SJ). The Jacob CAIRS Cutomizer™ (Epsilon Instruments, USA) helps to exquisitely and accurately customize the segments manually to any desired shape. Customization with the femtosecond laser is currently being developed by Ziemer Ophthalmic Systems AG (Sweden) in collaboration with the author (SJ) and Shady Awwad, MD (Lebanon). Under topical medication, the tunnel for the implantation of CAIRS segment in the recipient's eye can be made using the femtosecond laser or can be manually dissected at the mid periphery at mid stromal depth without disturbing the central optical zone of the cornea. We prefer creating broad mid-stromal channels with an inner diameter of about 4.6 mm since unlike INTACS, CAIRS does not cause glare or haloes. CAIRS are inserted using a push-through technique using a curved Y-rod and a curved reverse Sinskey making sure the segments are not twisted. Progressive cases are combined with collagen cross-linking (CXL) or thin cornea cross-linking techniques such as the contact lens assisted corneal cross-linking (CACXL) based on the corneal thickness as mentioned already (Figs. 21.3 and 21.4; Video 21.1) [17, 18].

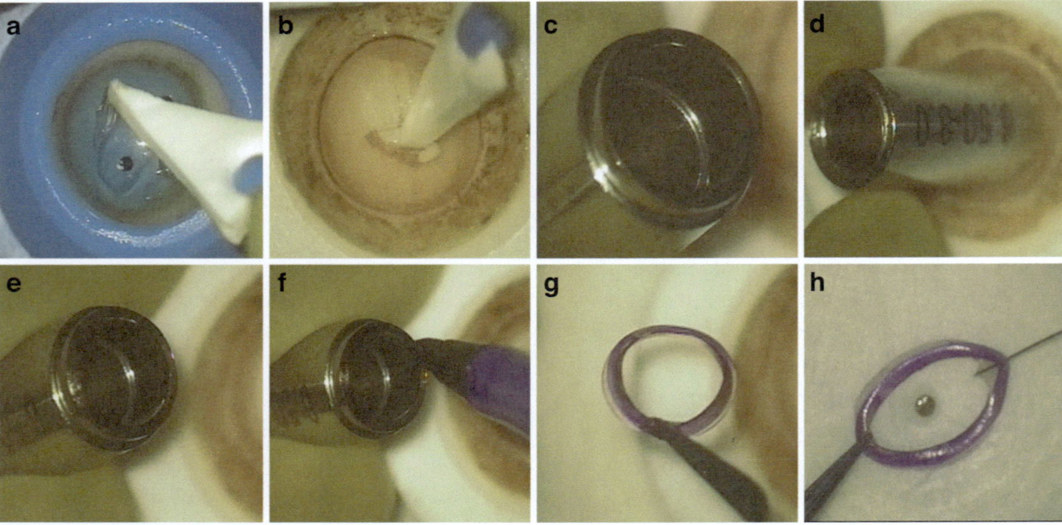

Fig. 21.3 Preparing CAIRS. (**a**, **b**) Scraping off the epithelium and endothelium from the donor corneal button; (**c**) Jacob CAIRS double bladed trephine™ (Madhu Instruments, New Delhi) is used to punch out the corneal stroma with precise sharp edges; (**d**) punching out the tissue with the special trephine; (**e**, **f**) marking of the Bowman's mebrane side of the punched out donor corneal stroma in the trephine; (**g**, **h**) ring of corneal stromal tissue and CAIRS segments are prepared by cutting the ring to the appropriate sized segments

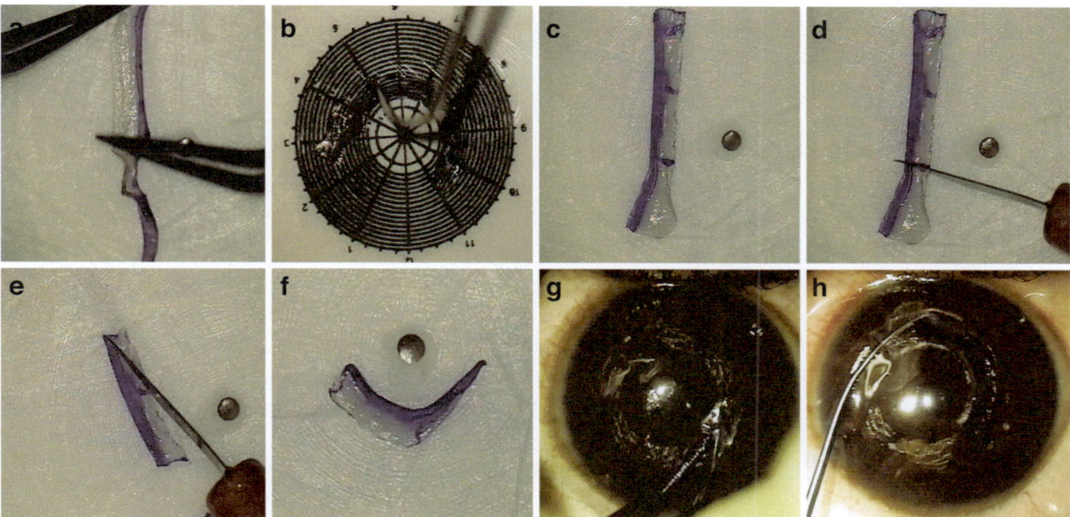

Fig. 21.4 Preparation of a customized CAIRS segment. (**a**) CAIRS segment is spread out; (**b**) the length of the segment to be implanted is marked intraoperatively as per the preoperative topographic plan after positioning it on the sterile Jacob CAIRS Customizer™ (Epsilon Instrumemts, USA); (**c**, **d**) appropriate lengths of the segments are marked and prepared for the length and taper; (**e**, **f**) custom-ization of the segment based on the topographic need is done by preparing a segment with superior tapering (the area that requires less flattening); (**g**) the segment is pushed through using a curved Y-rod into a channel already made using the femtosecond laser; (**h**) the segment is implanted without any twists and pulled through the other end using a reverse Sinskey hook, and finally, the segment is ironed out

The location of CAIRS is defined by the location of the cone. A single segment is placed in case of a decentered cone, the arc length being sufficient to enclose the area of steepness. A single segment generally suffices to correct comatose aberrations, flatten the cone and centralize it. For already centered cones, two 150° segments are placed for flattening it. Asymmetric segments may also be placed. Smaller segments at a slightly larger optic zone are placed for correcting cylindrical errors. Thicker CAIRS segments prepared using the 6.5/8 mm diameter Jacob CAIRS trephine are used for higher refractive errors, whereas for low refractive errors, the 7.75/8.75 mm diameter trephines are used. The 8/9.5 mm trephines are used for very advanced keratoconus [19, 20].

Postoperative Medications

A quick and short tapering course of antibiotic plus steroid drops in conjunction with lubricants are used over a period of 5 weeks. If combined with cross-linking, ultraviolet protective glasses are advised for 6 months when outside. Follow-up includes uncorrected and spectacle-corrected visual acuity, regular topographic evaluation to assess all parameters and to analyze stability, and anterior segment OCT to monitor segment thickness and depth on follow-ups.

Benefit of CAIRS in Advanced Cases

CAIRS has a wide range of applications from early to advanced stages of keratoconus. In advanced cases, for instance, with steep corneal curvatures >58 D and thin pachymetry <400–450 μm, placing a synthetic segment at 70–80% depth is associated with risks and complications. The mid-stromal placement of CAIRS is safer without the risk of stromal melt, migration, intrusion or extrusion. It therefore covers a wide range of candidates who can undergo the procedure and a wide range of thicknesses, arc lengths and customization can be attained by the surgeon on table with CAIRS while synthetic implants may need FDA approval for different thicknesses and different arc lengths.

Though deep anterior lamellar keratoplasty provides satisfactory outcomes in advanced cases, the risk of complications such as irregular astigmatism, rejection, secondary glaucoma, graft failure, Urrets Zavalia syndrome, loosening of sutures, incitement of neovascularization etc. exist. CAIRS on the other hand has a simple learning curve with low risk of any intra-operative complication. It is helpful in avoiding or at least delaying the need for corneal transplantation. In the scenario of progression post-CAIRS and CXL, DALK can still be performed safely.

Customized CAIRS

A standard ICRS device has uniform thickness along its length. The idea of asymmetric ICRS is to help achieve the necessary flattening where it is required and to create less effect on areas which are less severely affected. Similar to asymmetric synthetic ICRS, customized CAIRS can be easily fashioned with different thicknesses, width, arc lengths, diameters, etc. and with specific shapes in order to tailor-make the CAIRS according to the individual patient's topography [21]. Such customized correction for asymmetric keratoconus targets better correction of higher order aberrations and is more helpful for achieving a better quality of vision. Pair segments with different thickness, arc lengths, or widths are also possible as is an arc length of up to 360° Customization in case of CAIRS is possible to amuch larger degree than is possible with asymmetric synthetic ICRS (Video 21.2).

Combined Procedures

CAIRS may be combined with corneal cross-linking or thin cornea cross-linking techniques such as contact lens assisted collagen cross-linking for progressive cases. They may also be combined as bioptics with topography- guided photorefractive keratectomy, phakic IOL placement, refractive lens exchange, conductive keratoplasty, etc. The advantage of CAIRS is reversibility and adjustability—they can be exchanged, adjusted, or customized post-surgery if required.

Stability of the CAIRS Segments

Serial scans of anterior segment OCT showed no significant change in segment thickness in our initial analysis, though larger studies are needed to confirm this. The mid stromal placement and the combined cross-linking could be some of the factors contributing to the stability of the segments (Fig. 21.5).

Results

To date, about 600 cases have been performed by us including customized CAIRS. In the published

Fig. 21.5 AS-OCT showing a customised CAIRS segment with one end tapered and placed at 50% depth in the corneal stroma

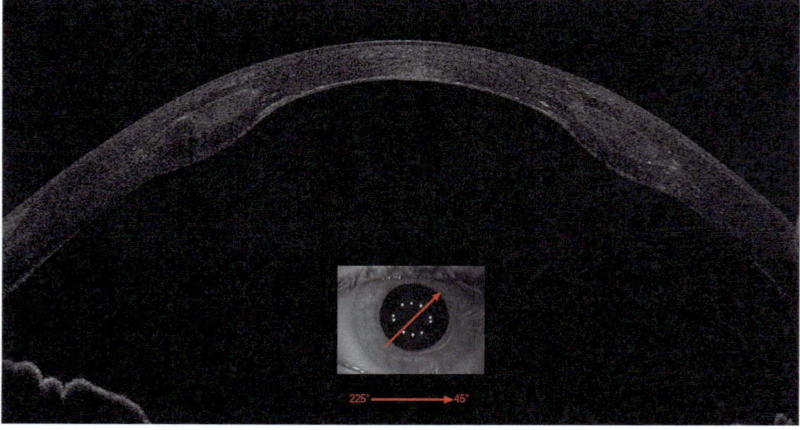

pilot study conducted by Jacob et al. [7], for a period of 1 year between March 2016 and March 2017, 24 eyes of 20 keratoconus patients who underwent CAIRS had a significant improvement in almost all postoperative parameters including the visual outcome and the topographic parameters. Significant improvement was observed in both UCVA and BCVA with reduced topographic astigmatism and an improvement in the mean power in both 3 and 5 mm zones.

On follow-up ranging from 6 to 18 months, there was an improvement in UCVA within a range of 0–8 lines, mean improvement of 2.79 ± 2.65 lines. There was also an improvement in CDVA by a mean of 1.29 ± 1.33 lines. The depth of the implantation was at an average of 314.4 ± 61 μm. The central corneal thickness as measured by ASOCT-Pachymetry did not show any statistically significant change when compared pre and postoperatively. On follow-up, no significant progression was observed as measured with Kmax/Steep K >0.75 D. CAIRS segments were well positioned and remained stable in thickness during the entire follow up.

Take Home Notes

- CAIRS is superior to synthetic segments as biocompatible allogenic material is used, thereby reducing complications.
- Significant improvements are seen in visual and topographic parameters.
- Customization according to the topographic pattern of the patient can further improve visual outcome.

Financial Disclosure Soosan Jacob has a patent for special trephines, devices and processes used to create these segments as well as for the CAIRS segments and various types of shaped corneal segments; Madhu; Ziemer.

References

1. Rabinowitz YS. Keratoconus. Surv Ophthalmol. 1998;42(4):297–319.
2. Millodot M, Ortenberg I, Lahav-Yacouel K, Behrman S. Effect of ageing on keratoconic corneas. J Opt. 2016;9(2):72–7.
3. Gordon-Shaag A, Millodot M, Shneor E, Liu Y. The genetic and environmental factors for keratoconus. Biomed Res Int. 2015;2015:795738.
4. Kwitko S, Severo NS. Ferrara intracorneal ring segments for keratoconus. J Cataract Refract Surg. 2004;30(4):812–20.
5. Barraquer JI. Modification of refraction by means of intracorneal inclusions. Int Ophthalmol Clin. 1966;6(1):53–78.
6. Burris TE, Baker PC, Ayer CT, et al. Flattening of central corneal curvature with intrastromal corneal rings of increasing thickness: an eye-bank eye study. J Cataract Refract Surg. 1993;19(Suppl): 182–7.
7. Jacob S, Patel SR, Agarwal A, Ramalingam A, Saijimol AI, Raj JM. Corneal Allogenic Intrastromal Ring Segments (CAIRS) combined with corneal cross-linking for keratoconus. J Refract Surg. 2018;34(5):296–303.
8. Carpal EF, Santilli C, Maltry A. Long-term viability of allogenic donor stroma. Indian J Ophthalmol. 2020;68(12):3057–9.
9. Dapena I, Parker JS, Melles GRJ. Potential benefits of modified corneal tissue grafts for keratoconus: Bowman layer 'inlay' and 'onlay' transplantation, and allogenic tissue ring segments. Curr Opin Ophthalmol. 2020;31(4):276–83.
10. Parker JS, Dockery PW, Jacob S, Parker JS. Preimplantation dehydration for corneal allogenic intrastromal ring segment implantation. J Cataract Refract Surg. 2021;47(11):e37–9.
11. Parker JS, Dockery PW, Parker JS. Flattening the curve: manual method for corneal allogenic intrastromal ring segment implantation. J Cataract Refract Surg. 2021;47(11):e31–3.
12. Parker JS, Dockery PW, Parker JS. Trypan blue-assisted corneal allogenic intrastromal ring segment implantation. J Cataract Refract Surg. 2021;47(1):127.
13. Jarade E, Issa M, Chanbour W, Warhekar P. Biologic stromal ring to manage stromal melting after intrastromal corneal ring segment implantation. J Cataract Refract Surg. 2019;45(9):1222–5.
14. Kozhaya K, Mehanna CJ, Jacob S, Saad A, Jabbur NS, Awwad ST. Management of anterior stromal necrosis after polymethylmethacrylate ICRS: explantation versus exchange with corneal allogenic intrastromal ring segments. J Refract Surg. 2022;38(4):256–63.
15. Gunn D. New keratoconus treatment Australia: CAIRS - corneal allogenic intrastromal ring segments. https://www.drdavidgunn.com.au/blog/cairs-keratoconus-treatment. Accessed 19 Jul 2022.
16. Dockery P, Parker JS, Parker JS. Corneal allogenic intrastromal ring segments can be implanted with manual technique. https://www.healio.com/news/ophthalmology/20201029/corneal-allogenic-intrastromal-ring-segments-can-be-implanted-with-manual-technique. Accessed 19 Jul 2022.
17. Kumar DA, Jacob S, Agarwal A. Contact lens-assisted corneal cross-linking. J Refract Surg. 2015;31(7):496.

18. Srivatsa S, Jacob S, Agarwal A. Contact lens assisted corneal cross linking in thin ectatic corneas - a review. Indian J Ophthalmol. 2020;68(12):2773–8.
19. Jacob S. CAIRS. A new technique for keratoconus and corneal ectasias. https://youtu.be/qF 9ycSQPq8. Accessed 19 Jul 2022.
20. Jacob S. CAIRS (Corneal Allogeneic Intrastromal Ring Segments) for keratoconus, ectasias & irregular corneas. https://www.youtube.com/watch?v=SkxLwgP8cXA. Accessed 19 Jul 2022.
21. Jacob S. Customised CAIRS. https://www.youtube.com/watch?v=_iiGZqNz-ig&t=9s. Accessed 19 Jul 2022.

Kunal A. Gadhvi and Bruce D. Allan

Key Points

- Endothelial rejection and decompensation, the leading cause of penetrating keratoplasty (PK) failure.
- Deep anterior lamellar keratoplasty (DALK) in conditions with intact endothelium improves graft survival by eliminating endothelial rejection.
- DALK is a difficult surgery with a high intraoperative conversion rate to PK.
- Automating stages of DALK with a femtosecond laser significantly reduce the risk of conversion to PK.
- Minimizing the diameter of Descemet baring to within the confines of the pre-Descemet layer with a mushroom DALK configuration reduces the risk of intraoperative perforation.

Supplementary Information The online version contains supplementary material available at https://doi.org/10.1007/978-3-031-32408-6_22.

K. A. Gadhvi (✉)
Department of Corneal and External Diseases, Liverpool University Hospitals NHS Foundation Trust, Liverpool, UK
e-mail: kunal.gadhvi1@nhs.net

B. D. Allan
Department of Corneal and External Eye Diseases, Moorfields Eye Hospital, London, UK
e-mail: bruce.allan1@nhs.net

Background

Anterior lamellar keratoplasty was first published in 1914, only 9 years after the first penetrating keratoplasty (PK) [1]. It was another 50 years before a deep dissection of the stroma demonstrated that Descemet membrane could be bared, giving rise to deep anterior lamellar keratoplasty (DALK) in 1965 [2].

DALK is a technique of corneal grafting whereby anterior corneal tissue is selectively removed, down to the Descemet or pre-Descemet layer. This can be achieved by a layer-by-layer dissection or more recently, the "Big Bubble" pneumatic or visco-dissection techniques. The benefit of DALK over a full-thickness PK is maintenance of the host endothelium, the rejection of which remains the leading cause of graft failure after PK [3].

Prior to the adoption of contemporary techniques like Melles air reflection or the "Big Bubble," the outcomes of DALK were deemed to be inferior to PK in British and Australian registry studies [4, 5]. DALK was associated with poorer visual outcomes and higher failure rates.

The UK graft registry demonstrates that during the early adoption of DALK with contemporary techniques, failure within 3 years of surgery was twice as likely compared to PK in keratoconus [4]. However, 19% of these early failures were reported within 30 days of surgery with equal survival beyond this time point, demonstrating that surgical technique and management of early post-operative complications were the dominant reasons. Poorer visual outcomes following DALK were related to residual pre-Descemetic stroma of greater than 80 microns [6].

As a result of these factors, the uptake of DALK has lagged compared to the uptake of other forms of lamellar corneal surgery [7]. DALK currently still trails behind PK in the management of keratoconus worldwide.

However, since the wider adoption of modern Descemet baring techniques, it has become easier to remove the stroma and bare the pre-Descemet layer [8]. With these contemporary techniques, visual outcomes and survival for DALK are now similar to PK for common etiologies such as keratoconus [9].

Despite these advances in technique, DALK remains a challenging operation to perform. The risk of perforation of the Descemet membrane and intraoperative conversion from DALK to PK remain high, at 0–24% [9].

Most intraoperative perforations occur in peripheral rather than central corneal dissection. Understanding the anatomy of the posterior cornea may be the key to designing a more reliable technique. In the next section, we will explore the natural cleavage plane in the posterior cornea with a focus on the pre-Descemet layer to demonstrate why the diameter of exposure is important.

Role of the Pre-Descemet layer in DALK

When a pneumatic separation of the posterior cornea with the "Big Bubble" technique is successful, the cleavage plane develops in two potential zones, between the pre-Descemet layer and the stroma (Type 1 bubble- approximately 80% of bubbles) or the Descemet and pre-Descemet/posterior stroma (type 2 bubble—approximately 20% of bubbles) [10]. Type 1 bubbles propagate from the center outward terminating before the limbus (see Fig. 22.1a).

A type 2 bubble is highly unpredictable and frequently bursts intraoperatively because of the fragility of the Descemet layer (see Fig. 22.1b).

The type 1 bubble is stronger because of the presence of the pre-Descemet layer. The pre-Descemet layer is a robust acellular layer in the posterior stroma, impervious to air and conferring a significant strength to the eye. Air trapped between the pre-Descemet and posterior stroma in a type 1 bubble has an average burst pressure of 1.45 bar compared to 0.6 bar in a type 2 bubble [11].

The pre-Descemet layer measures 10.15 +/−3.6 microns thick and is made of predominantly type 1 collagen bundles in 5–11 lamellae in long transverse, longitudinal, and oblique bundles. This layer terminates central to the Descemet layer, inserting into the stroma at 6-9 mm diameter. Consequently, separation of the pre-Descemet from stroma pneumatically is limited to a maximum of 8-9 mm, at which point a white ring will form from stromal emphysema [11]. This diameter, however, is dependent on individ-

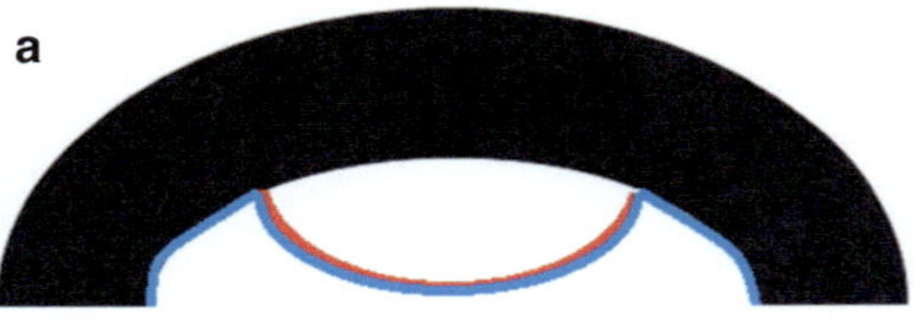

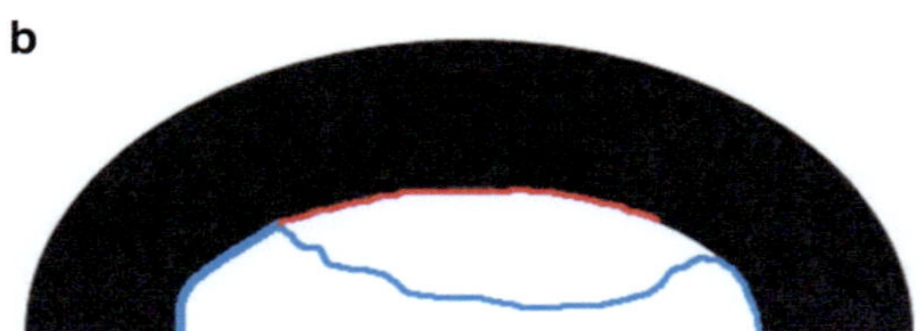

Fig. 22.1 (a) Type 1 bubble. The black dome represents corneal stroma with air trapped between the pre-Descemet in red and the posterior stroma representing the location of a type 1 bubble. Note the abrupt termination of the red Descemet layer and type 1 bubble. (b) Type 2 bubble. Here air is trapped between the Descemet in blue and the pre-Descemet representing the location of a type 2 bubble. The Descemet extends further into the periphery than the pre-Descemet

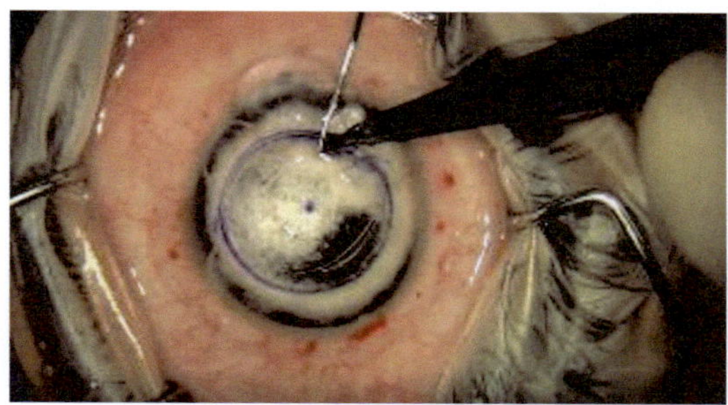

Fig. 22.2 Bubble rupture following visco-expansion of a type 1 bubble

ual anatomy and the maximal diameter of the bubble and will not always match the trephination diameter in cases of DALK. DALK is often converted to PK because the Descemet tears when a type 1 bubble bursts or during peripheral baring of the Descemet (Fig. 22.2).

Reducing the diameter of deep dissection in DALK to 6 mm and respecting the natural anatomy of the pre-Descemet layer should reduce the risk of perforation and subsequent conversion to PK. This is the theory behind the "mini-bubble" DALK/.

A 6 mm DALK would not treat wider stroma pathology such as in keratoconus adequately. However, the mushroom configuration (6 mm diameter deep posterior stromal dissection, large diameter mid/anterior stromal dissection) combines deep central dissection with wider removal of the anterior corneal stroma. Manually, a mushroom pattern dissection is difficult to achieve. But automation using femtosecond laser technology makes mushroom pattern dissection easy and safe.

Use of Femtosecond lasers in Keratoplasty/DALK

Femtosecond lasers have the capacity to deliver complex three-dimensional cut patterns within the cornea through the process of photo-disruption at predetermined depths based on information from optical coherence tomography (OCT) mapping of the corneal dimensions either preoperatively or intraoperatively. The automation of surgery can improve the safety and reproducibility of the trephination steps of keratoplasty.

Different techniques for the use of femtosecond lasers in DALK surgery have been described for over a decade. In 2009, Price and Farid and Steinert et al. [12, 13] demonstrated that the precise determination of cut depth using femtolaser-assisted dissection improved canula placement for pneumatic dissection and enhanced stromal removal in layer-by-layer stromal dissection, helping surgeons to achieve a deep, predetermined depth in the posterior stroma.

Additionally, 3D femtosecond laser-assisted cut profiles can improve tissue apposition by enhancing the surface area of contact between the donor and recipient. Alio et al. report using a femtosecond laser-created mushroom configuration where the amount of visible scar tissue between host and donor is comparatively greater in this configuration compared to conventional vertical trephination [14]. This suggested the presence of enhanced healing which might allow earlier suture removal and protect against late remodeling of the graft host junction in keratoconus (see Fig. 22.3).

A variation of the mushroom pattern is utilized for minibubble femtosecond laser-assisted DALK (F-DALK) combining a large anterior cap (9 mm diameter), removing abnormal corneal stroma in keratoconus over a wide area, with a small diameter posterior optical zone (6 mm) which respects the pre-Descemet layer insertion into the anterior stroma [11] (see Fig. 22.4). This technique more than triples the surface area of contact between the donor and host and reduces the area of Descemet bearing by a factor of 1.8 (see Fig. 22.5). It was hypothesized that a larger anterior cap diameter might also reduce post-keratoplasty astigmatism.

Fig. 22.3 (**a**) Scheimpflug image of manual DALK in cross section 1 year and 10 years postoperative. The recurrence of ectasia outside of the host and remodeling of the graft- host junction are demonstrated. (**b**) This corresponds to an increase in irregular anterior corneal curvature over the same period

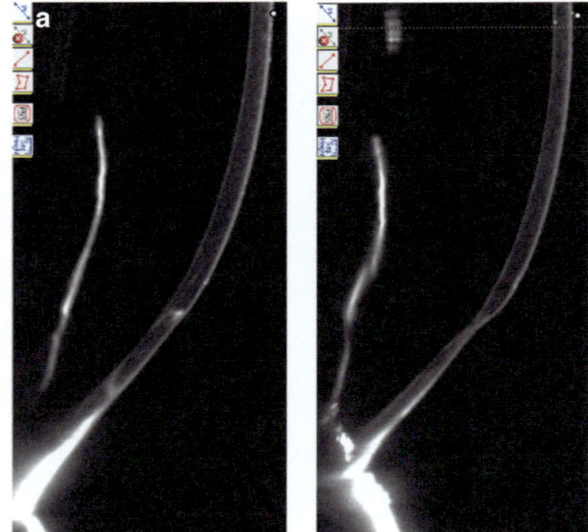

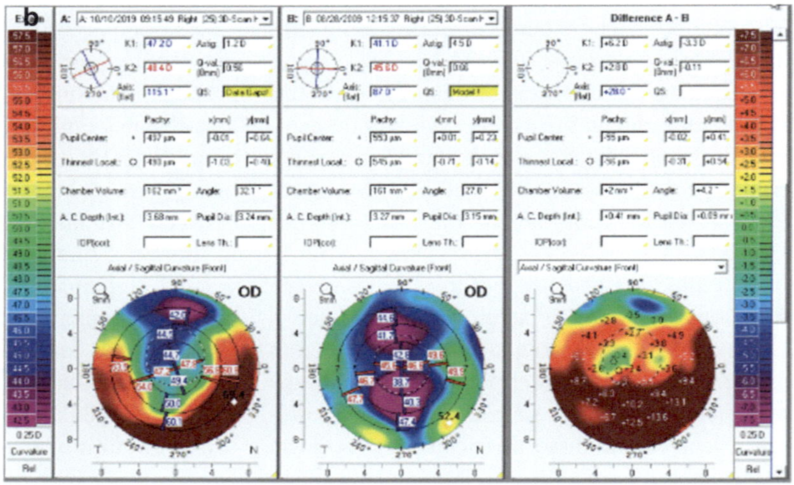

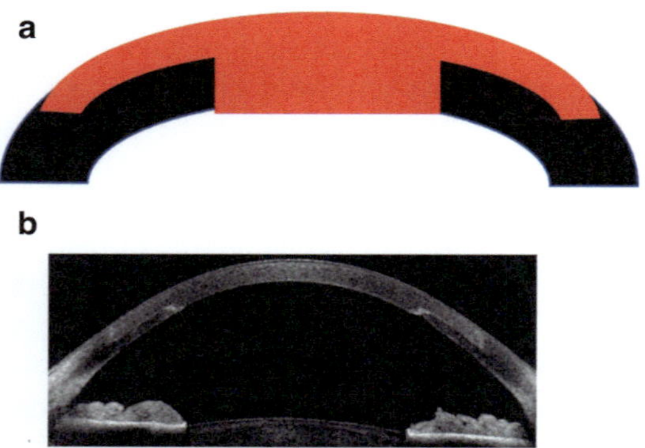

Fig. 22.4 (**a**) Configuration of F-DALK in diagrammatic cross section. (**b**) Postoperative anterior segment OCT of Mushroom pattern Femto-DALK (Casia SS-1000, Tomey, Nagoya, Japan)

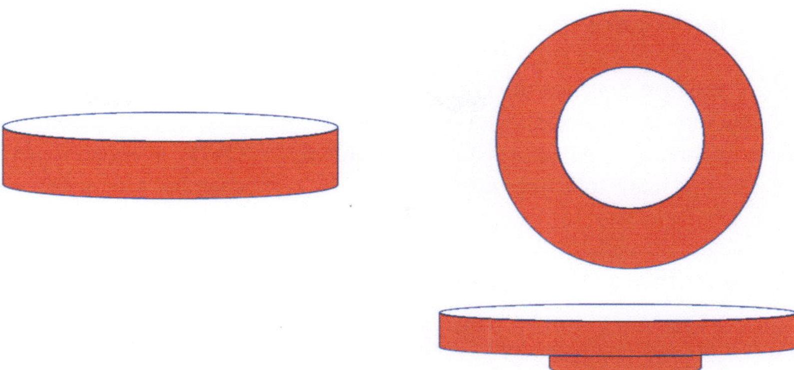

Fig. 22.5 The contact area between donor and host corneal stroma (in red) is over three-fold greater with a mushroom DALK configuration (52mm²) compared to conventional manual DALK (16mm²))

Technique for Mini Bubble mushroom Femto DALK Surgery

In the following section, we will describe a technique for mini-bubble mushroom F-DALK developed at Moorfields Eye Hospital to combine the benefits of a wide anterior stroma removal and a small 6 mm central zone of deep dissection.

Preoperative Planning

Preoperatively, it is important to identify how deep the posterior ring cut of the mushroom keratoplasty needs to be set to allow a deep dissection without perforating the host Descemet membrane. This is achieved by using an optical coherence tomography (OCT) device for mapping of the host cornea to identify the thinnest point at a 6 mm diameter around the corneal vertex (see Fig. 22.6) .

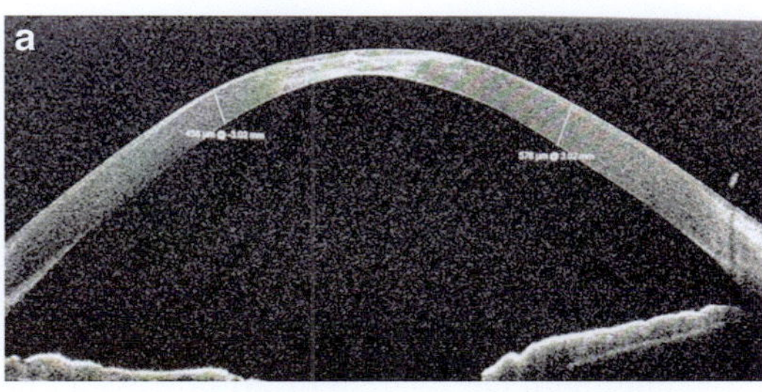

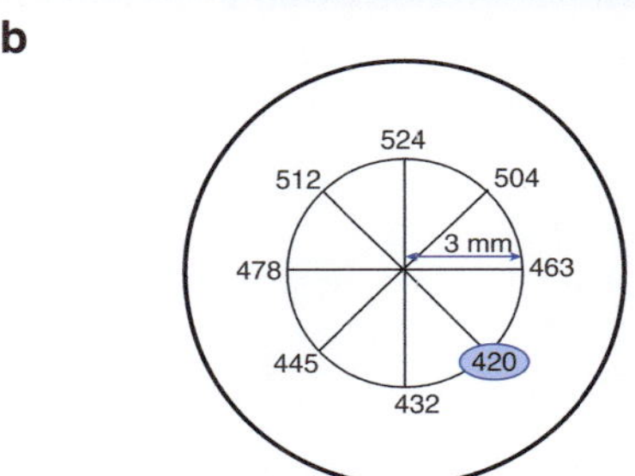

Fig. 22.6 (a) OCT image of keratoconus cornea in cross section. Corneal thickness assessed 3 mm wither side of the corneal vertex at 8 different points. (b) Thinnest point at 6 mm identified and utilized for programming of host femtosecond deep trephination

Laser Setting

A mushroom-cut pattern is programmed in both donor and host corneas using the desired femtosecond Laser device. Some lasers now come with bespoke software; others require the manual programming of parameters.

How to Prepare the Host Cornea

The geometric center of the host cornea needs to be marked as a reference for the forthcoming femtosecond cuts. All cuts are centered in reference to this mark following applanation.

Programming the Host Cut

A 6 mm diameter posterior side-cut is programmed. This is in reference to the minimum thickness measured on OCT at 6 mm minus 70 μm.

The depth of the lamellar ring cut (horizontal cut between 6 and 9 mm) should set as the maximum depth of the posterior side cut minus 50 μm.

The diameter of the anterior side is at 9 mm for most cases, with a reduction to 8.7 mm where the minimum white-to-white measurement is less than 11 mm (estimated on the slit lamp).

A minimum cut overlap of 20 μm should be programmed in all directions to ensure intersection of all cuts (see Fig. 22.7).

How to Prepare the Donor Cornea

The donor corneal button is prepared on an artificial anterior chamber. A thin layer of cohesive OVD covers the anterior surface of the artificial chamber mount to protect the endothelium.

Applanation must be performed with a firm supporting pressure within the artificial anterior chamber. Filtered air is used to bring the chamber to a firm physiological pressure once the locking ring has been engaged symmetrically over the donor corneal limbus. The use of air is important. Air (gas) is compressible during femtosecond applanation even at supraphysiological pressure, whereas balanced salt solution or viscoelastics are not. Air support in the artificial anterior chamber facilitates wide applanation without softening the chamber and is particularly important for clean lamellar dissection using femtosecond lasers with a flat applanation interface.

Once the subcorneal pressure has been checked, the corneal epithelium can be irrigated gently with BSS, then dried carefully around the edges, so that a clear image of a thin meniscus at

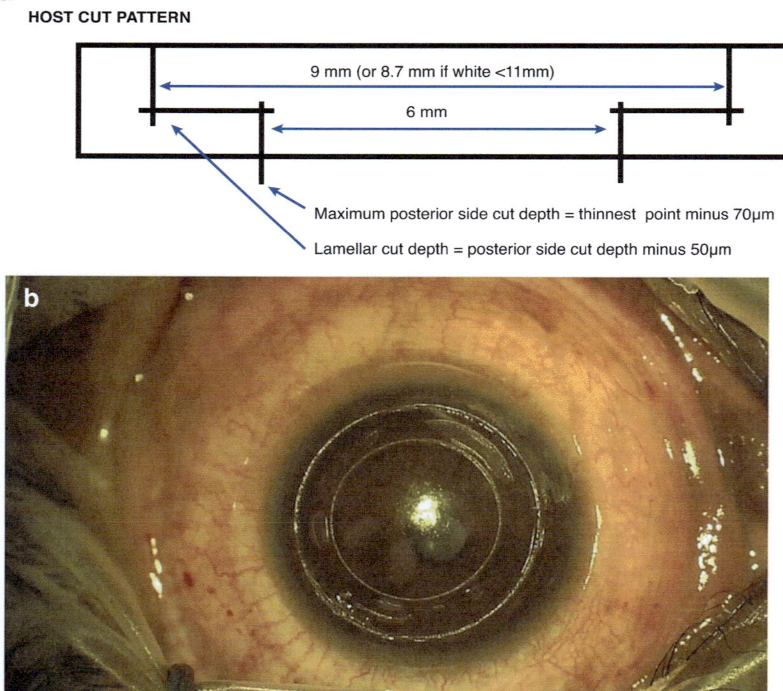

Fig. 22.7 (**a**) Schematic of femtosecond laser cut pattern we used in host corneas based on preoperative OCT measurements of the host cornea. All cuts were programmed to intersect by a minimum of 20 μm. (**b**) Color image of host cornea immediately following femtosecond cut. 6 mm inner and 9 mm outer ring cuts visible

the edge of the applanation is clearly seen during laser docking. Excessive fluid should be avoided, as fluid may become trapped by capillary action between the applanation glass and the cornea giving a false meniscus—a risk factor for an incomplete anterior side cut. The meniscus should be concentric with and just outside the guide marker for maximum cut diameter prior to laser cutting.

Wherever possible, larger diameter donor corneas without extensive peripheral lipid deposition (arcus) should be used. Smaller diameter corneas are no problem for DMEK, but can make dissection of a larger anterior cap in F-DALK difficult. Eye Banks should be aware of this emerging trend in tissue selection preferences.

Laser Parameters for Donor

For the donor cornea, a reciprocal mushroom cut pattern is programmed into the laser. The setting for the anterior side cut diameter is equal to the host diameter plus 0.3 mm (a marginal oversizing). The posterior side cut diameter remains 6 mm, and the lamellar ring cut depth is that of the host depth plus 20 μm. This allows for donor tissue deturgescence post-transplantation. The posterior depth of the donor tissue should be set to maximum to ensure complete anterior chamber penetration (see Fig. 22.8).

After the donor cut is completed, the culture medium should be infused gently through the artificial anterior chamber, to expel air from beneath the donor corneal endothelium. This marks the end of the preparatory stage before the transplantation procedure.

Transplantation Procedure

DALK surgery is usually performed under general anaesthesia or local anaesthesia with sedation. When performing this surgery, the recommended approach is to use a variation of the "Big-Bubble" technique described by Anwar and Teichman [8].

1. Identifying the Inner 6 mm Zone: The first step is blunt dissecting the lamellar cut and marking the inner edge of the lamellar cut 360° with gentian violet. Following the injection of air, surgical emphysema may make this 6 mm diameter posterior side cut harder to identify—the ink will help with this.
2. Creating a channel for the air cannula: The deep aspect of the posterior side cut is identified and dried with a surgical sponge. A small sharp dissection using a bent 27-gauge needle, similar to a Paufique dissector, is made at this level as a deep stromal entry point for a

DONOR CUT PATTERN

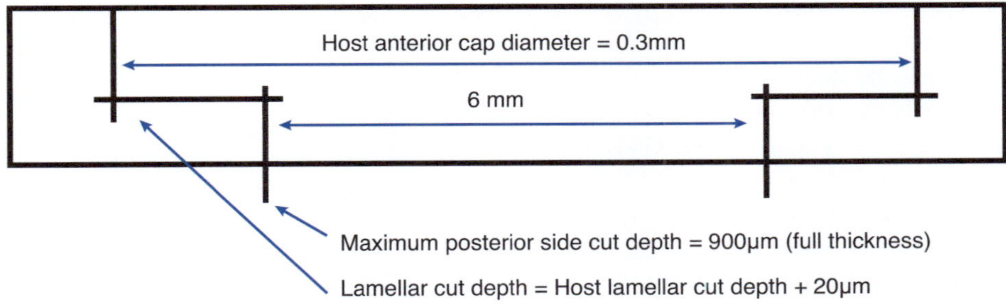

Fig. 22.8 Schematic of femtosecond laser cut pattern we used in donor corneas based on preoperative OCT measurements of the host cornea. All cuts were programmed to intersect by a minimum of 20 μm

blunt trochar to form the track for the air cannula.

The blunt trocar is passed, dissecting as closely as possible to the Descemet membrane (see Fig. 22.9).

3. Pneumatic dissection: A blunt 27-gauge Fontana cannula (Surgistar, Vista, CA) is then advanced down this channel to the center of the cornea for air dissection. Air is injected with the aim of forming a big bubble which will enable dissection down to the pre-Descemet layer in the 6 mm central optical zone (see Fig. 22.10). The bubble should not be expanded much beyond 6mm in order to respect the anatomy of the pre-Descemet layer and minimize the risk of bubble rupture.

4. Checking you have a bubble and removal of stroma: Following attempted air-dissection, the small-bubble technique is used to confirm the presence of a big bubble [15]. A small bubble is introduced to the anterior chamber through a paracentesis and the eye is rolled to ensure that the small bubble remains visible in the anterior chamber periphery. If the small bubble moves into the center of the anterior chamber, this indicates that a big bubble separation of the pre-Descemet layer has not been achieved.

   Where a big bubble is present, it is recommended to proceed as described by Anwar and Teichman to expose the pre-Descemet layer using blunt scissors to clear residual posterior corneal stromal tissue within the 6 mm zone (see Fig. 22.11).

5. Where no bubble is identified: Where no big bubble is achieved, the next stage is visco-dissection with cohesive OVD [16]. If this fails, or if air was injected directly into the anterior chamber, layer-by-layer manual dissection is required to clear the posterior stroma within the optical zone (see Fig. 22.12). Various DALK blunt lamellar dissectors are available for this process. If a micro-perforation develops, then air can be injected via a paracentesis and the dissection continued distal to the site of the perforation. It is often then possible to save the posterior lamella and

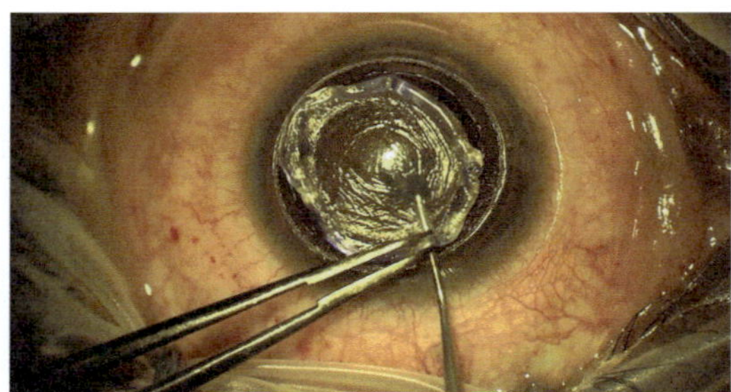

Fig. 22.9 Blunt trochar used to create channel in deep posterior stroma

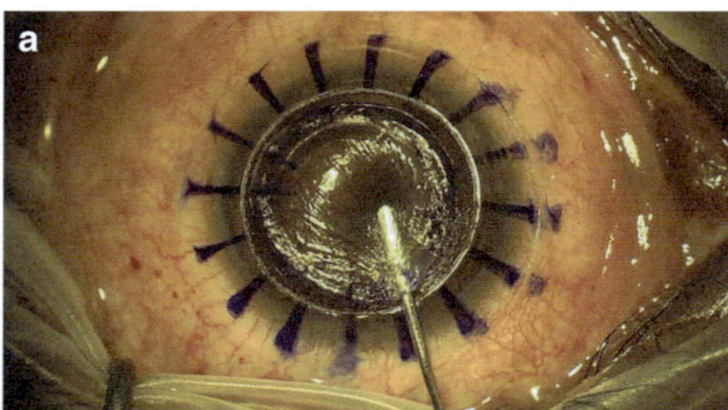

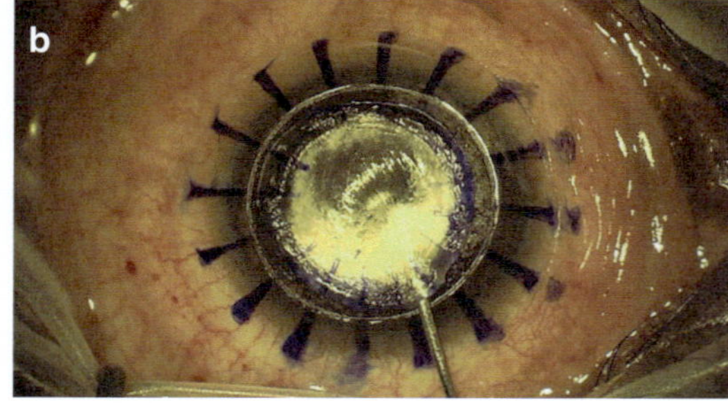

Fig. 22.10 (**a**) Fontana cannula passed through the channel created with the trochar. (**b**) Air injected and mini bubble forms between posterior stroma and pre-Descemet

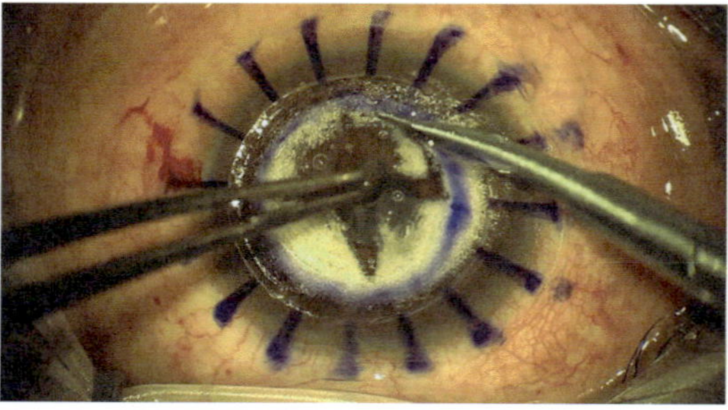

Fig. 22.11 Exposing the pre-Descemet layer following successful big bubble

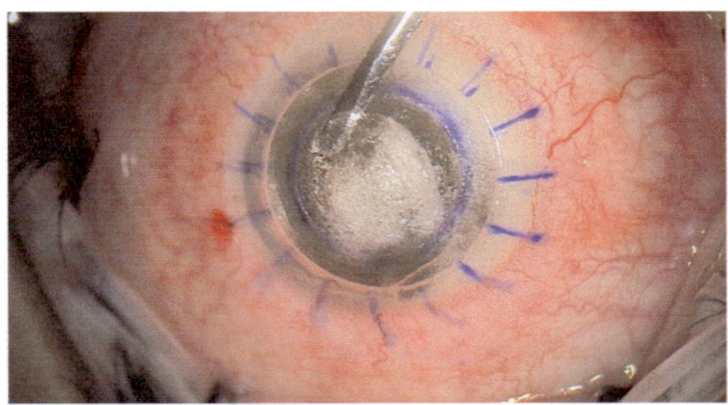

Fig. 22.12 Manual layer-by-layer dissection to clear posterior stroma within the optical zone

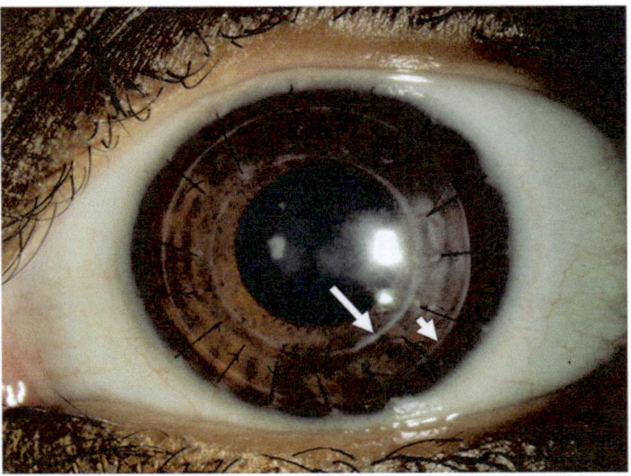

Fig. 22.13 Early postoperative slit lamp image of F-DALK with mushroom configuration. Small white arrow indicates superficial lamellar interface. Large white arrow indicates deep Descemet bearing 6 mm interface

tamponade with air postoperatively, as for endothelial keratoplasty rather than convert to PK. If air tamponade is used, strong pupil dilation must be maintained in the early postoperative period to avoid pupil block.

6. Securing the donor cornea Following host dissection, the predissected donor cornea is peeled from the mounted corneoscleral button. The donor Descemet membrane is removed with semi-dry arrow tip sponges. The donor is then washed in BSS and secured to the host with 16 interrupted 10–0 nylon sutures (see Fig. 22.13). Continuous sutures should be used with caution because of the higher risk of cheese wiring of the nylon through the thinner mushroom cap (typically approximately 350 μm depth). (Video 22.1).

Outcomes of the Mini Bubble mushroom DALK and Contemporary Technique

Perforation and Conversion

In comparison with standard 8 mm manual DALK techniques, we found that minibubble F-DALK resulted in significant reductions in intraoperative perforation of the Descemet layer (25% vs. 45%) and fewer conversions to PK (3% vs. 25%). Our review of 58 consecutive patients found no failures with this technique after 3 years of follow-up. Moorfields Eye Hospital is a multi-surgeon setting in which over 50% of DALK cases are performed by surgeons in training operating under supervision. In these circumstances, in particular, improvements in the safety and technical ease of DALK surgery are important.

Promising outcomes have been reported for other F-DALK techniques. Soulouti et reported a 1/860 perforation rate over 10 years with femtosecond laser-assisted trephination and full-width deep dissection using a variation in Melles air reflection technique, with good visual outcomes at 1 year (CDVA 0.17 ± 0.12) [17]. It remains to be seen whether such promising results can be replicated in a multi-surgeon setting. But this extremely low perforation rate suggests that partial automation using femtosecond laser assistance may enhance safety in DALK.

Big Bubble Success

F-DALK gives enhanced control over trephination depth, but placement of the dissection track for air injection remains poorly controlled with the technique we describe, and we did not observe any benefit for F-DALK in comparison with standard manual DALK in relation to the rate of Type I bubble formation (61 vs. 58%). Other groups have reported similar rates of big bubble formation in manual and F-DALK. Alio et al. observed a "Big Bubble" success rate of 84% with F-DALK and 80% in manual surgery utilizing a mushroom F-DALK configuration with an 8 mm cap and

Table 22.1 Astigmatic outcomes of contemporary F-DALK studies

Study	Laser model	Applanation	n	Diameter (Cut pattern)	Astigmatism (D)	CDVA (LogMAR)
Espandar et al. 2016 [21]	Femtec 520F	Curved	24	9.25 mm (decagonal cut)	1.82 ± 0.67	0.26 ± 0.16
Salouti et al. 2019 [17]	Femtec 520F	Curved	391	9.3–9.5 (mushroom or decagonal)	3.34 ± 1.88	0.09 ± 0.09
Alio et al. 2015 [14]	Intralase iFS	Flat	25	8 mm (mushroom)	5.43 ± NR[#]	0.26 ± NR
Li et al. 2016 [19]	Wavelight FS200	Flat	94	8.2 mm (button)	5.35 ± 1.73	0.08 ± 0.07
Gadhvi et al. 2020 [20]	Intralase iFS	Flat	58	9.17 ± 0.21 (mushroom)	5.00 ± 3.76*	0.16 ± 0.20

6 mm deep optical zone reaching 80% of the thinnest corneal pachymetry [14].

Automating the deep placement of the dissection track for the air injection cannula in big-bubble F-DALK may result in more consistent big bubble formation. Buzzonetti et al. demonstrated positive results using the IntraLase femtosecond laser (Intra-Lase FS Laser; Abbott Medical Optics, Inc., Santa Ana, CA) and a metal mask with a 0.7 mm channel to create a tunnel 100 microns above the thinnest pachymetric point. Cannula placement within this tunnel resulted in successful big bubble formation in 9/10 consecutive eyes in their series [18].

Recent advances, in particular the integration of OCT imaging with femtosecond laser systems, may make variations of this approach more accessible. Liu et al., utilizing the Ziemer LDV Z8 laser (Ziemer Ophthalmic System, Port, Switzerland) used intraoperative OCT guidance and cut programming to create a tunnel cut 3 mm in length, 80 μm in width, at a 60° downward angle to the applanated horizontal plane. This tunnel terminated 50 μm from Descemet membrane. They reported successful big bubble formation after placement of the air dissection canula within this pre-cut dissection track in 14 consecutive cases of F-DALK [19].

Vision outcomes and Refractive Outcomes

In F-DALK with a mushroom profile visual outcomes remain similar to manual DALK surgery despite large graft diameters in the F-DALK technique described. Larger diameter grafts are usually associated with better corneal regularization reflected by reductions in surface irregularity and asymmetry. Consequently, we would have expected that there would be better BSCVA in F-DALK comparative to the smaller diameter manual DALK. We found that 87% of patients undergoing F-DALK achieved BSCVA of 20/40 or better, similar to that of manual DALK surgery at 1 year postoperative [20]. On refraction F-DALK was associated with similar astigmatic outcomes to manual DALK with a mean refractive astigmatism of −5 ± 3.76D following suture removal using the technique described.

The explanation for the absence of improved BSCVA or reduced astigmatism with F-DALK likely arises from the flat applanation of an irregular cornea when creating all cuts with a femtosecond laser. Flat applanation results in distortion and resultant noncircular anterior side cut in irregular corneas, for example, in keratoconus eyes. F-DALK studies using curved applanators show a trend toward lower astigmatism (See Table 22.1).

Future Development

Avenues for further investigation include utilizing liquid interfaces for corneal surgery where applanation can avoided to reduce strain on the cornea and improve the cutting process. At present, this technique is available on the Ziemer LDV Z8 femtosecond laser (Ziemer Ophthalmic System, Port, Switzerland) and has only been utilized in studies of PK [22] and is yet to demonstrate an improvement in circularity of the corneal ex vivo [23] with clinical studies lacking in this area. Additionally liquid interface keratoplasty cut profile is limited to vertical or oblique at present with no mushroom profile programable.

Excimer laser keratoplasty could similarly help improve trephination regularity. In a mixed study of 35 eyes undergoing trephination with an excimer laser (Zeiss Meditec MEL70 excimer laser) and 34 eyes with a femtosecond laser with flat applanation (60-kHz IntraLase™ femtosecond laser) Tóth et al demonstrated a lower post suture removal astigmatism and better BSCVA were achieved in the excimer group inferring less irregular astigmatism [24]. Obviously, the drawback of the excimer laser is the absence of 3-D profiles however this could be overcome by combining with femtosecond assistance for lamellar cuts with the final anterior cap cut made with the excimer laser.

Surgical Pearls

Filling the artificial chamber with air during the applanation phase of donor preparation makes applanation at a supraphysiological pressure easier as air is compressible while liquids or viscoelastics are not.

The large diameter of the anterior cap in F-DALK necessitates large donor corneas without peripheral arcus or opacity which may otherwise interfere with the donor cutting. Do communicate this with your eyebank.

Because of the larger graft with sutures being placed close to the limbus in F-DALK, we found the incidence of loose sutures to be greater. As a result, interrupted sutures or a double running suture provide an added level of security over a single continuous.

Although the endothelium is not transplanted in DALK and rejection more than 2 years after DALK is unusual there is still a significant risk within the first 2 years of surgery and we advise keeping patients on some topical immune suppression, preferably a low dose steroid, during this period.

Take Home Notes

- Mushroom DALK with Femtosecond laser has a lower perforation and conversion rate in multisurgeon settings compared to manual DALK.
- Mushroom configurations reduce the diameter of the Descemet baring which may contribute to this.
- "Mini" type 1 bubble avoids expansion of the bubble to the termination of the pre Descemet. This may reduce bubble rupture rate.
- Flat applanating Femtosecond laser may contribute to higher-than-expected astigmatism despite large graft caps. Future development in curved and liquid interfaces may mitigate this.

References

1. Singh NP, Said DG, Dua HS. Lamellar keratoplasty techniques. Indian J Ophthalmol. 2018;66(9):1239–50.
2. Brown SI, Dohlman CH, Boruchoff SA. Dislocation Of descemet's membrane during keratoplasty. Am J Ophthalmol. 1965;60:43–5.
3. Borderie VM, Sandali O, Bullet J, Gaujoux T, Touzeau O, Laroche L. Long-term results of deep anterior lamellar versus penetrating keratoplasty. Ophthalmology. 2012;119(2):249–55. Feb [cited 2020 Feb 21]. http://www.ncbi.nlm.nih.gov/pubmed/22054997.
4. Jones MNA, Armitage WJ, Ayliffe W, Larkin DF, Kaye SB, NHSBT Ocular Tissue Advisory Group and Contributing Ophthalmologists (OTAG audit study 5). Penetrating and deep anterior lamellar keratoplasty for keratoconus: a comparison of graft outcomes in the United Kingdom. Invest Ophthalmol Vis Sci. 2009;50(12):5625–9. Dec [cited 2020 Feb 21]. http://www.ncbi.nlm.nih.gov/pubmed/19661238.
5. Coster DJ, Lowe MT, Keane MC, Williams KA. Australian corneal graft registry contributors. A comparison of lamellar and penetrating keratoplasty outcomes: a registry study. Ophthalmology. 2014;121(5):979–87. http://www.ncbi.nlm.nih.gov/pubmed/24491643.
6. Ardjomand N, Hau S, McAlister JC, Bunce C, Galaretta D, Tuft SJ, et al. Quality of vision and graft thickness in deep anterior lamellar and penetrating corneal allografts. Am J Ophthalmol. 2007;143(2):228–35.
7. Keenan TDL, Jones MNA, Rushton S, Carley FM. Trends in the indications for corneal graft surgery in the United Kingdom: 1999 through 2009. Arch Ophthalmol. 2012;130(5):621–8.

8. Anwar M, Teichmann KD. Deep lamellar keratoplasty: surgical techniques for anterior lamellar keratoplasty with and without baring of descemet's membrane. Cornea. 2002;21(4):374–83.

9. Gadhvi KA, Romano V, Fernández-Vega Cueto L, Aiello F, Day AC, Allan BD. Deep anterior lamellar Keratoplasty for keratoconus: multisurgeon results. Am J Ophthalmol. 2019;201:54–62.

10. Dua HS, Faraj LA, Kenawy MB, AlTaan S, Elalfy MS, Katamish T, et al. Dynamics of big bubble formation in deep anterior lamellar keratoplasty by the big bubble technique: in vitro studies. Acta Ophthalmol. 2018;96(1):69–76.

11. Dua HS, Faraj LA, Said DG, Gray T, Lowe J. Human corneal anatomy redefined: a novel pre-Descemet's layer (Dua's layer). Ophthalmology. 2013;120(9):1778–85.

12. Farid M, Steinert RF. Deep anterior lamellar keratoplasty performed with the femtosecond laser zigzag incision for the treatment of stromal corneal pathology and ectatic disease. J Cataract Refract Surg. 2009;35(5):809–13.

13. Price FWJ, Price MO, Grandin JC, Kwon R. Deep anterior lamellar keratoplasty with femtosecond-laser zigzag incisions. J Cataract Refract Surg. 2009;35(5):804–8.

14. Alio JL, Abdelghany AA, Barraquer R, Hammouda LM, Sabry AM. Femtosecond laser assisted deep anterior lamellar Keratoplasty outcomes and healing patterns compared to manual technique. Biomed Res Int. 2015;2015:1.

15. Parthasarathy A, Por YM, Tan DTH. Use of a "small-bubble technique" to increase the success of Anwar's "big-bubble technique" for deep lamellar keratoplasty with complete baring of descemet's membrane. Br J Ophthalmol. 2007;91(10):1369–73.

16. Shimmura S, Shimazaki J, Omoto M, Teruya A, Ishioka M, Tsubota K. Deep lamellar keratoplasty (DLKP) in keratoconus patients using viscoadaptive viscoelastics. Cornea. 2005;24(2):178–81.

17. Salouti R, Zamani M, Ghoreyshi M, Dapena I, Melles GRJ, Nowroozzadeh MH. Comparison between manual trephination versus femtosecond laser-assisted deep anterior lamellar keratoplasty for keratoconus. Br J Ophthalmol. 2019;103(12):1716–23.

18. Buzzonetti L, Petrocelli G, Valente P, Iarossi G, Ardia R, Petroni S, et al. The big-bubble full femtosecond laser-assisted technique in deep anterior lamellar Keratoplasty. J Refract Surg. 2015;31(12):830–4.

19. Liu Y-C, Wittwer VV, Yusoff NZM, Lwin CN, Seah XY, Mehta JS, et al. Intraoperative optical coherence tomography-guided femtosecond laser-assisted deep anterior lamellar keratoplasty. Cornea. 2019;38(5):648–53.

20. Gadhvi KA, Romano V, Fernández-Vega Cueto L, Aiello F, Day AC, Gore DM, et al. Femtosecond laser-assisted deep anterior lamellar Keratoplasty for keratoconus: multi-surgeon results. Am J Ophthalmol. 2020;220:191–202.

21. Espandar L, Mandell JB, Niknam S. Femtosecond laser-assisted decagonal deep anterior lamellar keratoplasty. Can J Ophthalmol. 2016;51(2):67–70.

22. Boden KT, Schlosser R, Boden K, Januschowski K, Szurman P, Rickmann A. Novel liquid Interface for femtosecond laser-assisted penetrating Keratoplasty. Curr Eye Res. 2020;45(9):1051–7.

23. Donner R, Schmidinger G. Effects of femtosecond laser-assisted trephination on donor tissue in liquid interface as compared to applanated interface. Acta Ophthalmol. 2022;100(2):e409–13.

24. Tóth G, Szentmáry N, Langenbucher A, Akhmedova E, El-Husseiny M, Seitz B. Comparison of excimer laser versus femtosecond laser assisted trephination in penetrating Keratoplasty: a retrospective study. Adv Ther. 2019;36(12):3471–82.

Large Diameter Deep Anterior Lamellar Keratoplasty

Angeli Christy Yu and Massimo Busin

Key Points

- Deep anterior lamellar keratoplasty (DALK) involves selective replacement of diseased corneal stroma while preserving normal healthy endothelium.
- Despite several well-recognized advantages, DALK has failed to gain widespread popularity among corneal surgeons.
- Compared to conventional DALK, large 9.0-mm diameter DALK can provide superior visual outcomes at higher levels of Snellen BSCVA and significantly lower degrees of astigmatism without an increased risk of immune rejection and graft failure.
- Large diameter DALK with limited stromal clearance within the 6.0-mm optical zone optimizes visual and refractive outcomes while minimizing the risk of complications.

Supplementary Information The online version contains supplementary material available at https://doi.org/10.1007/978-3-031-32408-6_23.

A. C. Yu · M. Busin (✉)
Department of Translational Medicine University of Ferrara, Ferrara, Italy

Introduction

Deep anterior lamellar keratoplasty (DALK) involves targeted replacement of diseased corneal stroma while preserving healthy unaffected endothelium. Although the concept of lamellar grafting was first introduced more than 150 years ago by von Walther and Mühlbauer, DALK has gained renewed interest in recent years [1].

Specifically, various surgeons have developed several techniques for deep lamellar dissection including pneumatic dissection by Archila [2], the big-bubble technique by Anwar and Teichmann [3], hydrodelamination by Sugita and Kondo [4], and viscoelastic-assisted DALK by Maloney and associates [5]. Of these methods, big-bubble DALK has emerged as the most popular approach [2]. Basically, the original technique described by Anwar et al. involves partial thickness trephination followed by angled centripetal advancement of a needle and forceful intrastromal injection of air to obtain the so-called "big-bubble" [2].

One of the main challenges with the big-bubble technique is the need to reach the central cornea while relying on subjective signs of the appropriate cannular depth [6]. However, based on empirical evidence, what is most critical for successful pneumatic dissection is not the radial distance of the tip of the cannula to the center of the cornea but the depth at which air is injected within the corneal stroma [7, 8]. Thus, when the tip of the cannula is inserted within 100 μm from the posterior corneal surface, big-bubble formation can exceed 90% even with minimal centripetal advancement of the cannula [9].

Recent advances in corneal imaging and surgical instrumentation have driven significant improvements in the surgical procedure. Anterior segment optical coherence tomography (OCT) provides accurate measurements of the exact area of interest. Adjustable guarded trephines can be calibrated to the desired depth. It is our preference to set the trephine within 100 μm from the thinnest pachymetry value at the 9 mm zone so that the base of the deep trephination can be used to guide subsequent insertion of the air injection cannula [7]. Instead of trying to reach the proper depth during advancement of the cannula toward the center of the cornea, the insertion of the cannula can be initiated at the base of a deep trephination with minimal centripetal advancement by approximately 2 mm [7]. Using deep trephination during large-diameter DALK, the success rate of pneumatic dissection has been demonstrated to approach up to 85% [10]. Logistic regression analyses of consecutive DALK surgeries have likewise affirmed that both increased trephination diameter and depth positively influence successful big-bubble formation [10–12].

Despite significant advances in the surgical technique and instrumentation, DALK has failed to gain widespread popularity among corneal surgeons [3]. This is probably because the safety benefits of DALK including eliminating the risk of immune endothelial rejection and avoiding progressive endothelial cell loss become fully evident only several years postoperatively. Consequently, most surgeons do not feel sufficiently compelled to face the learning curve in performing this procedure. Instead, an improvement in visual and refractive outcomes, which are directly perceived by patients soon after suture removal, could provide the same surgeons with a greater incentive to transition to DALK.

It is commonly believed that increasing the graft size can improve postoperative visual rehabilitation by minimizing refractive astigmatism. However, with PK, an increase in graft size beyond the conventional 8.0–8.5-mm diameter must be weighed against the higher risk of immunologic endothelial rejection and consequent graft failure. On the other hand, large diameter 9.0-mm DALK has demonstrated excellent visual outcomes, especially at higher levels of Snellen BSCVA without an increased risk of complications.

Indications

The most common indication for DALK is keratoconus (KC), which accounts for more than half of cases. Other surgical indications include traumatic or infective corneal scarring, corneal stromal dystrophy and degeneration, postrefractive surgery ectasia, and scarring due to various causes including severe ocular surface disease with limbal stem cell deficiency, Stevens–Johnson syndrome, ocular cicatricial pemphigoid, and chemical or thermal burns. ALK can also be performed for tectonic indications including pellucid marginal degeneration and sterile Mooren's ulcer.

Keratoconus

Keratoconus is a degenerative corneal disease characterized by progressive corneal thinning and scarring. In its early stages, keratoconus can be managed adequately by spectacle or contact lens correction. However, in cases of reduced visual acuity secondary to corneal scarring and contact lens intolerance due to high degree irregular astigmatism, a surgical intervention would often be required. Since keratoconus cases present with isolated anterior pathology, DALK is an ideal procedure to retain the healthy endothelium and thereby obviate the risk of endothelial graft rejection [13]. In big bubble DALK, advanced stages of keratoconus with high mean K values and lower pachymetry values are associated with more frequent intraoperative complications [10]. The presence of scarring and older age are also significant predictors of type 2 bubble formation which in turn confers an increased risk of complications such as conversion to full-thickness keratoplasty [14, 15].

Corneal Scarring Secondary to Trauma or Infection

In response to an injury or infection, the cornea undergoes a complex process of wound healing involving inflammation, cell proliferation, and tissue fibrosis ultimately leading to stromal scarring. For proper preoperative assessment, anterior segment optical coherence tomography (AS-OCT) is valuable for assessment of the depth and extent of scarring. When possible, the corneal endothelium should also be evaluated by specular microscopy. Given that traumatic and post-infective corneal scars are often associated with otherwise functional endothelium and that most of these patients frequently have an emmetropic fellow eye, DALK should be initially attempted. In cases with a macroperforation or unsatisfactory clearance within the optical zone because of a full-thickness opacity, DALK can be converted to full-thickness keratoplasty.

For cases of scarring due to HSV keratitis, DALK should be contemplated only after the eyes have remained quiescent without episodes of reactivation or inflammation for a period of 6 months or longer. Initial high-dose antiviral prophylaxis with extended taper is recommended to reduce the risk of disease recurrence [16].

Other Indications

DALK can also be adapted for challenging cases with intracorneal ring segments [17], previous radial keratotomy [18], anterior lamellar keratoplasty [19], and even previous DSAEK surgery [20, 21].

Pneumatic dissection can also be achieved in post-PK eyes. However, it is often challenging to prevent expansion of the air bubble beyond the PK wound [22]. Alternatively, stromal exchange can be accomplished through stromal peeling along a natural plane of separation [23]. Ultrastructural alterations in the stromal microarchitecture allow stromal peeling of grafted corneas along a deep natural plane of separation without any type of dissection [23, 24]. The natural plane occurs along a continuous layer of keratocytes separating the overlying anterior stroma from a thin layer of pre-Descemet membrane stroma, which consisted of poorly organized collagen lamellae [24].

Surgical Technique

In 2013, Busin and associates introduced large diameter (9 mm) DALK with limited deep stromal clearance of the 6-mm optical zone [9]. Standardization of the large diameter DALK technique (Fig. 23.1) has substantially simplified the procedure and allowed high success rates independent of surgical experience [25]. Initial partial thickness deep trephination is carried out by a guarded trephine calibrated within 100 μm from the thinnest anterior segment OCT pachymetry value at the 9 mm zone [26]. In cases with significant asymmetry in corneal thickness, peripheral intrastromal hydration with BSS can be performed in zones with relative thinning to safely allow deep trephination [27].

A blunt probe is then inserted 1 mm centripetally from the base of the trephination. The blunt probe is then replaced by a cannula, which is advanced 1 mm further along the same track created by the probe, before attempting pneumatic dissection. Often, significant intrastromal air accumulation in the cornea precludes visualization of the circular silvery sheen of the bubble. In such cases of extensive emphysema, one can ascertain whether big bubble formation has been achieved based on lateral displacement of an air bubble injected intracamerally [28].

Correct identification and management of the type of bubble achieved during pneumatic dissection are instrumental in minimizing complication rates. Depending on the movement of air injected within the corneal stroma, pneumatic dissection can occur along physiologic cleavage planes. A type 1 bubble is a well-circumscribed central dome-shaped elevation that results from a separation between the deep stroma from the pre-Descemet layer while a type 2 bubble is a large, thinner-walled elevation at the level of Descemet membrane [29]. Since the residual bed consists of a thin Descemet's membrane-endothelium

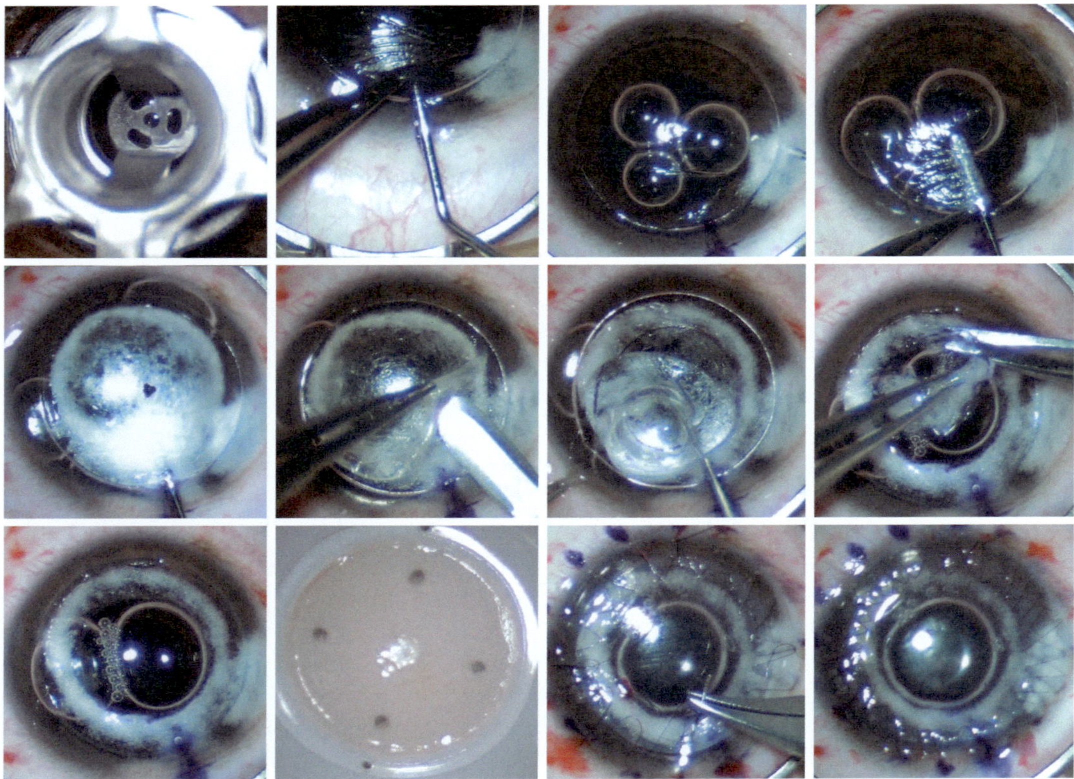

Fig. 23.1 Intraoperative steps of large diameter (9 mm) big bubble deep anterior lamellar keraotplasty with stromal clearance limited to the 6 mm optical zone

complex, a type 2 bubble is associated with a lower bursting pressure and is therefore more fragile [30].

After en bloc anterior keratectomy is performed starting from the base of deep trephination, the central 6 mm of the bubble roof is removed by baring the optical zone at the level of the pre-Descemet's layer or Descemet's membrane (DM), depending on the plane of dissection achieved [9].

Since a type 1 bubble is often limited within 7–8 mm optical zone, we prefer to combine large-diameter keratoplasty with limited stromal clearance within the central 6 mm [9]. Several investigators have likewise employed limited stromal clearance for femtosecond laser-assisted DALK [31, 32]. By respecting the anatomy of the pre-Descemet layer, restricting the deep dissection to the central cornea has been shown to reduce the risk of Descemet's membrane perfora-

tion and conversion to PK [9]. The presence of a peripheral stromal shoulder also protects the recipient bed during suturing, which has been reported to cause up to 21% of intraoperative Descemet's membrane perforations during conventional DALK surgery [33]. Over time, remodeling of the corneal stromal architecture with progressive disappearance of the posterior step at the edge of the 6 mm zone has also been observed (Figs. 23.2 and 23.3) [13].

A 9-mm anterior lamellar graft is then prepared by means of a 400-µm microkeratome head and sutured into place. The donor cornea is initially fixed with four cardinal 10–0 nylon sutures at 3, 6, 9, and 12 o'clock. Interrupted or double-running 10–0 nylon sutures can be used depending on the primary pathology and presence of neovascularization [9].

Although baring of the Descemet's membrane can be attempted in cases with a type 2 bubble,

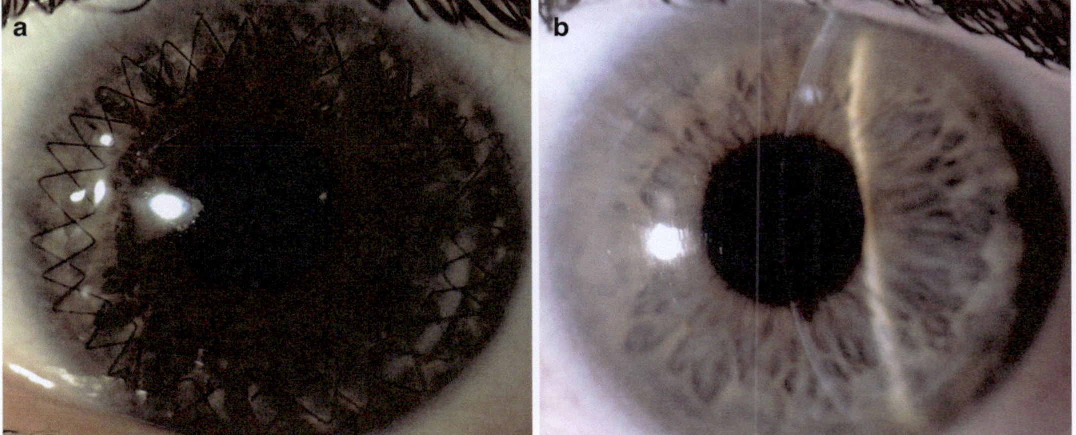

Fig. 23.2 Slit lamp photos taken 1 month (**a**) and 5 years (**b**) after large diameter DALK

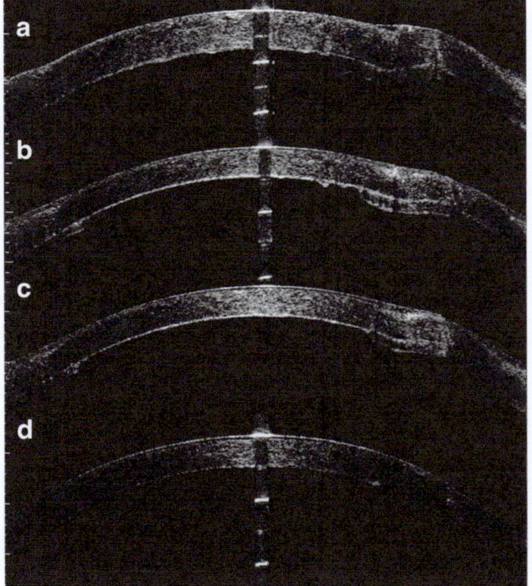

Fig. 23.3 Anterior segment optical coherence tomography showing the transition between the 6-mm central zone and the 9 mm outer zone with the residual recipient stroma. One day postoperatively a peripheral stromal shoulder is clearly visible (**a**) but eventually disappears through spontaneous stromal thinning and remodeling of posterior corneal curvature 1 month (**b**), 1 year (**c**), and 2 years (**d**) after surgery

manual or viscoelastic-assisted dissection techniques are often preferred in order to avoid inadvertent Descemet's membrane perforation [34]. Type 2 bubble formation is the strongest independent risk factor for double anterior chamber formation and conversion to PK [14, 15]. A mixed type 1 and 2 bubble is typically managed as in a type 1 bubble, allowing the type 2 bubble to resorb spontaneously [13].

Even with the current surgical technique, the overall success rate of pneumatic dissection still ranges between 60 and 85% [1]. In the event of failed big-bubble formation, other lamellar dissection techniques can be employed to salvage DALK surgery. Through the so-called microbubble incision technique, additional air can be injected into the corneal stroma. The presence of emphysematous tissue can then be used to guide layer-by-layer dissection, which is aimed at achieving a smooth recipient bed while removing as much residual corneal stroma as possible [35].

Since manual dissection is particularly tedious and is a significant risk factor for conversion to PK, we prefer sequential viscoelastic-assisted dissection in cases of failed pneumatic dissection and consider manual dissection only when all else fails [13, 36]. Even in cases of failed pneumatic dissection, the success of visco-bubble formation approaches 90% [36]. Although retained viscoelastic is initially associated with visually significant interface haze, the effect on visual acuity is transient and final outcomes are comparable with those of big-bubble DALK (Video 23.1) [37].

Optimizing Visual Outcomes

In the past, success following corneal transplantation was defined by the presence of a clear corneal graft [38]. Today, however, visual acuity is considered the primary criteria for surgical success. Based on some earlier comparative studies, visual outcomes were apparently worse following DALK due to inclusion of cases, which were not reflective of the contemporary surgical technique, and, thus, were likely associated with irregular or incomplete lamellar dissection [39–41]. Currently used surgical techniques, which exploit physiologic cleavage planes, result in a clear graft host-interface compatible with satisfactory visual outcomes, comparable with PK [26, 42]. Although prospective clinical trials are ideally required to make statistically valid comparisons, randomizing patients to PK over DALK could no longer be justified especially in view of the disproportionately higher risk for potentially severe complications following PK. Nevertheless, empiric evidence from large interventional case series has thus far validated the clinical benefits of DALK [26, 43, 44].

From a refractive standpoint, the use of large-diameter grafts for DALK has been shown to provide superior visual outcomes with lower degrees of myopia and astigmatism [36, 45]. In a large series of 346 eyes, 9 mm DALK is associated with excellent outcomes with up to 94% of cases achieving Snellen vision ≥20/40 and up to 89% with refractive astigmatism <4.5 diopters [26]. Unlike PK, large-diameter DALK does not pose an increased risk of immune-mediated stromal rejection, which in any case can be managed medically [16]. Additionally, performing large-diameter keratoplasty maximizes the removal of the diseased stroma, thereby preventing disease recurrence [46].

Managing Complications

The use of larger grafts conceivably provokes apprehension among some surgeons due to the potential need of conversion to full-thickness keratoplasty in cases of a significant perforation.

In our practice, should such complications occur during large-diameter DALK, the procedure is converted to 2-piece mushroom PK, as first described in 2004, instead of a full-thickness PK [9]. Minimal endothelial transplantation in mushroom PK combines excellent visual and survival outcomes with a lower risk of immune rejection related to less antigenic load [47].

The most frequent complication encountered during DALK is Descemet's membrane perforation [1]. If limited to a micro-perforation, the surgery can still be successfully completed as per standard technique by filling the anterior chamber with air. In cases with a macroperforation or unsatisfactory clearance within the optical zone because of a full-thickness opacity, DALK can be converted to full-thickness keratoplasty. A mushroom-shaped wound configuration for full-thickness keratoplasty whether obtained through microkeratome- or femtosecond laser-assisted techniques can be considered in order to combine the advantages of a large anterior refractive surface with minimal endothelial transplantation [9, 32].

Double anterior chamber formation is another complication following DALK. Inadvertent perforation of DM, even if surgery is still successfully completed without the need for conversion to PK, has been described to lead to an increased risk of early postoperative detachment of the recipient bed and consequent double anterior chamber formation. This has been found to occur without a perforation detected intraoperatively, while, on the other hand, an intraoperative perforation does not necessarily lead to the formation of a double anterior chamber. Corneal scarring, perforation, and the occurrence of a type 2 bubble are known independent risk factors for double anterior formation following DALK. Although there are reports of spontaneous resolution, this complication usually requires rebubbling with air or gas to be managed successfully. Complete AC air fill is maintained for 2 h before release of air at the slit lamp to achieve a fluid level at the height of the inferior pupillary border, thereby eliminating the risk of pupil block [15].

One of the leading causes of limited visual recovery after DALK is high astigmatism especially when greater than 4.5 D. With refraction after DALK stabilizing approximately 6 months after complete suture removal, refractive surgery can be subsequently performed to reduce residual postoperative astigmatism. Residual refractive errors after DALK can be managed through corneal or lens-based procedures. Astigmatic keratotomy, either manual or femtosecond laser-assisted, has been found to reduce astigmatism, although generally with unpredictable results [48]. Deeper, longer, and more central incisions are often required to achieve a greater treatment effect. An advantage to DALK with limited central stromal clearance would be the ability to create deep arcuate blunt relaxing incisions within the graft–host interface which result in satisfactory outcomes with minimal risk of perforation [49]. In the presence of a cataract, lens extraction with implantation of monofocal or even toric intraocular lenses can also be contemplated [50, 51]. For IOL power calculation, it must be considered that a tendency toward a myopic refractive shift is often observed in post-DALK eyes. Although the SRK/T, Kane, EVO, and Hoffer QST formulas tend to provide more accurate outcomes, the predictability of refractive outcomes following cataract surgery remains lower than in virgin eyes [52].

Other complications of DALK include persistent epithelial defect, corneal neovascularization, glaucoma, high astigmatism, cataract formation, and interface infection [13, 53].

Automated solutions have been explored to further address the technical challenges associated with DALK. Cross-sectional imaging can reduce the surgeon's dependence on subjective cues during the critical depth-dependent steps. Intraoperative OCT platform provides direct visualization and allows instantaneous quantitative analysis of acquired OCT scans for intraoperative planning based on patient-specific corneal anatomy [54–56]. Thus far, however, most of the proposed applications of intraoperative OCT during DALK are primarily qualitative [54, 55]. Based on our initial experience with a microscope-integrated intraoperative OCT with a built-in caliper tool, trephination depth can be used to assist decision-making on whether to proceed with pneumatic dissection or extend the trephination groove, which in turn can be used to guide subsequent placement of the air injection cannula [56]. Further work is still needed to establish and achieve the full potential of intraoperative OCT for intraoperative guidance of lamellar surgery.

Several investigators have also explored femtosecond laser-assisted DALK surgery [57–63]. As in stepped PK wounds, customized trephination patterns created using the femtosecond laser confer the advantage of an increased donor-host junction surface area, which theoretically can provide superior wound strength, induce faster wound healing, and allow earlier suture removal [57]. The femtosecond laser system can also be employed to create a deep intrastromal tunnel for the air injection cannula for pneumatic dissection [58]. However, one of the main drawbacks of femtosecond laser DALK is the poor laser penetration through opacified and neovascularized corneal tissue, which can result in incomplete or irregular dissection [64]. Although Li et al. demonstrated better visual outcomes following femtosecond laser-assisted DALK, visual performance in the manual DALK group was poorer due to greater residual bed thickness obtained in diamond knife-assisted lamellar dissection [63]. Moreover, all other published studies comparing manual and femtosecond laser-assisted DALK, thus far, consistently find no significant differences in terms of final visual acuity [58–62]. In general, the internal validity of these comparative studies is affected by the retrospective design [58–62], heterogenous study populations [59, 60], unequal sample sizes [60, 61, 63], or varied surgical protocols for lamellar dissection [59, 62, 63], graft sizing [59, 60, 63], and even suture techniques [59]. Randomized controlled trials based on sufficient sample size and standard protocol would be necessary to allow direct comparison and assessment of the true benefit of femtosecond laser technology for DALK.

Take Home Notes

- With its superior safety profile and favorable postoperative outcomes, current evidence supports that DALK outperforms PK for the management of anterior corneal pathology sparing the endothelium.

- Recent advances in corneal imaging and available instrumentation have led to the standardization of the big-bubble DALK technique.
- Regardless of the success of big-bubble formation, other lamellar dissection techniques can be employed sequentially as an alternative to pneumatic dissection.
- Since the unaffected host endothelium is retained, DALK provides the opportunity to use large-diameter grafts, which can more reliably achieve maximum visual potential without an increased risk of immune-mediated stromal rejection.

References

1. Yu AC, Spena R, Pellegrini M, et al. Deep anterior lamellar keratoplasty: current status and future directions. Cornea. 2022;41(5):539–44.
2. Archila EA. Deep lamellar keratoplasty dissection of host tissue with intrastromal air injection. Cornea. 1984;3(3):217–8.
3. Anwar M, Teichmann KD. Big-bubble technique to bare descemet's membrane in anterior lamellar keratoplasty. J Cataract Refract Surg. 2002;28(3):398.
4. Sugita J, Kondo J. Deep lamellar keratoplasty with complete removal of pathological stroma for vision improvement. Br J Ophthalmol. 1997;81:184–8.
5. Manche EE, Holland GN, Maloney RK. Deep lamellar keratoplasty using viscoelastic dissection. Arch Ophthalmol. 1999;117(11):1561–5.
6. Scorcia V, Lucisano A, Pietropaolo R, et al. Red reflex-guided big-bubble deep anterior lamellar keratoplasty: a simple technique to judge dissection depth. Cornea. 2015;34(9):1035–8.
7. Busin M, Scorcia V, Leon P, et al. Outcomes of air injection within 2 mm inside a deep trephination for deep anterior lamellar keratoplasty in eyes with keratoconus. Am J Ophthalmol. 2016;164:6–13.
8. Scorcia V, Busin M, Lucisano A, et al. Anterior segment optical coherence tomography-guided big-bubble technique. Ophthalmology. 2013;120(3):471–6.
9. Busin M, Leon P, Nahum Y, et al. Large (9 mm) deep anterior lamellar keratoplasty with clearance of a 6-mm optical zone optimizes outcomes of keratoconus surgery. Ophthalmology. 2017;124(7):1072–80.
10. Scorcia V, Giannaccare G, Lucisano A, et al. Predictors of bubble formation and type obtained with pneumatic dissection during deep anterior lamellar keratoplasty in keratoconus. Am J Ophthalmol. 2020;212:127–33.
11. Borderie VM, Touhami S, Georgeon C, et al. Predictive factors for successful type 1 big bubble during deep anterior lamellar keratoplasty. J Ophthalmol. 2018;2018:4685406. https://doi.org/10.1155/2018/4685406.
12. Feizi S, Javadi MA, Daryabari SH. Factors influencing big-bubble formation during deep anterior lamellar keratoplasty in keratoconus. Br J Ophthalmol. 2016;100(5):622–5.
13. Yu AC, Mattioli L, Busin M. Optimizing outcomes for keratoplasty in ectatic corneal disease. Curr Opin Ophthalmol. 2020;21(4):268–75.
14. Myerscough J, Friehmann A, Bovone C. Evaluation of the risk factors associated with conversion of intended deep anterior lamellar keratoplasty to penetrating keratoplasty. Br J Ophthalmol. 2020;104(6):764–7.
15. Myerscough J, Bovone C, Mimouni M, et al. Factors predictive of double anterior chamber formation following deep anterior lamellar keratoplasty. Am J Ophthalmol. 2019;205:11–6.
16. Giannaccare G, Weiss JS, Sapigni L, et al. Immunologic stromal rejection after deep anterior lamellar keratoplasty with grafts of a larger size (9 mm) for various stromal diseases. Cornea. 2018;37(8):967–72.
17. Ravera V, Bovone C, Scorcia V, et al. Deep anterior lamellar Keratoplasty in eyes with intrastromal corneal ring segments. Cornea. 2019;38(5):642–4.
18. Einan-Lifshitz A, Belkin A, Sorkin N, et al. Evaluation of big bubble technique for deep anterior lamellar keratoplasty in patients with radial keratotomy. Cornea. 2019;38(2):194–7.
19. Yu AC, Myerscough J, Galante G, et al. Pneumatic dissection for large-diameter (9-mm) deep anterior lamellar keratoplasty in eyes with previous anterior lamellar keratoplasty. Cornea. 2021;40(9):1098–103.
20. Gutfreund S, Leon P, Graffi S, et al. Deep anterior lamellar keratoplasty after descemet stripping automated endothelial keratoplasty. Am J Ophthalmol. 2017;175:129–36.
21. Busin M, Beltz J. Deep anterior lamellar keratoplasty after descemet stripping automated endothelial keratoplasty. Cornea. 2011;30(9):1048–50.
22. Scorcia V, Beltz J, Busin M. Small-bubble deep anterior lamellar keratoplasty technique. JAMA Ophthalmol. 2014;132:1369–71.
23. Bovone C, Nahum Y, Scorcia V, et al. Stromal peeling for deep anterior lamellar keratoplasty in post-penetrating keratoplasty eyes. Br J Ophthalmol. 2022;106(3):336–40.
24. Busin M, Bovone C, Scorcia V, et al. Ultrastructural alterations of grafted corneal buttons: the anatomic basis for stromal peeling along a natural plane of separation. Am J Ophthalmol. 2021;231:144–53.
25. Myerscough J, Bovone C, Scorcia V, et al. Deep trephination allows high rates of successful pneumatic dissection for DALK independent of surgical experience. Cornea. 2019;38(5):645–7.
26. Myerscough J, Roberts H, Yu AC, et al. Five-year outcomes of converted mushroom keratoplasty from intended deep anterior lamellar keratoplasty

(DALK) mandate 9-mm diameter DALK as the optimal approach to keratoconus. Am J Ophthalmol. 2020;220:9–18.

27. Bovone C, Myerscough J, Friehmann A, et al. Peripheral intrastromal hydration facilitates safe, deep trephination in corneas of irregular thickness. Cornea. 2020;39(2):207–9.

28. Parthasarathy A, Por YM, Tan DTH. Using a "small bubble technique" to aid in success in Anwar's "big bubble technique" of deep lamellar keratoplasty with complete baring of descemet's membrane. Br J Ophthalmol. 2008;92(3):422.

29. Dua HS, Faraj LA, Kenawy MB. Dynamics of big bubble formation in deep anterior lamellar keratoplasty by the big bubble technique: in vitro studies. Acta Ophthalmol. 2018;96(1):69–76.

30. AlTaan SL, Mohammed I, Said DG. Air pressure changes in the creation and bursting of the type-1 big bubble in deep anterior lamellar keratoplasty: an ex vivo study. Eye (Lond). 2018;32(1):145–51.

31. Shehadeh-Mashor R, Chan CC, Bahar I, et al. Comparison between femtosecond laser mushroom configuration and manual trephine straight-edge configuration deep anterior lamellar keratoplasty. Br J Ophthalmol. 2014;98:35–9.

32. Gadhvi KA, Romano V, Cueto LFV, et al. Femtosecond laser-assisted deep anterior lamellar keratoplasty for keratoconus: multi-surgeon results. Am J Ophthalmol. 2020;220:191–202.

33. Huang OS, Htoon HM, Chan AM, et al. Incidence and outcomes of intraoperative Descemet membrane perforations during deep anterior lamellar keratoplasty. Am J Ophthalmol. 2019;199:9–18.

34. Myerscough J, Friehmann A, Bovone C, et al. Management of type 2 bubble formed during big bubble deep anterior lamellar keratoplasty (letter to the editor). Cornea. 2019;38:e20.

35. Riss S, Heindl LM, Bachmann BO, et al. Microbubble incision as a new rescue technique for big-bubble deep anterior lamellar keratoplasty with failed bubble formation. Cornea. 2013;32(2):125–9.

36. Scorcia V, De Luca V, Lucisano A, et al. Results of viscobubble deep anterior lamellar keratoplasty after failure of pneumatic dissection. Br J Ophthalmol. 2018;102(9):1288–92.

37. Scorcia V, De Luca V, Lucisano A, et al. Comparison of corneal densitometry between big-bubble and visco-bubble deep anterior lamellar keratoplasty. Br J Ophthalmol. 2019;104:336–40.

38. Cornea Donor Study Investigator Group. The effect of donor age on corneal transplantation outcome results of the cornea donor study. Ophthalmology. 2008;118(4):620–6.

39. Shimazaki J, Shimmura S, Ishioka M, et al. Randomized clinical trial of deep lamellar keratoplasty vs penetrating keratoplasty. Am J Ophthalmol. 2002;134:159–65.

40. Funnell CL, Ball J, Noble BA. Comparative cohort study of the outcomes of deep lamellar keratoplasty and penetrating keratoplasty for keratoconus. Eye (Lond). 2006;20:527–32.

41. Ardjomand N, Hau S, McAlister JC, et al. Quality of vision and graft thickness in deep anterior lamellar and penetrating corneal allografts. Am J Ophthalmol. 2007;143:228–35.

42. Han DC, Mehta JS, Por YM, et al. Comparison of outcomes of lamellar keratoplasty and penetrating keratoplasty in keratoconus. Am J Ophthalmol. 2009;148:744–51.

43. Arundhati A, Chew MC, Mehta JS, et al. Comparative study of long-term graft survival between penetrating keratoplasty and deep anterior lamellar keratoplasty. Am J Ophthalmol. 2021;224:207–16.

44. Borderie VM, Sandali O, Bullet J, et al. Long-term results of deep anterior lamellar versus penetrating keratoplasty. Ophthalmology. 2012;119(2):249–55.

45. Huang T, Hu Y, Gui M, et al. Large-diameter deep anterior lamellar keratoplasty for keratoconus: visual and refractive outcomes. Br J Ophthalmol. 2015;99:1196–200.

46. Yu AC, Franco E, Caruso L, et al. Ten-year outcomes of microkeratome-assisted lamellar keratoplasty for keratoconus. Br J Ophthalmol. 2021;105(12): 1651–5.

47. Yu AC, Spena R, Fusco F, et al. Long-term outcomes of two-piece mushroom Keratoplasty for traumatic corneal scars. Am J Ophthalmol. 2022;236:20–31.

48. Kubaloglu A, Coskun E, Sari ES, et al. Comparison of astigmatic keratotomy results in deep anterior lamellar keratoplasty and penetrating keratoplasty in keratoconus. Am J Ophthalmol. 2011;151:637–43.

49. Elkadim M, Myerscough J, Bovone C, et al. A novel blunt dissection technique to treat modified deep anterior lamellar keratoplasty (DALK)-associated high astigmatism. Eye (Lond). 2020;34(8):1432–7.

50. Scorcia V, Lucisano A, Savoca V, et al. Deep anterior lamellar keratoplasty followed by toric lens implantation for the treatment of concomitant anterior stromal diseases and cataract. Ophthalmol Point Care. 2017;1:oapoc.0000008.

51. Pellegrini M, Furiosi L, Yu AC, et al. Outcomes of cataract surgery with toric intraocular lens implantation after keratoplasty. J Cataract Refract Surg. 2022;48(2):157–61.

52. Pellegrini M, Furiosi L, Salgari N, et al. Accuracy of intraocular lens power calculation for cataract surgery after deep anterior lamellar keratoplasty. Clin Exp Ophthalmol. 2022;50(1):17–22.

53. Pellegrini M, Scorcia V, Giannaccare G, et al. Corneal neovascularisation following deep anterior lamellar keratoplasty for corneal ectasia: incidence, timing and risk factors. Br J Ophthalmol. 2021;106:1363. https:// doi.org/10.1136/bjophthalmol-2021-319339.

54. De Benito-Llopis L, Mehta JS, Angunawela RI, et al. Intraoperative anterior segment optical coherence tomography: a novel assessment tool during deep anterior lamellar keratoplasty. Am J Ophthalmol. 2014;157(2):334–41.

55. Steven P, Le Blanc C, Lankenau E, et al. Optimising deep anterior lamellar keratoplasty (DALK) using intraoperative online optical coherence tomography (iOCT). Br J Ophthalmol. 2014;98(7):900–4.

56. Santorum P, Yu AC, Bertelli E, Busin M. Microscope-integrated intraoperative optical coherence tomography-guided big-bubble deep anterior lamellar keratoplasty. Cornea. 2022;41(1):125–9.
57. Farid M, Steinert RF. Deep anterior lamellar keratoplasty performed with the femtosecond laser zigzag incision for the treatment of stromal corneal pathology and ectatic disease. J Cataract Refract Surg. 2009;35(5):809–13.
58. Lucisano A, Giannaccare G, Pellegrini M, et al. Preliminary results of a novel standardized technique of femtosecond laser-assisted deep anterior lamellar Keratoplasty for keratoconus. J Ophthalmol. 2020;2020:5496162. https://doi.org/10.1155/2020/5496162.
59. Shehadeh-Mashor R, Clan C, Yeung SN, et al. Long-term outcomes of femtosecond laser-assisted mushroom configuration deep anterior lamellar keratoplasty. Cornea. 2013;32(4):390–5.
60. Salouti R, Zamani M, Ghoreyshi M, et al. Comparison between manual trephination versus femtosecond laser-assisted deep anterior lamellar keratoplasty for keratoconus. Br J Ophthalmol. 2019;103(12):1716–23.
61. Bleriot A, Martin E, Lebranchu P, et al. Comparison of 12-month anatomic and functional results between Z6 femtosecond laser-assisted and manual trephination in deep anterior lamellar keratoplasty for advanced keratoconus. J Fr Ophthalmol. 2017;40(6):e193–200.
62. Alio JL, Abdelghany AA, Barraquer R, et al. Femtosecond laser assisted deep anterior lamellar keratoplasty outcomes and healing patterns compared to manual technique. Biomed Res Int. 2015;2015:397891.
63. Li S, Wang T, Bian J, et al. Precisely controlled side cut in femtosecond laser-assisted deep lamellar keratoplasty for advanced keratoconus. Cornea. 2016;35(10):1289–94.
64. Yu AC, Friehmann A, Myerscough J, et al. Initial high-dose prophylaxis and extended taper for mushroom keratoplasty in vascularized herpetic scars. Am J Ophthalmol. 2020;217:212–23.

Regenerative Surgery of the Corneal Stroma for Advanced Keratoconus

24

Mona El Zarif, Jorge L. Alió del Barrio, and Jorge L. Alió

Key Ponits

- Previous studies have demonstrated, in the animal model, the capacity of human stem cells (implanted within the corneal stroma) to alleviate corneal scars, improve corneal transparency, generate new organized collagen within the corneal host stroma, and with immunosuppressive and immunomodulatory properties.
- Autologous extraocular stem cells do not require a healthy contralateral eye and they do not involve any ophthalmic procedure for their isolation. Mesenchymal stem cells have been the most widely assessed and have a high potential to differentiate into functional adult keratocytes in vivo and in vitro.

- Advanced stem cell therapy of the corneal stroma, with implantation of autologous ADASCs with or without decellularized human corneal stroma, showed good preliminary results for the treatment of advanced keratoconus in the first clinical trial recently published.

Introduction

Keratoconus is the most common corneal dystrophy with a diverse prevalence in the population from 0.05 to 2.3%. Being a relatively prevalent disease, it is more observed today than before due to the more advanced diagnostic tools that are available for the diagnosis of early keratoconus [1]. Moreover, a recent meta-analysis found that keratoconus is prevalent in 1.38 per 1000 of the world's population (95% CI: 1.14–1.62 per 1000) [2]. It is characterized by progressive thinning, bulging, and distortion of the cornea and causes progressive changes in vision with increased myopia and myopic astigmatism, corneal irregularity, and visual loss [3].

The corneal stroma constitutes more than 90% of the corneal thickness. Many features of the cornea including its strength, morphology, and transparency are attributable to the anatomy and properties of the corneal stroma [4]. The extracellular matrix of the corneal stroma is composed of collagen, which forms more than 70% of the weight of the dehydrated cornea, the most abun-

Supplementary Information The online version contains supplementary material available at https://doi.org/10.1007/978-3-031-32408-6_24.

M. El Zarif
Optica General, Saida, Lebanon

Division of Ophthalmology, Universidad Miguel Hernández, Alicante, Spain

Lebanese University, Doctoral School of Sciences and Technology, Beirut, Lebanon

J. L. A. del Barrio · J. L. Alió (✉)
Vissum Miranza, Miguel Hernández University, Alicante, Spain
e-mail: jlalio@vissum.com

dant being type I (75%), and proteoglycans including keratan sulfate which is the most abundant (65%) whose protein nucleus is composed of lumican, keratocan, and mimecan [4]. Keratocan is expressed only in the corneal stroma; therefore, it is considered in tissue engineering as a specific marker of keratocytic differentiation [5]. The cellular component of the corneal stroma occupies only 2–3% of the stromal volume, and in it, the largest cells are keratocytes, which are distributed among the collagen lamellae, mesenchymal cells derived from the neural crest. In the normal corneal keratocytes are in a quiescent state, and they are responsible for the continuous replacement of the stromal extracellular matrix through the production of collagen, which is very essential for the maintenance of corneal transparency. When keratocytes have an activated metabolism, they transdifferentiate into fibroblasts and myofibroblasts and participate in the corneal stroma's healing. The renewal capacity of stromal keratocytes is due to precursor cells in the anterior limbal corneal stroma, which expresses adult stem cell markers [6].

Keratoconus is characterized by a progressive loss of keratocytes: their number decreases from anterior to posterior stroma [7], leading to the progressive thinning of the stroma [1, 7] and a decrease in corneal strength [8]. This definition is valid for most patients with keratoconus, although some variations in the phenotypic expression of the disease might be present [9]. Most keratoconus cases have thin corneas and a weak mechanical resistance related to the progressive loss of keratocyte density [10]. Apoptosis of keratocytes [7, 11] or enzymes is thought to be the cause of keratocyte loss and consequently loss of corneal stroma over time [7, 11]. The proportion of the corneal keratocytes is decreased with the progression of the disease [7]. In the end stages of keratoconus, the clinical aspects of the thin and debilitated cornea are associated with a sharp decrease in the number of keratocytes. A severe corneal deformation is observed [7], and an alteration in the location of the corneal apex is obtained [12], causing a severe visual loss.

The prevalence and progressive character of keratoconus have led to the suggestion of different alternative therapies, such as collagen crosslinking (**CXL**), intracorneal rings and segments, corneal transplantation, and more recently, Bowman's membrane (**BM**) implantation [3]. Meanwhile, advanced corneal ectasias require penetrating or lamellar corneal transplantation techniques to enhance visual rehabilitation, which presents several drawbacks such as failure, graft rejection, and slow visual recovery due to high levels of induced postoperative astigmatism related to the sutures [3]. Also, it should be considered that in several countries, access to donor corneal tissue is limited, approximately 53% of the world's population has no access to corneal transplantation [13]. Therefore, the demand for adequate donor corneas is increasing faster than the number of donors, leaving thousands of curable patients around the world waiting for possible treatment [14, 15]. The quantification of the great shortage of corneal graft tissue showed that a cornea is only available for 70 cases needed [13].

To solve the global health problem, recent research studies have focused on developing in the laboratory corneal substitutes that could mimic human cornea features in vivo, and subsequently could be a substitute to human donor tissue, to find an alternative to classical corneal transplantation, but this has not yet been achieved due to the extreme difficulty of mimicking the ultrastructure of the highly complex corneal stroma, obtaining substitutes that no achieve sufficient transparency or resistance [16, 17]. Furthermore, synthetic scaffolds have raised some important concerns, such as strong inflammatory responses induced in their biodegradation, or non-specific chronic inflammatory responses [18]. On the other hand, several corneal decellularization techniques have recently been performed, which provide an acellular corneal matrix (**ECM**) [19]. These scaffolds have gained great interest as they provide an ideal natural environment for cell growth and differentiation (either transplanted donor cells or migratory host cells) [20]. Also, components of the **ECM** are generally preserved among species, and the removal of all immunogenic cellular components could open the field of xenotransplantation to human recipients by using porcine donor tissue, which shares important similarities with the human cornea [21].

In the last few years, cellular therapy of the corneal stroma has been gaining interest as a potential alternative treatment option for corneal stroma diseases such as corneal scarring, dystrophies, and ectasias. Such diseases induce distortion of the anatomy and physiology of the cornea and lead to loss of its transparency and subsequent loss of vision. Using mesenchymal stem cells (**MSCs**) from either ocular or extraocular sources has gained a lot of importance; studies showed that **MSCs** are capable of differentiating into adult keratocytes in vitro and in vivo [4]. Numerous authors, including reports from our research group, have proved [18, 20, 22] that these stem cells can not only survive and differentiate into adult human keratocytes in xenogeneic scenarios without inducing an inflammatory reaction but also produce new collagen within the corneal stroma [22, 23], and modulated the preexisting scars [24, 25], and improving the corneal transparency in animal models [26–29]. MSCs have also shown immunomodulatory properties in syngeneic, allogeneic, and even xenogeneic scenarios [29, 30]. Early clinical data on the safety and preliminary efficacy of corneal stromal cell therapy from Phase 1 human clinical trials are now available for up to 3-year outcomes [31, 32], which may soon provide a real alternative treatment option for corneal diseases.

Considering existing scientific evidence, it seems that all types of **MSCs** have similar behavior in vivo (Table 24.1), and thus can achieve keratocyte differentiation and modulate the corneal stroma with immunomodulatory properties [33]. It has also been newly reported that **MSCs** secrete paracrine factors such as vascular endothelial growth factor (**VEGF**), platelet-derived growth factor (**PDGF**), hepatocyte growth factor (**HGF**), and transforming growth factor-beta 1 (**TGFβ1**). Although the precise actions of the different growth factors for cornea wound healing are not fully understood, overall, they seem to promote cell migration, keratocyte survival by apoptosis inhibition, and upregulate the expression of the **ECM** component genes in keratocytes, subsequently enhancing corneal re-epithelialization and stromal wound healing [34]. **MSCs** can be acquired from many human tissues, including adipose tissue, umbilical cord, placenta, bone marrow, dental pulp, gingiva, hair follicle, and cornea [35, 36]:

1. Corneal stromal stem cells (**CSSCs**) are a promising source for cellular therapy as the isolation technique and culture methods have been optimized and refined [37]; presumably, they should be efficient in differentiating into keratocytes as they are already committed to the corneal lineage. On the other hand, isolating **CSSCs** autologously is more technically demanding considering the small amount of tissue that they are obtained from. Furthermore, this technique still requires a contralateral healthy eye, which is not always available (bilateral disease). Therefore, these drawbacks may limit its use in clinical practice. Allogeneic **CSSC** use requires living or cadaveric donor corneal tissue.

2. Human adult adipose tissue is a good source of autologous extraocular stem cells as it satisfies many requirements: easy accessibility to the tissue, high cell retrieval efficiency, and

Table 24.1 Stem cells assessed for corneal stroma regeneration: evidence of keratocyte or keratocyte-like differentiation and their potential autologous application

	BM-MSCs	CSSCs	UMSCs	ESCs	ADASCs	iPSCs
Keratocyte differentiation in vitro demonstrated	Yes	Yes	Yes	Yes	Yes	Yes
Keratocyte differentiation in vivo demonstrated	Yes	Yes	Yes	No	Yes	No
Possible autologous use	Yes	Yes/no	Yes/no	No	Yes	Yes

BM-MSCs bone marrow mesenchymal stem cells, *CSSCs* corneal stromal stem cells, *MSCs* mesenchymal stem cells, *UMSCs* umbilical MSCs, *(ESCs)* embryonic stem cells, *ADASCs* adipose-derived adult stem cells, *iPSCs,* induced pluripotent stem cells

the ability of its human adipose-derived adult stem cells (**h-ADASCs**) to differentiate into multiple cell types (keratocytes, osteoblasts, chondroblasts, myoblasts, hepatocytes, neurons, etc) [22]. This cellular differentiation occurs due to the effect of very specific stimulating factors or environments for each cell type, avoiding the mix of multiple kinds of cells in different niches.

3. Bone marrow **MSCs** (**BM-MSCs**) are the most widely studied **MSCs**, presenting a similar profile to adipose-derived adult stem cells (**ADASCs**), but their extraction requires a bone marrow puncture, which is a complicated and painful procedure requiring general anesthesia.

4. Umbilical **MSCs** (**UMSCs**) present an attractive alternative, but their autologous use is currently limited as the umbilical cord is not generally stored after birth.

5. Embryonic stem cells (**ESCs**) have great potential, but also present important ethical issues. However, the use of induced pluripotent stem cells (**iPSCs**) technology [38] could solve such problems, and their capability to generate adult keratocytes has already been proven in vitro [39].

Finally, it is important to remark that the therapeutic effect of **MSCs** in a damaged tissue is not always related to the potential differentiation of the **MSCs** in the host tissue as multiple mechanisms might contribute simultaneously to this therapeutic action, for example, secretion of paracrine trophic, and growth factors capable of stimulating resident stem cells, reduction of tissue injury and activation of immunomodulatory effects, in which case the direct cellular differentiation of the **MSCs** might not be relevant and could even be non-existent [33, 40–42].

Background: Translational Regenerative Surgery

In the last few years, interest in cellular therapy of the corneal stroma using MSCs from either ocular or extraocular sources has gained a lot of interest; studies show that MSCs are capable of differentiating into adult keratocytes in vitro and in vivo [4]. Several authors, including reports from our research group, have demonstrated [18, 20, 22] that these stem cells can not only survive and differentiate into adult human keratocytes in xenogeneic scenarios without inducing an inflammatory reaction but also: (1) produce new collagen within the host stroma [22, 23], (2) modulate preexisting scars by corneal stroma remodeling [24, 25], and (3) improve corneal transparency in animal models for corneal dystrophies by collagen reorganization as well as in animal models for metabolopathies by the catabolism of accumulated proteins [26–29].

The use of autologous human keratocytes in cell therapy of the corneal stroma is a promising therapeutic approach, but it has many disadvantages, such as causing damage to the donor's cornea, insufficient cells, and inefficient cell subculture [43]. On the other hand, based on previous successful animal studies performed in part by our team, it has been investigated an extraocular source of abundant and more accessible cells for this purpose [22, 23]. The adipose tissue has shown to be an ideal source of autologous stem cells, known as "human adipose-derived adult stem cells" (**h-ADASCs**), that can differentiate into different cell lineages [22, 43]. Moreover, these cells have shown immunomodulatory properties even in xenogeneic scenarios [18, 20]. We found that human **ADASCs** transplanted into damaged rabbit corneas were able to differentiate in corneal keratocytes and produce corneal collagens and keratocan that are representative of the human corneal stroma [22]. Besides, the corneal decellularized matrices provide a more natural environment for the growth and differentiation of cells compared to synthetic scaffolds, it has been demonstrated the efficiency of Sodium dodecyl sulfate (**SDS**) decellularization on the human cornea. In our study, we used decellularized human corneal laminas alone, or repopulated by **h-ADASCs**, which have been shown excellent results during the follow-up, the corneal transparency has been completely preserved without any signs of scarring [20]. We have been able to demonstrate that the **h-ADASCs** transplanted into a human decellularized lamina survives at least 12 weeks after transplantation in vivo in the animal model, and they also differentiate into human keratocytes, Therefore, with this model, we could potentially be able to obtain an autologous graft using adipose tissue from the patient and an allogeneic donor cornea, theoretically avoiding the risk of stromal rejection associated with allogenic lamellar transplant options [20]. Also, the advantage of our protocol is the possibility of obtaining several grafts from a unique allogeneic donor, increasing the availability of donor tissue, and shortening waiting lists.

The goal of this research line is to translate the research done by our group and apply it to human patients suffering from keratoconus. A simple procedure of liposuction and a nontransplantable donor cornea can provide an optically transparent autologous stromal graft, with excellent demonstrated biocompatibility. With the new noninvasive surgical technique, many complications associated with the usual techniques can be avoided, improving the visual parameters and the quality of life of patients.

These experimental studies opened the translational of this concept into the therapy of human corneal diseases, using the advanced keratoconus disease as the model for this type of advanced therapy. This study aims to build a stem cell therapy alternative to the classic corneal transplantation techniques to regenerate the corneal stroma, avoiding the complications and limitations commonly observed with existing techniques.

Clinical Human Surgery in Advanced Keratoconus

Recently, our group performed the implantation of **ADASCs** and decellularized/recellularized laminas in 14 patients with advanced keratoconus (Video 24.1). This clinical experience opens a new and exciting line of research therapy. The production of new **ECM** by the implanted **MSCs** was demonstrated in previous animal studies, although was not quantitatively enough to be able to restore the thickness of a severely diseased human cornea such as keratoconus. Meanwhile,

the implantation of decellularized/recellularized laminas could restore the corneal thickness and the keratometric parameters (Video 24.2). Nevertheless, the direct injection of stem cells may provide a promising treatment modality for corneal dystrophies, corneal stroma opacification, and the modulation of corneal scarring.

Study Design, and Subjects

This investigation was a prospective interventional randomized, nonmasked consecutive series of cases. The study was conducted in strict adherence to the tenets of the Declaration of Helsinki and it was registered in *ClinicalTrials.gov* (Code: NCT02932852).

Fourteen patients were enrolled in the study and were randomly distributed into three study groups: Group 1 (G-1) patients received ADASCs implantation ($n = 5$ patients); group 2 (G-2) received decellularized human corneal stroma implantation ($n = 5$ patients); and group 3 (G-3) sreceived autologous ADASCs-recellularized human corneal stroma implantation ($n = 4$ patients).

Thirteen patients completed the clinical follow-up, only one patient from G-1 was lost after the first postoperative month because of inability to attend further follow-up for motives unrelated to the study.

Inclusion and exclusion criteria were defined in previous publications [31, 32, 44, 45]. As well clinical follow-up of the patients was established at 1, 3, 6, 12, and 36 months for the clinical outcomes of the investigation and to survey implant safety for a long time.

Methodology

Autologous ADASC Isolation, Characterization, and Culture

Patients underwent standard liposuction. Approximately 250 mL of fat mixed with local anesthesia were obtained from each patient. The adipose tissue processing was performed according to the procedures described in the previous articles [22, 31, 46–48].

Laminas

The human corneal stroma of donor corneas with negative viral serology, but with nonviable endothelium was used. The corneas were provided by the eye bank. The quality and safety standards for donation, procurement, testing, processing, conservation, storage, and testing of human cells and tissues were followed. Donor corneas were dissected with IntraLase iFS femtosecond laser (AMO, Santa Ana, CA), 2–3 consecutive laminas of 120 (µm) thick, and 9.0 mm in diameter were obtained. The decellularization protocol was based on previous publications [19, 20, 32, 49]. The recellularized tissue was placed 24 h before implantation in tissue culture wells for recellularization with autologous ADASCs (0.5 × 106 cells per 1 mL of PBS were cultured on each side of the laminas). Then the laminas were immersed in PBS at room temperature and transported to implantation [32, 44, 45].

Surgical Procedure

Autologous ADASC Implantation

The method for the implantation of ADASCs has been previously described [30]. Topical anesthesia was used. 60 kHz IntraLase iFS femtosecond laser (AMO Inc., Irvine, CA) was used in a single-pass mode for the recipient corneal lamellar dissection. An intrastromal laminar cut of 9.5 mm in diameter was created at a medium depth of the thinnest preoperative pachymetry point measured by the Visant OCT (Carl Zeiss, Germany). Three million autologous ADASCs contained in 1 mL PBS were injected into the pocket.

Lenticule Implantation

Topical anesthesia was applied with oral sedation for all surgeries, and the 60-kHz IntraLase iFS femtosecond laser was used in single-pass mode. Assisted corneal dissection was done with a 50° anterior cut. After opening the corneal intrastro-

mal pocket, the lamina was inserted, centered, and unfolded through gentle tapping and massaging from the epithelial surface of the host. Also before implantation, a temporary limbal paracentesis was performed to reduce intraocular pressure. In those cases, which received a recellularized lamina (G-3), to compensate for the cellular damage expected by the implantation process, the pocket was irrigated immediately before and after insertion with a solution containing an additional one million autologous ADASc in 1 mL of PBS with a 25G cannula. The incision was then closed with an interrupted 10/0 nylon suture [19, 32, 44, 45].

Postoperative Care and Follow-Up Schedule

Postoperatively, the patients were followed at 1 day, 1 week, and at 1, 3, 6, 12, and 36 months for the evaluation of clinical parameters: unaided distance visual acuity (UDVA), corrected distance visual acuity (CDVA), rigid contact lens distance visual acuity (CLDVA) in (decimal equivalent to the logMar scale), refractive sphere (Rx Sphr) in diopters (D), and refractive cylinder (Rx Cyl) (D). Central corneal thickness (CCT) (µm) was measured by (AS-OCT) (Visante, Carl Zeiss). Scheimpflug corneal topography thinnest point (Thinnest point) (µm), cornea volume (CV) (mm^3), corneal aberrometry, anterior mean keratometry (anterior Km) (D), posterior mean keratometry (posterior Km) (D), maximum keratometry (Kmax) (D), topographic cylinder (Topo Cyl) (D), and corneal densitometry (CD) (Pentacam; Oculus Inc., Wetzlar, Germany). Slit-lamp biomicroscopy, fundoscopy, intraocular pressure (Goldmann applanation tonometry IOP) (mmHg), and endothelial cell density (ECD) ($cells/mm^2$) by specular microscopy (Nidek, Aichi, Japan). The confocal microscopy study was completed up to 12 months using the confocal microscope HRT3 RCM (Heidelberg) with Rostock Cornea Module.

Results

Slit Lamp Biomicroscopy and AS-OCT Results

No complications were observed during the 3-year follow-up. No adverse events, such as haze or infection, were obtained. All corneas did not show any posterior stromal or predescemetic scars and presented a fully transparent visual axis (Figs. 24.1, 24.2, 24.3, and 24.4). Full corneal transparency was recovered within the first postoperative day in all patients of G-1 (Fig. 24.1a, b) At the level of the stromal pocket, a neo-collagen production was observed as patchy hyperreflective areas (Fig. 24.2a, b) [31, 44, 45]. Meanwhile,

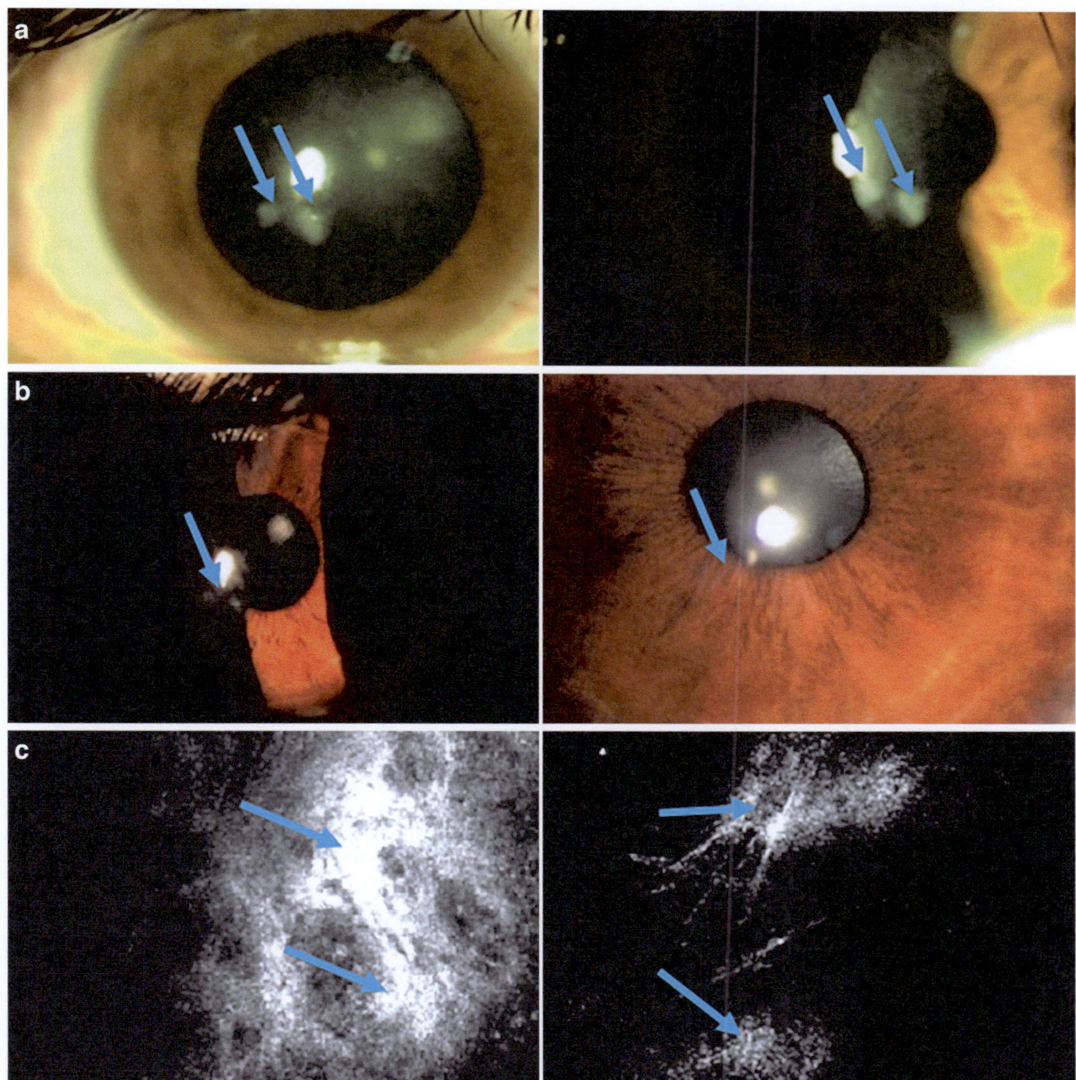

Fig. 24.1 Biomicroscopic changes among the preoperative and up to 36 months postoperative, confocal microscopy findings till 12 months postoperative in G-1, case-2. (**a**) Observe the presence of paracentral scars (blue arrows) at the preoperative level (left) and 1 month postoperative (right). (**b**) Notice the marked improvement of the paracentral scars (blue arrows), at 12 months (left), and 36 months (right). (**c**) Confocal microscopy findings in the same Case-2: notice the high reflective deposits and fibrotic tissue in the anterior stroma of the corneal at the preoperative level (blue arrows; left), that corresponded to the paracentral scars. At 12 months (right), an improvement of the anterior stroma fibrotic tissue could be noticed (blue arrows)

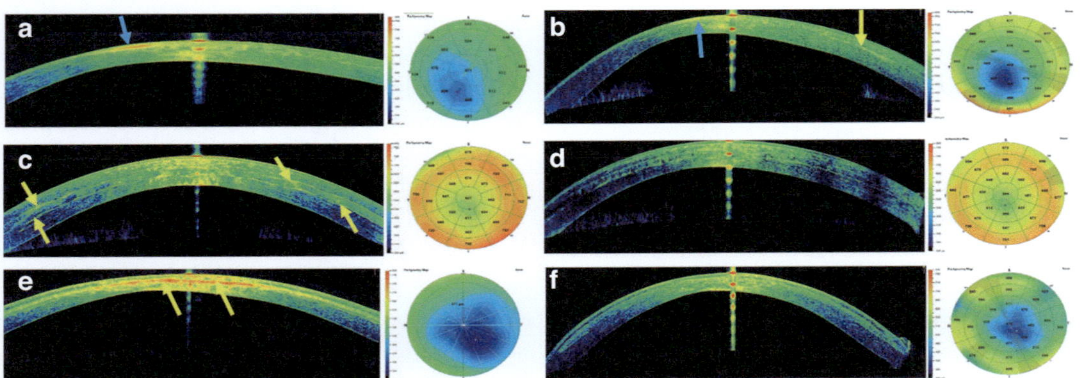

Fig. 24.2 Corneal anterior segment OCT sections and pachymetric maps (Visante) in G-1, G-2 & G-3. (**a**) G-1, (case-2) at 1 month postoperative: observe the reflective paracentral scar (blue arrow). (**b**) The same patient after 36 months: shows low reflectance of the band of neocollagen (yellow arrow), the reflective paracentral scar has disappeared (bleu arrow). (**c**) G-2, (case-6) at 6 months: observe the high reflectance of the implanted lamina (yellow arrows) and the restoration of the corneal thickness. (**d**) Same patient after 36 months: observe the improvement in the integration of the implanted lamina in the host stoma, and the stability of the pachymetric map. (**e**) G-3, (case-11) at 1 month: observe the high reflectance of the implanted lamina (yellow arrows). (**f**) Same patient as (**e**) at 36 months: notice the integration of the implanted tissue in the host stroma and the enhancement in corneal densitometry

the implanted laminas in G-2, and G-3 showed a mild early haziness during the first postoperative month. This issue was related to mild lenticular edema. Corneal full transparency was observed within the third postoperative month in all patients (Figs. 24.2c–f, 24.3a, b, 24.4a, b) [32, 44, 45].

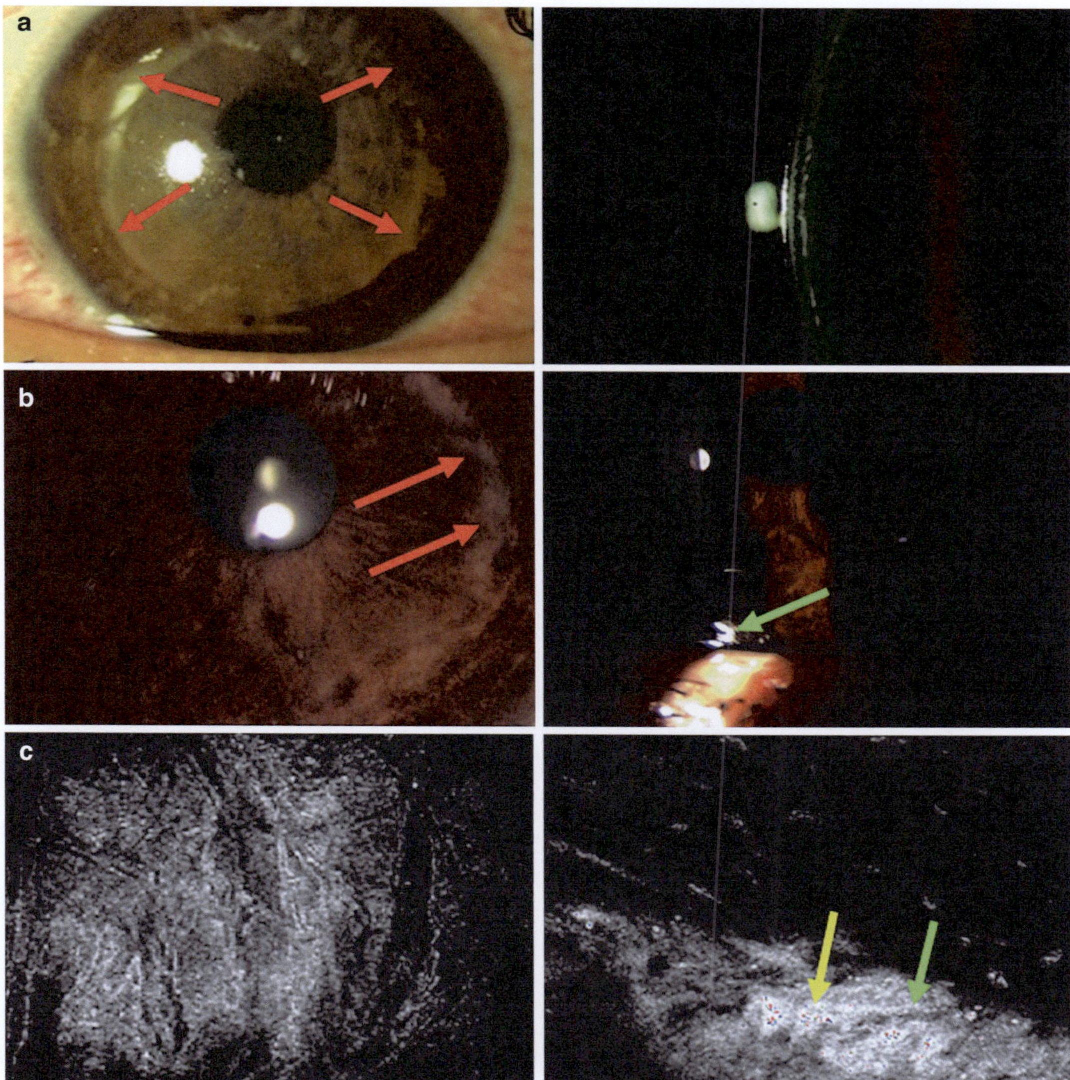

Fig. 24.3 Biomicroscopic changes between the preoperative and up to 36 months postoperative, confocal microscopy findings till 12 months post-op in G-2, case-5. (**a**) At 1 day postoperative (left and right): reduced transparency due to edema of the implanted lamina. (Red arrows) show the borders of the lamina. (**b**) Improvement in the transparency of the implanted tissue at 36 months (red arrows). Paracentral fibrotic tissue at the surgical plane (green arrow; right). (**c**) Confocal microscopy finding at 1 month (left) we can observe the acellular anterior surface of the decellularized lamina. After 12 months (right), we can notice in the periphery of the lamina migrating keratocytes nuclei from the host stroma toward the posterior surface of the decellularized lamina (yellow arrow), and the presence of some paracentral fibrotic tissue (green arrow)

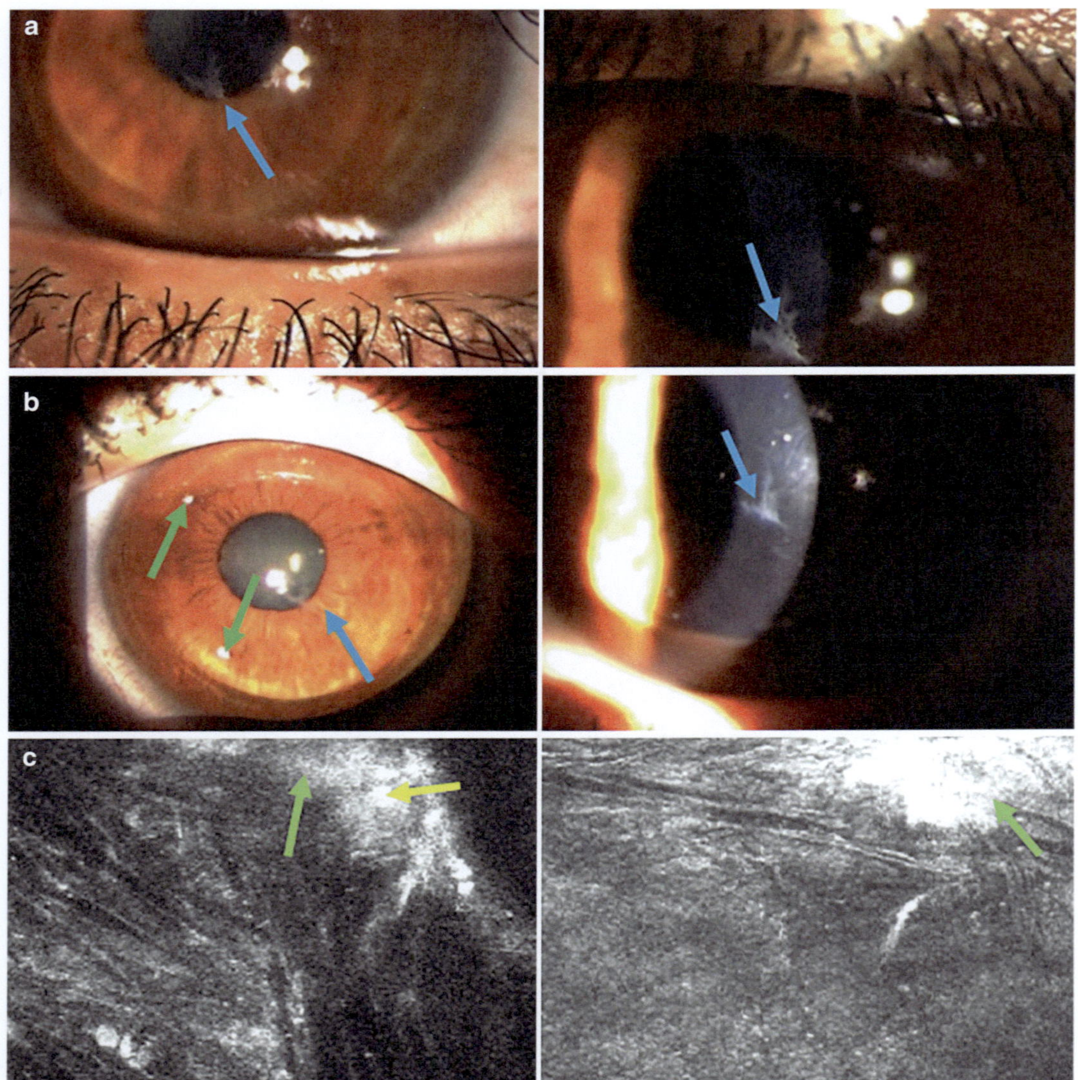

Fig. 24.4 Biomicroscopy changes in G-3, case-11 from preoperative until 36 months postoperative. (**a**) Preoperative. (Blue arrows) shows the presence of a paracentral scar (right, and left). (**b**) Observe the improvement of the paracentral opacification at 36 months (blue arrows). (Green arrows) shows the presence of fibrotic anterior tissue. (**c**) Confocal microscopy in G-3 case-11: (yellow arrow) an accumulation of migrating keratocytes on the periphery of the posterior surface of the recellularized lamina is noticed (left), while the (green arrow) shows the presence of some fibrotic tissue. 12 months later (left), a highly reflective fibrotic tissue (green arrow) in the anterior surface of the recellularized lamina is observed

Visual Parameter Results

No patient lost lines of visual acuity. All cases presented an improvement in their visuals parameters measured in decimal equivalent to LogMar scale. The unaided distance visual acuity (**UDVA**) results for all groups presented an improvement in mean values ranging between [0.08 and 0.14] (Fig. 24.5a; Table 24.2). Also, corrected distance visual acuity (**CDVA**) showed an enhancement in mean values results for all groups ranging

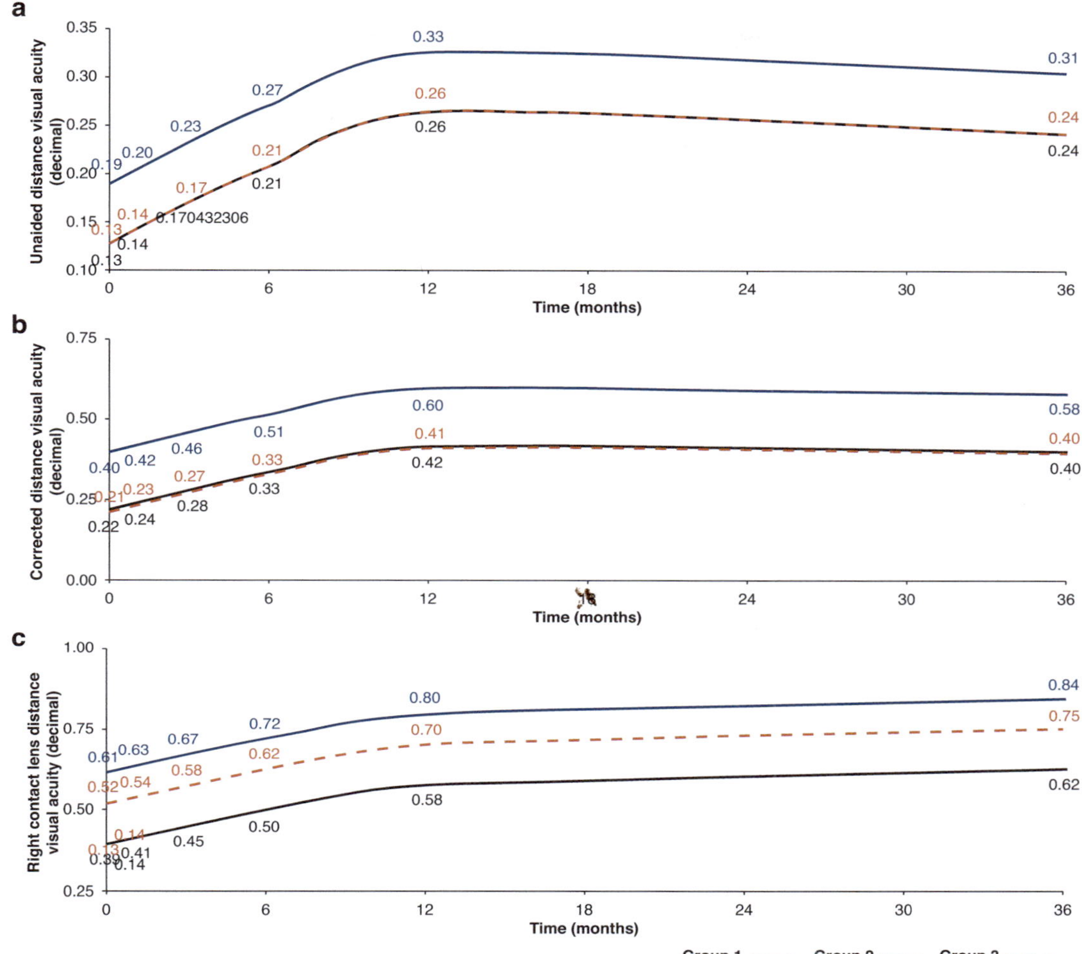

Fig. 24.5 Visual outcomes in G-1, G-2, and G-3 up to 36 months after surgery in (decimal equivalent to LogMar scale). (**a**) Unaided distance visual acuity. (**b**) Corrected distance visual acuity. A statistically significant worsening was obtained in mean values in G-2 & G-3 compared to the G-1. (**c**) Rigid contact lens visual acuity. A statistically significant worsening was obtained in G-2 when compared to G-1 & G-3

between [0.11 and 0.2] (Fig. 24.5b; Table 24.2), and rigid contact lens visual acuity (**CLDVA**) improvement results were ranged between [0.1–0.23] (Fig. 24.5c; Table 24.2) at 36 months of follow-up [45].

Results of central corneal thickness (**CCT**) (μm) measured by **AS-OCT** (Fig. 24.2, 24.6a; Table 24.2), Scheimpflug corneal topography thinnest point (**Thinnest point**) (μm), and cornea volume (**CV**) (mm^3) (Fig. 24.6b, c, 24.7, 24.8, 24.9) presented an increase in mean values in all patients of all the different groups of 30 μm, 31 μm, and 2–3 mm^3, respectively, at 36 months of follow-up [45]. The authors found a statistical significance difference improvement at 36 months in **CCT, thinnest point,** and **CV** when comparing the mean values among G-2/ G-1 and G-3/G-1 (Table 24.2) [45].

Table 24.2 Difference in Mean Values of all the variables of the study among (G-1)–(G-2), (G-1)–(G-3), and (G-2)–(G-3)

	(G-1)–(G-2)	(G-1)–(G-3)	(G-2)–(G-3)
UDVA	0.07	0.07	0.00
CDVA	0.18[a]	0.19[a]	0.01
CLDVA	0.22[a]	0.10	−0.12[a]
Visante CCT (μm)	−44.00[a]	−77.00[a]	−33.00
Thinnest point (μm)	−51.00[a]	−65.00[a]	−14.00
CV (mm³)	−5.00[a]	−5.00[a]	0.00
Kmax (D)	0.00	2.00	2.00
Anterior km (D)	−3.00	1.00	4.00
Posterior km (D)	1.3[a]	0.2	−1.1[a]
Topo Cyl (D)	1.1	0.9	−0.2
3rd order RMS	4.65[a]	3.54[a]	−1.11
4th order RMS	1.28	−0.17	−1.45[a]
HOA RMS	4.9	2.78	−2.12
LOA RMS	−3.87[a]	1.32[a]	5.19
Rx Sphr (D)	0.10	−0.10	−0.20
Rx Cyl (D)	−1.00[a]	−0.60[a]	0.40

[a] Indicates a statistically significant difference between the compared groups

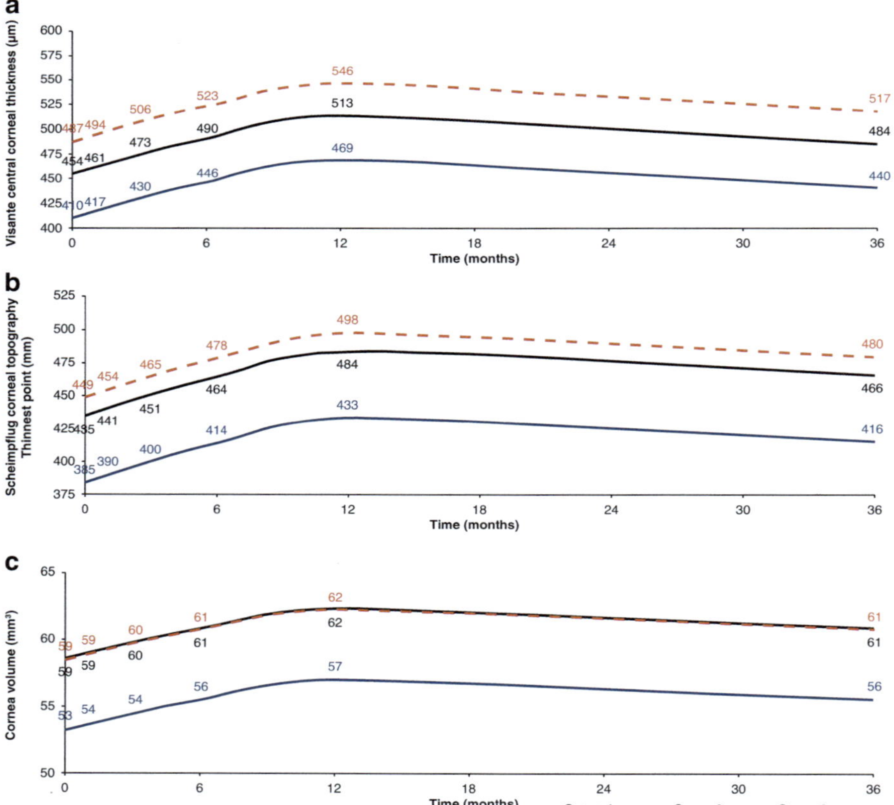

Fig. 24.6 (**a**) Central corneal thickness was measured with AS-OCT Visante (μm). (**b**) Scheimpflug corneal topography thinnest point (μm). (**c**) Cornea volume was measured with Pentacam (mm³). CCT, thinnest point, and CV showed significant improvement in the mean values at 3-year in G-2 & G-3 when compared to G-1

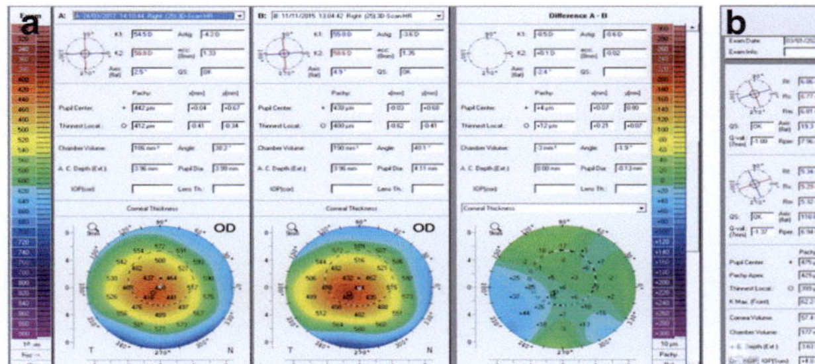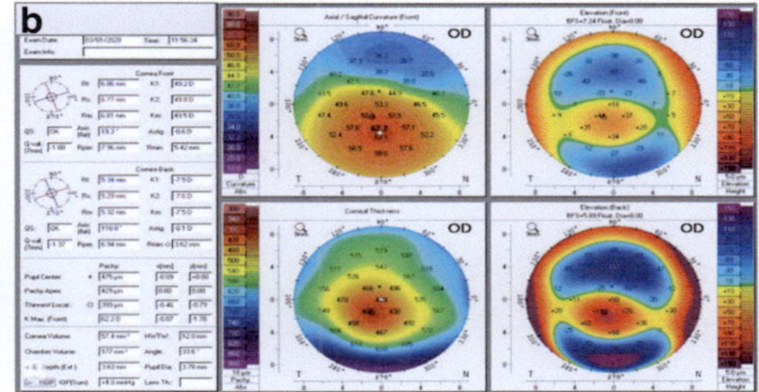

Fig. 24.7 Corneal topography (Pentacam) comparison among preoperative, 12 and 36 months postoperative in G-1, case-1. (**a**) Preoperative versus 12 months postoperative: observe the minimal enhancement of the pachymetric parameters. (**b**) Four maps corneal topography with the same case at 36 months postoperative: no significant increase of the pachymetric or keratometric parameters was obtained

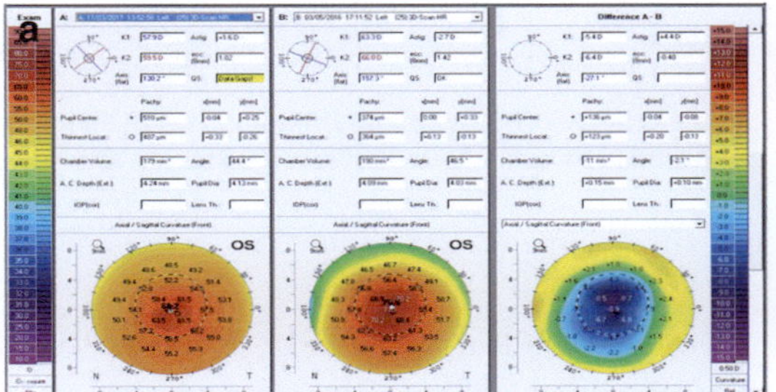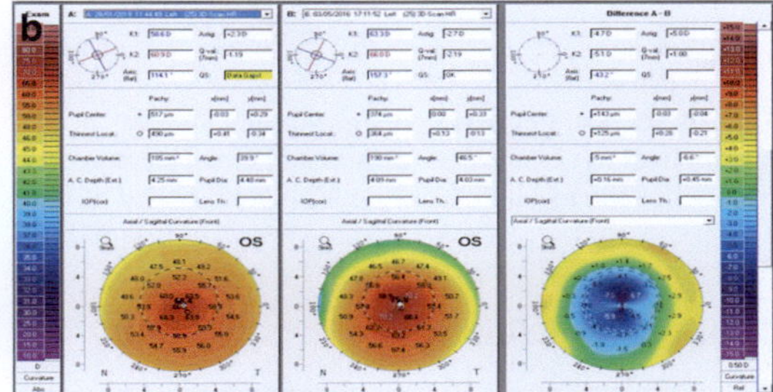

Fig. 24.8 Corneal topography (Pentacam) comparison among preoperative, 12 and 36 months postoperative in G-2, case-7. (**a**) Preoperative versus 12 months, and (**b**) Preoperative versus 36 months: notice the keratometric improvement

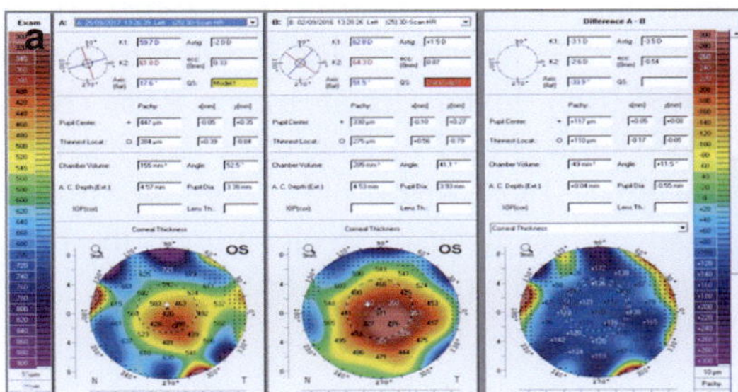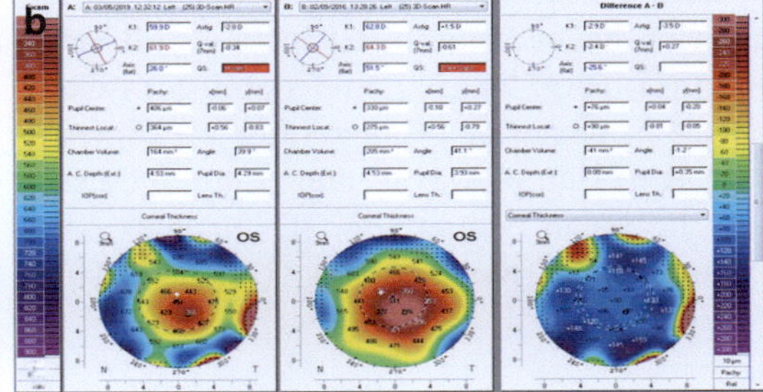

Fig. 24.9 Corneal topography (Pentacam) comparison between preoperative, 12 and 36 months postoperative in G-3, case 11. (**a**) Preoperative versus 12 months postoperative, and (**b**) Preoperative versus 3-year postoperative: notice the keratometric improvement and the noticeable increase in the pachymetric parameters

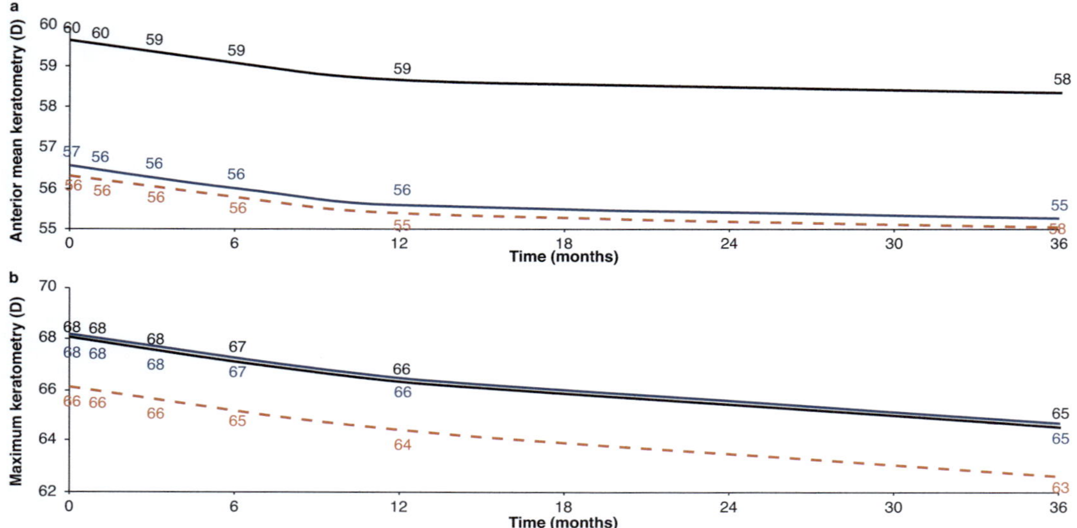

Fig. 24.10 Keratometric outcomes after 3 years of follow-up in G-1, G-2 & G-3. (**a**) Anterior mean keratometry (D): notice the mean improvement of two diopters of flattening at 3-year. (**b**) Maximum keratometry (D): there was a mean flattening of three diopters of flattening at 3-year

Topographic Results

The refractive sphere (**Rx Sphr**) (D) presented an improvement of 1.1 myopic diopters at 36 months. Meanwhile, the refractive cylinder (**Rx Cyl**) (D) presented an increase of 0.5D until 36 months postoperative [45]. Also, the authors detected at 36 months postoperative a modest improvement of 2D in the anterior mean keratometry values (**anterior Km**) (D) (Fig. 24.10a), and stability in mean values of posterior mean keratometry (**posterior Km**) (D). However, they found a flattening in mean values of 3D in maximum keratometry (**Kmax**) (D) (Fig. 24.10b).

Finally, the topographic cylinder (**Topo Cyl**) (D) remained stable [45].

Corneal Aberrometry Results

As well, an improvement in mean values was obtained at 36 months follow-up in third-order aberration RMS (**third-order RMS**) (μm), fourth-order aberration RMS (**fourth- order RMS**) (μm), high-order aberration RMS (**HOA RMS**) (μm) (Fig. 24.11), and low-order aberration RMS (**LOA RMS**) [45]. More information about the comparative results among the three groups is summarized in Table 24.2.

a

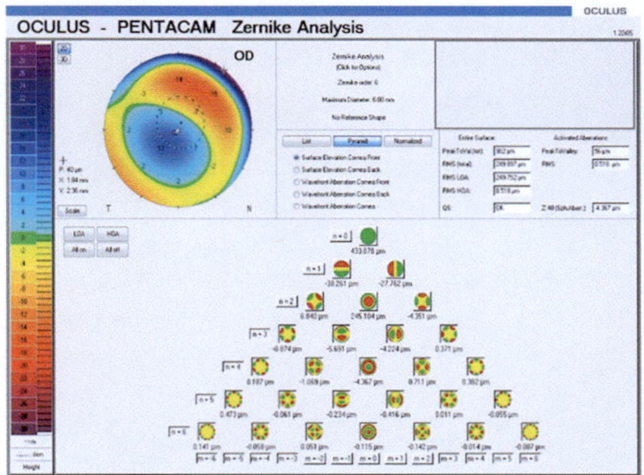

b

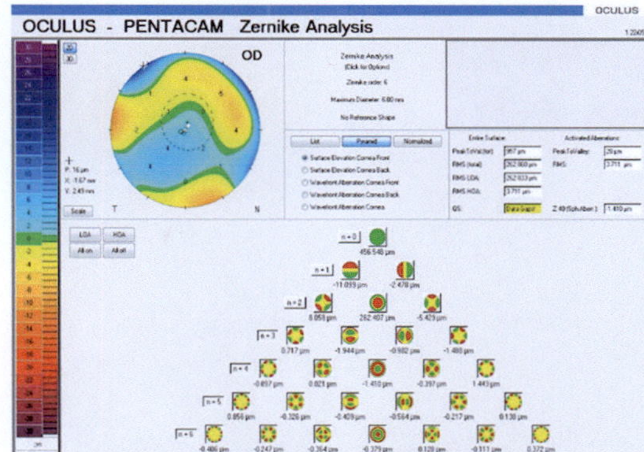

Fig. 24.11 Corneal high-order aberration RMS (HOA RMS) (μm) comparison, notice the improvement among the preoperative (**a**), and 36 months (**b**) in G-2 case-9

Corneal Densitometry (CD) Results

The authors studied the CD at the annular zones centered on the corneal apex (0–2 mm, 2–6 mm, and 6–10 mm), resulting in the following outcomes:

Anterior CD

In G-1, a decrease in all CD mean values was obtained up to 36 months regarding the preoperative values. Meanwhile, in G-2 and G-3, there was an increase in the CD mean values at 1 month. Then, mean values reached the same preoperative level (or below them) up to 36 months [50].

Central and Total CD

In G-1, the CD mean values had a slight increase at 1 month. Then, these values decreased progressively up to 36 months until they reached the same (or below) preoperative level. However, in G-2, and G-3, the CD mean values increased more notably than in ADASCs group at 1 month, noting that the increase in G-3, was more marked than in G-1 and G-2. Then, the CD mean values decreased progressively in G-2 and G-3 till getting somehow above the preoperative mean values (Table 24.3) [50].

Table 24.3 Average differences of corneal densitometry among the G-1, G-2, and G-3

	G2–G1		G3–G1		G3–G2	
Central						
0–2 mm	3.29[a]	0.004	6.58[a]	0.000	3.44[a]	0.002
2–6 mm	2.08[a]	0.001	3.00[a]	0.000	1.78[a]	0.000
6–10 mm	0.93[a]	0.019	1.18[a]	0.004	0.23	0.564
Total						
0–2 mm	2.54[a]	0.030	3.59[a]	0.003	1.17	0.259
2–6 mm	1.57[a]	0.000	2.09[a]	0.000	0.70	0.010
6–10 mm	0.81[a]	0.000	0.72[a]	0.000	−0.05	0.833

[a]Statistically significant differences among the compared groups

Posterior CD

There were slight variations in the mean values of the CD between preoperative and 36 months' postop values in all the groups [50].

Confocal Microscopy Results

Morphological Results

The confocal microscopy resulted in morphological findings showing that ADASCs in G-1 is more rounded, voluminous, more luminous, and refringent compared to the host keratocytes (Fig. 24.12a). However, the shape of ADASCs

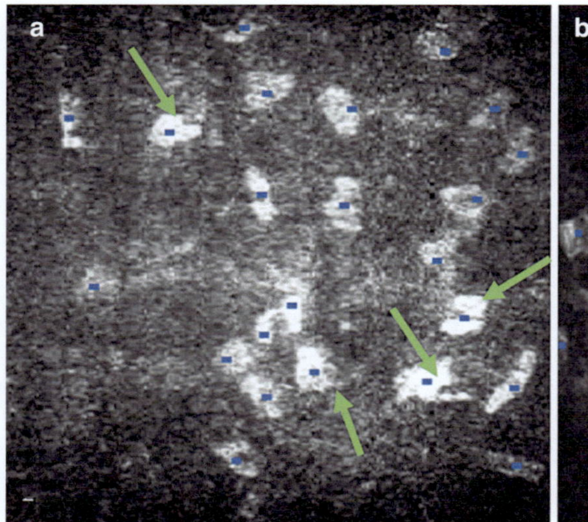
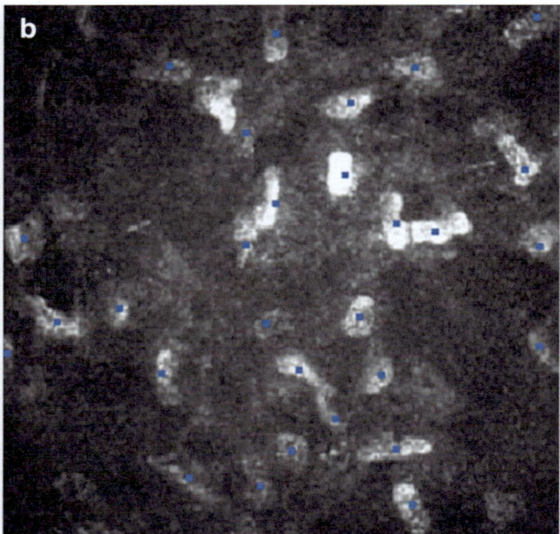

Fig. 24.12 ADASCs morphological changes in G-1, case-1: (**a**) The implanted ADASCs at 1 month have a rounded shape, larger, more refringent, and more lumi- nous than the host keratocytes (green arrows). (**b**) At 1 year after implantation, all corneal stromal cells assimi- late a similar morphology to the host keratocytes

changed from round to fusiform after 6 months from implantation (Fig. 24.12b) [31, 44, 45, 51]. Meanwhile, the decellularized laminas appeared acellular within the first few months (Fig. 24.13a), unlike the recellularized ones that showed in some determined areas similar structures to cor- neal keratocytes (Fig. 24.13b). The number of cells increased gradually during the 12 months follow-up in the decellularized and recellularized laminas in G-2, and G-3 and became more colo- nized by keratocyte-type cells until they showed similar morphology of normal corneal kerato- cytes (Fig. 24.13c, d) [31, 44, 45, 51].

Statistical Results

The confocal microscopy statistical density mean values showed a gradual and statistically significant increase in the cellularity in the ante- rior and posterior stroma of patients in G-1, G-2, and G-3 a year after the surgery in com- parison with the preoperative cell density mean values. In G3, the results in cell density were the highest, followed by G-2 and then G-1. Also, results in cellular densities at the mid-corneal stroma in G-1 showed a significant increase a 12 months postoperative. Similar results were obtained at the anterior and posterior surfaces and within the implanted laminas in G-2 and G-3 [51].

On the other hand, we detected the formation of a few fibrotic tissue areas in some cases of G-1, while a somehow stronger formation of such fibrotic tissue areas was observed in almost all cases of G-2 and G-3. Nevertheless, we did not find a direct and significant association between the recellularization of the implanted laminas and the presence of such fibrotic tissue [51].

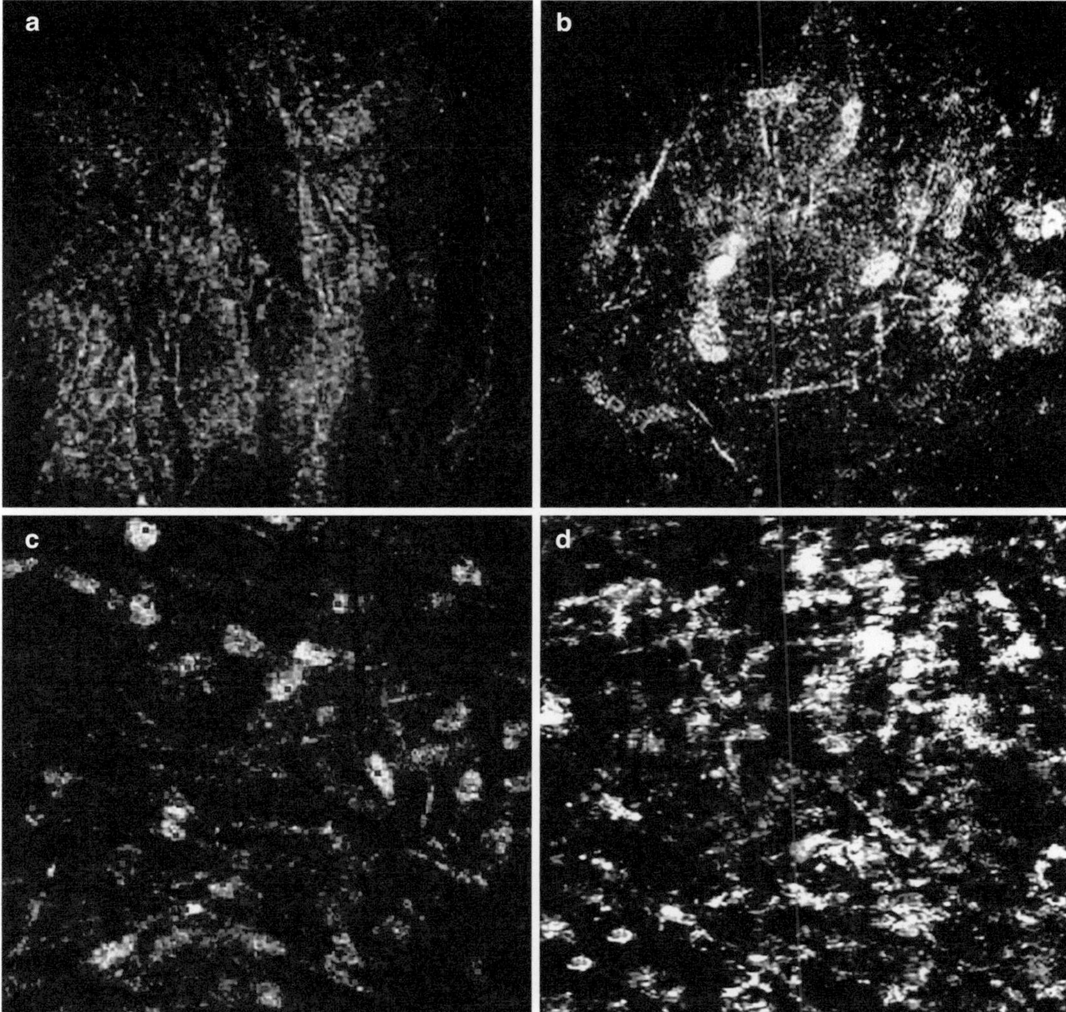

Fig. 24.13 Morphological changes in decellularized and recellularized laminas in G-2, and G-3. (**a**) G-2, case-9, the anterior surface of a decellularized lamina appears without cells 1 month after surgery. (**b**) The posterior surface of the recellularized lamina in G-3, case-13 at one-month postoperative, notice the presence of few ADASCs, similar in morphology to keratocytes-type cells. (**c**) In the same case-9, the decellularized lamina is observed with the presence of cells assimilate to the host 1 year after the surgery. (**d**) The posterior surface of the recellularized lamina with the same case-13 at 12 months postoperative, notice the high number of cells similar to the host corneal stroma

Discussion and Conclusions

Our research group demonstrated for the first time the feasibility of the implantation of ADASCs into the corneal stromal pocket in cases of advanced keratoconus, they confirmed the appearance of new collagen in the injected areas, this new collagen could be useful for repairing the corneal dystrophies, scars and increase slightly the corneal thickness, but this improvement is not enough to reestablish the corneal disease in advanced keratoconus [31, 44, 45].

Also, we confirmed for the first time that decellularized human corneal stromal laminas, colonized or not by autologous ADASCs, can be implanted for a clinical basis in the corneal stroma for therapeutic purposes. Also, such clinical application showed the safety and the feasibility of the use of femtosecond laser to dissect the cornea in the middle of the corneal stroma with advanced keratoconus, even when a large 9.5 mm corneal pocket was performed [32, 44, 45]. After 3-year postoperative, no patient showed inflammation, rejection, or any evidence of scarring or haze (Figs. 24.1, 24.2, 24.3 and 24.4). Moreover; there was an improvement with all the cases after 3-year follow-up in all the visual parameters with 1–2 lines in decimal equivalent to LogMar scale (Fig. 24.5). A significant increase in thinnest corneal point, in central corneal thickness, and corneal volume was obtained (Fig. 24.6), and the mean value results were statistically significantly better with the groups with implanted decellularized/recellularized laminas with ADASCs when comparing with the group of implanted ADASCs alone (Table 24.2). There was also an improvement in all the corneal aberrations (Fig. 24.11) and stability or improvement of corneal topographic parameters (Figs. 24.7, 24.8, 24.9 and 24.10) [45].

Besides, our study showed that the CD behavior significantly differed among the different studied groups (Table 24.3) [50]. Clinically, in G-1, corneal transparency fully recovered within 24 h postoperatively and was maintained throughout the follow-up period. The changes in CD were obtained at the central cornea, increasing slightly the mean values at 1 month, this fact is possibly related to the surgical intervention itself, the implantation of ADASCs increased cell density in the surgical interface, or with the subtle deposit of neo-collagen [50]. While, with G-2, and G-3 patients clinically showed an early haziness during the first postoperative month, this fact was related with a mild lenticule edema, then progressively improving throughout the follow-up period, demonstrating total corneal transparency by the third postoperative month [32, 44, 45, 50], this clinical result was directly related to the increase produced in central DC, presenting a spike between months 1 and 3, and then improving during the 36-month follow-up. This increase was greater in G-3 than in G-2 and may be pro-

duced by the interaction between the seeded ADASCs and the collagenous tissue of the lamina, obtaining in this group permanent increase in CD values up to 36 postoperative months (Table 24.3) [50].

Confocal microscopy was a necessary tool for the evaluation and monitoring in "in vivo" of the evolution of the ADASCs nuclei and their morphological changes, being rounded cells and highly refractive up to 6 months, changing to fusiform shaped structures, and less refringent nuclei up to 12 months. These findings demonstrate in the human clinical model that the ADASCs implanted in the corneal human pocket have survived and have been able to differentiate into keratocytes (Fig. 24.12) [51, 52]. Such findings were confirmed previously in animal studies in which the post-mortem analysis demonstrated the survival of these human cells, and their capacity to produce human collagen in the corneal rabbit [18, 22]. Also, confocal microscopy allowed to monitor the morphological changes that occurred in the decellularized and recellularized laminas, it assisted in determining the change in the cell density in the implanted tissue, as well as in all the corneal stroma [51, 52]. The ADASCs implantation increased significantly the cellularity at 12 months (Figs. 24.12b). In addition, the implantation of decellularized or recellularized laminas increased significantly the level of the stromal cells when compared with the groups of implanted ADASCs. Besides, this increase was larger with corneal laminas impregnated with ADASCs than that observed when acellular corneal laminas are implanted (Fig. 24.13c, d) [51, 52].

In conclusion, cellular therapy of the corneal stroma is a novel treatment modality for stromal diseases, which even though further studies are still mandatory with larger sample sizes to establish its safety and efficacy for different corneal stromal diseases, the initial results obtained from the pilot clinical trials are encouraging. Corneal thickness improvement in the corneas only with ADASCs implantation seems to be insufficient to restore normal corneal thickness, while the implantation of corneal laminas demonstrated the best result regarding corneal thickness restoration with a significant increase in cell density in the group implanted with recellularized laminas. The total absence of complications, the corneal transparency restoration, the reestablishment of the CD, and the modest, but significant visual and refractive enhancements obtained confirm the achievability of this therapeutic approach as a possible novel technique for the treatment of keratoconus and other corneal dystrophies. Future studies with larger samples in less advanced keratoconus cases will guarantee the therapeutic potential of this new regenerative surgery.

Take Home Notes

- Cellular therapy of the corneal stroma is a novel treatment modality for corneal stroma diseases, which initial results obtained from a pilot clinical trial are encouraging.
- Nevertheless, further studies with larger samples and other treated diseases different from keratoconus are still necessary in order to stablish its efficacy and safety profiles and so its clinical usefulness.
- ADASC corneal thickness improvement seems to be insufficient to restore severely thinned corneas, while the implantation of decellularized corneal stroma laminas enhances such thickness restoration.
- Enhanced corneal stromal remodeling is observed by confocal microscopy in those cases receiving ADASC within the corneal stroma.

References

1. Alio J. In: Alió JL, editor. Keratoconus: recent advances in diagnosis and treatment. Cham: Springer; 2017.
2. Hashemi H, Heydarian S, Hooshmand E, Saatchi M, Yekta A, Aghamirsalim M, et al. The prevalence and risk factors for keratoconus: a systematic review and meta-analysis. Cornea. 2020;39(2):263–70.
3. Arnalich-Montiel F, Alió Del Barrio J, Alió J. Corneal surgery in keratoconus: which type, which technique, which outcomes? Eye Vis (Lond). 2016;3:2.
4. De Miguel MP, Casaroli-Marano RP, Nieto-Nicolau N, Martínez-Conesa EM, Alió del Barrio JL, Alió JL, et al. Frontiers in regenerative medicine for cornea and ocular surface. In: Rahman A, Anjum S, editors. Frontiers in stem cell and regenerative medicine research. 1st ed. Sharjah: Bentham Publisher; 2015. p. 92–138.
5. Carlson EC, Liu C-Y, Chikama T, Hayashia Y, Kao CW-C, Birk DE, et al. Keratocan, a cornea-specific keratan sulfate proteoglycan, is regulated by lumican. J Biol Chem. 2005;280:25541–7.
6. Du Y, Funderburgh M, Mann M, Sundar Raj N, Funderburgh J. Multipotent stem cells in human corneal stroma. Stem Cells. 2005;23(9):1266–75.
7. Ku J, Niederer R, Patel D, Sherwin T, McGhee C. Laser scanning in vivo confocal analysis of keratocyte density in keratoconus. Ophthalmology. 2008;115(5):845–50.
8. Piñero DP, Alió JL, Barraquer RI, Michael R, Jiménez R. Corneal biomechanics, refraction, and corneal aberrometry in keratoconus: an integrated study. Invest Ophthalmol Vis Sci. 2010;51: 1948–55.
9. Alió J, Piñero D, Alesón A, Teus M, Barraquer R, Murta J, et al. Keratoconus-integrated characterization considering anterior corneal aberrations, internal astigmatism, and corneal biomechanics. J Cataract Refract Surg. 2011;37(3):552–68.
10. Mastropasqua L, Nubile M. Normal corneal morphology. In: Mastropasqua L, Nubile M, editors. Confocal microscopy of the cornea. Thorofare, NJ: SLACK; 2002. p. 7–16.
11. Ali Javadi M, Kanavi M, Mahdavi M, Yaseri M, Rabiei H, Javadi A, et al. Comparison of keratocyte density between keratoconus, post-laser in situ keratomileusis keratectasia, and uncomplicated post-laser in situ keratomileusis cases. A confocal scan study. Cornea. 2009;28(7):774–9.
12. Edmund C. Assessment of an elastic model in the pathogenesis of keratoconus. Acta Ophthalmol. 1987;65(5):545–50.
13. Gain P, Jullienne R, He Z, Aldossary M, Acquart S, Cognasse F, et al. Global survey of corneal transplantation and eye banking. JAMA Ophthalmol. 2016;134(2):167–73.
14. Griffith M, Alarcon EI, Brunette I. Regenerative approaches for the cornea. J Intern Med. 2016;280(3):276–86.
15. Fagerholm P, Lagali N, Merrett K, Jackson W, Munger R, Liu Y, et al. A biosynthetic alternative to human donor tissue for inducing corneal regeneration: 24-month follow-up of a phase 1 clinical study. Sci Transl Med. 2010;2(46):46ra61.
16. Isaacson A, Swioklo S, Connon CJ. 3D bioprinting of a corneal stroma equivalent. Exp Eye Res. 2018;173:188–93.
17. Ruberti J, Zieske J. Prelude to corneal tissue engineering—gaining control of collagen organization. Prog Retin Eye Res. 2008;27(5):549–77.
18. Alió del Barrio J, Chiesa M, Ferrer GG, Garagorri N, Briz N, Fernandez-Delgado J, et al. Biointegration of corneal macroporous membranes based on poly(ethyl

acrylate) copolymers in an experimental animal model. J Biomed Mater Res A. 2015;103(3):1106–18.

19. Lynch A, Ahearne M. Strategies for developing decellularized corneal scaffolds. Exp Eye Res. 2013;108:42–7.

20. Alio del Barrio J, Chiesa M, Garagorri N, Garcia-Urquia N, Fernandez-Delgado J, Bataille L, et al. Acellular human corneal matrix sheets seeded with human adipose-derived mesenchymal stem cells integrate functionally in an experimental animal model. Exp Eye Res. 2015;132:91–100.

21. Hara H, Cooper DKC. Xenotransplantation—the future of corneal transplantation? Cornea. 2011;30(4):371–8.

22. Arnalich-Montiel F, Pastor S, Blazquez-Martinez A, Fernandez-Delgado J, Nistal M, Alio J, De Miguel M. Adipose-derived stem cells are a source for cell therapy of the corneal stroma. Stem Cells. 2008;26(2):570–9.

23. Espandar L, Bunnell B, Wang G, Gregory P, McBride C, Moshirfar M. Adipose-derived stem cells on hyaluronic acid-derived scaffold: a new horizon in bioengineered cornea. Arch Ophthalmol. 2012;130(2):202–8.

24. Mittal SK, Omoto M, Amouzegar A, Sahu A, Alexandra R, Katikireddy KR, et al. Restoration of corneal transparency by mesenchymal stem cells. Stem Cell Rep. 2016;7(4):583–90.

25. Demirayak B, Yüksel N, Çelik O, Subaşı C, Duruksu G, Unal Z, et al. Effect of bone marrow and adipose tissue-derived mesenchymal stem cells on the natural course of corneal scarring after penetrating injury. Exp Eye Res. 2016;151:227–35.

26. Du Y, Carlson E, Funderburgh M, Birk D, Pearlman E, Guo N, et al. Stem cell therapy restores transparency to defective murine corneas. Stem Cells. 2009;27(7):1635–42.

27. Liu H, Zhang J, Liu C-Y, Wang I-J, Sieber M, Chang J, et al. Cell therapy of congenital corneal diseases with umbilical mesenchymal stem cells: lumican null mice. PLoS One. 2010;5(5):e10707.

28. Coulson Thomas VJ, Caterson B, Kao W. Transplantation of human umbilical mesenchymal stem cells cures the corneal defects of mucopolysaccharidosis VII mice. Stem Cells. 2013;31(10):2116–26.

29. Winston W-YK, Vivien J. CT Cell therapy of corneal diseases. Cornea. 2016;35(Suppl 1):S9–S19.

30. De Miguel M, Fuentes-Julián S, Blázquez-Martínez A, Pascual C, Aller M, Arias J, et al. Immunosuppressive properties of mesenchymal stem cells: advances and applications. Curr Mol Med. 2012;12(5):574–91.

31. Alió Del Barrio J, El Zarif M, De Miguel M, Azaar A, Makdissy N, Harb W, et al. Cellular therapy with human autologous adipose-derived adult stem cells for advanced keratoconus. Cornea. 2017;36(8):952–60.

32. Alió Del Barrio J, El Zarif M, Azaar A, Makdissy N, Khalil C, Harb W, et al. Corneal stroma enhancement with decellularized stromal laminas with or without stem cell recellularization for advanced keratoconus. Am J Ophthalmol. 2018;186:47–58.

33. Harkin D, Foyn L, Bray L, Sutherland A, Li F, Cronin B. Concise reviews: can mesenchymal stromal cells differentiate into corneal cells? A systematic review of published data. Stem Cells. 2015;33(3):785–91.

34. Jiang Z, Liu G, Meng F, Wang W, Hao P, Xiang Y, et al. Paracrine effects of mesenchymal stem cells on the activation of keratocytes. Br J Ophthalmol. 2017;101(11):1583–90.

35. Hendijani F. Explant culture: an advantageous method for isolation of mesenchymal stem cells from human tissues. Cell Prolif. 2017;50(2):e12334.

36. Górski B. Gingiva as a new and the most accessible source of mesenchymal stem cells from the oral cavity to be used in regenerative therapies. Postepy Hig Med Dosw (Online). 2016;70(0):858–71.

37. Basu S, Hertsenberg AJ, Funderburgh ML, Burrow MK, Mann MM, Du Y, Lathrop KL, Syed-Picard FN, Adams SM, et al. Human limbal biopsy-derived stromal stem cells prevent corneal scarring. Sci Transl Med. 2014;6(266):266ra172.

38. Takahashi K, Yamanaka S. Induction of pluripotent stem cells from mouse embryonic and adult fibroblast cultures by defined factors. Cell. 2006;126(4):663–76.

39. Naylor RW, Charles NJM, Cowan CA, Davidson AJ, Holm TM, Sherwin T. Derivation of corneal keratocyte-like cells from human induced pluripotent stem cells. PLoS One. 2016;11(10):e0165464.

40. Yao L, Bai H. Review: mesenchymal stem cells and corneal reconstruction. Mol Vis. 2013;19:2237–43.

41. Caplan AI. Mesenchymal stem cells: time to change the name! Stem Cells Transl Med. 2017;6(6):1445–51.

42. Alió JL, El Zarif M, Alió del Barrio JL. Cellular therapy of the corneal stroma: a new type of corneal surgery for keratoconus and corneal dystrophies a translational research experience. 1st ed. Amsterdam: Elsevier; 2020.

43. De Miguel M, Alio J, Arnalich-Montiel F, Fuentes-Julian S, de Benito-Llopis L, Amparo F, Bataille L. Cornea and ocular surface treatment. Curr Stem Cell Res Ther. 2010;5(2):195–204.

44. Alió J, Alió Del Barrio J, El Zarif M, Azaar A, Makdissy N, Khalil C, et al. Regenerative surgery of the corneal stroma for advanced keratoconus: 1-year outcomes. Am J Ophthalmol. 2019;203:53–68.

45. El Zarif M, Alió J, Alió del Barrio J, Abdul Jawad K, Palazón-Bru A, Abdul Jawad Z, et al. Corneal stromal regeneration therapy for advanced keratoconus: long-term outcomes at 3 years. Cornea. 2021;40(6):741–54.

46. Zuk P, Zhu M, Mizuno H, Huang J, Futrell J, Katz A, et al. Multilineage cells from human adipose tissue: implications for cell-based therapies. Tissue Eng. 2001;7(2):211–28.

47. Zuk PA, Zhu M, Ashjian P, De Ugarte D, Huang J, Mizuno H, et al. Human adipose tissue is a source of multipotent stem cells. Mol Biol Cell. 2002;13(12):4279–95.

48. Bourin P, Bunnell B, Casteilla L, Dominici M, Katz A, March K, et al. Stromal cells from the adipose tissue-derived stromal vascular fraction and culture expanded adipose tissue-derived stromal/stem cells:

a joint statement of the International Federation for Adipose Therapeutics and Science (IFATS) and the international Society for Cellular Therapy (ISCT). Cytotherapy. 2013;15(6):641–8.

49. Ponce Márquez S, Martínez V, McIntosh Ambrose W, Wang J, Gantxegui N, Schein O, et al. Decellularization of bovine corneas for tissue engineering applications. Acta Biomater. 2009;5(6):1839–47.

50. El Zarif M, Alió del Barrio J, Mingo D, Abdul Jawad K, Alió J. Corneal stroma densitometry evolution in a clinical model of cellular therapy for advanced keratoconus. Cornea. 2022;42:332.

51. El Zarif M, Abdul Jawad K, Alió del Barrio J, Abdul Jawad Z, Palazón-Bru A, De Miguel M, et al. Corneal stroma cell density evolution in keratoconus corneas following the implantation of adipose mesenchymal stem cells and corneal laminas: an in vivo confocal microscopy study. Invest Ophthalmol Vis Sci. 2020;61(4):22.

52. El Zarif M, Abdul Jawad K, Alió JL. Confocal microscopy of the cornea in a clinical model of corneal stromal expansion using adipose stem cells and corneal decellularized laminas in patients with keratoconus. In: Alió JL, Alió del Barrio JL, Arnalich-Montiel F, editors. Corneal regeneration therapy and surgery. 1st ed. Essentials in ophthalmology. Cham: Springer; 2019. p. 363–86.

Part V

Endothelial Keratoplasty

Endothelial Keratoplasty. Historical Review and Current Outcomes

Farideh Doroodgar, Hassan Hashemi, Sana Niazi, Sepehr Feizi, and Mohammad Ali Javadi

Key Points

- Corneal endothelial dysfunction is treated using EK, which has been demonstrated to be more effective than PK.
- DSEK and its variations became the most popular EK approach because to its good surgical results.
- The new suggested details for DSEK, DSAEK, and DMEK need to be thoroughly evaluated.

Introduction

After more than a century of success with penetrating keratoplasty (PK), endothelial keratoplasty (EK) ushered in a paradigm shift in corneal transplantation surgery, with surgical processes and clinical outcomes that are constantly evolving. Because past review studies have fallen short of giving the most up-to-date information, we examine the history of EK evolution with a focus on the primary forms of EK, which include (1) Descemet stripping endothelial keratoplasty (DSEK) and its improvements, such as Descemet stripping automated endothelial keratoplasty (DSAEK) and ultrathin DSAEK, (2) Descemet membrane endothelial keratoplasty (DMEK), and (3) pre-Descemet's endothelial keratoplasty (PDEK) and address the indications, surgical techniques, risks, and prospects of various surgical treatments. (Fig. 25.1).

Supplementary Information The online version contains supplementary material available at https://doi.org/10.1007/978-3-031-32408-6_25.

F. Doroodgar (✉)
Negah Aref Ophthalmic Research Center, Shahid Beheshti University of Medical Science, Tehran, Iran

Translational Ophthalmology Research Center, Tehran University of Medical Sciences, Tehran, Iran
e-mail: f-doroodgar@farabi.tums.ac.ir

H. Hashemi
Noor Ophthalmology Research Center, Noor Eye Hospital, Tehran, Iran

Eye Research Center, Farabi Eye Hospital, Tehran University of Medical Sciences, Tehran, Iran
e-mail: hhashemi@noorvision.com

S. Niazi
Negah Aref Ophthalmic Research Center, Shahid Beheshti University of Medical Science, Tehran, Iran

Translational Ophthalmology Research Center, Tehran University of Medical Sciences, Tehran, Iran
e-mail: sananiazi@sbmu.ac.ir

S. Feizi · M. A. Javadi
Department of Opthalmology, Labbafinezhad Hospital, Shahid Beheshti University of Medical Sciences, Tehran, Iran

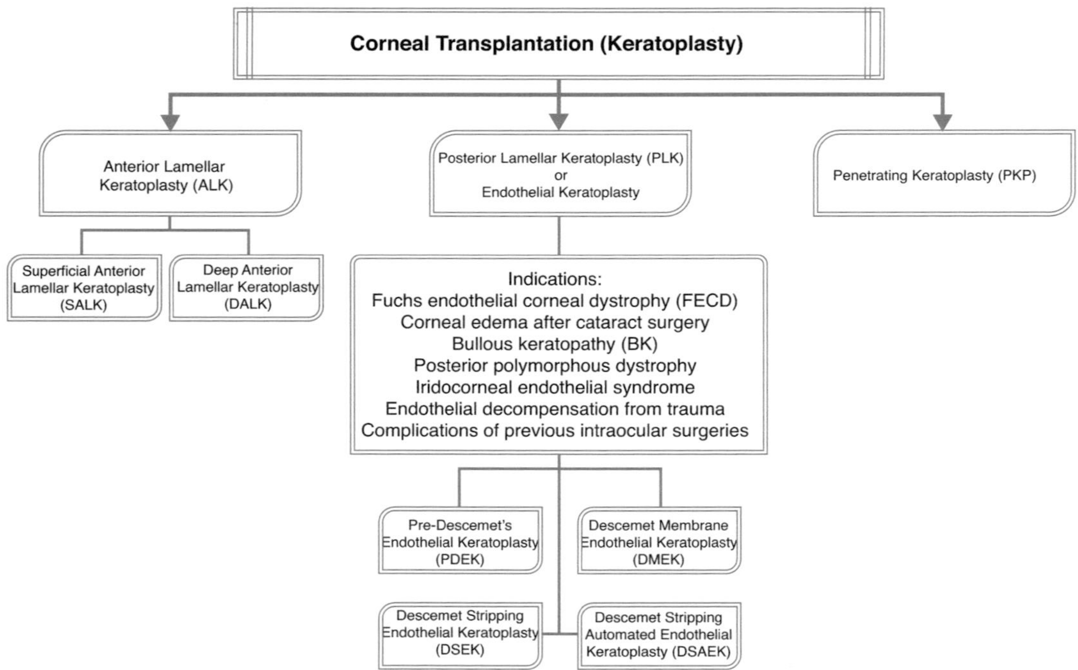

Fig. 25.1 The types of corneal transplantations

Evolution of EK

In 1906, the first successful human corneal transplant took place [1]. As the suggested procedures became more successful, the demand for cornea from cadavers grew, leading in the establishment of eye banking in the 1940s, which greatly expanded corneal transplantation in the United States and around the world [2]. Surgical procedures improved dramatically as knowledge of basic principles of the cornea, such as anatomy, physiology, immunology, tissue biology, and anesthetic, grew [2].

EK's origins can be traced back to studies on the selective replacement of damaged posterior corneal layers. Tillett used full-thickness grafts from donor endothelium to accomplish posterior lamellar keratoplasty (PLK) in 1956, which was the first effort to employ the cornea's inner layer. Glaucoma, endothelial damage, and poor donor–recipient apposition all contributed to the transplant's failure [3]. EK was developed as a result of research into the selective replacement of injured posterior corneal layers. In 1956, Tillett performed the first posterior lamellar keratoplasty (PLK) using full-thickness grafts from donor endothelium, which was the first attempt to use the cornea's inner layer. The transplant failed because of glaucoma, endothelial deterioration, and poor donor–recipient apposition [3]. The next attempts, such as the anterior approach, were likewise unsuccessful. Because the use of sutures for attachment of the donor graft to the recipient cornea was the main technical difficulty of these procedures, Melles and colleagues (1998) introduced a new modification in which air was used instead of sutures to attach the donor lenticule to the posterior recipient cornea, resulting in a better visual outcome [4]. They next lowered the corneal incision from 9 to 5 millimeters and placed a folded donor lenticule into the anterior chamber [5]. Deep lamellar endothelial keratoplasty (DLEK) was introduced to the United States by Terry and Ousley [6]. Unfortunately, the clinical outcomes were poor, and the surgical approach was difficult to duplicate, preventing the technique from becoming widely used and prompting the researchers to seek new alternatives.

Melles and colleagues (2004) simplified the procedure known as DSEK by removing the most difficult element of PLK/DLEK (i.e., dissection and excision of the recipient stroma) and replacing it with descemetorhexis. DSEK takes an internal method to remove the host's Descemet's membrane (DM) and endothelium, leaving a smooth surface [7]. Because of the smaller incision, this procedure quickly gained popularity, resulting in improved safety, a lower risk of postoperative complications, and faster visual rehabilitation [8]. Manual dissection of the donor cornea, like PLK/DLEK, resulted in a donor lenticule with a variable thickness profile; thus, Gorovoy (2006) modified this technique by dissecting donor corneas with a microkeratome and introducing DSAEK, which improved the visual outcome by smoothing the donor-recipient interface [9]. When compared to PK, the early research on DSAEK showed it to be a successful surgical technique with less problems, including as graft failure, and faster visual recovery with less astigmatism [10–12]. With the preparation of the donor tissue by the eye banks and the use of innovative techniques for tissue delivery, DSAEK acquired greater popularity; nonetheless, the visual acuity following DSAEK remained unsatisfactory [13].

Melles and colleagues (2006) presented another improvement of EK to improve visual acuity, known as DMEK, in which rolled DM and endothelium from the donor are inserted into the recipient's anterior chamber (AC) through a 3-mm incision and unfolded using air and balanced salt solution (BSS) [14]. When opposed to DSAEK, DMEK preserves corneal architecture and delivers superior visual results by replacing the defective layer of the recipient cornea with matching donor tissue [15–17]. Even after providing better tissue preparation procedures, such as 'no-touch' harvesting technique, the fundamental downside of this technology that has resulted in limited expansion of its application is technical difficulties in preparing donor tissue [18–20]. According to the Eye Bank Association of America's data, the number of DSAEK still outnumbers the number of DMEK (Fig. 25.1).

Neff and colleagues (2011) created ultrathin DSAEK grafts, thinner than 130 m, known as ultrathin DSAEK (UT-DSAEK), which led to superior postoperative visual results than normal DSAEK [21] in search of a more uniform surface [22]. The surgical outcome and best-corrected visual acuity (BCVA) of UT-DSAEK have been shown to be equivalent to [23, 24], or better than that of DMEK in later trials [25, 26]. However, a 32-month follow-up of patients who had DMEK, DSAEK, UT-DSAEK, nano-thin DSAEK (15–49 m), ultrathin DSAEK (50–99 m) revealed identical visual acuity, ruling out the influence of graft thickness and regularity on patient visual outcomes [27]. The contradictory findings highlight the need for additional standardized studies and meta-analysis in this area.

Agarwal and colleagues (2013) reported PDEK, a surgical method for EK in which the pre-Descemet stromal layer (Dua's layer; separated by an air bubble) is additionally transplanted with DM and endothelium [28]. The following publications all showed positive outcomes, suggesting that PDEK tissue preparation and unrolling is straightforward and repeatable [29]. In comparison to DMEK, PDEK grafts are 25–30 mm thick, which reduces postoperative graft-host interface haze and improves intraoperative tissue handling [30]. Furthermore, PDEK overcomes another drawback of DMEK by allowing surgeons to use corneal tissue from young donors [28]. In DMEK, the presence of a large number of hexagonal cells in the stromal layer of donors younger than 40 raises the likelihood of implant rejection, whereas PDEK lacks a full stromal layer and hence has no such concerns [30].

Indications

Patients with endothelial dysfunction, such as Fuchs endothelial corneal dystrophy (FECD), corneal edema after cataract surgery, bullous keratopathy (BK), posterior polymorphous dystrophy, iridocorneal endothelial syndrome, and endothelial decompensation from trauma, as well as complications of previous intraocular surgeries, are candidates for EK [31, 32]. DSAEK became the most popular form of EK utilized globally with the introduction of DSEK and subsequent modifications. When compared to DSAEK and PK, the next procedure presented, DMEK, resulted in better and quicker visual recovery as well as greater endothelium survival for patients with FECD and BK [33, 34]. Patients with FECD who had no corneal scar, preserved AC anatomy, and an intact lens/iris diaphragm had favorable results; additionally, patients with BK had a higher rate of endothelial damage than those with FECD, with endothelial failure occurring only in patients with concomitant ocular pathology [35, 36]. Despite these limitations, DMEK was not frequently utilized after its inception, and DSAEK remains the most common surgical approach of EK, especially in difficult situations [37], as discussed below.

The state of the crystalline lens is a crucial factor to consider when choosing a surgical procedure; individuals with cataracts require both cataract surgery and EK, which may be done simultaneously or in stages depending on the AC depth and the condition of the anterior corneal surface [38]. In phakic eyes left without cataract surgery for 2 years, DSEK has been reported to hasten cataract formation, but DMEK has been proven to be safe with great visual results in these circumstances without removing the crystalline lens [39–41].

A history of unsuccessful keratoplasty, either PK or EK, is another reason for EK. However, in this situation, the choice of surgical technique is debatable; some suggest the safety and favorable outcomes of DSAEK, with graft dislocation rates comparable to primary DSAEK [42], while others have reported favorable visual outcomes for DMEK after failed PK, with relatively good long-term outcomes [43, 44]; however, in cases complicated by glaucoma or AC intraocular lens (IOL), DMEK was associated with higher graft detachment and reb [45, 46]. DMEK following a failed DSAEK has also been proven to improve the visual quality of patients to a level equivalent to initial DMEK [47, 48]. When comparing the results of DMEK for failed PK with a repeat PK, it was discovered that DMEK resulted in greater wound stability and fewer suture-related problems [49]. Furthermore, the total failure rate of

DSAEK and DMEK following failed PK was equal [50].

Patients who have had previous glaucoma surgery, such as trabeculectomy and implantation of a glaucoma shunt device, have an additional hurdle with EK, which can result in bleb-related problems, tissue loss, and graft displacement. Furthermore, owing to mechanical strain of the glaucoma device [43], the DMEK donor graft may be injured during unfolding [51]. Although additional considerations are necessary during surgery to ensure a full air fill at the conclusion of surgery and relocating the glaucoma device, DSAEK is regarded a suitable surgical approach for patients with concurrent glaucoma or a history of glaucoma surgery [52]. Additionally, narrow angels in glaucoma patients and Asians, resulting in peripheral anterior synechiae and shallow ACs, provide a significant problem that necessitates EK method changes [53].

In aphakic individuals and those with iris anomalies such aniridia, EK might be difficult. In such circumstances, DSAEK can be done with additional surgical modifications, such as donor lenticule suturing to the recipient cornea, to lessen the chance of posterior graft dislodgment [54]. Obviously, this change cannot be made during DMEK. In situations with corneal endothelium dysfunction necessitating EK, the presence of an AC IOL poses an additional obstacle; for whom the IOL to be replaced, this operation can be done in stages or all at once. Although visual acuity was poorer than with DSAEK alone, evidence suggests that concurrent IOL exchange with DSAEK does not increase the risks of dislocation, primary graft failure, donor endothelial cell loss, or pupillary block [55]. In patients with an AC IOL, DMEK is recommended as a viable procedure, but IOL removal is recommended in individuals with a high risk of postoperative problems [46]. Overall, DSAEK is preferred over DMEK in difficult cases due to its greater adaptability and predictability, which includes a wider range of graft insertion techniques, the ability to secure the lenticule to the overlying stroma, and direct interface fluid evacuation, as well as the more robust nature of the DSAEK lenticule itself [56]. However, the present literature has a poor level of evidentiary certainty, and further research is needed to establish the best surgical approach for these purposes [57].

It's also been claimed that UT-DSAEK can be done on any eye that's been diagnosed as needing DSAEK. In terms of postoperative BCVA, endothelial cell density, and survival rate, UT-DSAEK and DMEK had similar outcomes [58, 59]. However, there is a paucity of data about the superiority of surgical procedures in certain situations, and additional research is needed before definitive conclusions can be drawn. PDEK suffers from a greater lack of data, since most studies have focused on surgical procedures and overall results rather than particular purposes or comparisons with other techniques [30]. Despite the fact that the surgical approaches are comparable to those used in DMEK, data shows that surgeons prefer DSAEK in the majority of cases.

Surgical Procedures

Table 25.1 summarizes the four endothelial keratoplasty surgical procedures, with more specific information provided in the following sections. (Also, in Fig. 25.2, you can see the procedures together.)

DSEK/DSAEK

DSEK, as well as its subsequent modifications DSAEK, is the most frequent technique performed today, and it is suitable for practically all patients. On the recipient eye, a 3–5 mm incision (corneal/scleral or limbal) is made. Then, utilizing air, fluid, or viscoelastic, descemetorhexis is conducted, and recipient DM is removed. In DSEK, donor preparation is done by hand, but in DSAEK, lamellar dissection is done with a microkeratome, which makes donor preparation easier and results in a smoother interface (Video 25.1). The clinical results of precut tissues from eye banks are positive and comparable to those of surgeon-cut tissues [60, 61]. To avoid AC angle closure, the donor cornea is sliced with a trephine 3 mm smaller than the recipient horizontal cornea diameter after lamellar dissection [62]. The recipient's AC receives the trephined donor posterior lenticule. To limit endothelial cell loss, many procedures for donor insertion have been created, including forceps (taco technique), glides (including Busin glide, Sheets glide, Tan EndoGlide), and inserters [9, 43]. To avoid pupillary obstruction, a peripheral iridotomy may be required before donor implantation in some situations [43]. The air bubble is utilized to approxi-

Table 25.1 The distinctions between the four endothelial keratoplasty surgical procedures

	DSAEK/DSEK/ UT-DSAEK	DMEK	PDEK
Surgical layers	Stroma, DM, and endothelium	DM and endothelium	Predescemet, DM, and endothelium
Microkeratome	Yes	No	No
Artificial anterior chamber	Required	N/A	N/A
Type of procedure	Tissue additive	Tissue neutral	Minimal tissue additive
Technical difficulty	Easy	Difficult	Moderate
Graft unrolling	Easy	Difficult	Moderate
Tissue handling	Good	Difficult	Good
Eye bank prepared donor tissue	Yes	Yes	Yes
Induced hyperopia	Yes	No	No
Corneal thickness	Increased	Normal	Minimal
Intrastromal interface	Yes	No	Minimal
Type of big bubble	N/A	Type 2	Type 1
Donor tissue loss	Negligible	Yes	Yes
Cost	Costly	Cost effective	Cost effective
Visual recovery	Slow	Fast	Fast

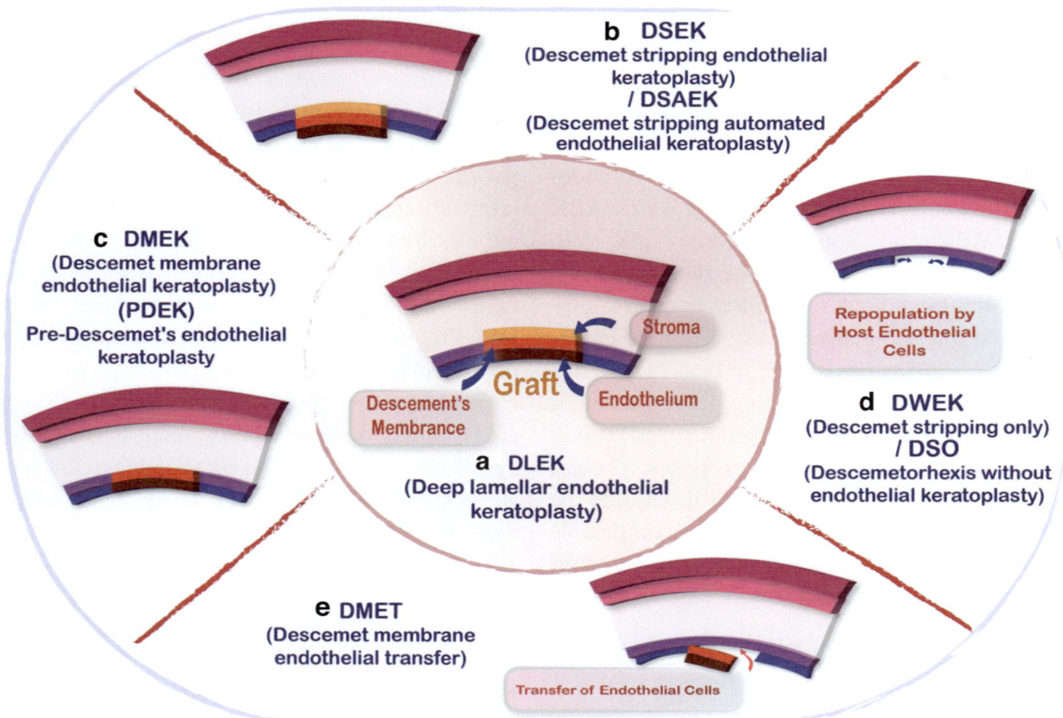

Fig. 25.2 Illustration of Endothelial Keratoplasty techniques. (**a**) In DLEK, a posterior stromal pocket in the patient's cornea is created for placement of a partial-thickness graft. (**b**) In DSEK/DSAEK, only the pathologic tissue is removed via a descemetorhexis, and a graft with a thin layer of stroma, created manually or with a microkeratome, is used to replace the removed tissue. (**c**) DMEK is the replacement of pathologic Descemet's membrane and endothelium with a graft prepared by a descemetorhexis technique. (**d**) PDEK grafts include the pre-Descemet layer prepared using pneumodissection. (**e**) DWEK/DSO is descemetorhexis alone of the patient's cornea, relying on primary intention healing. (**f**) DMET is a proposed technique involving a focally attached graft that acts as a source for endothelial cells. (*Courtesy of Moshirfar & Thomson* This figure is distributed under the terms of the Creative Commons Attribution 4.0 International License (http://creativecommons.org/licenses/by/4.0/), which permits use, duplication, adaptation, distribution, and reproduction in any medium or format)

mate the donor lenticule to the recipient cornea's posterior stroma after correct unfolding. In complex circumstances, such as aphakic eyes, full-thickness sutures can also be utilized to secure donor corneas.

UT-DSAEK

UT-DSAEK is a DSAEK variant in which the central donor thickness is less than 130 m. An RCT found that UT-DSAEK had better visual outcomes than DSAEK [22, 23]. When UT-DSAEK was compared to DMEK, the results were mixed; although some studies found similar results [23, 24], others found that DMEK resulted in better visual outcomes [25, 26]. A microkeratome can be used to prepare the UT-DSAEK tissue in a single- or double-pass procedure. The double-pass approach has been linked to a greater risk of endothelial injury and donor tissue perforation in several studies. To lessen the danger of donor perforation, hydration of the grafts after the first incision and the use of a low-pulse high-frequency femtosecond laser have been recommended [63–65].

DMEK

By removing the stromal layer, DMEK was able to overcome the key drawbacks of DSEK, such as interface haziness and hyperopic shift. As a result, DMEK produces a better visual result than DSEK/DSAEK. Donor DM is removed in order to prepare DMEK donor tissue (Video 25.2). Several strategies for tissue preparation have been introduced. In the SCUBA technique, DM is grasped (using a nontoothed forceps) and slowly stripped away from the stroma approximately halfway to the center; then, the central part is separated by central partial-thickness trephination (SCUBA technique), while other techniques such as manual peeling, forceps peeling, combined manual delamination, and hydro dissection, as well as a trend toward a no-touch technique, have also been suggested [66, 67]. Another suggested approach for DMEK tissue production is pneumatic dissection, in which the pre-Descemet stromal layer remains linked to the DM was, in reality, supplying PDEK tissue (described below). Eye banks also supply pre-stripped tissues for DMEK, which have proved to have similar cell viability to surgeon-prepared tissues [68], and preloaded DMEK tissues have also exhibited superior visual results than pre-loaded DSAEK tissues [69].

The insertion of the donor tissue, which is the most difficult aspect of all types of EK, comes next after tissue preparation and recipient cut. Melles and colleagues first utilized a glass pipette to implant DMEK tissue [14], but other approaches, such as the use of IOL injectors such as the STAAR microinjector, Alcon B cartridge, Jones tube, and Bonfadini-Todd injector, have also been proposed. Each insertion approach causes endothelial cell death at a variable rate [70–72], and there is no consensus on the best and safest procedure. After insertion, the donor tissue should be unfolded using a variety of techniques, including a combination of air and BSS, the Yoeruek no-touch technique with a double roll, the Dirisamer technique (carpet unrolling while fixing graft edge), the Dapena maneuver (small air bubble-assisted unrolling), mechanical tapping, and the single sliding cannula maneuver [73]. After unfolding the donor tissue in the proper orientation, such as with DSAEK, air is injected to attach the graft to the recipient cornea; some surgeons remove the air after a few hours to avoid pupillary block, while others maintain a complete air fill and routinely perform a peripheral iridotomy.

PDEK

In addition to DM and endothelium, EK's recent invention advises retaining the prelayer Descemet's composite, resulting in a graft with a diameter of 7.5–8.5 mm, which has demonstrated good outcomes. PDEK tissue is simpler to handle and unroll in AC since it scrolls less. It also enables for the harvesting of transplant tissue from young donors [28, 74, 75]. Intrastromal injection of air is used to generate a type 1 large bubble (BB) with a diameter of 7–8 mm for donor tissue preparation [30]. The donor tissue is next trephined or manually incised at the intersection of the bubble wall and the corneal stroma with MicroVannas scissors [30]. After stripping the recipient's DM and endothelium, the graft is injected or pulled into the AC and unfurled following the procedures outlined before. PDEK tissue is simpler to handle than DMEK tissue, making the treatment easier to complete [29]. More research is needed to discover the optimum insertion and unfolding strategies, as well as endothelial cell loss and visual results following the use of this EK approach [62, 76–78].

DWEK

Descemetorhexis without endothelial kerato-plasty (DWEK) is a proposed term to describe the surgical removal of Descemet membrane (DM) without subsequent endothelial transplantation (Video 25.3) [79]. DWEK was based on several case reports of spontaneous resolution of corneal edema after iatrogenic (during intraocular surgery) and deliberate removal of DM in patients with FECD [80–83]. This potential for endothelial "rejuvenation" in FECD contrasts with bullous keratopathy, thought to be an endothelial depletion disease [84]. Presence of central guttae, clear peripheral cornea with an endothelial cell count >1000 cells/mm2 on confocal or specular microscopy, phakic or pseudophakic, and patient's preference are indications of FECD, while advanced corneal stromal edema, peripheral endothelial cell count <1000 cells/mm^2, presence of secondary corneal pathology, and history of herpes simplex virus or cytomegalovirus keratitis are the contraindications. Complications include descemetorhexis decentration, descemet membrane detachment, posterior stromal opacities at the margin of the descemetorhexis, abnormal corneal topography and irregular corneal astigmatism [85], and persistent corneal edema (apart from Arbelaez [86], which had issues with DMEK detachments, successful DMEK and DSAEK procedures were described in these cases [87, 88]).

DSEK, DSAEK, UT-DSAEK, DMEK, and PDEK Visual Results

DSEK has been proven to provide rapid and consistent visual recovery, with BCVAs of 20/40 or better reported in 38–100% of patients 3 months after surgery, and 20/33 to 20/60 3–30 months after surgery [89, 90]. However, when compared to DSAEK, a larger number of patients had a BCVA of 20/200 following PK [43]. BCVA varies according on the reason for EK, with eyes with PK having a better visual result than those with FECD [91, 92]. DMEK has been demonstrated to produce the quickest and finest visual recovery, with 82% and 89% of patients, respectively, reaching a BCVA of 20/25, 5, and 10 years after surgery [93].

One year following DSAEK and DMEK, a single surgeon's experience with more than 200 patients revealed BCVAs of 20/50 and 20/125, respectively [94]. DMEK demonstrated a superior BCVA (mean difference of 20/16) after 1 year [57] and a better BSCVA (mean difference of 20/13.5) after 6 months in comparative meta-analysis studies compared to DSEK/DSAEK [95].

When comparing DMEK to DSAEK, Zhu and colleagues found that BCVA was superior, with more patients having a BCVA of 20/25 and 20/20 [26]. Other meta-analysis studies have also demonstrated that DMEK improves visual accuracy over DSEK/DSAEK [96, 97].

Clinical results following UT-DSAEK and PDEK were investigated and compared in a smaller number of trials. BSCVA of 20/20 in 36.3%, 37.4%, 46.4%, and 53.4% of eyes 1 year, 2 years, 3 years, and 5 years after UT-DSAEK, and 20/40 in 95.5%, 95.3%, 96.0%, and 96.6% of eyes 1 year, 2 years, 3 years, and 5 years after UT-DSAEK, respectively [58]. With improved results following UT-DSAEK vs. DSAEK, the quicker and better visual recovery has been observed [22]. Droutsas and colleagues, on the other hand, found that DSAEK had much better results than UT-DSAEK [98]. Similarly, comparing the visual outcomes of UT-DSAEK and DMEK revealed mixed findings; some researchers claim that UT-DSAEK is equal to DMEK [23, 24, 99], while others claim that BCVA after DMEK is higher [25, 26].

Despite the technical benefits of PDEK, few research have looked into patients' postoperative visual acuity [30]. As a result, additional research is needed to establish the results of various EK approaches after surgery.

Graft Survival of DSEK, DSAEK, UT-DSAEK, DMEK, and PDEK

The 5-year graft survival after DSEK has been compared to that after PK [100, 101]; however, DSAEK was shown to be superior than PK (79.4% vs. 66.5%, respectively) [102]. Unsatisfactory visual outcomes following DSAEK, on the other hand, lead to a greater probability of repeat EK [103]. DSEK/DSAEK survival rates have been reported to range from 55 to 100% [43]. This large range reflects a variety of variables that affect graft survival, including the severity of intraoperative trauma, which is directly related to the surgeon's experience. In addition, the patient's underlying ocular disorders have a role; 5-year graft survival is 95% in FECD, 76%

in pseudophakic or aphakic bullous keratopathy, and 40% in eyes with a glaucoma shunt or a history of trabeculectomy [101]. After 1, 2, 3, and 5 years, UT-DSAEK graft survival was reported to be 99.1%, 96.2%, 94.2%, and 94.2%, respectively [58], and endothelial cell loss was observed to be equivalent to DSAEK [22].

Despite the fact that DMEK is associated with a decreased graft survival rate, some authors have observed greater 5- and 10-year survival rates following DMEK [93, 104]. Price and colleagues found that DSEK and DMEK graft survival was equivalent after 5 years [105]. The authors ascribed this result to DMEK's reduced rate of immunologic rejection, which compensates for the technique's higher rate of intraoperative cell loss [105]. As a result, additional research is needed to demonstrate DMEK's advantage over DSEK/DSAEK in terms of graft failure [106]. More research on the long-term effects of PDEK is needed.

Complications

Graft displacement, graft rejection, and idiopathic primary graft failure are some of the most common postoperative complications described for various kinds of EK (IPGF). According to Maier and colleagues, graft dislocation was 0–82% in DSAEK and 31–81% in DMEK, IPGF was 0–29% in DSAEK, 0–9% in DMEK, and 0–3% in PK, and the probability of rejection was 4% in DSAEK, 1–3% in DMEK, and 0.5–23.3% in PK [107]. The broad range of complication rates alludes to the variations in attributing variables between experiments. To identify the pooled analysis findings of the pure rates of complications, as well as a comparison of the complication rates between the EK techniques, meta-analysis studies are necessary.

Graft dislocation can occur if donor tissue is not adhered properly. To reduce postoperative wound leakage and hypotony, precise wound construction is essential. Complete fluid removal from the interface and full AC air fill are two further methods. It is also a good idea to tell the patient not to touch his or her eyes [108]. Partially separated lenticules may spontaneously recon-

nect, whereas the complete dislocated graft can be reattached using air injection or rebubbling. However, this technique may result in a greater loss of endothelial cells [109]. DMEK and DSAEK done by competent surgeons had identical graft dislocation rates, according to Philips and colleagues [110]. A review of nonrandomized trials found that DMEK had a greater risk of graft dislocations and rebubbling than DSAEK, but the evidence was of insufficient quality to draw firm conclusions [57].

Endothelial graft rejection is less common after EK than it is after PK. At the same time, race, glaucoma history, and corticosteroid-induced ocular hypertension have all been found as significant variables to transplant failure [111]. After 2 years, the rejection rates of DSEK, DMEK, and PK were significantly different (12%, 1%, and 18%, respectively), indicating that DMEK is a key priority in this regard [112]. Other research verified that DMEK has the lowest rejection rate when compared to DSAEK and PK [113]. Modern lamellar procedures, which result in a lower immune response, are thought to be the most important element in lowering the graft rejection rate following DSAEK and DMEK [114]. Only one incidence of graft rejection was recorded in a study of 72 individuals (144 eyes) who received DSAEK in one eye followed by DMEK in the other, indicating that this complication is not a worry with these surgical techniques [57]. More research on the long-term effects of PDEK and UT-DSAEK is needed.

IPGF has documented a rare PK consequence (3%), but DSAEK and DMEK have reported greater rates (0–29% and 0–9%, respectively) [107]. IPGF is caused by the donor's endothelial function being inadequate, which might be related to poor donor quality or surgical stress. A retrospective comparison between DSAEK and DMEK revealed that DMEK had a higher IPGF rate [115], which might be attributable to surgeons' lack of competence with the newer procedure [116].

Glaucoma, cataract, endophthalmitis, microbial keratitis, suture-related problems, suprachoroidal hemorrhage, and DM separation from the donor graft are some of the less frequent consequences [117].

Future of EK

EK techniques are always changing. Several innovative surgical approaches are proposed, including the use of a hydrogel scaffold [118], a preloaded transport cartridge [119], and a DMEK surgery marking technique [120]. For improved vision [121] and predicting the visual prognosis following surgery, new technologies and procedures are being developed [122]. As a result, the new recommended details for the aforementioned surgical kinds, such as DSEK, DSAEK, and DMEK, must be extensively evaluated for their reliability and application. Furthermore, the two EK procedures examined in this study, UT-DSAEK and PDEK, are relatively novel techniques, with few major randomized clinical trials examining their long-term surgical results. PDEK, which is simpler and more adaptable than DMEK, may be the next generation of the most often used EK. More research is needed to compare the long-term surgical results of PDEK with other EK methods.

Conclusion

EK has been found to be superior to PK in treating corneal endothelial dysfunction and is now the therapy of choice. DSEK and its variations became the most extensively utilized EK approach after its inception, owing to its positive surgical results. The eye banks' precut tissues play an important role in the widespread usage of this technology. However, because of the long visual recovery and danger of problems like as graft rejection, another approach, DMEK, was developed, which demonstrated a quicker and better visual recovery. Despite this, DMEK's surgical problems prevented it from being widely used. PDEK's innovation may be able to overcome DMEK's constraints, such as technological difficulties and the age restriction for donor selection. However, because PDEK is a novel approach, further research is needed to assess long-term clinical outcomes and compare it to other procedures.

Literature Search

We used PubMed, MEDLINE, EMBASE, ISI, and the Cochrane Central Register of Controlled Trials (CENTRAL) to conduct an electronic database search, following the PRISMA (Preferred Reporting Items for Systematic Review and Meta-Analyses) statement's widely accepted technique standards. "Endothelial keratoplasty," "corneal" and "transplantation," "Descemet stripping endothelial keratoplasty," "Descemet membrane endothelial keratoplasty," "Descemet stripping automated endothelial keratoplasty," "Descemet stripping automated endothelial keratoplasty," "Descemet stripping automated endothelial keratoplasty," "Desc "DSEK" vs. "DMEK," "DSEK" vs. "DSAEK," "ultrathin Descemet stripping automated endothelial keratoplasty," "UT-DSAEK" vs. "DSAEK," "UT-DSAEK" vs. "DMEK," "pre-endothelial descemet's keratoplasty," "eye bank," or "eye banking" and "endot." From 2010 to 2021, one researcher examined the journals and retrieved studies published in English. This review did not include any non-English articles. Conference abstracts, complete texts without raw data retrieval, duplicate publications, case reports, and letters were all removed. The whole text of the publications chosen by the first researcher was then evaluated by all writers, who meticulously scrutinized the articles. Any relevant references listed in the publications were also reviewed and incorporated in the research during the careful examination of the complete text of the articles. The final form of the literature review described above was agreed upon by all authors. Articles were chosen for inclusion depending on their importance and limits.

Take Home Notes

- PDEK may be the next generation of the most widely used EK because it is easier and more applicable than DMEK.
- More research is needed to compare the long-term surgical outcomes of PDEK with other EK methods.

References

1. Zirm E. Eine erfolgreiche totale Keratoplastik. Graefes Arhiv für Ophthalmologie. 1906;64(3):580–93.
2. Güell JL, El Husseiny MA, Manero F, Gris O, Elies D. Historical review and update of surgical treatment for corneal endothelial diseases. Ophthalmol Therapy. 2014;3(1–2):1–15.
3. Tillett CW. Posterior lamellar keratoplasty. Am J Ophthalmol. 1956;41(3):530–3.
4. Melles G, Eggink F, Lander F, Pels E, Rietveld F, Beekhuis WH, Binder PS. A surgical technique for posterior lamellar keratoplasty. Cornea. 1998;17(6):618–26.
5. Melles GR, Lander F, Nieuwendaal C. Sutureless, posterior lamellar keratoplasty: a case report· of a modified technique. Cornea. 2002;21(3):325–7.
6. Terry MA, Ousley PJ. Deep lamellar endothelial keratoplasty in the first United States patients: early clinical results. Cornea. 2001;20(3):239–43.
7. Melles GR, Wijdh RH, Nieuwendaal CP. A technique to excise the Descemet membrane from a recipient cornea (descemetorhexis). Cornea. 2004;23(3):286–8.
8. Price FW, Price MO. Descemet's stripping with endothelial keratoplasty in 50 eyes: a refractive neutral corneal transplant. J Refract Surg. 2005;21(4):339–45.
9. Gorovoy MS. Descemet-stripping automated endothelial Keratoplasty. Cornea. 2006;25(8):886–9.
10. Koenig SB, Covert DJ, Dupps WJ Jr, Meisler DM. Visual acuity, refractive error, and endothelial cell density six months after Descemet stripping and automated endothelial keratoplasty (DSAEK). Cornea. 2007;26(6):670–4.
11. Bahar I, Sansanayudh W, Levinger E, Kaiserman I, Srinivasan S, Rootman D. Posterior lamellar keratoplasty—comparison of deep lamellar endothelial keratoplasty and Descemet stripping automated endothelial keratoplasty in the same patients: a patient's perspective. Br J Ophthalmol. 2009;93(2):186–90.
12. Covert DJ, Koenig SB. Descemet stripping and automated endothelial keratoplasty (DSAEK) in eyes with failed penetrating keratoplasty. Cornea. 2007;26(6):692–6.
13. Chen ES, Shamie N, Terry MA, Hoar KL. Endothelial keratoplasty: improvement of vision after healthy donor tissue exchange. Cornea. 2008;27(3):279–82.
14. Melles GR, San Ong T, Ververs B, van der Wees J. Descemet membrane endothelial keratoplasty (DMEK). Cornea. 2006;25(8):987–90.
15. Price MO, Giebel AW, Fairchild KM, Price FW Jr. Descemet's membrane endothelial keratoplasty: prospective multicenter study of visual and refractive outcomes and endothelial survival. Ophthalmology. 2009;116(12):2361–8.
16. Dapena I, Ham L, Melles GR. Endothelial keratoplasty: DSEK/DSAEK or DMEK-the thinner the better? Curr Opin Ophthalmol. 2009;20(4):299–307.
17. Bhandari V, Reddy JK, Relekar K, Prabhu V. Descemet's stripping automated endothelial keratoplasty versus Descemet's membrane endothelial keratoplasty in the fellow eye for fuchs endothelial dystrophy: a retrospective study. Biomed Res Int. 2015;2015:1.
18. Price MO, Feng MT, Price FW Jr. Endothelial Keratoplasty update 2020. Cornea. 2021;40(5):541–7.
19. Eye OAS. Standardized "no-touch" technique for Descemet membrane endothelial keratoplasty. Arch Ophthalmol. 2011;129(1):88–94.
20. Kruse FE, Laaser K, Cursiefen C, Heindl LM, Schlötzer-Schrehardt U, Riss S, Bachmann BO. A stepwise approach to donor preparation and insertion increases safety and outcome of Descemet membrane endothelial keratoplasty. Cornea. 2011;30(5):580–7.
21. Neff KD, Biber JM, Holland EJ. Comparison of central corneal graft thickness to visual acuity outcomes in endothelial keratoplasty. Cornea. 2011;30(4):388–91.
22. Dickman MM, Kruit PJ, Remeijer L, van Rooij J, Van der Lelij A, Wijdh RH, van den Biggelaar FJ, Berendschot TT, Nuijts RM. A randomized multicenter clinical trial of ultrathin Descemet stripping automated endothelial keratoplasty (DSAEK) versus DSAEK. Ophthalmology. 2016;123(11):2276–84.
23. Busin M, Madi S, Santorum P, Scorcia V, Beltz J. Ultrathin Descemet's stripping automated endothelial keratoplasty with the microkeratome double-pass technique: two-year outcomes. Ophthalmology. 2013;120(6):1186–94.
24. Mencucci R, Favuzza E, Marziali E, Cennamo M, Mazzotta C, Lucenteforte E, Virgili G, Rizzo S. Ultrathin Descemet stripping automated endothelial keratoplasty versus Descemet membrane endothelial keratoplasty: a fellow-eye comparison. Eye. 2020;7:1–9.
25. Chamberlain W, Lin CC, Austin A, Schubach N, Clover J, McLeod SD, Porco TC, Lietman TM, Rose-Nussbaumer J. Descemet endothelial thickness comparison trial: a randomized trial comparing ultrathin Descemet stripping automated endothelial keratoplasty with Descemet membrane endothelial keratoplasty. Ophthalmology. 2019;126(1):19–26.
26. Zhu L, Zha Y, Cai J, Zhang Y. Descemet stripping automated endothelial keratoplasty versus descemet membrane endothelial keratoplasty: a meta-analysis. Int Ophthalmol. 2018;38(2):897–905.
27. Tourabaly M, Chetrit Y, Provost J, Georgeon C, Kallel S, Temstet C, Bouheraoua N, Borderie V. Influence of graft thickness and regularity on vision recovery after endothelial keratoplasty. Br J Ophthalmol. 2020;104(9):1317–23.

28. Agarwal A, Dua HS, Narang P, Kumar DA, Agarwal A, Jacob S, Agarwal A, Gupta A. Pre-Descemet's endothelial keratoplasty (PDEK). Br J Ophthalmol. 2014;98(9):1181–5.

29. Ross AR, Said DG, Gisoldi RAC, Nubile M, El-Amin A, Gabr AF, Abd M, Mencucci R, Pocobelli A, Mastropasqua L. Optimizing pre-Descemet endothelial keratoplasty technique. J Cataract Refract Surg. 2020;46(5):667–74.

30. Narang P, Agarwal A. Pre-Descemet's endothelial keratoplasty. Indian J Ophthalmol. 2017;65(6):443.

31. Park CY, Lee JK, Gore PK, Lim C-Y, Chuck RS. Keratoplasty in the United States: a 10-year review from 2005 through 2014. Ophthalmology. 2015;122(12):2432–42.

32. Mohamed A, Chaurasia S, Murthy SI, Ramappa M, Vaddavalli PK, Taneja M, Garg P, Chinta S, Basu S, Rathi VM. Endothelial keratoplasty: a review of indications at a tertiary eye care Centre in South India. Asia Pac J Ophthalmol. 2014;3(4):207–10.

33. Woo J-H, Ang M, Htoon HM, Tan D. Descemet membrane endothelial keratoplasty versus Descemet stripping automated endothelial keratoplasty and penetrating keratoplasty. Am J Ophthalmol. 2019;207:288–303.

34. Green M, Wilkins MR. Comparison of early surgical experience and visual outcomes of DSAEK and DMEK. Cornea. 2015;34(11):1341–4.

35. Baydoun L, Ham L, Borderie V, Dapena I, Hou J, Frank LE, Oellerich S, Melles GR. Endothelial survival after Descemet membrane endothelial keratoplasty: effect of surgical indication and graft adherence status. JAMA Ophthalmol. 2015;133(11):1277–85.

36. Birbal RS, Baydoun L, Ham L, Miron A, Van Dijk K, Dapena I, Jager MJ, Böhringer S, Oellerich S, Melles GR. Effect of surgical indication and pre-operative lens status on Descemet membrane endothelial keratoplasty outcomes. Am J Ophthalmol. 2020;212:79–87.

37. Veldman PB, Terry MA, Straiko MD. Evolving indications for Descemet's stripping automated endothelial keratoplasty. Curr Opin Ophthalmol. 2014;25(4):306–11.

38. Price FW Jr, Price MO. Combined cataract/DSEK/DMEK: changing expectations. Asia Paci J Ophthalmol. 2017;6(4):388–92.

39. Chaurasia S, Price FW Jr, Gunderson L, Price MO. Descemet's membrane endothelial keratoplasty: clinical results of single versus triple procedures (combined with cataract surgery). Ophthalmology. 2014;121(2):454–8.

40. Parker J, Dirisamer M, Naveiras M, Tse WHW, van Dijk K, Frank LE, Ham L, Melles GR. Outcomes of Descemet membrane endothelial keratoplasty in phakic eyes. J Cataract Refract Surg. 2012;38(5):871–7.

41. Trindade BLC, Eliazar GC. Descemet membrane endothelial keratoplasty (DMEK): an update on safety, efficacy and patient selection. Clin Ophthalmol. 2019;13:1549.

42. Clements JL, Bouchard CS, Lee WB, Dunn SP, Mannis MJ, Reidy JJ, John T, Hannush SB, Goins KM, Wagoner MD. Retrospective review of graft dislocation rate associated with descemet stripping automated endothelial keratoplasty after primary failed penetrating keratoplasty. Cornea. 2011;30(4):414–8.

43. Anshu A, Price MO, Tan DT, Price FW Jr. Endothelial keratoplasty: a revolution in evolution. Surv Ophthalmol. 2012;57(3):236–52.

44. Schrittenlocher S, Schlereth SL, Siebelmann S, Hayashi T, Matthaei M, Bachmann B, Cursiefen C. Long-term outcome of descemet membrane endothelial keratoplasty (DMEK) following failed penetrating keratoplasty (PK). Acta Ophthalmol. 2020;98(7):e901–6.

45. Liarakos VS, Satué M, Livny E, van Dijk K, Ham L, Baydoun L, Dapena I, Melles GR. Descemet membrane endothelial keratoplasty for a decompensated penetrating keratoplasty graft in the presence of a long glaucoma tube. Cornea. 2015;34(12):1613–6.

46. Liarakos VS, Ham L, Dapena I, Tong CM, Quilendrino R, Yeh R-Y, Melles GR. Endothelial keratoplasty for bullous keratopathy in eyes with an anterior chamber intraocular lens. J Cataract Refract Surg. 2013;39(12):1835–45.

47. Weller JM, Tourtas T, Kruse FE, Schlötzer-Schrehardt U, Fuchsluger T, Bachmann BO. Descemet membrane endothelial keratoplasty as treatment for graft failure after descemet stripping automated endothelial keratoplasty. Am J Ophthalmol. 2015;159(6):1050–7. e2

48. Agha B, Shajari M, Slavik-Lencova A, Kohnen T, Schmack I. Outcome of Descemet membrane endothelial keratoplasty for graft failure after Descemet stripping automated endothelial keratoplasty. Clin Ophthalmol. 2019;13:553.

49. Mitry D, Bhogal M, Patel AK, Lee BS, Chai SM, Price MO, Price FW, Jun AS, Aldave AJ, Mehta JS. Descemet stripping automated endothelial keratoplasty after failed penetrating keratoplasty: survival, rejection risk, and visual outcome. JAMA Ophthalmol. 2014;132(6):742–9.

50. Einan-Lifshitz A, Mednick Z, Belkin A, Sorkin N, Alshaker S, Boutin T, Chan CC, Rootman DS. Comparison of Descemet stripping automated endothelial keratoplasty and Descemet membrane endothelial keratoplasty in the treatment of failed penetrating keratoplasty. Cornea. 2019;38(9):1077–82.

51. Bonnet C, Ghaffari R, Alkadi T, Law SK, Caprioli J, Yu F, Deng SX. Long-term outcomes of Descemet membrane endothelial keratoplasty in eyes with prior glaucoma surgery. Am J Ophthalmol. 2020;218:288–95.

52. Aldave AJ, Chen JL, Zaman AS, Deng SX, Yu F. Outcomes after DSEK in 101 eyes with previous trabeculectomy and tube shunt implantation. Cornea. 2014;33(3):223–9.

53. Mehta JS, Parthasarthy A, Por Y-M, Cajucom-Uy H, Beuerman RW, Tan D. Femtosecond laser-assisted endothelial keratoplasty: a laboratory model. Cornea. 2008;27(6):706–12.

54. Eguchi H, Miyamoto T, Hotta F, Tomida M, Inoue M, Mitamura Y. Descemet-stripping automated endothelial keratoplasty for vitrectomized cases with traumatic aniridia and aphakic bullous keratopathy. Clin Ophthalmol. 2012;6:1513.

55. Shah AK, Terry MA, Shamie N, Chen ES, Phillips PM, Hoar KL, Friend DJ, Davis-Boozer D. Complications and clinical outcomes of Descemet stripping automated endothelial keratoplasty with intraocular lens exchange. Am J Ophthalmol. 2010;149(3):390–7. e1

56. Sharma N, Maharana PK, Singhi S, Aron N, Patil M. Descemet stripping automated endothelial keratoplasty. Indian J Ophthalmol. 2017;65(3):198.

57. Stuart AJ, Romano V, Virgili G, Shortt AJ. Descemet's membrane endothelial keratoplasty (DMEK) versus Descemet's stripping automated endothelial keratoplasty (DSAEK) for corneal endothelial failure. Cochrane Database Syst Rev. 2018;6(6):CD012097.

58. Madi S, Leon P, Nahum Y, D'Angelo S, Giannaccare G, Beltz J, Busin M. Five-year outcomes of ultrathin Descemet stripping automated endothelial keratoplasty. Cornea. 2019;38(9):1192–7.

59. Dunker SL, Dickman MM, Wisse RP, Nobacht S, Wijdh RH, Bartels MC, Tang ML, van den Biggelaar FJ, Kruit PJ, Nuijts RM. Descemet membrane endothelial keratoplasty versus ultrathin Descemet stripping automated endothelial keratoplasty: a multicenter randomized controlled clinical trial. Ophthalmology. 2020;127(9):1152–9.

60. Yamazoe K, Yamazoe K, Shinozaki N, Shimazaki J. Influence of the precutting and overseas transportation of corneal grafts for Descemet stripping automated endothelial keratoplasty on donor endothelial cell loss. Cornea. 2013;32(6):741–4.

61. Price MO, Baig KM, Brubaker JW, Price FW Jr. Randomized, prospective comparison of precut vs surgeon-dissected grafts for descemet stripping automated endothelial keratoplasty. Am J Ophthalmol. 2008;146(1):36–41. e2

62. Singh NP, Said DG, Dua HS. Lamellar keratoplasty techniques. Indian J Ophthalmol. 2018;66(9):1239.

63. Phillips PM, Phillips LJ, Saad HA, Terry MA, Stolz DB, Stoeger C, Franks J, Davis-Boozer D. "Ultrathin" DSAEK tissue prepared with a low–pulse energy, high-frequency femtosecond laser. Cornea. 2013;32(1):81–6.

64. Sikder S, Nordgren RN, Neravetla SR, Moshirfar M. Ultra-thin donor tissue preparation for endothelial keratoplasty with a double-pass microkeratome. Am J Ophthalmol. 2011;152(2):202–8. e2

65. Boynton GE, Woodward MA. Eye-bank preparation of endothelial tissue. Curr Opin Ophthalmol. 2014;25(4):319.

66. Birbal RS, Sikder S, Lie JT, Groeneveld-van Beek EA, Oellerich S, Melles GR. Donor tissue preparation for Descemet membrane endothelial keratoplasty: an updated review. Cornea. 2018;37(1):128–35.

67. Maharana PK, Sahay P, Singhal D, Sharma N, Titiyal JS. Donor preparation in Descemet membrane endothelial keratoplasty. New Front Ophthalmol. 2018;5:1–6.

68. Romano V, Kazaili A, Pagano L, Gadhvi KA, Titley M, Steger B, Fernández-Vega-Cueto L, Meana A, Merayo-Lloves J, Diego P. Eye bank versus surgeon prepared DMEK tissues: influence on adhesion and re-bubbling rate. Br J Ophthalmol. 2020;106:177.

69. Romano V, Pagano L, Gadhvi KA, Coco G, Titley M, Fenech MT, Ferrari S, Levis HJ, Parekh M, Kaye S. Clinical outcomes of pre-loaded ultra-thin DSAEK and pre-loaded DMEK. BMJ Open Ophthalmol. 2020;5(1):e000546.

70. Ighani M, Karakus S, Eghrari AO. Clinical outcomes of Descemet membrane endothelial keratoplasty using the Bonfadini-Todd injector for graft insertion. Clin Ophthalmol. 2019;13:1869.

71. Shen E, Fox A, Johnson B, Fárid M. Comparing the effect of three Descemet membrane endothelial keratoplasty injectors on endothelial damage of grafts. Indian J Ophthalmol. 2020;68(6):1040.

72. Droutsas K, Lazaridis A, Kymionis G, Chatzistefanou K, Moschos M, Koutsandrea C, Sekundo W. Comparison of endothelial cell loss and complications following DMEK with the use of three different graft injectors. Eye. 2018;32(1):19–25.

73. Liarakos VS, Dapena I, Ham L, van Dijk K, Melles GR. Intraocular graft unfolding techniques in Descemet membrane endothelial keratoplasty. JAMA ophthalmol. 2013;131(1):29–35.

74. Dua HS, Termote K, Kenawy MB, Said DG, Jayaswal R, Nubile M, Mastropasqua L, Holland S. Scrolling characteristics of pre-Descemet endothelial keratoplasty tissue: an ex vivo study. Am J Ophthalmol. 2016;166:84–90.

75. Pereira NC, dos Santos FA, Maluf RCP, Dua HS. Pre-Descemet's endothelial keratoplasty: a simple, Descemet's membrane scoring technique for successful graft preparation. Br J Ophthalmol. 2021;106:786–9.

76. Dua H, Said D. Pre-descemets endothelial keratoplasty: the PDEK clamp for successful PDEK. Eye. 2017;31(7):1106–10.

77. Saint-Jean A, Soper M, Den Beste K, Iverson S, Price MO, Price FW. Technique for ensuring type I bubble formation for pre-descemet endothelial keratoplasty preparation. Cornea. 2019;38(10):1336–8.

78. Altaan SL, Gupta A, Sidney LE, Elalfy MS, Agarwal A, Dua HS. Endothelial cell loss following tissue harvesting by pneumodissection for endothelial keratoplasty: an ex vivo study. Br J Ophthalmol. 2015;99(5):710–3.

79. Kaufman AR, Nosé RM, Roberto Pineda I. Descemetorhexis without endothelial keratoplasty (DWEK): proposal for nomenclature standardization. Cornea. 2018;37:e20–1.

80. Moloney G, et al. Descemetorhexis without grafting for Fuchs endothelial dystrophy—supplementation with topical ripasudil. Cornea. 2017;36:642–8.

81. Dirisamer M, Ham L, Dapena I, van Dijk K, Melles GR. Descemet membrane endothelial transfer:"free-floating" donor Descemet implantation as a potential alternative to "keratoplasty". Cornea. 2012;31:194–7.

82. Shah RD, Randleman JB, Grossniklaus HE. Spontaneous corneal clearing after descemet's stripping without endothelial replacement. Ophthalmology. 2012;119:256–60.

83. Moloney G, et al. Descemetorhexis for fuchs' dystrophy. Can J Ophthalmol. 2015;50:68–72.

84. Borkar DS, Veldman P, Colby KA. Treatment of Fuchs endothelial dystrophy by Descemet stripping without endothelial keratoplasty. Cornea. 2016;35:1267–73.

85. Iovieno A, Neri A, Soldani AM, Adani C, Fontana L. Descemetorhexis without graft placement for the treatment of fuchs endothelial dystrophy: preliminary results and review of the literature. Cornea. 2017;36:637–41.

86. Arbelaez JG, Price MO, Price FW Jr. Long-term follow-up and complications of stripping descemet membrane without placement of graft in eyes with fuchs endothelial dystrophy. Cornea. 2014;33:1295–9.

87. Bleyen I, Saelens IE, van Dooren BT, van Rij G. Spontaneous corneal clearing after Descemet's stripping. Ophthalmology. 2013;120:215.

88. Koenig SB. Planned descemetorhexis without endothelial keratoplasty in eyes with Fuchs corneal endothelial dystrophy. Cornea. 2015;34:1149–51.

89. Heinzelmann S, Shanab WA, Böhringer D, Maier P, Reinhard T. Prediction of visual acuity after Dsaek from oct images. Invest Ophthalmol Vis Sci. 2012;53(14):43.

90. Li JY, Terry MA, Goshe J, Davis-Boozer D, Shamie N. Three-year visual acuity outcomes after Descemet's stripping automated endothelial keratoplasty. Ophthalmology. 2012;119(6):1126–9.

91. Lanza M, Boccia R, Ruggiero A, Melillo P, Bifani Sconocchia M, Simonelli F, Sbordone S. Evaluation of donor and recipient characteristics involved in Descemet stripping automated endothelial Keratoplasty outcomes. Front Med. 2021; 8:421.

92. Wacker K, Bourne WM, Patel SV. Effect of graft thickness on visual acuity after Descemet stripping endothelial keratoplasty: a systematic review and meta-analysis. Am J Ophthalmol. 2016;163:18–28.

93. Vasiliauskaitė I, Oellerich S, Ham L, Dapena I, Baydoun L, van Dijk K, Melles GR. Descemet membrane endothelial keratoplasty: ten-year graft survival and clinical outcomes. Am J Ophthalmol. 2020;217:114–20.

94. Jansen C, Zetterberg M. Descemet membrane endothelial keratoplasty versus descemet stripping automated keratoplasty–outcome of one single surgeon's more than 200 initial consecutive cases. Clin Ophthalmol. 2021;15:909.

95. Singh A, Zarei-Ghanavati M, Avadhanam V, Liu C. Systematic review and meta-analysis of clinical outcomes of descemet membrane endothelial keratoplasty versus Descemet stripping endothelial keratoplasty/descemet stripping automated endothelial keratoplasty. Cornea. 2017;36(11):1437–43.

96. Pavlovic I, Shajari M, Herrmann E, Schmack I, Lencova A, Kohnen T. Meta-analysis of postoperative outcome parameters comparing descemet membrane endothelial keratoplasty versus Descemet stripping automated endothelial keratoplasty. Cornea. 2017;36(12):1445–51.

97. Li S, Liu L, Wang W, Huang T, Zhong X, Yuan J, Liang L. Efficacy and safety of Descemet's membrane endothelial keratoplasty versus Descemet's stripping endothelial keratoplasty: a systematic review and meta-analysis. PLoS One. 2017;12(12):e0182275.

98. Droutsas K, Petrelli M, Miltsakakis D, Andreanos K, Karagianni A, Lazaridis A, Koutsandrea C, Kymionis G. Visual outcomes of ultrathin-descemet stripping endothelial keratoplasty versus Descemet stripping endothelial keratoplasty. J Ophthalmol. 2018;2018:1.

99. Torras-Sanvicens J, Blanco-Domínguez I, Sánchez-González J-M, Rachwani-Anil R, Spencer J-F, Sabater-Cruz N, Peraza-Nieves J, Rocha-de-Lossada C. Visual quality and subjective satisfaction in ultrathin descemet stripping automated endothelial keratoplasty (UT-DSAEK) versus descemet membrane endothelial Keratoplasty (DMEK): a fellow-eye comparison. J Clin Med. 2021;10(3):419.

100. Li ALW, Kwok RPW, Kam KW, Young AL. A 5-year analysis of endothelial vs penetrating keratoplasty graft survival in Chinese patients. Int J Ophthalmol. 2020;13(9):1374.

101. Price MO, Fairchild KM, Price DA, Price FW Jr. Descemet's stripping endothelial keratoplasty: five-year graft survival and endothelial cell loss. Ophthalmology. 2011;118(4):725–9.

102. Ang M, Soh Y, Htoon HM, Mehta JS, Tan D. Five-year graft survival comparing DESCEMET stripping automated endothelial keratoplasty and penetrating keratoplasty. Ophthalmology. 2016;123(8):1646–52.

103. Letko E, Price DA, Lindoso EM, Price MO, Price FW Jr. Secondary graft failure and repeat endothelial keratoplasty after Descemet's stripping automated endothelial keratoplasty. Ophthalmology. 2011;118(2):310–4.

104. Birbal RS, Dhubhghaill SN, Bourgonje VJ, Hanko J, Ham L, Jager MJ, Böhringer S, Oellerich S, Melles GR. Five-year graft survival and clinical outcomes of 500 consecutive cases after Descemet membrane endothelial keratoplasty. Cornea. 2020;39(3):290–7.

105. Price DA, Kelley M, Price FW Jr, Price MO. Five-year graft survival of Descemet membrane endothelial keratoplasty (EK) versus Descemet stripping EK and the effect of donor sex matching. Ophthalmology. 2018;125(10):1508–14.

106. Patel SV. Graft survival and endothelial outcomes in the new era of endothelial keratoplasty. Exp Eye Res. 2012;95(1):40–7.
107. Maier P, Reinhard T, Cursiefen C. Descemet stripping endothelial keratoplasty—rapid recovery of visual acuity. Dtsch Arztebl Int. 2013;110(21):365.
108. Deshmukh R, Nair S, Ting DSJ, Agarwal T, Beltz J, Vajpayee RB. Graft detachments in endothelial keratoplasty. Br J Ophthalmol. 2021;106:1.
109. Gerber-Hollbach N, Baydoun L, López EF, Frank LE, Dapena I, Liarakos VS, Schaal S-C, Ham L, Oellerich S, Melles GR. Clinical outcome of rebubbling for graft detachment after descemet membrane endothelial keratoplasty. Cornea. 2017;36(7):771–6.
110. Phillips PM, Phillips LJ, Muthappan V, Maloney CM, Carver CN. Experienced DSAEK surgeon's transition to DMEK: outcomes comparing the last 100 DSAEK surgeries with the first 100 DMEK surgeries exclusively using previously published techniques. Cornea. 2017;36(3):275–9.
111. Price MO, Jordan CS, Moore G, Price FW. Graft rejection episodes after Descemet stripping with endothelial keratoplasty: part two: the statistical analysis of probability and risk factors. Br J Ophthalmol. 2009;93(3):391–5.
112. Anshu A, Price MO, Price FW Jr. Risk of corneal transplant rejection significantly reduced with Descemet's membrane endothelial keratoplasty. Ophthalmology. 2012;119(3):536–40.
113. Heinzelmann S, Böhringer D, Eberwein P, Reinhard T, Maier P. Outcomes of Descemet membrane endothelial keratoplasty, Descemet stripping automated endothelial keratoplasty and penetrating keratoplasty from a single Centre study. Graefes Arch Clin Exp Ophthalmol. 2016;254(3):515–22.
114. Hos D, Matthaei M, Bock F, Maruyama K, Notara M, Clahsen T, Hou Y, Le VNH, Salabarria A-C, Horstmann J. Immune reactions after modern lamellar (DALK, DSAEK, DMEK) versus conventional penetrating corneal transplantation. Prog Retin Eye Res. 2019;73:100768.
115. Hamzaoglu EC, Straiko MD, Mayko ZM, Sáles CS, Terry MA. The first 100 eyes of standardized descemet stripping automated endothelial keratoplasty versus standardized descemet membrane endothelial keratoplasty. Ophthalmology. 2015;122(11):2193–9.
116. Dapena I, Ham L, van Luijk C, van der Wees J, Melles GR. Back-up procedure for graft failure in descemet membrane endothelial keratoplasty (DMEK). Br J Ophthalmol. 2010;94(2):241–4.
117. Zafar S, Wang P, Woreta FA, Aziz K, Makary M, Ghous Z, Srikumaran D. Postoperative complications in Medicare beneficiaries following endothelial keratoplasty surgery. Am J Ophthalmol. 2020;219:1–11.
118. Daniell M, Brown KD, Gurr P, Scheerlinck J-P, Dusting G, Sawant O, Titus M, Qiao G. Use of novel hydrogel scaffold to assist Descemet's membrane endothelial keratoplasty (DMEK) surgery. Invest Ophthalmol Vis Sci. 2020;61(7):3601.
119. Rickmann A, Wahl S, Hofmann N, Knakowski J, Haus A, Börgel M, Szurman P. Comparison of preloaded grafts for Descemet membrane endothelial keratoplasty (DMEK) in a novel preloaded transport cartridge compared to conventional precut grafts. Cell Tissue Bank. 2020;21:1–9.
120. Or L, Krakauer Y, Sorkin N, Knyazer B, Ashkenazy Z, Gushansky K, Dubinsky-Pertzov B, Gazit I, Einan-Lifshitz A. A novel marking technique for descemet membrane endothelial graft using an ophthalmic viscoelastic device. Cornea. 2021;40(4):529–32.
121. Fogla R. A novel device to visualize Descemet membrane during donor preparation for descemet membrane endothelial keratoplasty. Indian J Ophthalmol. 2021;69(6):1609–13.
122. Khalid M, Khan FS. Nonlinear DSEK model: a novel mathematical model that predicts stability in ocular parameters after Descemet's stripping endothelial Keratoplasty. Punjab Univ J Mathematics. 2020;52(4):1–14.

Endothelial Keratoplasty: Current State of the Art

Anjulie Gang, Francis W. Price, and Marianne O. Price

Key Points

- EK offers a significantly better risk/benefit ratio than PK.
- The primary methods of EK are DSAEK/DSEK and DMEK.
- DMEK provides the most rapid visual improvement, least refractive change, and least risk of rejection and the need for topical corticosteroids.
- DSEK is more advantageous in eyes with large iris defects or aphakia.
- Trifolded EK grafts unfold easier and are advantageous in the complicated eye with previous pars planna vitrectomy, aphakia, or iris defects.

Supplementary Information The online version contains supplementary material available at https://doi.org/10.1007/978-3-031-32408-6_26.

A. Gang · F. W. Price
Price Vision Group, Indianapolis, IN, USA
e-mail: anjuliegang@pricevisiongroup.net;
fprice@pricevisiongroup.net

M. O. Price (✉)
Cornea Research Foundation, Price Vision Group,
Indianapolis, IN, USA
e-mail: mprice@cornea.org

Introduction

The advent of selective endothelial replacement (EK) has revolutionized treatment of corneal endothelial dysfunction, a leading indication for corneal transplantation, because EK can be performed through a small (2-mm) incision, is a closed eye procedure, and provides faster recovery and more predictable visual outcomes than penetrating keratoplasty (PK). Moreover, just as in cataract surgery, the smaller incision provides protection against wound/eye rupture from minor trauma which is a life-long risk after PK or other large incision surgery like intracapsular cataract surgery. The smaller EK incisions also preserve corneal innervation and therefore do not produce the neurotrophic issues and secondary dry eye problems often see after PK. The improved benefit-to-risk ratio with EK allows earlier intervention in the disease process.

The two EK techniques in widespread use are Descemet membrane endothelial keratoplasty (DMEK) and Descemet stripping automated endothelial keratoplasty (known as DSAEK or DSEK). Both typically involve the removal of dysfunctional endothelium and Descemet membrane from the central 8 to 9 mm of the recipient cornea and replacement with healthy donor tissue. With DMEK the donor tissue consists of endothelium and Descemet membrane, thus exactly replacing the layers removed from the host cornea. DSAEK includes a thin layer of posterior donor stroma along with Descemet membrane and endothelium. Although the thinner DMEK tissue was initially more challenging to handle when the technique was first introduced by Melles in 2006 [1], with subsequent advances, DMEK has become the preferred EK technique worldwide and is a viable option even in difficult eyes with various ocular comorbidities. Compared with PK and DSAEK, DMEK has the lowest rejection rate [2], requires the smallest incision, and provides the fastest visual recovery [3]. However, DSAEK can be advantageous in certain situations, particularly in eyes with challenging ocular co-morbidity.

PDEK is a variation of EK with a slightly thicker donor than DMEK [4]. The PDEK donor tissue is produced by performing a type-1 bubble and then excising the bubble (DMEK is essentially a thinner layer as achieved with a type-2 bubble). Current limitations of PDEK are the donor prep is more difficult and the size of the bubble is limited to 7–8 mm in diameter. However, recent studies have suggested techniques to produce 8–9 mm donor diameters for PDEK and that may allow more widespread use of this technique.

Indications

Endothelial keratoplasty is the gold standard for treating all types of visually significant corneal endothelial dysfunction. The leading indications in Europe, America, and Australia are Fuchs endothelial corneal dystrophy (FECD), corneal decompensation following cataract and/or glaucoma surgery, and failure of a prior corneal transplant. In Asia, FECD is less prevalent and endothelial dysfunction is more often associated with trauma from surgery or laser procedures in eyes with anatomically narrow angles and a shallow anterior chamber. Less common conditions amenable to treatment with EK include iridocorneal endothelial syndrome (ICE) syndrome, posterior polymorphous dystrophy (PPMD), and corneal endotheliitis (in the absence of visually significant stromal scarring).

Penetrating keratoplasty can be a better option than EK for visual rehabilitation of eyes with endothelial dysfunction accompanied by visually significant stromal scarring or opacification because PK replaces all layers of the cornea. However, if the goal is simply to alleviate edema and painful bullae, EK is a less invasive option.

In eyes with a dislocated intraocular lens (IOL) or anterior chamber (AC) IOL, we only perform EK after the lens anomaly is treated first as either a staged or combined procedure. In eyes with significant iris abnormalities, aniridia and/or aphakia, DSAEK is generally a better choice than DMEK because the thicker DSAEK tissue can be suture-fixated to the recipient cornea to prevent dislocation into the posterior chamber, and the pressure changes in the unicameral eye when DMEK donors are manipulated can easily lead to loss of the donor into the posterior portion of the eye. For both DMEK or DSAEK, pull-through techniques are advantageous in aphakic eye or eyes with large iris defects.

Among patient characteristics to consider, essential blepharospasm or chronic eye rubbing could impede EK attachment because indenting the cornea can lead to graft detachment in the early post-operative period. Obesity or thyroid orbitopathy could increase the posterior pressure during surgery. Finally, it was long thought that supine positioning for at least the initial 24 h was necessary to ensure DMEK attachment, but that is problematic for some patients. Recent studies have suggested that prolonged supine positioning may not be necessary after all, especially if the patient is discharged with a large residual air or gas bubble to hold the graft in place.

Surgical Technique

DSAEK Tissue Preparation

Both DMEK and DSAEK donor tissue can be prepared by the surgeon or by an eye bank technician, and it can be prepared at the time of surgery or up to several days ahead of time. Occasionally, the endothelium may be damaged excessively during tissue preparation, so preparing the tissue ahead of time can prevent uncertainty and save time on the day of surgery.

DSAEK/DSEK tissue is usually prepared by mounting a donor corneal-scleral rim on an artificial anterior chamber and dissecting it with microkeratome. Thinner tissue is associated with better visual outcomes so various single- and double-pass techniques have been devised to produce very thin tissue while minimizing the risk of perforation. A microkeratome is expensive, so it can make sense for an eye bank to purchase one and prepare tissue for multiple surgeons. This approach also allows the eye bank to absorb the cost of any tissue lost in preparation. The rate of donor loss increases as thinner cuts are attempted with a microkeratome. Manual dissection can be done instead of using a microkeratome and was the original way the donor was prepared, but a microkeratome generally produces a more uniform dissection plane. We are not aware of anyone who has tried an anterior peel technique (as used in deep anterior lamellar keratoplasty (DALK) for donor preps, which if feasible would provide a very thin uniform dissection plane [5].

Femtosecond laser dissection has been tried, but tissue applanation is usually required and this produces compression folds in the posterior cornea, resulting in undulating dissection plane after the applanation is released. Also, the laser dissection plane is not as regular or smooth as that achieved with a microkeratome because of the collagen fiber arrangement in the posterior cornea. Thus, the visual outcomes tend to be disappointing.

DMEK Tissue Preparation

Direct peeling from the posterior surface of the donor is the most widely used method of separating the donor endothelium and Descemet membrane (DM) from the stroma [6–8]. This approach does not require any expensive instrumentation and can be readily implemented in any part of the world. Alternatives include hydro- or pneumo-dissection producing either type-1 or 2 bubbles, but these can result in more endothelial cell dam-age, higher failure rates, or with type-1 bubbles limitations on donor diameter (PDEK).

Multiple variations of direct peeling exist. In the SCUBA technique [7, 8], a Y- hook, or other instrument, with a blunt smooth tip is used to score the peripheral Descemet membrane just inside the trabecular meshwork and Schwalbe's line for the full circumference of the donor cornea. Trypan blue dye appropriate for ocular use (i.e. Vision Blue 0.6 mg/mL, DORC) is applied for about 30 s to mark the scored edges and reveal any areas incompletely scored. Trypan blue stains exposed stroma and DM but not intact endothelium. Prolonged exposure to trypan blue at high concentrations should be avoided because it can be toxic to the endothelium.

The donor tissue is submerged in corneal storage solution, and an olive-tipped micro-finger (Moria, Antony, France) is glided under the outer edge of DM to lift and free it from the underlying stroma. As the DM edge is lifted, any tags or tears are removed with small tiers to prevent tears from extending further centrally. After completely lifting the edges, the DM is grasped with forceps and carefully peeled in quadrants towards the center. It is important to watch for localized areas of strong adhesion, which appear as horse-shoe shaped tears. These start small and, when detected promptly, can be gently lifted free with the micro-finger instrument. Alternatively, peeling can be attempted from the opposite direction to free localized adhesions without propagating larger tears. After each quadrant is freed, it is floated back down onto the stroma. After peeling all four quadrants, the donor cornea is transferred to a cutting block. An 8- to 9-mm diameter trephine is used to cut through DM and partially into the stroma with the donor endothelial side up. The trephine is gently tapped to perforate DM with only shallow penetration into the stroma. We typically leave the donor attached in a small area centrally, and one of three options can be taken. The first traditional option is to peel the donor completely and load it endothelial side out in the desired inserting instrument. The second option is to leave it attached and place the whole donor corneal scleral rim back into the storage solution to be peeled the next day at surgery. The final option is to fold it into a trifold configuration and then peel it completely and load it into an IOL injector (Fig. 26.1a–g).

Tissue Orientation Marks

The final orientation of the donor graft in the eye is critical, and the endothelium needs to be facing the iris; if it is facing the stroma the graft will be nonfunctional. Therefore, with both DSAEK and DMEK, many surgeons like to have a Gentian violet orientation mark, such as an "S", stamped on the non-endothelial side during donor tissue preparation, although this can cause some endothelial damage [9]. Asymmetric orientation marks can also be cut along the edge of the tissue during preparation. Orientation marks help the surgeon ensure that the tissue is correctly oriented inside the recipient eye with the donor endothelium facing toward the host iris. However, such marks are not needed if the surgeon has access to intraoperative optical coherence tomography (OCT) because it provides a cross-sectional image of the graft configuration, and in our practice, we have not used orientation marks [10].

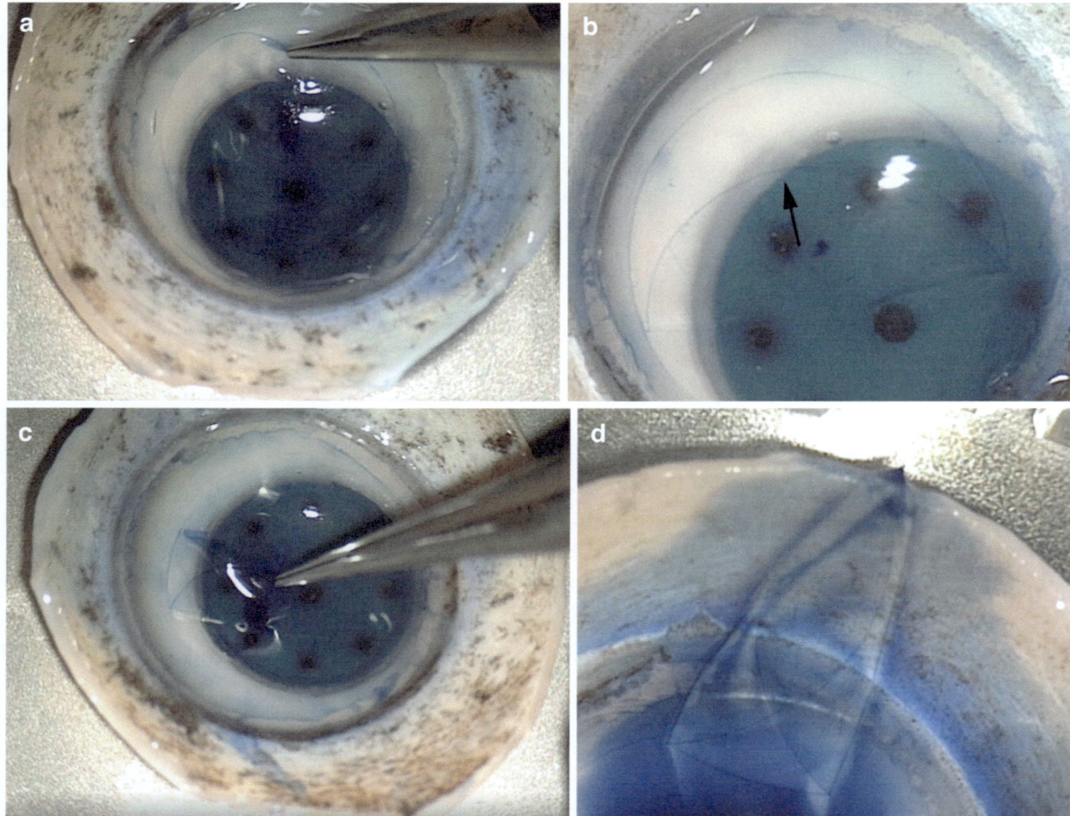

Fig. 26.1 DMEK tissue preparation and insertion using the trifold configuration. (**a**) After the donor tissue was punched to the desired diameter, typing forceps were used to grasp one edge of the tissue and fold it over with the endothelium facing inward. (**b**) An arrow shows where one-third of the tissue was folded over; also, the corneal-scleral rim was rotated 180°. (**c**) The opposite side was folded over to create a trifold. (**d**) Both sides of the tissue were folded into a trifold with the endothelium facing inward, and the tissue was pulled to the edge of the scleral button. (**e**) The blue-stained DMEK trifold was pulled into IOL cartridge. (**f**) The IOL cartridge tip was filled with fresh storage solution, and the DMEK trifold was pulled into the tip using 23-gage intraocular forceps. (**g**) The blue-stained DMEK trifold was inserted into the recipient eye; the inset at the lower right shows the corresponding intraoperative OCT image

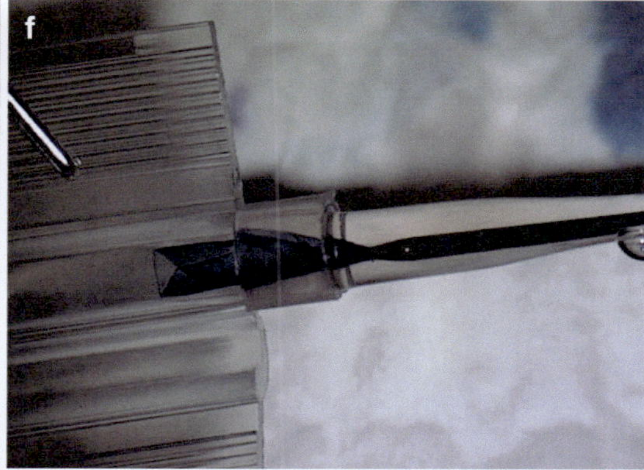

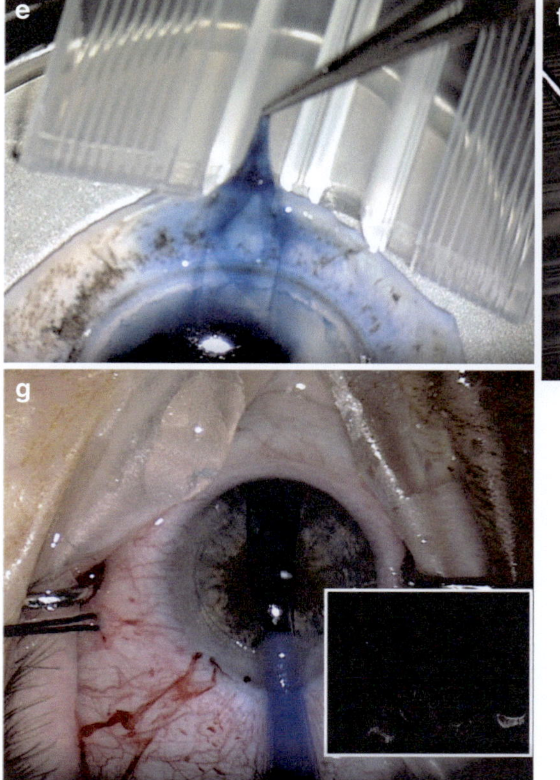

Fig. 26.1 (continued)

Recipient Preparation

We prescribe topical nonsteroidal anti-inflammatory eye drops for 3 days before surgery. At the time of surgery, pilocarpine nitrate 2% eye drops are instilled to constrict the pupil, or carbachol 0.01% can be instilled if EK is not being combined with either cataract surgery or pars planna vitrectomy. Pupil constriction helps prevents contact between the graft endothelium and the crystalline or intraocular lens during graft unfolding and positioning and decreases the likelihood of the graft being inserted posterior to the iris. Also, it can help minimize the risk of vitreous prolapse in pseudophakic eyes with previous YAG-laser capsulotomies.

We almost always perform EK with topical anesthesia supplemented with intracameral lidocaine and intravenous sedation, thereby avoiding the risks associated with a local block or general anesthesia. We place 4–0 silk scleral traction sutures superiorly and inferiorly to aid with eye positioning.

With both DMEK (Video 26.1) and DSAEK (Video 26.2), we mark the recipient epithelium with a trephine of the same diameter as that used for the donor graft to provide a reference for removal of host DM and endothelium. When EK is combined with cataract surgery, we use a temporal 2.0–2.8 mm clear corneal incision. With non-cataract cases we use a 2.0-mm scleral tunnel incision temporally. All cases have 2 short self-sealing paracenteses 45° to each side of the main incision made with 15° super sharp paracentesis blades.

Next, the dysfunctional endothelium and Descemet membrane are removed from the central recipient cornea. Use of air or viscoelastic in the anterior chamber (AC) improves visualization and helps prevent corneal edema from increasing during the DM stripping process. In cases with combined cataract surgery, stripping occurs after the IOL is in place and viscoelastic fills the anterior chamber. A reverse Price-Sinskey hook (Moria, Antony, France) is introduced through the paracentesis and used first to score DM along the epithelial reference mark, then to strip DM from the planned graft area and discard it. If viscoelastic was used in the AC it must be thoroughly evacuated at this point with phaco-emulsification bi-manuals, because retained viscoelastic at the graft/host interface impedes attachment and impairs vision. Trypan blue dye is injected into the AC and then irrigated out after about 30 s to help show any residual strands of DM, loose stromal fibers, or areas of incomplete stripping. Exposed DM stains dark blue, exposed stroma stains light blue, and areas with attached DM will have little to no staining. Loose residual tags of DM can be removed with phacoemulsification bi-manuals and loose stromal fibers with intraocular 23-gage scissors.

With DMEK it is common to create an inferior peripheral iridotomy (PI) to minimize the risk of pupillary block with prolonged use of an air or gas bubble to hold the graft in place. The PI can be created with micro-scissors, followed by aspiration of posterior residual iris pigment using the bi-manual aspiration tip of the bi-manuals to ensure patency. Alternatively, a PI can be created ahead of time with a laser. Hydration is used to seal the paracenteses.

Graft Insertion and Positioning

DSAEK grafts are typically folded into a 60/40 taco or a trifold endothelium-inward configuration for insertion. The tissue can be pulled into the eye with forceps with single- or multiuse devices specifically designed for this purpose, pulled in with sutures, pushed/inserted with a needle or forceps, or inserted with specially designed injectors. Certain bimanual techniques involve pulling the tissue through a device that causes it to curl, using micro-forceps introduced from the opposite side of the eye (Busin glide (Moria); Endoglide (Coronet)). This allows the surgeon to hold onto the tissue until an air bubble can be injected beneath it to press it against the recipient cornea, which can be helpful in cases of aphakia with large pupils, large iris defects, or aniridia.

DMEK tissue naturally tends to curl into a single or double scroll configuration with the endothelium facing outward when submerged in fluid (whereas in air it crumples up). The scrolled tissue can be sucked into a glass tube or loaded into a plastic intraocular lens cartridge or other insertion device for injection into the recipient eye. Alternatively, the tissue can be folded into a trifold configuration (like a pamphlet folded into thirds) with the endothelium facing inward to facilitate unfolding after insertion.

During graft insertion, it is important to be aware of the graft orientation and preferable to insert the tissue with the endothelium facing downward (toward the recipient iris). Graft orientation can be ascertained by looking at an orientation mark that was added during donor preparation, or it can be determined by viewing the graft configuration in cross-section using a hand-held slit beam or intraoperative OCT [10, 11], because a DMEK graft always curls with endothelium facing outward. If the graft is not correctly oriented in the eye, it can be flipped or rotated with short bursts of balanced salt solution (BSS) aimed slightly under the graft to create a fluid wave.

An advantage of the trifold configuration is that it tends to open naturally as the AC is gradually deepened by injection of BSS to provide space for the leaflets to unfold, and for a short time there is often some memory to the trifold, so the graft does not immediately revert to an endothelium-outward scroll configuration. Deepening the AC too quickly or too much should be avoided as this can allow the trifold to revert to a scroll or double scroll configuration.

To uncurl scrolled DMEK tissue short bursts of BSS are used. Long continuous injections of fluid are avoided, because that would raise the pressure in the eye and extrude the graft out of the incision. As the graft is uncurled, the orientation is checked to make sure it is unscrolling endothelium down and DM up. If the graft is upside down, then short bursts of BSS under the graft will flip it over. Once correct orientation is confirmed, the AC is shallowed, and a small air bubble is placed beneath the tissue with a 30-gauge needle to hold the graft open and in the correct orientation while it is centered on the area of recipient stripping. A cannula is used to tap the recipient corneal surface at the edges of the scroll to open it. The graft is centered by gently stroking the corneal surface with a cannula (like swinging a golf club) to induce fluid waves that shift the tissue in the desired direction.

After the tissue is centered and unfolded, air or gas, such as 10% C_3F_8 or 20% SF_6 [12], is injected at the limbus with a 30-gauge needle, bevel facing up, to achieve a 90% air/gas fill. Care should be taken not to increase the pressure to the point of compromising the optic nerve or its blood supply. This can be confirmed by asking the patient if they can see the microscope light come and go as the surgeon waves a hand beneath it, and if they can see any photopsia. Fluid and air levels in the AC can be adjusted as needed to achieve the appropriate fill.

Postoperative Management

If the eye is left nearly full of air/gas at the end of the case, as is common with DMEK, the patient should have a slit lamp exam and intraocular pressure (IOP) measurement about an hour later, to ensure there is no pupillary block [13]. Patients should be advised not to rub or push on the eye because that could dislocate the graft.

Topical antibiotic eye drops are typically prescribed for a week and topical corticosteroids (beginning 4 times daily and tapering to once daily) are prescribed indefinitely to prevent graft rejection. It is common to start patients on a relatively strong topical corticosteroid, such as prednisolone acetate 1% or dexamethasone. Studies have shown that after DMEK it is safe to switch Caucasian patients to a weaker topical steroid, such as fluorometholone 0.1% or loteprednol etabonate 0.5% after the first month. This significantly reduces the risk of steroid-induced ocular hypertension or glaucoma [14, 15]. Patients with darkly pigmented irises may be more prone to inflammation and graft rejection, and therefore, we recommend tapering topical corticosteroids more slowly [16].

Resumption of daily activities depends on incision size and contour. Like cataract surgery, normal activities can be resumed within a couple of weeks with small corneal incisions or self-sealing scleral tunnel incisions.

Visual rehabilitation is so rapid with DMEK that patients with bilateral endothelial dysfunction can have the second eye treated within a week of the first eye, with or without combined cataract surgery [17]. Rapid sequential DMEK has not been found to increase the risk of immunologic rejection. The typical postoperative appearance at 1 day, 5 days, and 1 month after DMEK is shown in (Fig. 26.2a–e).

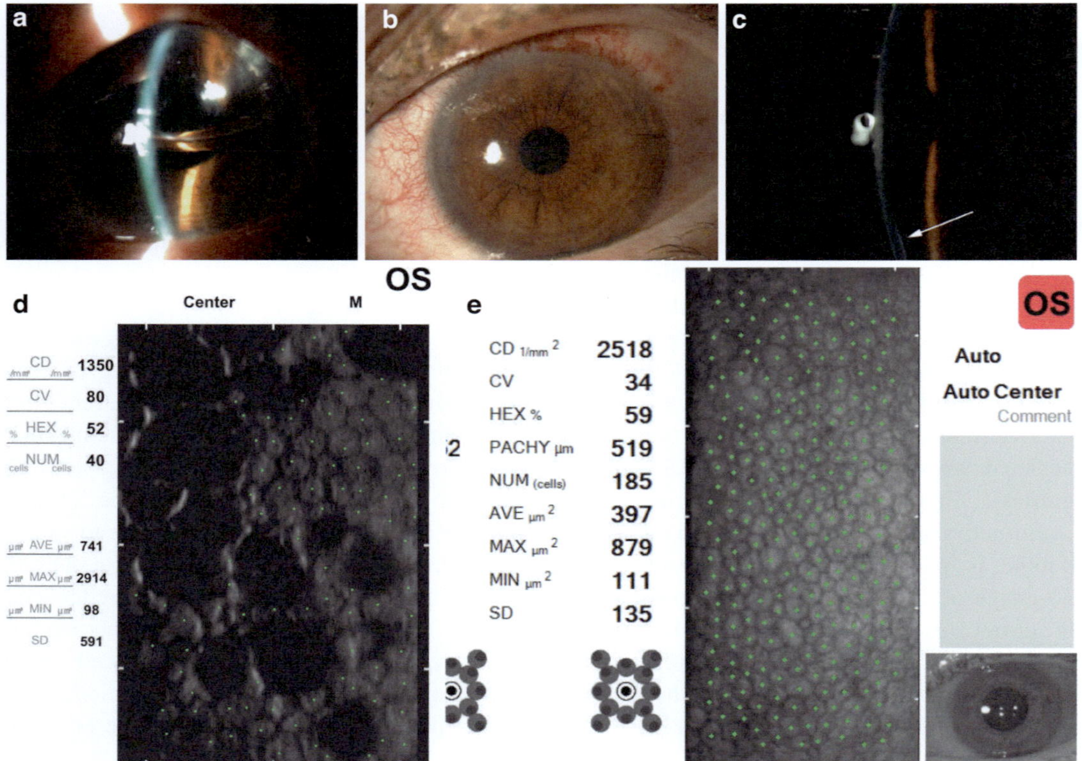

Fig. 26.2 DMEK postoperative images. (**a**) A postoperative day 1 slit lamp image showed that a residual air bubble filled approximately 50% of the anterior chamber with the patient sitting upright. (**b**) A postoperative day 5 slit lamp image showed no residual air remaining in the anterior chamber. (**c**) A postoperative day 5 slit beam image showed the central cornea was compact and clear, and there was a small inferior edge detachment with corresponding mild inferior corneal edema. The uncorrected distance visual acuity was 20/50 at day 5. (**d**) A preoperative specular microscopy image showed dark areas of guttae, characteristic of Fuchs dystrophy. (**e**) At 1-month, specular microscopy showed the central DMEK endothelial cell density was 2518 cells/mm²; also, the corrected distance visual acuity was 20/20 Snellen

Complications

Intraoperative Bleeding and Fibrin Formation

Heme in the AC can occur at any step of the case: during surgical peripheral iridotomy creation, from iatrogenic iris damage/iridodialysis during insertion of instruments or insertion of the donor tissue, or from blood entering from the main wound. To address blood in the AC, the first step is to stop active bleeding by temporarily increasing IOP for several minutes. Filling the AC with viscoelastic or a full air fill is an alternative way to tamponade active intraocular bleeding. Next, the AC should be thoroughly washed out with BSS to remove any remaining heme, fibrin, viscoelastic, or air. If bleeding recurs, the above steps should be repeated. It is important to wait until the bleeding is controlled before inserting the graft.

Fibrin can sometimes develop in the anterior chamber making it difficult to unfold or manipulate the graft, as can blood. Fibrin is not visible. Use of an anterior chamber maintainer helps washout any heme as well as minimizing the chance of fibrin accumulation in the eye with insertion of the graft. We remove the anterior chamber maintainer once the graft is in the eye.

Graft Detachment

Graft detachment is the most common early postoperative complication. It is usually detected by slit lamp examination and can be confirmed with anterior segment OCT imaging. Strategies to reduce the risk of DMEK or DSAEK detachment include ensuring a firm gas or air tamponade, careful wound construction to preclude wound leaks, and reminding patients to avoid rubbing the eye.

Strategies specifically designed to promote DSAEK attachment include massaging the surface of the host cornea to remove residual fluid from the host/graft interface, creation of small venting incisions in the mid-periphery of the host cornea to allow fluid escape, and scraping the periphery of the host corneal bed. Intraoperative OCT aids in detecting pockets of residual interface fluid. With DSAEK, partial detachments can be watched and usually seal down over time without intervention.

DMEK grafts do not adhere well to host DM, so the graft is typically slightly undersized relative to the host stripped area. Partial edge detachments are more common with DMEK than DSAEK. Partial detachments can be treated by reinjecting an air or gas bubble at the slit lamp or in a minor procedure room. It is easiest to add air or gas to an existing residual bubble because this ensures that the new bubble is not being injected between the graft and host cornea. Determining when to reinject air is very subjective with different surgeons. Typical criteria for DMEK re-bubbling are when the detachment affects more than one-third of the graft area, is increasing in size, or seems to be affecting vision. Full DMEK detachments are usually taken back to the operating room for repositioning and attachment.

Graft Failure

Early graft failure is defined as initial failure to clear and can be caused by surgical trauma, graft detachment, upside-down positioning, or be attributable to the donor tissue. Secondary graft failure is corneal decompensation after initial clearing and can be caused by immunologic rejection or endothelial decompensation.

It is straightforward to remove and replace a failed EK graft and best to do so promptly, before long-term edema results in stromal changes that could impair vision [18].

Immunologic Rejection

Immunologic rejection of an EK graft is characterized by AC cell reaction, corneal edema, a rejection line, or keratic precipitates. Immunologic rejection rates vary with the amount of donor tissue implanted. Rejection rates are lowest with DMEK (1% within 2 years), somewhat higher with DSAEK, and highest with PK (20% within 2 years) [2]. Compared with PK rejection episodes, EK rejection episodes tend to be milder and less likely to result in graft failure [19]. Treatment consists of increased topical corticosteroid use.

Less Common Complications

Other complications may include cystoid macular edema, subcapsular lens opacities, cataract progression, posterior synechiae, pupillary abnormalities, iris ischemia, fungal infections from donor tissue, and calcification of hydrophilic IOLs.

Anatomy-Related Challenges and Technique Adaptations

Crystalline Lens

In patients with endothelial dysfunction and visually significant lens opacity, EK can be combined with or staged before or after cataract surgery. Many patients prefer the convenience of a single, combined procedure. To achieve the best refractive outcomes and uncorrected vision, EK can be combined with implantation of an IOL that can be adjusted postoperatively, or EK can be staged first to eliminate the corneal edema before IOL selection [20].

Patients under 50 years of age without a visually significant cataract and an adequately deep anterior chamber are generally good candidates for phakic DMEK. A shallow anterior chamber makes donor positioning and manipulation difficult and increases the risk of iatrogenic cataract formation with intraocular surgery. Pilocarpine eye drops are instilled preoperatively to provide miosis and to protect the crystalline lens. Scoring and stripping are done under viscoelastic to provide increased anterior chamber stability and decrease the risk of premature cataract formation. Patients over 50 years of age are more likely to experience cataract formation and progression after EK or any other type of intraocular surgery, so the pros and cons of a staged vs. combined approach should be carefully discussed with them.

Post YAG-Capsulotomy

Preoperative examination should include evaluation of the posterior capsule for signs of a capsulotomy. An open capsule, especially a large posterior capsulotomy, can increase the chance of vitreous prolapse into the AC during surgery. If pupil peaking or vitreous to the wounds is observed during EK and vitreous prolapse is suspected, a thorough anterior vitrectomy should be completed prior to graft insertion because vitreous in the AC will interfere with graft manipulation and unfolding.

Post-Vitrectomy

In eyes with a posterior vitrectomy, an AC air bubble has a tendency to move posteriorly into the large vitreous cavity, in accordance with Laplace's law. This is especially a problem in eyes with large iris defects or aniridia. It is important to have the eye relatively firm prior to injecting air to decrease the tendency of the air going posteriorly.

Also, for DMEK where we often rely on anterior chamber shallowing to hold the donor open after it is unfolded, post-vitrectomy eyes may not shallow at all. Therefore, pull-in techniques are helpful and with a trifold, air can be injected under the graft before letting go of the graft once it is pulled in.

Figure 26.3a–c show DMEK in a 63-year-old female with a history of aphakia after cataract surgery. A pars plana victrectomy with placement of a secondary IOL using the Yamane intrascleral haptic fixation technique was staged 1 month before DMEK.

Severe Host Corneal Edema

Severe corneal edema or severe anterior stromal or subepithelial scarring can limit the view during surgery increasing the risk of complications. Intraoperative OCT is particularly helpful because it can image through a cloudy cornea. Removing the epithelium can help improve the view into the eye, but we typically do not remove

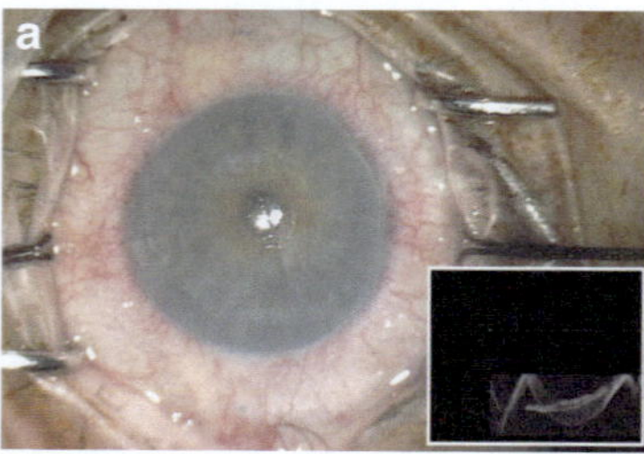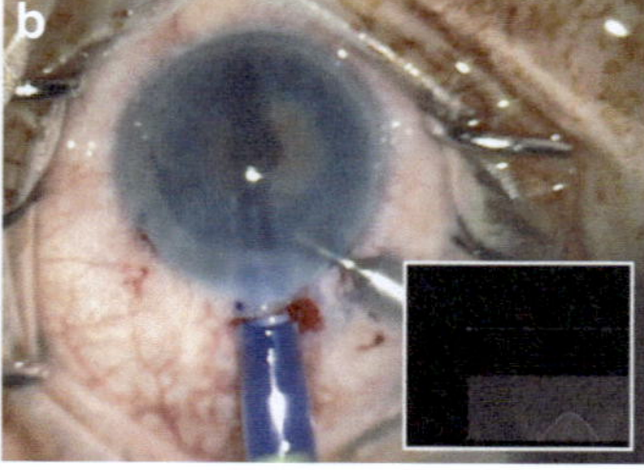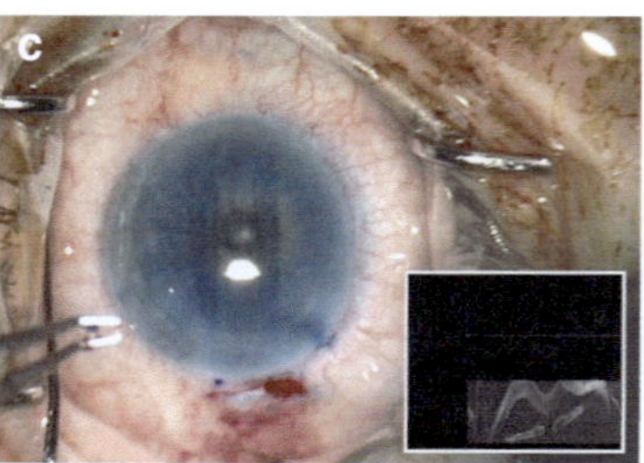

Fig. 26.3 Intraoperative images of DMEK in an eye with bullous keratopathy and a previous pars plana victrectomy. (**a**) Image showing the hazy cornea at the start of the case. (**b**) Image showing insertion of the blue-stained DMEK trifold. (**c**) Image showing unfolding of the DMEK tissue. The previous victrectomy made it difficult to sufficiently shallow the anterior chamber, so the central cornea was indented to help unfold and hold the DMEK tissue open; the indentation of the central cornea is more readily apparent in the OCT image (inset lower right)

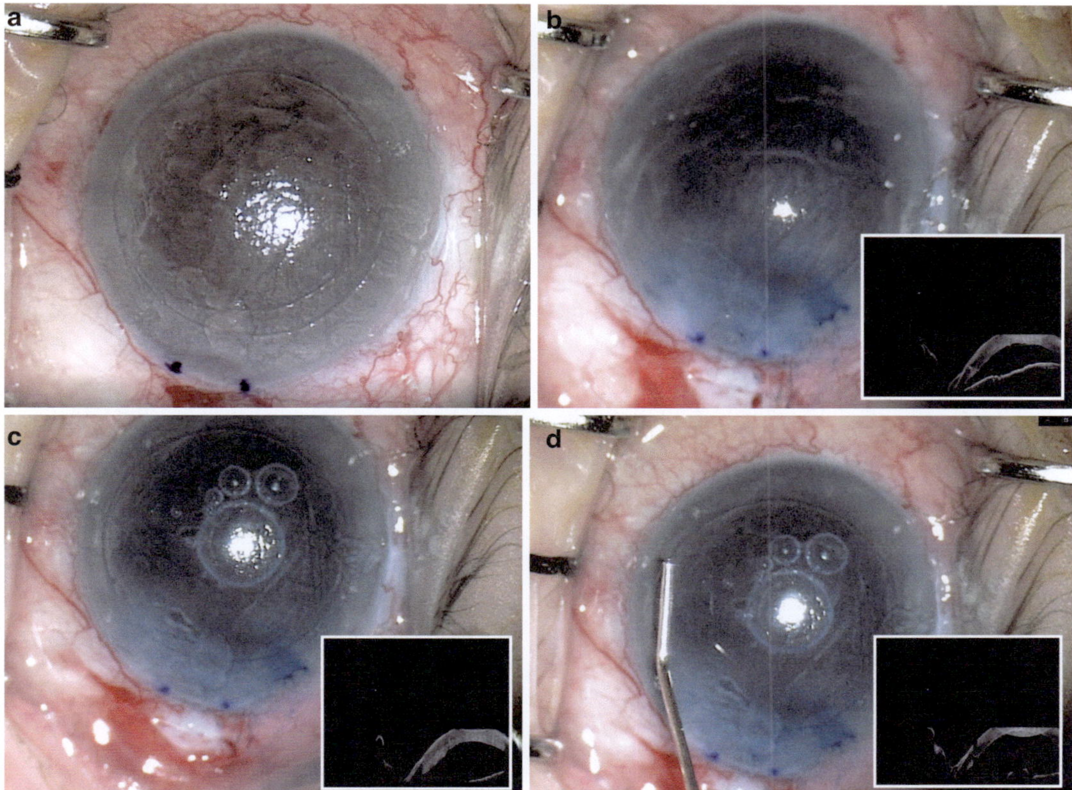

Fig. 26.4 Intraoperative images of a DMEK procedure in an eye with severe corneal edema. (**a**) Image showing the severe corneal edema and diffuse bullae at the start of the case. (**b**) Image taken immediately after insertion of the DMEK trifold into the host anterior chamber. The corresponding intraoperative OCT image (inset lower right) showed that the left side of the graft was scrolled up toward the host cornea and the right third was still folded under in the trifold configuration, indicating that the graft was correctly oriented with the donor endothelium facing the host iris. (**c**) Next, a small air bubble was injected beneath the graft to help hold it open in the correct orientation. The inset OCT image was used to reconfirm correct orientation and centration before increasing the bubble size. (**d**) The shadow cast on the OCT image, by the cannula used to inject balanced salt solution, was used to help check whether the graft edges were centered on the previously scored and stripped area of the recipient cornea. Centration could be adjusted by gently stroking the corneal surface with the cannula to induce fluid waves to shift the tissue in the desired direction

any epithelium until the donor is in the eye to minimize the chance of dragging some recipient epithelium into the eye during graft insertion.

Poor visualization while scoring and stripping the host DM increases the risk of disrupting the posterior stroma, which may impair DMEK attachment, whereas roughened posterior stroma does not affect DSAEK attachment. Poor visualization also makes it difficult to discern orientation marks on the graft and impedes assessment of graft orientation. With DMEK, use of a trifold configuration with a pull-through technique is helpful in such eyes because this approach minimizes the need for graft manipulation in the AC. Ensuring that the tissue is thoroughly stained with trypan blue is helpful, and intraoperative OCT is helpful for confirming graft orientation and centration as shown in (Fig. 26.4a–d).

Lens, Iris, or Anterior Chamber Abnormalities

Tamponade with an intracameral bubble is required for EK adherence. The bubble and graft are normally retained in the anterior chamber by the lens/iris diaphragm. When this diaphragm is compromised, it may not be possible to adequately create or maintain the bubble, and precautions should be taken to prevent escape of the stripped host DM and/or graft to the posterior chamber. Replacement or repositioning of a dislocated IOL, treatment of aphakia with implantation of a sulcus- or scleral-fixated IOL, and treatment of iris abnormalities with iridoplasty, pupilloplasty, or iris reconstruction should be considered before performing EK.

DSAEK is usually preferable to DMEK in aphakic eyes or eyes with significant iris openings. With DSAEK, host DM does not need to be stripped unless it has guttae or scarring. The DSAEK graft can be inserted over a glide that covers the iris or it can be pulled into the eye with micro-forceps, which allow the surgeon to hold onto the graft until it is secured with a bubble. Also, a temporary fixation suture should be placed in a DSAEK graft at 12 o'clock to secure it to the host cornea during the early postoperative period when there are large iris defects or fixed pupils. Finally, pupillary block is not a concern in eyes with large iris defects, so the AC can be left completely full of air or gas at the end of the case to promote attachment.

In eyes with a shallow or crowded AC, the AC can be filled with viscoelastic to improve stability prior to stripping host DM. DMEK grafts tend to be easier to unfold in a relatively shallow AC. On the other hand, with DSAEK, continuous infusion with an AC maintainer helps keep the AC formed during graft insertion, and use of glide insertion techniques have been associated with better outcomes in Asian eyes, which are more likely to have a shallow AC and iris prolapsing [21].

Any preoperative anterior synechiae should be lysed before inserting EK tissue. Postoperative anterior synechiae may develop in overly shallow eyes after DMEK and especially after DSAEK because it is thicker.

In eyes with an AC IOL, some surgeons prefer to leave the lens in place if it is correctly positioned and the AC depth is sufficient. However, other surgeons prefer to exchange the lens for an iris- or scleral-fixated lens either ahead of time or in combination with EK.

Previous Failed PK

EK provides significantly faster visual rehabilitation than a PK regraft and is the preferred approach if the refractive outcomes were acceptable with the original PK. The 6-month median corrected distance vision was 20/30 Snellen with DMEK and 20/50 Snellen with DSAEK in series performed to rescue failed PK grafts [22].

The principal considerations for EK planning are that the PK incision has limited wound strength, and the host posterior corneal surface may be irregular along the PK incision. Preoperative assessment with anterior segment OCT helps reveal irregularities and step offs that may affect graft unfolding and attachment.

With DSAEK, it is not necessary to strip the host DM unless irregularities that could affect vision, such as guttae or scarring, are present because DSAEK will easily adhere to host DM. With DMEK in primary cases, it has been observed that the DMEK graft does not adhere well to unstripped areas of DM, so in early series for treatment of failed PK, it was standard practice to strip DM when placing a DMEK graft. However, stripping DM in post PK eyes can be difficult, leaving shreds of DM that must be removed with forceps and/or disturbing the posterior stroma. One option is to use a femtosecond laser to do the scoring, so there is a more precise demarcation between the area of DM removed and that which is left [23]. Another option is to not strip DM from the prior PK; this approach should leave a smoother posterior surface and works well when combined with use of long-acting gas to help the donor stay in contact with the PK DM until it attaches [12, 24, 25]. In fact, we recommend always using a long-acting gas with DMEK after failed PK, whereas we use air for most other DMEK cases. We have also found that keeping the DMEK graft diameter somewhat smaller than that of the previous PK facilitates attachment [22].

Previous Glaucoma Surgery

EK provides better visual outcomes and faster visual rehabilitation than PK in eyes with prior glaucoma surgery. In eyes with a glaucoma tube shunt, the proximity of the tube to the cornea should be assessed preoperatively because a long tube could pose challenges during EK manipulation and centration and damage the donor endothelium. The tube can be trimmed to an appropriate length with micro-scissors during EK surgery if the tube placement is acceptable. However, in cases where the tube needs to be repositioned, we prefer to do that a month ahead of time to give the eye time to heal and get past the risk of hypotony that sometimes occurs with repositioning tubes to posterior chamber or pars planna insertions.

The presence of a superior glaucoma tube shunt or trabeculectomy can allow air to escape from the eye as the AC is being filled, and further outflow can occur when the patient sits up. To help promote graft attachment, the AC can be left almost completely full of air or gas in eyes with an aqueous shunt. Trabeculectomies are a bit more complicated, because sometimes the air can block the filtration site leading to increased IOP or loss of the bleb. The IOP should be checked 1–2 h afterward to ensure adequate filtration and the bubble should be reduced if needed. Use of a long-acting gas, such as 10% C_3F_8 instead of air, can also help promote attachment. When necessary to prevent bubble escape, an aqueous tube can be temporarily plugged with viscoelastic, which will spontaneously fall away when the patient sits up.

Conclusions

In conclusion, EK has revolutionized treatment of corneal endothelial dysfunction and is currently the gold standard treatment. Appropriate technique modifications allow successful use in eyes with various ocular comorbidities.

Take Home Notes
- Topical anesthesia is the preferred method for EK surgery.
- The risk of rejection is least with DMEK.
- The need for topical corticosteroids is least with DMEK leading to less steroid-induced glaucoma.
- EK works well for failed PK, leading to faster visual recovery, less tissue damage, and less risk of rejection compared to repeat PK, if the original PK has acceptable ocular surface characteristics.

References

1. Melles GR, Ong TS, Ververs B, van der Wees J. Descemet membrane endothelial keratoplasty (DMEK). Cornea. 2006;25:987–90.
2. Anshu A, Price MO, Price FW Jr. Risk of corneal transplant rejection significantly reduced with Descemet's membrane endothelial keratoplasty. Ophthalmology. 2012;119:536–40.
3. Chamberlain W, Lin CC, Austin A, Schubach N, Clover J, McLeod SD, Porco TC, Lietman TM, Rose-Nussbaumer J. Descemet endothelial thickness comparison trial: a randomized trial comparing ultrathin Descemet stripping automated endothelial keratoplasty with Descemet membrane endothelial keratoplasty. Ophthalmology. 2019;126:19–26.
4. Agarwal A, Dua HS, Narang P, Kumar DA, Agarwal A, Jacob S, Agarwal A, Gupta A. Pre-Descemet's endothelial keratoplasty (PDEK). Br J Ophthalmol. 2014;98:1181–5.
5. Malbran E, Stefani C. Lamellar keratoplasty in corneal ectasias. Ophthalmologica. 1972;164:59–70.
6. Lie JT, Birbal R, Ham L, van der Wees J, Melles GR. Donor tissue preparation for Descemet membrane endothelial keratoplasty. J Cataract Refract Surg. 2008;34:1578–83.
7. Price MO, Giebel AW, Fairchild KM, Price FW Jr. Descemet's membrane endothelial keratoplasty: pro-

spective multicenter study of visual and refractive outcomes and endothelial survival. Ophthalmology. 2009;116:2361–8.

8. Tenkman LR, Price FW, Price MO. Descemet membrane endothelial keratoplasty donor preparation: navigating challenges and improving efficiency. Cornea. 2014;33:319–25.

9. Veldman BP, Dye PK, Holiman JD, Mayko ZM, Sales CS, Straiko MD, Galloway JD, Terry MA. The S-stamp in Descemet membrane endothelial keratoplasty safely eliminates upside-down graft implantation. Ophthalmology. 2016;123:161–4.

10. Price FW Jr. Intraoperative optical coherence tomography: game-changing technology. Cornea. 2021;40:675–8.

11. Burkhart ZN, Feng MT, Price MO, Price FW. Handheld slit beam techniques to facilitate DMEK and DALK. Cornea. 2013;32:722–4.

12. Guell JL, Morral M, Gris O, Elies D, Manero F. Comparison of sulfur hexafluoride 20% versus air tamponade in Descemet membrane endothelial keratoplasty. Ophthalmology. 2015;122:1757–64.

13. Gonzalez A, Price FW Jr, Price MO, Feng MT. Prevention and management of pupil block after Descemet membrane endothelial keratoplasty. Cornea. 2016;35:1391–5.

14. Price MO, Price FW Jr, Kruse FE, Bachmann BO, Tourtas T. Randomized comparison of topical prednisolone acetate 1% versus fluorometholone 0.1% in the first year after Descemet membrane endothelial keratoplasty. Cornea. 2014;33:880–6.

15. Price MO, Feng MT, Scanameo A, Price FW Jr. Loteprednol etabonate 0.5% gel vs. prednisolone acetate 1% solution after Descemet membrane endothelial keratoplasty: prospective randomized trial. Cornea. 2015;34:853–8.

16. Price MO, Jordan CS, Moore G, Price FW Jr. Graft rejection episodes after Descemet stripping with endothelial keratoplasty: part two: the statistical analysis of probability and risk factors. Br J Ophthalmol. 2009;93(93):391–5.

17. McKee Y, Price MO, Gunderson L, Price FW Jr. Rapid sequential endothelial keratoplasty with and without combined cataract extraction. J Cataract Refract Surg. 2013;39:1372–6.

18. Letko E, Price DA, Lindoso EM, Price MO, Price FW Jr. Secondary graft failure and repeat endothelial keratoplasty after Descemet's stripping automated endothelial keratoplasty. Ophthalmology. 2011;118:310–4.

19. Price MO, Price FW Jr. Descemet stripping endothelial keratoplasty: fifteen-year outcomes. Cornea. 2022;42:449–55.

20. Price MO, Pinkus D, Price FW Jr. Implantation of presbyopia-correcting intraocular lenses staged after Descemet membrane endothelial keratoplasty in patients with Fuchs dystrophy. Cornea. 2020;39:732–5.

21. Mehta JS, Por YM, Poh R, Beuerman RW, Tan D. Comparison of donor insertion techniques for Descemet stripping automated endothelial keratoplasty. Arch Ophthalmol. 2008;126:1383–8.

22. Pasari A, Price MO, Feng MT, Price FW Jr. Descemet membrane endothelial keratoplasty for failed penetrating keratoplasty: visual outcomes and graft survival. Cornea. 2019;38:151–6.

23. Sorkin N, Mimouni M, Santaella G, Trinh T, Cohen E, Einan-Lifshitz A, Chan CC, Rootman DS. Comparison of manual and femtosecond laser-assisted Descemet membrane endothelial keratoplasty for failed penetrating keratoplasty. Am J Ophthalmol. 2020;214:1–8.

24. Alió Del Barrio JL, Montesel A, Ho V, Bhogal M. Descemet membrane endothelial keratoplasty under failed penetrating keratoplasty without host Descemetorhexis for the management of secondary graft failure. Cornea. 2020;39:13–7.

25. Alió Del Barrio JL, Bhogal M, Ang M, Ziaei M, Robbie S, Montesel A, Gore DM, Mehta JS, Alió JL. Corneal transplantation after failed grafts: options and outcomes. Surv Ophthalmol. 2021;66:20–40.

Corneal Endothelial Cell Transfer

Shigeru Kinoshita, Morio Ueno, and Chie Sotozono

Historical Pathway Leading to Endothelial Cell Transfer

Due to recent developments in corneal endothelial transplantation strategies, the methods applied for the treatment of corneal endothelial dysfunction and failure are evolving and are now beginning to shift away from penetrating corneal transplantation to corneal endothelial transplantation [1, 2]. Current transplantation procedures include Descemet stripping automated endothelial keratoplasty (DSAEK) [3–5] and Descemet membrane endothelial keratoplasty (DMEK) [6, 7], and more recently, Descemet stripping only (DSO). Of those, DSO is a novel procedure that strips away the Descemet membrane with corneal guttae in the central region of the cornea and has been found to be somewhat effective for treating cases afflicted with mild Fuchs endothelial cor-

Supplementary Information The online version contains supplementary material available at https://doi.org/10.1007/978-3-031-32408-6_27.

S. Kinoshita (✉)
Department of Frontier Medical Science and Technology for Ophthalmology, Kyoto Prefectural University of Medicine, Kyoto, Japan

M. Ueno · C. Sotozono
Department of Ophthalmology, Kyoto Prefectural University of Medicine, Kyoto, Japan
e-mail: mueno@koto.kpu-m.ac.jp; csotozon@koto.kpu-m.ac.jp

neal dystrophy, a non-inflammatory sporadic, or autosomal dominant disorder that can ultimately lead to blindness if left untreated [8]. Moreover, a clinical trial was recently initiated to investigate the safety and efficacy of topically applying Rho-associated protein kinase (ROCK)-inhibitor eye drops for the promotion of corneal endothelial wound healing post DSO [9, 10].

As an alternative to corneal transplantation or DSO, groundbreaking corneal regenerative-medicine strategies have now introduced the next generation of state-of-the-art therapeutic pathways for the treatment of corneal endothelial dysfunction and endothelial failure. To that end, and in concert with the latest biological knowledge of human corneal endothelial cells (CECs) (HCECs) and cutting-edge cell-culture technology, cell-based therapy has been developed for corneal endothelial dysfunction and failure. One such innovative pathway involves the surgical transfer of cultured HCECs (cHCECs), termed "HCEC-Injection Therapy," a regenerative-medicine therapeutic concept that provides several advantages, such as being minimally invasive, the ability to intraoperatively supply possibly less-damaged nonaged CECs to the posterior surface of the cornea, and a vastly improved optical quality of the cornea post surgery due to no additional corneal tissue being implanted [11, 12]. Since the CECs obtained from just one donor eye can be used to subsequently create enough cHCECs to treat a large number of patients, another benefit of the procedure is that it holds the promise of ultimately ending the worldwide shortage of donor corneas, a problem that persists annually [13].

CEC Failure and Repair

Corneal endothelium comprises of a single layer of CECs that lines the posterior surface of the cornea [14]. In normal healthy eyes, CECs are arrested in the G1-phase of the cell cycle and rarely proliferate due to cell-to-cell contact inhibition and the high concentration of transforming growth factor beta 2 (TGF-β2) in the aqueous humor [15]. Thus, in cases in which CECs migrate and/or enlarge, it is more likely that the migration and enlargement is in response to wound healing than cell division [16]. In corneal endothelium, the CEC density slowly decreases with age, even in normal healthy subjects [17]. Corneal endothelial dysfunction occurs due to an impairment of pump and barrier function resulting from the abnormality of CECs with guttae formation and/or a decrease of CEC density in response to a wide variety of diseases, such as Fuchs endothelial corneal dystrophy [18], pseudoexfoliation syndrome [19], and cytomegalovirus corneal endothelitis [20], as well as intraoperative corneal endothelial trauma that can occur and ultimately lead to complete corneal endothelial failure in cases undergoing laser-iridotomy ophthalmic surgery [21], cataract surgery [22], glaucoma surgery [23], and vitreo-retinal surgery [24]. Thus, in cases afflicted with corneal endothelial dysfunction and failure resulting from corneal endothelial disease, there are several different "soils" in the anterior chamber environment [25, 26]. Although the existence of stem/progenitor cells in in vivo HCECs has yet to be proven, it is theorized that these endothelial cells likely retain their proliferative ability in vitro [15]. Furthermore, studies have shown that in cases of corneal endothelial failure, corneal endothelial transplantation using a central-cornea donor graft can sufficiently restore corneal transparency for a substantial period of time.

Since the transplantation of cHCECs in vivo does not require constant cell proliferation, surgical strategies for treating corneal endothelial dysfunction must be considered differently from those used for the treatment of limbal deficiency that require an adequate supply of corneal epithelial stem cells [27].

HCEC-Injection Therapy Concept

Currently, there are at least two different regenerative-medicine cell-based therapeutic concepts applied for the treatment of damaged corneal tissue. One is the release of beneficial small molecules via the transfer of cHCECs to the damaged tissue, which promotes functional restoration of the healthy tissue via cell regeneration and reorganization. The other is a "true replacement" of damaged CECs via the surgical transfer of cHCECs. The novel HCEC-injection therapy that we recently developed aims at the latter concept of a regenerative-medicine cell-based therapeutic approach [11, 12]. One fundamental question that needs to be addressed is whether or not constant cell proliferation is essential for maintaining healthy corneal endothelial function following the transfer of the cHCECs. To our surprise, the answer to that question is "NO!," as corneal endothelial dysfunction results from the loss of the physiological function of the CEC layer due to a depletion or malfunction of the CECs themselves, and not due to endothelial stem-cell deficiency. Thus, our investigations have revealed that there is no need for stem or progenitor cells once the cHCECs are surgically transferred to the posterior surface of the cornea.

cHCECs for Clinical Use

Numerous previous studies have been conducted to investigate the laboratory procedures used for the culture of HCECs, as they are known to be difficult to proliferate in vitro. For

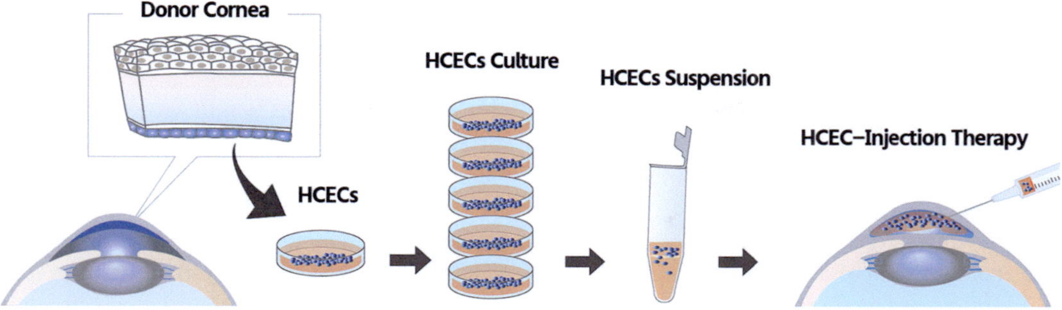

Fig. 27.1 Schematic presentation of the procedures from cell culture to cell transfer in HCEC-Injection Therapy

example, for the cHCECs used in our novel HCEC-injection therapy, we found that in order to closely mimic HCECs in vivo, it is essential to create cells with a high (i.e., 90%) purity rate of mature-differentiated cells to obtain the optimal surgical outcome and a higher postoperative CEC density [28]. For the creation of such cells, merely the expression of (Na$^+$- K$^+$)-ATPase and ZO-1 is not enough, as that is fundamental for defining cell maturation by cell density and several cell surface markers, etc. [29–40]. Thus, the mature-differentiated cHCECs created for use in our HCEC-injection therapy must express distinct cell-surface markers such as CD166+, CD44−/dull, CD24-, CD26-, and CD105−/dull to closely mimic in vivo HCECs [28].

In addition, in order to verify that the cHCECs are suitable for clinical application, it must be confirmed via bacterial testing, viral testing, and the findings of a low endotoxin concentration that there is no mycoplasma contamination of the cells and that the final culture media is completely sterile [11]. Since many cultured cells are prepared from a single donor cornea and are provided to many patients as "one lot," that single lot can bring not only effective clinical results but also adverse events if those strict safety guidelines are not followed. Thus, a great deal of care is required to assure safety. Incidentally, mature-differentiated cHCECs are not tumorigenic and have no chromosomal abnormalities [30, 41].

For practical application, donor corneas obtained from young donors are used in in vitro culture material and are cultured at a cell processing center under the standard operating procedure that conforms to the good manufacturing practices guidelines. Cell lots for clinical application are examined to verify that they meet the strict criteria for clinical application, and enzyme-linked immunosorbent assay (ELISA) and/or flow cytometric analysis are performed to verify the above-described biological characteristics of the cells. A sterile suspension of cHCECs is then prepared into a small container several hours prior to the HCEC-injection therapy being performed. Currently, the number of cHCECs to be injected in 300 μL of modified Opti-MEM™ I Reduced Serum Medium (Thermo Fisher Scientific) is supplemented with ROCK-inhibitor Y-27632 is 1.0×10^6 cells (Fig. 27.1) [11, 12, 28].

Surgical Procedure Used for HCEC-Injection Therapy

For patients undergoing HCEC-injection therapy, a 1.6-mm incision at the corneal limbus is first created under local anesthesia. Next, a silicone needle is used to remove abnormal extracellular matrix on the patient's Descemet membrane and/or degenerated CECs in an 8-mm-diameter area of the posterior surface of the cornea. Post removal and full collapse of the anterior chamber, all of the prepared cHCECs in the suspension are injected into the anterior chamber using a 26-gauge needle with a dead-spaced free syringe (Video 27.1). Immediately after post injection, the patients are placed in a "face-down" position for 3 h to enhance the adhesion of the injected cells [11].

Following surgery, all patients receive both systemic and topical administrations of steroids to inhibit acute innate immunity-related inflammation and/or immunological reaction, with antimicrobial agents also being administered as a prophylaxis to prevent infection under the drug regimen administered in standard corneal transplantation procedures [11].

Clinical Results

Based on the 5-year postoperative findings of the 11 cases treated in the initial clinical trial, HCEC-injection therapy has been found to be an overall safe and effective treatment for complete corneal restoration in patients afflicted with severe corneal endothelial failure (Fig. 27.2). Those clinical findings revealed that normal corneal thickness was achieved in 10 of the 11 treated eyes during the 5-year-postoperative follow-up period, with complete disappearance of corneal edema. The cHCECs produced by the first-generation culture protocol were successfully repopulated on the Descemet membrane and/or the bare posterior surface of the corneal stroma, thus illustrating that they are biologically functional with excellent longevity. Specular microscopy imaging performed at 5-years postoperative revealed a relatively high CEC density at the center of the posterior corneal surface in 10 of the 11 treated eyes (range,

601 to 2067 cells/mm^2), a decrease in the coefficient of variation, and an increase of cell hexagonality, thus indicating that at 5-years postoperative, the CECs at the posterior corneal surface tended to be more biophysically stable than those observed at the early postoperative period. Compared with the previously published data regarding the surgical outcomes of DSAEK and DMEK at 5-years postoperative, the findings in our pilot study showed that our novel HCEC-injection therapy seems to be equivalent, or even a bit superior, to the various previously reported clinical outcomes, including the findings related to corneal graft survival rate, immunological rejection rate, CEC density, and best-corrected visual acuity post surgery (Fig. 27.3) [11, 12].

The findings in our interventional study confirmed that although the number of cells injected into the anterior chamber, the surgical procedure applied, and the postoperative care administered were identical between the two groups in the study, HCEC-injection therapy using the second-generation cHCECs (i.e., a cell suspension with an over 90% higher population of the mature-differentiated cells) resulted in an even better corneal restoration in terms of CEC density than that resulting from the use of the first-generation cultured HCECs at both 24-weeks and 3-years postoperative (Figs. 27.4 and 27.5). In addition, use of the second-generation cHCECs resulted in a faster recovery of corneal thinning compared with the findings obtained using the first-generation cHCECs, probably due to the rapid functional recovery for corneal dehydration (Fig. 27.6). Specular microscopy images obtained at 3-years postoperative confirmed a higher CEC density at the central area of the cornea in the eyes treated with the second-generation cHCECs (range, 2182

a

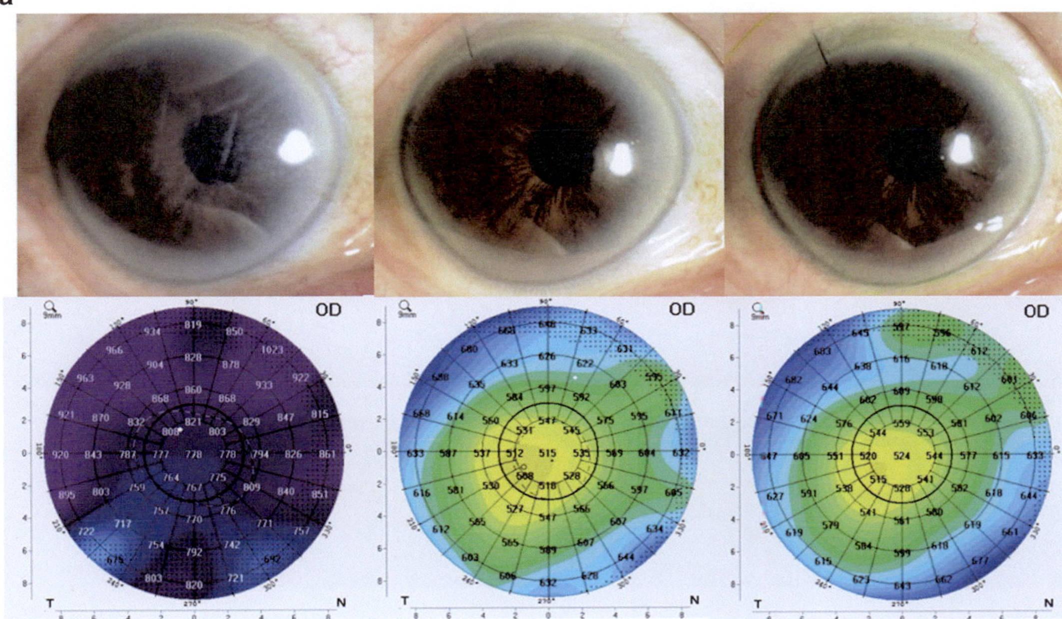

b

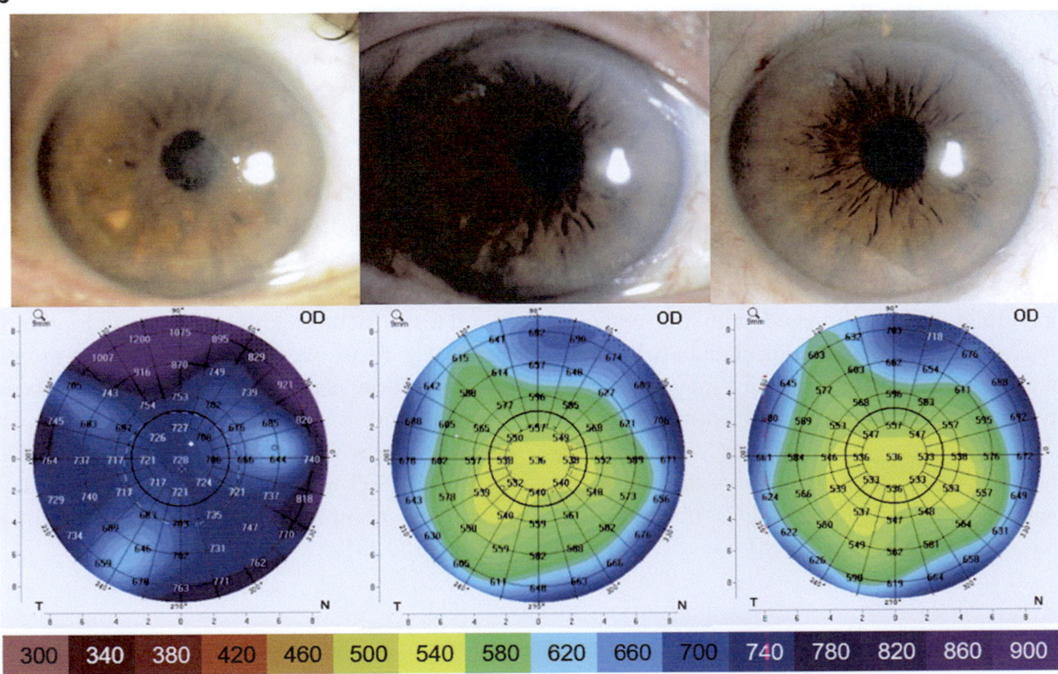

Fig. 27.2 Slit-lamp microscopy images (upper) and Scheimpflug camera images (lower) of two representative patients obtained at prior to surgery and at 3- and 5-years post HCEC-Injection Therapy with the first-generation cHCECs. (**a**) A patient with Fuchs endothelial corneal dystrophy (FECD), (**a**) a patient with argon-laser-iridotomy induced bullous keratopathy. Pre-surgery (left column), 3-years post injection (middle column), and 5-years post injection (right column). The color maps shown below each slit-lamp microscopy image (**a**) and Scheimpflug camera image (**b**) illustrate the corneal thickness at each representative area of the corneal image above. The color bar located below **b** indicates the approximate corneal thickness of each of the colors shown in the maps (cited from Fig. 2, Numa K, et al. *Ophthalmology* 2021;128:504–514)

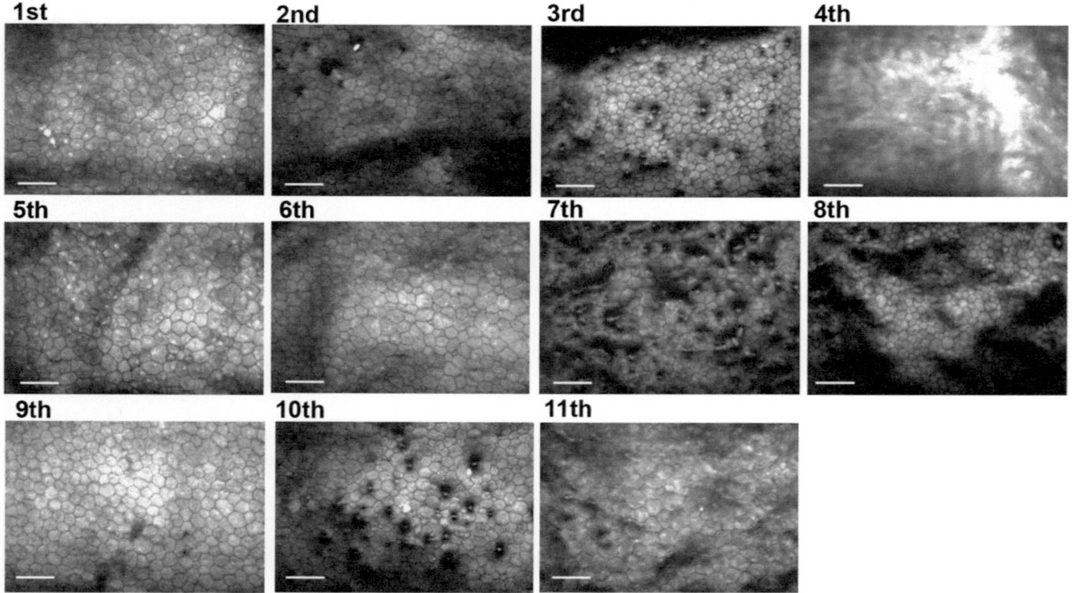

Fig. 27.3 Contact specular microscopy images of the central cornea in each of the 11 cases at 5-years postoperative. Scale bar: 100 µm. The endothelial cells are clearly visible, and a reasonable corneal endothelial cell density (ECD) can be seen in 10 of the 11 treated eyes. The image of the eye of Patient 4 shows some cells, yet not clear, thus suggesting that the eye was borderline corneal edema. FECD cases (Patients 2, 3, 5, 7, 8, 10, and 11) still show corneal guttae, however, the density of corneal guttae in those cases was found to have tended to be decreased (cited from Fig. 4, Numa K, et al. *Ophthalmology* 2021;128:504–514)

to 4417 cells/mm^2) than in the eyes treated with the first-generation cHCECs (range, 746 to 2104 cells/mm^2). Surprisingly, at 3-years post-injection, the CEC density of the eyes treated with the second-generation cHCECs was very high with only mild decay compared with the outcomes obtained from ordinary corneal endothelial transplantation. Those findings may suggest not only the long-term stability and integrity of the cHCECs post surgery but also excellent rejuvenation of the CEC layer when using the well-differentiated (i.e., mature) cHCECs obtained from young-age donor corneas [28].

In regard to safety, all eyes that underwent our HCEC-injection therapy showed no immunological rejection, uveitis, infection, or increase of intraocular pressure directly related to the cell product. It should be noted that blood tests, including blood cell and blood biochemistry tests, were performed at 1 month post injection, and that the findings in those examinations were almost within a normal range. Moreover, our doctor-initiated clinical trial of HCEC-injection therapy in Japan has now been completed with favorable clinical results [11, 28].

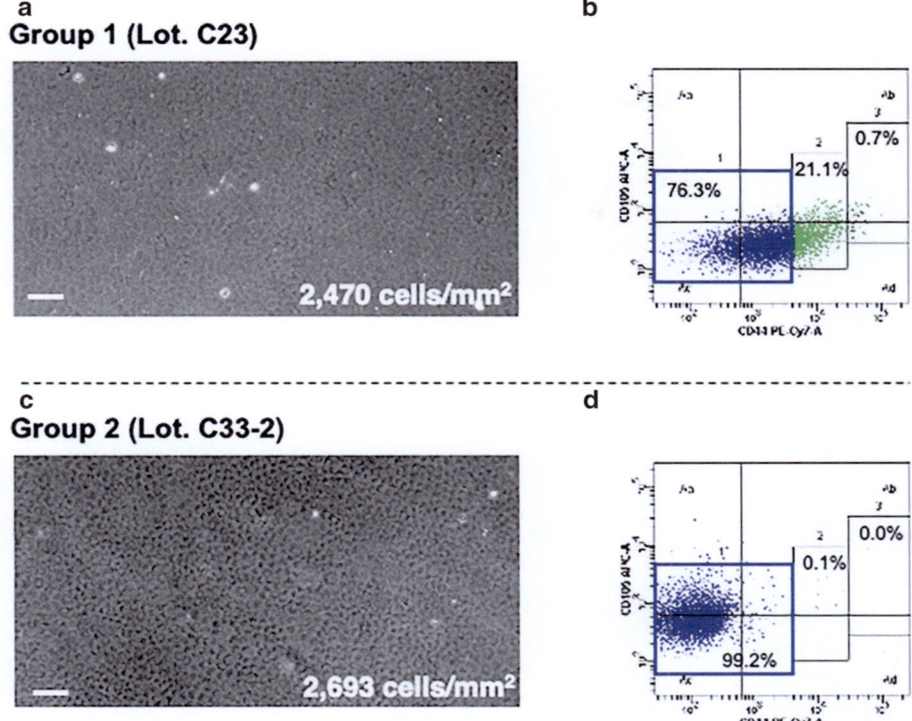

Fig. 27.4 Representative data of the cultured human corneal endothelial cells (hCECs) in Group 1 (Gr1) cell lots used for Patient 9 and Group 2 (Gr2) cell lots used for Patient 15. (**a, c**) Phase contrast microscopy images of the cultured hCECs used for the hCEC-injection therapy. Scale bars, 200 μm. (**b, d**) Fluorescence-activated cell sorting (FACS) analysis graphs of the cells shown in images **a** and **c** based on CD44 and CD105 to identify subpopulations (SPs). Mature-differentiated SP are indicated in blue and the E-ratio (the proportion of these blue cells) was calculated. (**a, b**) Cell Lot 23 in Gr1 showed 76.3% of E-ratio. (**c, d**) Cell Lot 33–2 in Gr2 showed 99.2% of E-ratio (cited from Fig. 1, Ueno M, et al. *Am J Ophthalmol* 2022;237:267–277)

Fig. 27.5 Clinical data of the corneal endothelial cell density (CECD) obtained from the contact specular microscopy images. Box and whisker plot of the CECD of the patients at 24-weeks and 3-years postoperative in Group 1 (Gr1) and Group 2 (Gr2). In the Gr1 treated eyes, a relatively lower proportion (0.1 to 76.3%) of mature cell SPs was administered, while in the Gr2 eyes, a relatively higher proportion (>90%) of mature cell SPs was administered. Box plots demonstrate the median (line) as well as lower and upper interquartile range (IQR; box), whiskers show the highest and lowest CECD values. There were marked significant differences in CECD at 24-weeks and 3-years postoperative between the two groups (*P < 0.001) (Wilcoxon rank-sum test) (cited from Fig. 2, Ueno M, et al. *Am J Ophthalmol* 2022;237:267–277)

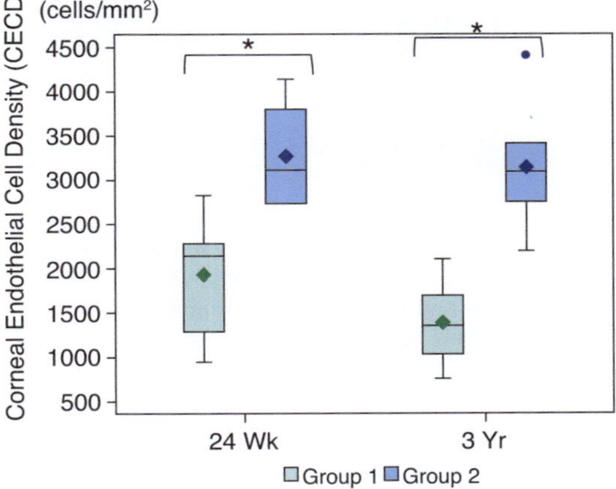

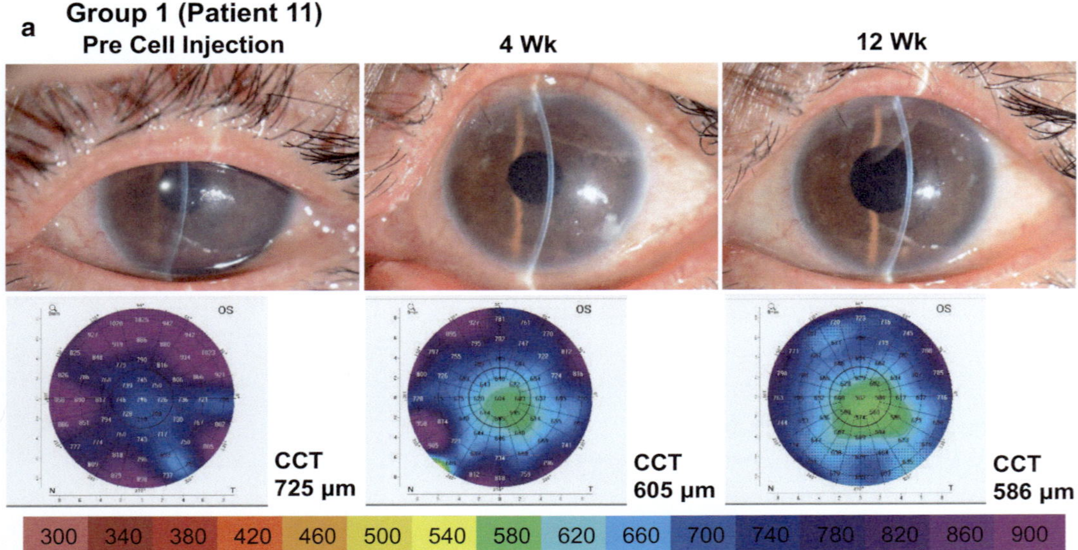

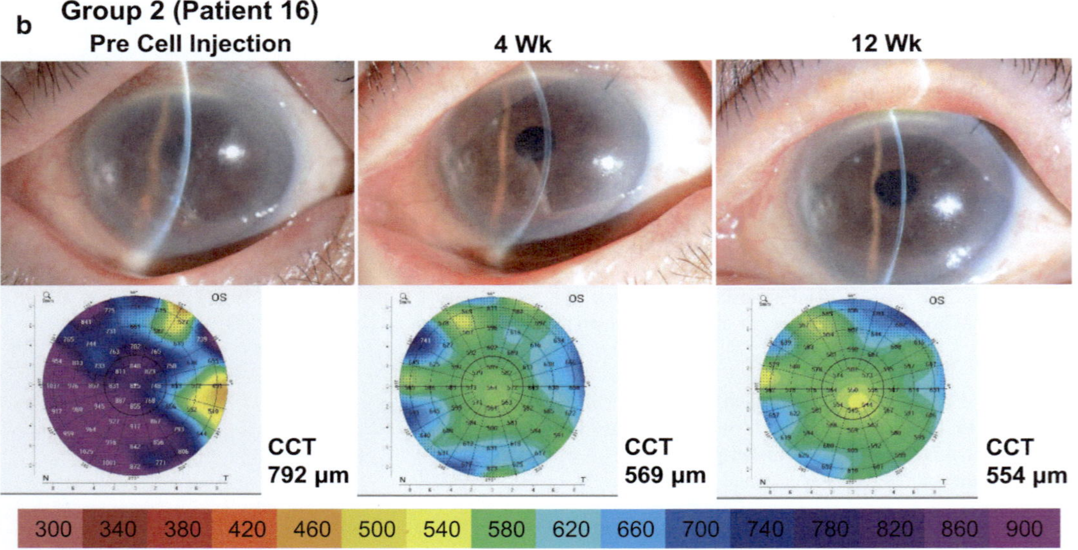

Fig. 27.6 Slit-lamp microscopy images (Upper) and Scheimpflug images (Lower) of representative patients in Group 1 (Gr1) and Group 2 (Gr2) obtained at prior to surgery and at 4- and 12-weeks post cultured human corneal endothelial cell (hCEC)-injection therapy. (**a**) Fuchs endothelial corneal dystrophy in a Gr1 patient (Patient 11). (**b**) Pseudophakic corneal endothelial failure in a Gr2 patient (Patient 16). Pre-surgery (Left column), 4-weeks post injection (Middle), and 12-weeks post injection (Right column). The central corneal thickness (CCT) is shown in each panel. The rapid decrease of CCT in the Gr2 patient is apparent by the two-dimensional corneal pachymetry images (cited from Fig. 6, Ueno M, et al. *Am J Ophthalmol* 2022;237:267–277)

Antigenicity of Allogeneic Cells and Fate of Escaped Cells from the Eye

Since cHCECs are created from allogeneic donor corneas, strict and thorough consideration must be made toward immunological reactions. In fact, corneal endothelial reaction occurs more often in cases undergoing penetrating keratoplasty [42], followed by cases undergoing DSAEK [43] and DMEK [44]. However, none of the eyes that have undergone HCEC-injection therapy have shown immunological reaction in the clinical setting. In fact, in mouse experiments, an immune tolerance was obtained by injecting allogeneic CECs into the anterior chamber, and similar results occurred when administered intravenously [45]. Moreover, Streilein and colleagues reported that an immunological privilege could be maintained via anterior chamber-associated immune deviation to protect allogeneic cells in the anterior chamber [46, 47]. Thus, it can be assumed that a minimal amount of immunological reaction occurs post cell injection therapy.

Furthermore, the expression of human leukocyte antigen class 1 in the cHCECs diminished in the cells with a higher degree of cell maturation [34], thus indicating that from the aspect of immunogenicity, mature-differentiated cells are ideal for clinical use. Moreover, the findings in the animal-model experiments have shown that a few cultured CECs or cellular components that escape from the anterior chamber into the circulatory system post injection produce no adverse events [11, 28, 41].

Future Directions

In the future, clinical feedback is needed to fully elucidate the relationship between the "seeds," i.e., in terms of cHCEC quality, and the "soil," i.e., in terms of corneal endothelial diseases and the anterior chamber environment, in order to optimize the indicative diseases for HCEC-injection therapy [25].

Over time, the understanding of CEC biology will broaden, and interest in the methods applied for acquiring an abundant cell expansion, an easy cell delivery procedure, and cryopreservation will flourish. In order to attain that groundbreaking apex, the cHCECs must be of the highest quality to be deemed ideal for use in the clinical setting. When this formidable barrier is eventually overcome, the clinical use of cHCECs will surely become the global standard for treating patients afflicted with severe corneal disorders. Now that it has been confirmed that cHCECs injected as a cell suspension into the anterior chamber can self-organize and reconstitute the endothelial cell layer with full corneal restoration, cutting-edge advancements in medical science and clinical applications are sure to arise in the near future.

References

1. Tan DT, Dart JK, Holland EJ, Kinoshita S. Corneal transplantation. Lancet. 2012;379(9827):1749–61.
2. Dana R. A new frontier in curing corneal blindness. N Engl J Med. 2018;378(11):1057–8.
3. Gorovoy MS. Descemet-stripping automated endothelial keratoplasty. Cornea. 2006;25(8):886–9.
4. Price MO, Calhoun P, Kollman C, Price FW Jr, Lass JH. Descemet stripping endothelial keratoplasty: ten-year endothelial cell loss compared with penetrating keratoplasty. Ophthalmology. 2016;123(7):1421–7.
5. Lass JH, Benetz BA, Patel SV, et al. Donor, recipient, and operative factors associated with increased endothelial cell loss in the cornea preservation time study. JAMA Ophthalmol. 2019;137(2):185–93.
6. Melles GR, Ong TS, Ververs B, van der Wees J. Preliminary clinical results of Descemet membrane endothelial keratoplasty. Am J Ophthalmol. 2008;145(2):222–7.
7. Tourtas T, Laaser K, Bachmann BO, Cursiefen C, Kruse FE. Descemet membrane endothelial keratoplasty versus descemet stripping automated endothelial keratoplasty. Am J Ophthalmol. 2012;153(6):1082–90.e2.
8. Weinstein JE, Weiss JS. Descemet membrane and endothelial dystrophies. In: Mannis JM, Holland EJ, editors. Cornea. 4th ed. Philadelphia, PA: Elsevier; 2017. p. 800–17.
9. Macsai MS, Shiloach M. Use of topical rho kinase inhibitors in the treatment of Fuchs dystrophy after Descemet stripping only. Cornea. 2019;38(5):529–34.
10. Moloney G, Garcerant Congote D, Hirnschall N, Arsiwalla T, Luiza Mylla Boso A, Toalster N, et al. Descemet stripping only supplemented with topical ripasudil for fuchs endothelial dystrophy 12-month outcomes of the sydney eye hospital study. Cornea. 2021;40(3):320–6.

11. Kinoshita S, Koizumi N, Ueno M, Okumura N, Imai K, Tanaka H, et al. Injection of cultured cells with a ROCK inhibitor for bullous keratopathy. N Engl J Med. 2018;378(11):995–1003.

12. Numa K, Imai K, Ueno M, Kitazawa K, Tanaka H, Bush JD, et al. Five-year follow-up of first 11 patients undergoing injection of cultured corneal endothelial cells for corneal endothelial failure. Ophthalmology. 2021;128(4):504–14.

13. Gain P, Jullienne R, He Z, Aldossary M, Acquart S, Cognasse F, Thuret G. Global survey of corneal transplantation and eye banking. JAMA Ophthalmol. 2016;134(2):167–73.

14. Dawson DG, Ubels JL, Edelhauser HF. Cornea and sclera. In: Adler's physiology of the eye. 11th ed. Philadelphia, PA: Elsevier; 2011. p. 96–104.

15. Joyce NC. Proliferative capacity of corneal endothelial cells. Exp Eye Res. 2012;95(1):16–23.

16. Matsuda M, Sawa M, Edelhauser HF, Bartels SP, Neufeld AH, Kenyon KR. Cellular migration and morphology in corneal endothelial wound repair. Invest Ophthalmol Vis Sci. 1985;26(4):443–9.

17. Ono T, Mori Y, Nejima R, Iwasaki T, Miyai T, Miyata K. Corneal endothelial cell density and morphology in ophthalmologically healthy young individuals in Japan: an observational study of 16842 eyes. Sci Rep. 2021;11(1):18224.

18. Krachmer JH, Purcell JJ Jr, Young CW, Bucher KD. Corneal endothelial dystrophy. A study of 64 families. Arch Ophthalmol. 1978;96(11):2036–9.

19. Miyake K, Matsuda M, Inaba M. Corneal endothelial changes in pseudoexfoliation syndrome. Am J Ophthalmol. 1989;108(1):49–52.

20. Koizumi N, Yamasaki K, Kawasaki S, Sotozono C, Inatomi T, Mochida C, et al. Cytomegalovirus in aqueous humor from an eye with corneal endotheliitis. Am J Ophthalmol. 2006;141(3):564–5.

21. Pollack IP. Current concepts in laser iridotomy. Int Ophthalmol Clin. 1984;24(3):153–80.

22. Ho JW, Afshari NA. Advances in cataract surgery: preserving the corneal endothelium. Curr Opin Ophthalmol. 2015;26(1):22–7.

23. Realini T, Gupta PK, Radcliffe NM, Garg S, Wiley WF, Yeu E, et al. The effects of glaucoma and glaucoma therapies on corneal endothelial cell density. J Glaucoma. 2021;30(3):209–18.

24. Matsuda M, Tano Y, Inaba M, Manabe R. Corneal endothelial cell damage associated with intraocular gas tamponade during pars plana vitrectomy. Jpn J Ophthalmol. 1986;30(3):324–9.

25. Forbes SJ, Rosenthal N. Preparing the ground for tissue regeneration: from mechanism to therapy. Nat Med. 2014;20(8):857–69.

26. Yamaguchi T, Higa K, Suzuki T, Nakayama N, Yagi-Yaguchi Y, Dogru M, et al. Elevated cytokine levels in the aqueous humor of eyes with bullous Keratopathy and low endothelial cell density. Invest Ophthalmol Vis Sci. 2016;57(14):5954–62.

27. Kinoshita S, Ueno M. Cultivated cells in the treatment of corneal diseases. In: Colby K, Dana R, editors. Foundations of corneal disease. Springer: Cham; 2020. p. 215–24.

28. Ueno M, Toda M, Numa K, Tanaka H, Imai K, Bush J, et al. Superiority of mature differentiated cultured human corneal endothelial cell injection therapy for corneal endothelial failure. Am J Ophthalmol. 2021;237:267–77.

29. Ueno M, Asada K, Toda M, Schlötzer-Schrehardt U, Nagata K, Montoya M, et al. Gene signature-based development of elisa assays for reproducible qualification of cultured human corneal endothelial cells. Invest Ophthalmol Vis Sci. 2016;57(10):4295–305.

30. Hamuro J, Ueno M, Toda M, Sotozono C, Montoya M, Kinoshita S. Cultured human corneal endothelial cell aneuploidy dependence on the presence of heterogeneous subpopulations with distinct differentiation phenotypes. Invest Ophthalmol Vis Sci. 2016;57(10):4385–92.

31. Ueno M, Asada K, Toda M, Nagata K, Sotozono C, Kosaka N, et al. Concomitant evaluation of a panel of exosome proteins and mirs for qualification of cultured human corneal endothelial cells. Invest Ophthalmol Vis Sci. 2016;57(10):4393–402.

32. Hamuro J, Ueno M, Asada K, Toda M, Montoya M, Sotozono C, et al. Metabolic plasticity in cell state homeostasis and differentiation of cultured human corneal endothelial cells. Invest Ophthalmol Vis Sci. 2016;57(10):4452–63.

33. Toda M, Ueno M, Yamada J, Hiraga A, Tanaka H, Schlötzer-Schrehardt U, et al. The different binding properties of cultured human corneal endothelial cell subpopulations to Descemet's membrane components. Invest Ophthalmol Vis Sci. 2016;57(11):4599–605.

34. Hamuro J, Toda M, Asada K, Hiraga A, Schlötzer-Schrehardt U, Montoya M, et al. Cell homogeneity indispensable for regenerative medicine by cultured human corneal endothelial cells. Invest Ophthalmol Vis Sci. 2016;57(11):4749–61.

35. Ueno M, Asada K, Toda M, Hiraga A, Montoya M, Sotozono C, et al. MicroRNA profiles qualify phenotypic features of cultured human corneal endothelial cells. Invest Ophthalmol Vis Sci. 2016;57(13):5509–17.

36. Toda M, Ueno M, Hiraga A, Asada K, Montoya M, Sotozono C, et al. Production of homogeneous cultured human corneal endothelial cells indispensable for innovative cell therapy. Invest Ophthalmol Vis Sci. 2017;58(4):2011–20.

37. Yamamoto A, Tanaka H, Toda M, Sotozono C, Hamuro J, Kinoshita S, et al. A physical biomarker of the quality of cultured corneal endothelial cells and of the long-term prognosis of corneal restoration in patients. Nat Biomed Eng. 2019;3(12):953–60.

38. Hamuro J, Numa K, Fujita T, Toda M, Ueda K, Tokuda Y, et al. Metabolites interrogation in cell fate decision of cultured human corneal endothelial cells. Invest Ophthalmol Vis Sci. 2020;61(2):10.

39. Hamuro J, Deguchi H, Fujita T, Ueda K, Tokuda Y, Hiramoto N, et al. Polarized expression of ion chan-

nels and solute carrier family transporters on heterogeneous cultured human corneal endothelial cells. Invest Ophthalmol Vis Sci. 2020;61(5):47.

40. Numa K, Ueno M, Fujita T, Ueda K, Hiramoto N, Mukai A, et al. Mitochondria as a platform for dictating the cell fate of cultured human corneal endothelial cells. Invest Ophthalmol Vis Sci. 2020;61(14):10.

41. Toda M, Yukawa H, Yamada J, Ueno M, Kinoshita S, Baba Y, et al. In vivo fluorescence visualization of anterior chamber injected human corneal endothelial cells labeled with quantum dots. Invest Ophthalmol Vis Sci. 2019;60(12):4008–20.

42. Vickers LA, Foulks GN, Gupta PK. Diagnosis and management of corneal allograft rejection. In: Cornea. 4th ed. Philadelphia, PA: Elsevier; 2011. p. 1687–96.

43. Lee WB, Jacobs DS, Musch DC, Kaufman SC, Reinhart WJ, Shtein RM. Descemet's stripping endothelial keratoplasty: safety and outcomes: a report by the American academy of ophthalmology. Ophthalmology. 2009;116(9):1818–30.

44. Deng SX, Lee WB, Hammersmith KM, Kuo AN, Li JY, Shen JF, et al. Descemet membrane endothelial keratoplasty: safety and outcomes: a report by the American academy of ophthalmology. Ophthalmology. 2018;125(2):295–310.

45. Yamada J, Ueno M, Toda M, Shinomiya K, Sotozono C, Kinoshita S, et al. Allogeneic sensitization and tolerance induction after corneal endothelial cell transplantation in mice. Invest Ophthalmol Vis Sci. 2016;57(11):4572–80.

46. Niederkorn JY. Immune privilege and immune regulation in the eye. Adv Immunol. 1990;48:191–226.

47. Streilein JW. Immune regulation and the eye: a dangerous compromise. FASEB J. 1987;1:199–208.

Ultrathin DSAEK

Angeli Christy Yu and Massimo Busin

Key Points

- Ultrathin Descemet stripping automated endothelial keratoplasty (UT-DSAEK) offers the potential to achieve the visual results of DMEK with the ease of handling and tissue preparation of conventional DSAEK.
- Quality control during donor tissue preparation for UT-DSAEK is mandatory in order to optimize postoperative outcomes.

Introduction

Over the past two decades, endothelial keratoplasty (EK) has become the gold standard for the surgical management of endothelial decompensation [1]. Modern EK procedures can broadly be divided into Descemet stripping automated endothelial keratoplasty (DSAEK) and Descemet membrane endothelial keratoplasty (DMEK) [1]. While DMEK provides faster visual rehabilitation and lower rate of immune rejection in comparison to DSAEK, DMEK is associated with technical challenges in graft preparation and delivery and increased frequency of postoperative complications both during and after surgery [2–4]. Moreover, the learning curve of DMEK is accompanied by a high rate of tissue loss (up to 16%), a high graft detachment rate of up to 63%, and a graft failure rate of up to 8% [5–7]. In eyes with complex anterior segment anatomy such as abnormalities of the iris-lens diaphragm or in eyes with previous glaucoma surgery or pars plana vitrectomy, poor control of the DMEK graft within the anterior chamber during unfolding increases the technical complexity of the procedure and often results in excess graft manipulation [8–11]. Currently, DSAEK is still the most popular EK technique performed worldwide [2, 3].

DSAEK involves replacement of Descemet membrane and the diseased endothelium with donor tissue composed of a thin layer of posterior stroma, Descemet membrane, and endothelium [1]. In 2006, Holland reported that the postoperative best-corrected visual acuity of DSAEK grafts thinner than 131 μm compared favorably to that of thicker grafts and even those DMEK. This data supported the correlation of postoperative vision to the morphologic characteristics of the DSAEK graft [12, 13]. Graft regularity has increasingly been recognized as a key determinant of the quality of DSAEK grafts [14]. Aberrations derived from substantial irregularities in lenticule shape and graft thickness have been also found to play a significant role in determining the final visual outcome [15, 16].

Supplementary Information The online version contains supplementary material available at https://doi.org/10.1007/978-3-031-32408-6_28.

A. C. Yu · M. Busin (✉)
Department of Translational Medicine, University of Ferrara, Ferrara, Italy

In an attempt to improve the postoperative outcomes of DSAEK, Busin introduced the concept of ultrathin DSAEK (UT-DSAEK) in 2009. UT-DSAEK employed grafts within 100 μm in thickness, thereby combining the visual outcomes of DMEK with the technical ease of DSAEK. Since then, double- and single-pass techniques have been used by surgeons and eye banks to reproducibly obtain DSAEK grafts of a predetermined thickness and planar profile, which have substantially improved the outcomes of DSAEK [17, 18].

Indications

UT-DSAEK shares the same indications of conventional DSAEK. Conditions requiring the procedure include patients with any type of endothelial dysfunction such as endothelial dystrophies including Fuchs endothelial dystrophy or posterior polymorphous dystrophy, pseudophakic or aphakic bullous keratopathy, iridocorneal endothelial syndrome and endothelial decompensation secondary to previous trauma, intraocular surgery, or failed previous grafts [19]. While DMEK is also feasible in complex eyes [20], UT-DSAEK can be more easily performed in the presence of ocular comorbidities such as aniridia, aphakia, extensive iris trauma, anterior chamber intraocular lenses, and previous glaucoma surgery [21–24]. However, when subsequent surgery of the host cornea can be anticipated, either because of stromal ulceration or fibrosis or because of high-degree refractive errors, a thicker DSAEK graft may be considered to avoid inadvertent penetration into the anterior chamber while performing the secondary anterior procedure.

Preoperative Planning

The first step of the preoperative evaluation involves eliciting a careful and detailed general and ophthalmic history. The presence of concomitant eye diseases such as amblyopia, glaucoma, optic neuropathy, and retinal disease must be explored. A history of previous operations or prior infections may require modifications of the surgical technique and perioperative management.

Complete ophthalmologic examination including slit-lamp examination, best spectacle-corrected visual acuity (BSCVA), manifest refraction, applanation tonometry, and funduscopy must also be performed. Endothelial cell function is assessed by specular or confocal microscopy of the central and peripheral cornea. Additionally, anterior segment OCT is useful to assess corneal curvature and pachymetry.

The decision to perform either combined or sequential EK and cataract surgery is dependent on several preoperative factors. A combined procedure is often considered in patients aged 50 years and older with signs of corneal decompensation, as the retained crystalline lens will otherwise invariably develop a cataract as a consequence of both surgical trauma and postoperative topical steroid treatment [21]. Phakic UT-DSAEK may be alternatively performed in younger patients with otherwise clear crystalline lens.

If a modern flexible open-loop anterior chamber intraocular lens (ACIOL) or an iris-fixated IOL is well-positioned and of appropriate size, it may be left in place [22, 23]. Otherwise, poorly positioned IOLs can be exchanged for a posterior chamber IOL (PCIOL) using transscleral suture fixation.

Finally, phakic IOLs causing progressive endothelial cell loss (ECL) may be removed at the time of a combined UT-DSAEK. Phacoemulsification and posterior chamber IOL implantation can then be sequentially performed to minimize the time required for visual rehabilitation [24].

Anesthesia Considerations

Selection of anesthesia should be individualized for every patient. In most cases, UT-DSAEK can be performed with local anesthesia such as peribulbar or retrobulbar anesthesia. Adjunct intravenous sedation can also be considered. Decompression with a Honan balloon or similar devices for at least 10 min allows vitreous dehydration and softening of the eye, thereby reducing the risk of excessive posterior pressure and anterior chamber shallowing.

Surgical Technique

Donor graft preparation is a very crucial step in the UT-DSAEK procedure. The first attempts at standardizing UT-DSAEK graft preparation by means of a pivoting microkeratome (Carriazo-Barraquer, Moria SA, Antony, France) have led to the development of the "double-pass" technique. The technique was based on the observation that the predictability of the dissection depth was inversely proportional to the width of the microkeratome head slit. In the double-pass technique, the donor cornea is mounted on an artificial anterior chamber (AAC) of the ALTK system (Moria, Antony, France). The central corneal thickness of the donor is measured using ultrasound pachymetry (SP-3000; Tomey GmbH). An initial debulking step is performed using 300 µm microkeratome head which would debulk the donor tissue to around 180–250 µm in thickness. After turning the dovetail of the AAC by 180°, a second microkeratome-assisted dissection (refinement cut) is carried out from the direction opposite to the one of the first cut. As microkeratome dissection is deepest at the beginning of the cut, dissecting twice from opposite directions not only prevents perforation but also equalizes peripheral graft thickness, thereby producing a regular lenticule with planar configuration and less optical aberrations. A thinner microkeratome head (90, 110, or 130 µm) is used in the refinement cut based on the Busin nomogram which was optimized to obtain a final central graft thickness within 100 µm. The pressure of the system is standardized to an ideal level of 80–90 mmHg by raising the infusion bottle to a height of 120 cm above the level of the AAC and then clamping the tubing at 50 cm from the entrance into the AAC. In order to obtain regular graft thickness, care must be taken in maintaining a slow uniform movement during manual microkeratome-dissection.

More recently, linear microkeratomes have been used for the creation of UT-DSAEK grafts.

The improved predictability of the current ALTK systems has allowed the use of single-pass techniques with microkeratome heads even up to 450 µm cutting depth. An additional advantage of the single-pass technique is that the dissection yields an anterior lamella thicker than that cut with the first dissection of the double-pass technique and can be more properly used for tectonic keratoplasty or also for deep anterior lamellar keratoplasty (DALK) (Video 28.1).

Before removing the tissue from the AAC, the stromal side is marked to facilitate correct intraoperative orientation of the graft. The posterior donor lamella is then placed on a punch with the endothelial side up and cut to the desired diameter (8.0–9.0 mm).

Recipient Preparation and Graft Delivery

The initial steps of UT-DSAEK (Fig. 28.1) do not differ from those of conventional DSAEK. Prior to commencing surgery, loose and edematous epithelium is removed from the recipient cornea to allow better intraoperative visualization and postoperative epithelialization. A small aliquot of aqueous is aspirated, and air is injected intracamerally. Descemet membrane-endothelium complex is scored and stripped using a 25-gauge needle or cannula, Descemet stripper, or reverse Sinskey hook. Gentle pressure is applied to the inner cornea, taking care not to press into corneal stroma in order to avoid creation of stromal tissue strands. Descemetorhexis under air improves visualization and obviates the need for viscoelastic or trypan blue. In cases with poor anterior chamber visualization, Descemet membrane may be left in situ in the absence of central guttae.

If not present, a peripheral iridotomy (PI) is created to avoid postoperative pupillary block. The authors prefer to perform a surgical inferior PI using guillotine micro-incision scissors under continuous irrigation from the anterior chamber maintainer.

While several glides have been developed, our preferred delivery device for UT-DSAEK is the modified Busin glide (mini-glide or Mini Busin

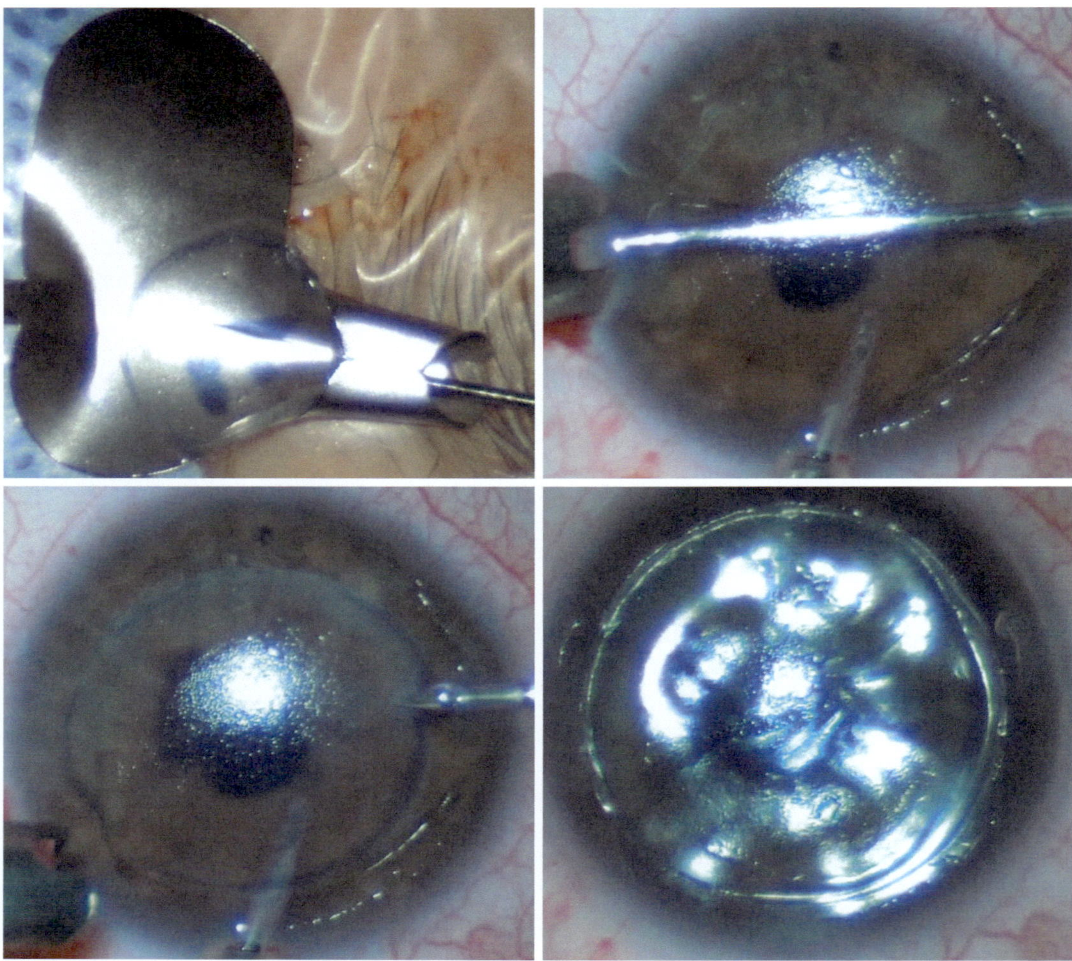

Fig. 28.1 Intraoperative steps of ultrathin Descemet stripping automated endothelial keratoplasty

Spatula, Moria SA, Antony, France). The modified Busin glide ensures proper graft delivery with correct orientation. The graft can also be trifolded before pulling it into the glide funnel, which can easily be inserted along the main incision at the nasal cornea. No viscoelastic substance is required during insertion. Using micro-incision forceps inserted through the temporal paracentesis, the UT-DSAEK graft is delivered bimanually under continuous, low-flow irrigation via an anterior chamber maintainer. Delivering the graft using the pull through technique provides total control throughout the procedure and allows spontaneous unfolding of the graft with minimal graft manipulation. Gentle tapping onto the surface of the anterior cornea allows spontaneous unfolding and centration of the UT-DSAEK graft.

Both the clear cornea tunnel and the side entry are sutured with interrupted 10–0 nylon sutures. The graft is attached to the posterior corneal surface by filling the anterior chamber with air injected. The authors prefer intracameral injection of air avoid due to concerns of potential endothelial toxicity of SF_6 and conflicting evidence of the latter's efficacy. Triamcinolone acetonide and gentamicin sulfate, 0.3%, are injected subconjunctivally at the end of the procedure.

Combined Surgeries

UT-DSAEK can be combined with other intraocular procedures such as phacoemulsification, IOL implantation, IOL exchange, secondary IOL implantation, pupilloplasty, and vitrectomy. These procedures are often performed immediately before insertion of the UT-DSAEK graft. Viscoelastic is also preferably avoided even in combined procedures. Continuous curvilinear capsulorhexis can be performed using a bent needle mounted on a syringe filled with saline to maintain a closed system, while a foldable IOL can be injected under continuous irrigation from an anterior chamber maintainer. IOLs should be of the hydrophobic type, as recent reports have pointed out the possibility of opacification of hydrophilic IOLs after DSAEK [25, 26]. Intracameral acetylcholine chloride is used to constrict the pupil after IOL implantation and prior to UT-DSAEK.

If use of viscoelastic is preferred, careful removal from the anterior chamber must be performed because retained material may hinder graft attachment or may result in interface opacities that can interfere with vision months after surgery. Intracameral acetylcholine is used to constrict the pupil after IOL implantation and prior to UT-DSAEK surgery (Fig. 28.2).

Postoperative Care

Subconjunctival antibiotic and corticosteroid injections may be administered immediately after completion of surgery. A fixed combination of topical antibiotic and steroid drops is initiated every 2 h daily and tapered off to 4 times daily over the first postoperative month. Subsequently, topical antibiotics is discontinued, while topical steroid is slowly tapered to once daily indefinitely. Steroid-induced ocular hypertension is treated with intraocular pressure lowering agents.

After the surgery, patients are instructed to lie supine for at least 2 h. Slit lamp exam is then performed to check for graft attachment. Air can be removed from one of the side entries using a blunt cannula, in order to avoid pupillary block. When the graft is detached, a rebubbling procedure is performed.

Results

Visual Outcomes

Visual recovery is faster and the proportion of eyes with final Snellen visual acuity of 20/20 is higher after UT-DSAEK than after conventional DSAEK, while no substantial difference is found with post-DMEK outcomes.

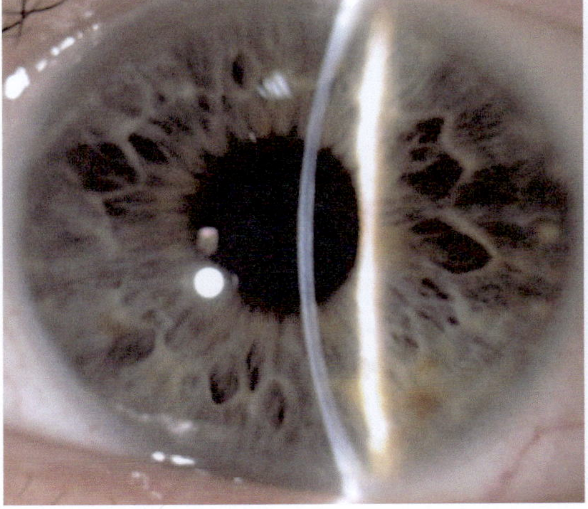
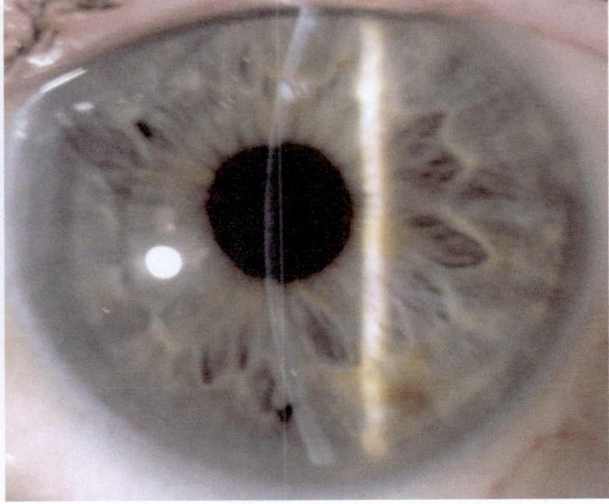

Fig. 28.2 Preoperative and postoperative images from a patient who underwent ultrathin Descemet stripping automated endothelial keratoplasty for Fuchs endothelial dystrophy

Recently published randomized controlled trials comparing provide discordant results with regard to visual outcomes. Unlike the DETECT study, Dunker et al. found no significant differences in visual acuity between DMEK and ultrathin DSAEK as early as 3 months and up to 1 year after surgery [19, 27]. No significant differences were also observed in terms of combined higher order aberrations, contrast sensitivity, straylight and vision-related quality of life [28–30]. Although 2-year results of DETECT seemed to suggest that DMEK provides superior visual outcomes, the results were inconclusive as the loss to follow-up may have affected the study findings [31]. A larger randomized clinical trial is warranted to further clarify differences in visual acuity after DMEK and ultrathin DSAEK.

Refractive Outcomes

Similar to DMEK, no significant change in astigmatism is seen after UT-DSAEK [17]. While a significant induced cylinder (up to 0.6 D) has been reported by several authors after conventional DSAEK, this is most probably a consequence of the different wound sizes employed for graft delivery [32]. UT-DSAEK grafts can be delivered through a 3 mm incision using the modified Busin glide.

Mild hyperopic shifts (0.78 ± 0.59 D) occur after UT-DSAEK procedures. Reversal of corneal edema after surgery can result in significant alterations in corneal curvature. Taking into account this shift during (IOL) calculations can minimize refractive surprises.

Endothelial Cell Density

Five years after UT-DSAEK, endothelial cell loss averaged 52%. This is similar to the values reported after conventional DSAEK by Price et al. (53%) [33], Wacker et al. (55%) [34], and Ang et al. (48.7%) [35] and with that of DMEK by Ham et al. (55%) [36] and by Vasiliauskaite et al. (59%) [37]. Randomized controlled trials comparing UT-DSAEK and DMEK likewise did not find significant differences in ECD and ECL [19, 27].

At 1 year, the ECL was comparable with that of conventional DSAEK, despite the the use of smaller (3.0-mm) incisions. After UT-DSAEK, ECD is significantly higher in glaucoma patients, as was previously reported after DSAEK [38].

Graft Survival

One-year graft survival for conventional DSAEK in series excluding the initial learning curve has been reported to vary between 94% and 100% [39, 40]. In our recent series on UT-DSAEK, Kaplan–Meier graft survival probability at 1, 2, 3, and 5 years was 99.1% (212/214 eyes), 96.2% (167/172 eyes), 94.2% (144/147 eyes), and 94.2% (105/105 eyes), respectively [41]. Price reported recently a conventional DSAEK graft survival rate at 5 years of 93%, with a significantly higher value for Fuchs patients (95%) than for patients with pseudophakic bullous keratopathy (76%) or previous glaucoma surgery (40%) [36]. Vasiliauskaite et al. reported a cumulative survival probability of 83% (95% confidence interval [CI], 0.75–0.92) 5 years following DMEK.

Immunologic rejection occurs less frequently after UT-DSAEK than after DSAEK, but still occurs more frequently over DMEK. Gender matching does not affect rates of immune rejection or graft failure [42].

Complications

The most common complication following UT-DSAEK is transient cystoid macular edema, which responds well to conservative treatment [43]. Graft detachment and graft failure are much less frequent than after conventional DSAEK or DMEK. In particular, the rate of rebubbling following UT-DSAEK is within 4%, which is lower than any DMEK statistic published to date. Total detachment is seen in most cases and generally successfully managed by rebubbling (with a single or double injection). Recent randomized controlled trials have shown higher rebubbling rates for DMEK compared to ultrathin DSAEK [19, 26]. Both studies report markedly similar rates of graft detachment (24%) in DMEK versus 4% in ultrathin DSAEK. Considering their absolute differences, the graft detachment rates after DMEK are appreciably higher than after ultrathin DSAEK.

Other complications of the procedure include pupillary block, persistent epithelial defect, persistent interface haze, interface infections, and cataract formation. Such adverse events do not seem to occur more or less frequently than after conventional DSAEK.

Take Home Notes
- UT-DSAEK still remains a valuable tool in the surgical armamentarium of any corneal specialist.
- Similar to conventional DSAEK, UT-DSAEK can be more easily performed in all eyes with complex anatomy and poor anterior chamber visualization.
- Unlike DMEK, the complication rates especially in terms of graft detachment are significantly lower following UT-DSAEK.
- Standardized graft preparation yields consistent graft quality, regularity, and thickness which in turn translates to excellent visual outcomes.

References

1. Deng SX, Barry Lee W, Hammersmith KM, et al. Descemet membrane endothelial keratoplasty: safety and outcomes. Ophthalmology. 2018;125(2):295–310.
2. 2019 Eye banking statistical report. Washington, DC: Eye Bank Association of America; https://restoresight.org/wp-content/uploads/2020/04/2019-EBAA-Stat-Report-FINAL.pdf. Accessed 23 May 2020.
3. Suryan DL, Armitage JW, Armitage M, et al. Outcomes of corneal transplantation in Europe: report by the European cornea and cell transplantation registry. J Cataract Refract Surg. 2021;47(6):780–5.
4. Zafar S, Parker JS, de Kort C, Melles G, Sikder S. Perceived difficulties and barriers to uptake of Descemet's membrane endothelial keratoplasty among surgeons. Clin Ophthalmol. 2019;13:1055–61.
5. Dapena I, Ham L, Droutsas K, van Dijk K, Moutsouris K, Melles GR. Learning curve in Descemet's membrane endothelial keratoplasty: first series of 135 consecutive cases. Ophthalmology. 2011;118(11):2147–54.
6. Rodríguez-Calvo-de-Mora M, Quilendrino R, Ham L, et al. Clinical outcome of 500 consecutive cases undergoing Descemet's membrane endothelial keratoplasty. Ophthalmology. 2014;20(14):161–4.
7. Gorovoy MS. DMEK complications. Cornea. 2014;33(1):101–4.
8. Aravena C, Yu F, Deng SX. Outcomes of Descemet membrane endothelial keratoplasty in patients with prior glaucoma surgery. Cornea. 2017;36/3:284–9.
9. Sorkin N, Mimouni M, Kisilevsky E, et al. Four-year survival of Descemet membrane endothelial keratoplasty in patients with previous glaucoma surgery. Am J Ophthalmol. 2020;218:7–16.
10. Santaella G, Sorkin N, Mimouni M. Outcomes of Descemet membrane endothelial keratoplasty in aphakic and aniridic patients. Cornea. 2020;39(11):1389–93.
11. Spaniol K, Holtmann C, Schwinde JH, Deffaa S, Guthoff R, Geerling G. Descemet-membrane endothelial keratoplasty in patients with retinal comorbidity-a prospective cohort study. Int J Ophthalmol. 2016;9(3):390–4.
12. Busin M, Albé E. Does thickness matter: ultrathin Descemet stripping automated endothelial keratoplasty. Curr Opin Ophthalmol. 2014;25(4):312–8.
13. Busin M, Yu A. The ongoing debate: Descemet membrane endothelial keratoplasty versus ultrathin Descemet stripping automated endothelial keratoplasty. Ophthalmology. 2020;127(9):1160–1.
14. Dickman MM, Cheng YY, Berendschot TT, et al. Effects of graft thickness and asymmetry on visual gain and aberrations after Descemet stripping automated endothelial keratoplasty. JAMA Ophthalmol. 2013;131:737e744.
15. Rudolph M, Laaser K, Bachmann BO, Cursiefen C, Epstein D, Kruse FE. Corneal higher-order aberrations after Descemet's membrane endothelial keratoplasty. Ophthalmology. 2012;119(3):528–35.
16. Ruzza A, Parekh M, Ferrari S, et al. Preloaded donor corneal lenticules in a new validated 3D printed smart storage glide for Descemet stripping automated endothelial keratoplasty. Br J Ophthalmol. 2015;99(10):1388–95.
17. Busin M, Madi S, Santorum P, Scorcia V, Beltz J. Ultrathin descemet's stripping automated endothelial keratoplasty with the microkeratome double-pass technique: two-year outcomes. Ophthalmology. 2013;120(6):1186–94.
18. Villarrubia A, Cano-Ortiz A. Development of a nomogram to achieve ultrathin donor corneal disks for Descemet-stripping automated endothelial keratoplasty. J Cataract Refract Surg. 2015;41(1):146–51.
19. Dunker SL, Dickman MM, Wisse RPL, et al. DMEK versus ultrathin DSAEK: a multicenter ran-

domized controlled clinical trial. Ophthalmology. 2020;127(9):1152–9.

20. Yu AC, Myerscough J, Spena R, et al. Three-year outcomes of tri-folded endothelium-in Descemet membrane endothelial keratoplasty with pull-through technique. Am J Ophthalmol. 2020;219:121–31.

21. Burkhart ZN, Feng MT, Price FW Jr, Price MO. One-year outcomes in eyes remaining phakic after Descemet membrane endothelial keratoplasty. J Cataract Refract Surg. 2014;40(3):430–4.

22. Elderkin S, Tu E, Sugar J, Reddy S, Kadakia A, Ramaswamy R, Djalilian A. Outcome of descemet stripping automated endothelial keratoplasty in patients with an anterior chamber intraocular lens. Cornea. 2010;29(11):1273–7.

23. Beltz J, Busin M. Descemet stripping automated endothelial keratoplasty in a case with a posteriorly fixated iris-claw intraocular lens. Cornea. 2012;31(1):96–7.

24. Nahum Y, Busin M. Quadruple procedure for visual rehabilitation of endothelial decompensation following phakic intraocular lens implantation. Am J Ophthalmol. 2014;158(6):1330–4.

25. Ahad MA, Darcy K, Cook SD, Tole DM. Intraocular lens opacification after descemet stripping automated endothelial keratoplasty. Cornea. 2014;33(12):1307–11.

26. Werner L, Wilbanks G, Nieuwendaal CP, Dhital A, Waite A, Schmidinger G, Lee WB, Mamalis N. Localized opacification of hydrophilic acrylic intraocular lenses after procedures using intracameral injection of air or gas. J Cataract Refract Surg. 2015;41(1):199–207.

27. Chamberlain W, Lin CC, Austin A, et al. Descemet endothelial thickness comparison trial: a randomized trial comparing ultrathin Descemet stripping automated endothelial keratoplasty with Descemet membrane endothelial keratoplasty. Ophthalmology. 2019;126:19e26.

28. Duggan MJ, Rose-Nussbaumer J, Lin CC, Austin A, Labadzinzki PC, Chamberlain WD. Corneal higher-order aberrations in Descemet membrane endothelial keratoplasty versus ultrathin DSAEK in the Descemet endothelial thickness comparison trial: a randomized clinical trial. Ophthalmology. 2019;126(7):946–57.

29. Ang MJ, Chamberlain W, Lin CC, Pickel J, Austin A, Rose-Nussbaumer J. Effect of unilateral endothelial keratoplasty on vision-related quality-of-life outcomes in the Descemet endothelial thickness comparison trial (DETECT): a secondary analysis of a randomized clinical trial. JAMA Ophthalmol. 2019;137(7):747–54.

30. Dunker SL, Dickman MM, Wisse RPL, Nobacht S, Wijdh RHJ, Bartels MC, Mei-Lie Tang NE, et al. Quality of vision and vision-related quality of life after Descemet membrane endothelial keratoplasty: a randomized clinical trial. Acta Ophthalmol. 2021;99:e1127. https://doi.org/10.1111/aos.14741; Epub ahead of print.

31. Rose-Nussbaumer J, Lin CC, Austin A, Liu Z, Clover J, McLeod SD, et al. Descemet endothelial thickness comparison trial: two-year results from a randomized trial comparing ultrathin Descemet stripping automated endothelial keratoplasty with Descemet membrane endothelial keratoplasty. Ophthalmology. 2020;128:1238. https://doi.org/10.1016/j.ophtha.2020.12.021; Epub ahead of print.

32. Koenig SB, Covert DJ. Early results of small-incision Descemet's stripping and automated endothelial keratoplasty. Ophthalmology. 2007;114(2):221–6.

33. Price MO, Fairchild KM, Price DA. Descemet's stripping endothelial keratoplasty: five-year graft survival and endothelial cell loss. Ophthalmology. 2011;118:725–9.

34. Wacker K, Baratz KH, Maguire LJ, et al. Descemet stripping endothelial keratoplasty for Fuchs' endothelial corneal dystrophy: five-year results of a prospective study. Ophthalmology. 2016;123:154–60.

35. Ang M, Soh Y, Htoon HM, et al. Five-year graft survival comparing Descemet stripping automated endothelial keratoplasty and penetrating keratoplasty. Ophthalmology. 2016;123:1646–52.

36. Ham L, Dapena I, Liarakos VS, et al. Midterm results of Descemet membrane endothelial keratoplasty: 4 to 7 years clinical outcome. Am J Ophthalmol. 2016;171:113–21.

37. Vasiliauskaite I, Oellerich S, Ham L, Dapena I, Baydoun L, van Dijk K, et al. Descemet membrane endothelial keratoplasty: ten-year graft survival and clinical outcomes. Am J Ophthalmol. 2020;217:114–20.

38. Quek DT, Wong T, Tan D, Mehta JS. Corneal graft survival and intraocular pressure control after descemet stripping automated endothelial keratoplasty in eyes with pre-existing glaucoma. Am J Ophthalmol. 2011;152(1):48–54.

39. Busin M, Bhatt PR, Scorcia V. A modified technique for descemet membrane stripping automated endothelial keratoplasty to minimize endothelial cell loss. Arch Ophthalmol. 2008;126(8):1133–7.

40. Price MO, Gorovoy M, Benetz BA, Price FW Jr, Menegay HJ, Debanne SM, Lass JH. Descemet's stripping automated endothelial keratoplasty outcomes compared with penetrating keratoplasty from the cornea donor study. Ophthalmology. 2010;117(3):438–44.

41. Madi S, Leon P, Nahum Y, et al. Five-year outcomes of ultrathin Descemet stripping automated endothelial keratoplasty. Cornea. 2019;38:1192–7.

42. Romano V, Parekh M, Virgili G, et al. Gender matching did not affect 2-year rejection or failure rates following DSAEK for Fuchs endothelial corneal dystrophy. Am J Ophthalmol. 2022;235:204–10.

43. Myerscough J, Roberts HW, Yu AC, et al. Factors predictive of cystoid macular oedema following endothelial keratoplasty: a single-Centre review of 2233 cases. Br J Ophthalmol. 2021;107:24. https://doi.org/10.1136/bjophthalmol-2020-318076.

Darren S. J. Ting and Marcus Ang

Key Points

- DMEK is emerging as an important lamellar keratoplasty technique for selective endothelial replacement to treat end-stage corneal endothelial diseases.
- Innovations in donor insertion for DMEK have led to development of devices that use injection (endothelium-out) or pull-through (endothelium-in) approaches.
- The use of intraoperative optical coherence tomography (iOCT) may enhance intraoperative visualisation of graft unfolding and attachment during DMEK surgery.
- Innovations in techniques, including safety-net suture, phakic collamer lens implantation and artificial iris implantation, have rendered DMEK possible for complex eyes such as those with shallow anterior chamber, aphakia and/or significant iris defect.

Supplementary Information The online version contains supplementary material available at https://doi.org/10.1007/978-3-031-32408-6_29.

D. S. J. Ting
Birmingham and Midland Eye Centre, Birmingham, UK

Academic Unit of Ophthalmology, Institute of Inflammation and Ageing, University of Birmingham, Birmingham, UK

Academic Ophthalmology, School of Medicine, University of Nottingham, Nottingham, UK

M. Ang (✉)
Singapore National Eye Center, Singapore Eye Research Institute, Singapore, Singapore

Department of Ophthalmology and Visual Sciences, Duke-NUS Medical School, Singapore, Singapore
e-mail: Marcus.Ang@singhealth.com.sg

Introduction

In recent decades, there has been a paradigm shift from penetrating keratoplasty to endothelial keratoplasty in treating end-stage corneal endothelial diseases, including Fuchs endothelial corneal dystrophy (FECD) and pseudophakic bullous keratopathy (PBK) [1–7]. Although the concept of endothelial keratoplasty (EK) for selective replacement of diseased corneal endothelium was first introduced as far back as 1950s by Charles Tillet [8], further modifications have led to the development of various techniques [8]. Currently, Descemet stripping automated endothelial keratoplasty (DSAEK) and Descemet membrane endothelial keratoplasty (DMEK) represent the two most widely performed EK techniques [9, 10].

DSAEK involves removal of the diseased Descemet membrane (DM) and endothelium, followed by grafting of a healthy donor cornea consisting of posterior stroma, DM and endothelium [11–13]. The preparation of the donor cornea is performed with the assistance of an automated microkeratome [6, 14]. This is currently a popular EK technique, supported by donor preparation by eye banks, though it may result in donor stroma and graft–host interface irregularity, which can negatively impact on visual outcomes [14–16]. In 2006, Melles et al. [17] introduced Descemet membrane endothelial keratoplasty (DMEK)—a like-to-like replacement of the diseased DM-endothelium with healthy donor DM-endothelium only. This technique helps minimise donor stroma–host interface irregularities, postoperative hyperopic shift and higher order aberrations associated with DSAEK. Most studies also report a faster recovery, lower graft rejection rate and reduced need for topical steroids (hence a lower risk of glaucoma) compared to DSAEK [10, 14, 18–20].

In addition, the preparation of the DMEK donor does not require a microkeratome unlike in DSAEK, which makes donor preparation more accessible. However, DMEK donor preparation, insertion and unfolding have a steeper learning curve than DSAEK [9, 19], which may account for the slower adoption of this technique in some centres. Thus, some centres have reported a higher rate of complications such as graft detachment requiring postoperative re-bubbling and primary graft failure in DMEK compared to DSAEK [14, 19, 21–23].

In view of the above-described challenges faced with DMEK, various improvement and modifications have been described to further refine the surgical techniques of DMEK, with an aim to reduce complications and improve clinical outcomes. Thus, we aim to provide an overview of recent innovations in DMEK, including donor insertion (endothelium-out) and pull-through (endothelium-in) devices, and novel techniques for DMEK in complex eyes. In each section, we also describe the original techniques and highlight the innovative measures that have been introduced.

Graft Preparation

In this section, we describe the main techniques and innovations related to DMEK donor preparation, which involves donor stripping and marking.

The DMEK surgery was original described using an endothelium-out, injection technique [17], though recent innovations have made both endothelium-out and endothelium-in techniques feasible with comparable clinical outcomes. For donor graft harvesting and marking, the steps are similar for both techniques. DMEK graft harvesting is usually initiated by a 360° peripheral scoring and stripping of the donor peripheral DM from the posterior stroma. Since the first description of its original technique using manual scoring with a Sinskey hook or fine non-toothed forceps, various techniques have been described for facilitate this step, including big and small trephines, big bubble technique and liquid bubble technique using a DMEK graft preparation device, DescePrep [9, 17, 24–27]. Femtosecond laser (FSL)-assisted graft preparation has also been described by McKee and Jhanji in three patients [28]. In this technique, the donor cornea is mounted on an artificial anterior chamber and a partial deep circular cut is fashioned with the use of FSL through the posterior stroma, DM and corneal endothelium.

During graft preparation, several vital dyes, including trypan blue or VisionBlue (D.O.R.C., Zuidland, The Netherland), Membrane Blue Dual (D.O.R.C., Zuidland, The Netherland) and Brilliant Blue G (Sigma-Aldrich, St. Louis, USA), can be used to enhance the visualisation of the thin DM-endothelium tissue [8, 9, 29, 30]. After the peripheral donor DM is completely detached from the posterior stroma, the DMEK graft is then peeled and harvested using the "submerged cornea using backgrounds away (SCUBA)" technique [31–33]. By using this technique, the DM can be peeled more easily without any tear or break, with >95% success rate in DMEK graft preparation.

In the original technique, the graft orientation was primarily ascertained based on the inherent endothelium-out scrolling pattern of the donor DM tissue. However, eyes with poor intraocular view or donor tissues with less scrolling (observed in older donors) may cause difficulty in determining the graft orientation, which can lead to inadvertent implantation of an upside-down graft and consequent primary DMEK graft failure [34, 35]. To address this, several innovations have been proposed and implemented for marking the graft to ensure its correct orientation [34, 36]. One of the most common methods is the use of a stromal window in marking the anterior part of the DM. In this technique, the donor DM-endothelium is partially peeled away from the stroma, followed by the creation of a small stromal window using a 3–4 mm diameter skin punch. The DM-endothelium is then completely placed back onto the stroma. After drying the excess fluid from the graft preparation bed (to ensure complete attachment between DM-endothelium and stroma), the donor cornea is then flipped to face epithelium-side up. The anterior part of the DM is then accessed via the stromal window and marked with a violet ink-stained "S" or "F" stamp [37]. The marked, incompletely detached DM-endothelium is then punched with a 7.5–8.0 mm trephine and completely released from the stroma, in preparation for graft loading.

While this technique produces consistent marking of the DMEK graft, the creation of a stromal window negates the possibility of using the remaining anterior portion of donor cornea for other types of transplantation such as anterior lamellar keratoplasty (ALK) and deep anterior lamellar keratoplasty (DALK). To increase the utility of the donor corneas for simultaneous DMEK and ALK/DALK (one donor cornea for two different recipients), a number of innovations have been described, which include asymmetry marking/cutting of the edge of the DMEK graft, use of ophthalmic viscoelastic device (OVD), and bandage contact lens interface technique [8, 36, 38, 39]. These marking techniques are particularly useful in the current era of corneal transplantations where there is persistent shortage of donor corneas globally, for which the issue has been further exacerbated by the recent COVID-19 pandemic [40].

To eliminate the risk of unsuccessful harvesting of the DMEK graft intraoperatively and to reduce the intraoperative time, there has been an increasing shift towards the use of eye bank-prepared pre-stripped and pre-loaded DMEK graft for clinical use [41]. Preparation of the donor tissue by the eye bank can also increase the consistency and quality of the graft as the eye bank technicians will have more access and experience in donor tissue preparation (compared to the surgeons who are likely to perform 1–2 DMEK per week or even less in some centres). The DMEK graft can be pre-loaded in the chosen injector either in an endothelium-out or endothelium-in fashion. Chen et al. [42] compared the endothelial cell viability between preloaded scrolled DM-endothelium (endothelium-out) and tri-folded DM-endothelium (endothelium-in) technique and demonstrated similar cell viability between the two techniques (86.3% vs. 85.2%) at 4 days post-loading into the injector. In a recent multi-centre study, Parekh et al. [43] reported the clinical outcomes of preloaded DMEK for FECD or PBK and found that the rate of graft detachment was around 40% and the mean endothelial cell loss was 46% and 48% at 3-month and 1-year post-DMEK surgery, respectively. Therefore, while pre-loaded DMEK has its inherent advantages, this needs to be balanced with the slightly higher rate of graft detachment and endothelial cell loss when compared to non-preloaded-DMEK [18, 29, 44, 45].

Graft Insertion and Unfolding

After the DMEK graft is marked and harvested, the free-floating graft has an inherent tendency to scroll with endothelium on the outer surface due to a relatively higher elastin content in the anterior part of the DM [46]. The scroll tightness of the donor DM-endothelium appears to increase with the decrease in donor age [47], which may lead to difficulties in unfolding the graft in the transplanted eye. That said, reduced scroll tightness observed in older donor may cause issue in identifying the correct orientation of the DMEK graft, highlighting the importance of graft marking during the harvesting process. Once the donor DM-endothelium graft has been prepared, it can be loaded into an injector or an insertor to

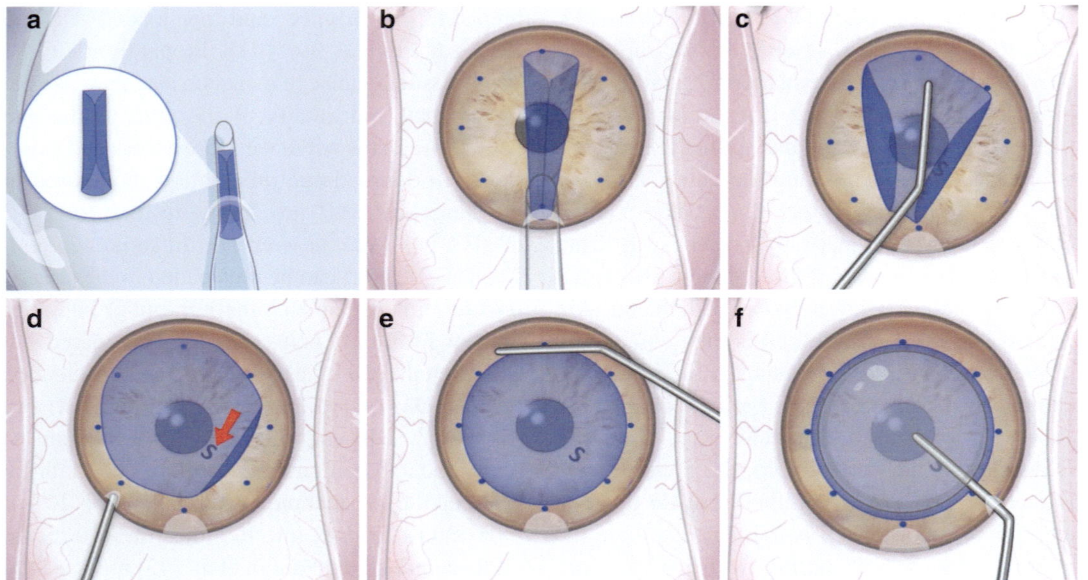

Fig. 29.1 An animated video demonstrating the surgical technique of an endothelium-out Descemet membrane endothelial keratoplasty (DMEK) surgery using a Geuder glass tube with injection technique. (**a**) A DMEK graft (stained with vital blue dye) is loaded into the Geuder glass tube in an endothelium-out fashion. (**b**) Insertion of the DMEK graft into the anterior chamber of the recipient. (**c**) Unfolding of the graft using the tapping method. (**d**) Complete unfolding of the DMEK graft in a correct orientation (confirmed by the "S" stamp). (**e**) Centration of the DMEK graft using the tapping method. (**f**) Air or gas tamponade of the DMEK graft against the recipient's posterior stroma

facilitate an endothelium-out (Fig. 29.1a–f) (Video 29.1) or endothelium-in DMEK (Fig. 29.2a–i).

Donor Injection (Endothelium-out) Technique

Different types of injectors, including glass injection devices and IOL cartridges, have been used for loading an endothelium-out DMEK graft [8, 34, 45, 48–51]. As the endothelium-out technique is associated with an inevitable contact between the donor endothelium and the luminal wall of the insertion device, it can cause undesirable and irreversible loss of corneal endothelial cells. Shen et al. [52] conducted an ex vivo study evaluating three different commercially available injectors for DMEK, namely the Geuder glass injector, modified Jones tube and the STAAR intraocular (IOL) injector. It was shown that Geuder cannula caused less iatrogenic damage to the donor endothelium (24%) compared to the other two injectors (37–38%). On the other hand, Droutsas et al. [53] conducted a large comparative clinical study evaluating the amount of endothelial cell loss of the DMEK graft among three commercially available glass injectors, namely the Melles DMEK injector (D.O.R.C., Zuidland, The Netherlands), the Szurmann DMEK injector (Geuder, Germany) and the Pasteur pipette, and found no statistically significant difference among them.

Once the graft is loaded into an injector, it is inserted into the anterior chamber of the recipient's eye and unfolded using a combination of techniques and manoeuvres. To facilitate the unfolding of DMEK graft, the majority of the described techniques require a relatively flattened anterior chamber. A series of controlled taps on the corneal surface or short burst of intracameral injection of water is then performed to

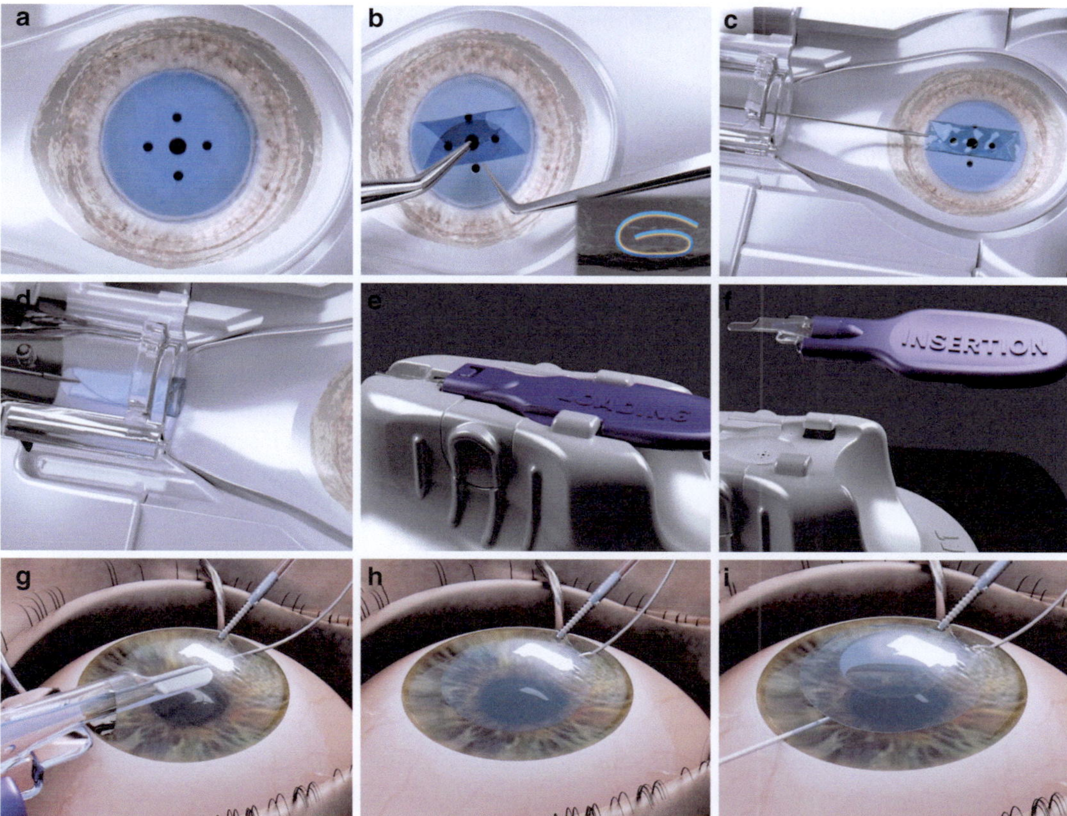

Fig. 29.2 An animated video demonstrating the surgical technique of an endothelium-in Descemet membrane endothelial keratoplasty (DMEK) surgery using a DMEK Endoglide (Network Medical Products, North Yorkshire, UK) with pull-through technique. (**a**) A DMEK graft (stained with vital blue dye) with complete detachment from the posterior stroma. (**b**) Preparation of the DMEK graft in a tri-folded, endothelium-in fashion. (**c**, **d**) After drying the excess fluid from the graft preparation bed, the DMEK graft is pulled into the DMEK Endoglide. (**e**) Securing of the DMEK graft in the loader with the "loading" mark facing up. (**f**) The DMEK Endoglide is turned around with the "insertion" mark facing up. (**g**) Insertion of the DMEK graft using a pull-through technique. (**h**) Complete unfolding of the DMEK graft while holding the graft with the curved forceps. (**i**) Air or gas tamponade of the DMEK graft against the recipient's posterior stroma

centralise and unfold the graft. Double-roll no-touch technique, Dirisamer technique (carpet unrolling while fixating 1 graft edge), Dapena manoeuvre (small air bubble-assisted unrolling) and single sliding cannula manoeuvre are some of the innovative techniques described in the literature [8, 54, 55]. Once the graft is fully unfolded and centred, intracameral injection of air or gas is performed to tamponade and attach the DMEK graft. However, such technique may be infeasible in eyes with deep anterior chamber, previous vitrectomy or aphakia where the anterior chamber cannot be sufficiently flattened to achieve effi-cient manipulation of the graft within the anterior chamber.

To overcome this, Hayashi et al. [56] and Parker et al. [57] described an innovative double-bubble technique to help unfold the graft in eyes with deep anterior chamber and/or previous vitrectomy. By using a small bubble over the graft to help partially unfold the graft, a slightly bigger bubble is injected under the graft to help float and fully unfold the graft. On the other hand, Saad et al. [58] described a relatively simple and reproducible technique (named Cornea Press or C-Press) to help unfolding the DMEK graft in vitrectomised eyes. During the graft unfolding, a cannula is inserted within the scrolled graft (DM side) and moved left and right to open the graft while irrigating with balanced salt solution. At the same time, another cannula is used to press on the corneal surface to artificially induce the shallowing of anterior chamber. After the graft is fully unfolded, intracameral injections of air/gas are performed underneath to tamponade the graft. The cannula over the corneal surface is released.

Furthermore, Kobayashi et al. [59] described an innovative technique using a 25-gauge graft manipulator to assist an endothelium-out DMEK surgery. After the graft was inserted into the anterior chamber using an injector, the graft was grasped throughout the unfolding and centration process, until the graft is fully attached and tamponaded with air or gas. This technique was shown to help reduce the intraoperative surgical time by around 16 min, with comparable clinical outcomes. Other technique such as the use of pars plana infusion to stabilise the anterior chamber during DMEK surgery in previously vitrectomised eyes has also been described [60].

Pull-Through (Endothelium-in) Donor Insertion Technique

In recent years, the endothelium-in DMEK technique has been gaining increasing popularity in view of the perceived advantages over the endothelium-out techniques [45, 61]. First, by having an endothelium-in graft, it reduces any undesirable touch of the donor corneal endothelium against the luminal wall of the injector. Second, as the scrolled donor DM-endothelium has a natural tendency to roll endothelium-outward, inserting the DMEK graft in an endo-

thelium-in manner (with DM side up) will allow the graft to unfold naturally. As this technique obviates the need for excessing tapping and manipulation of the graft within the AC, it helps reduce the risk of graft misorientation, the intraoperative time and the technical difficulty in challenging eyes (e.g., eyes with deep anterior chamber, previous vitrectomy or poor corneal clarity obscuring the intraoperative view; Fig. 29.3a–l).

Various devices, including the DMEK EndoGlide (Network Medical Products, North Yorkshire, UK) [45] and IOL cartridges [61], have been used to insert an endothelium-in DMEK graft using a pull-through technique. The graft is usually loaded into the devices in an endothelium tri-folded inward manner and inserted into the eye using a bimanual pull-through technique, similar to the technique used in DSAEK. A hybrid-DMEK technique has also been described, which involves using EndoGlide Ultrathin DSAEK pull-through donor insertion device and donor stroma as carrier [62]. In this technique, the DM is partially peeled from a thin, pre-cut DSAEK donor tissue graft (~150 µm thickness). After trephining through the donor DM, stroma and anterior cap, the remaining attached part of DM is then completely separated from the stroma. Subsequently, the anterior cap is removed and the DM-endothelium and thin stroma are transferred together into the EndoGlide and pulled towards the anterior opening of the glide to achieve a "double-coil" configuration, similar to a DSAEK graft. The donor DM-endothelium (without the donor stroma) is subsequently pulled through the corneal or corneoscleral tunnel into the anterior chamber, with endothelium side down. The graft is then allowed to open spontaneously, followed by a relatively full air or gas tamponade.

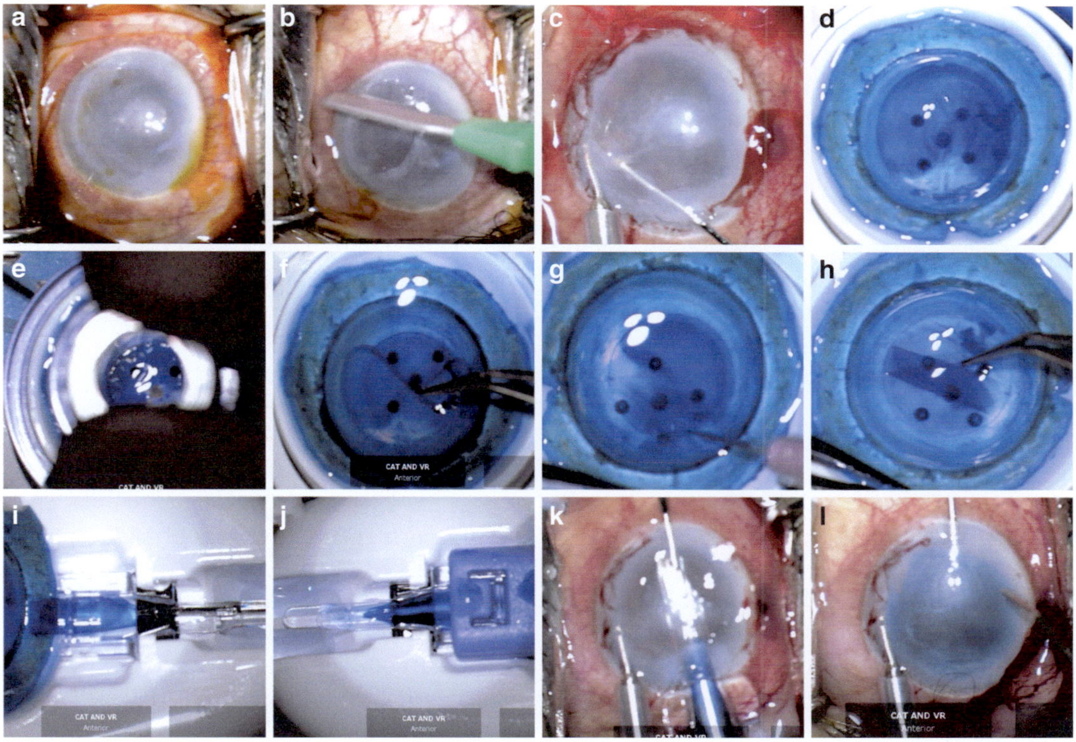

Fig. 29.3 Intraoperative snapshots of an endothelium-in Descemet membrane endothelial keratoplasty (DMEK) surgery in an eye with difficult view. (**a**) A decompensated cornea with significant corneal oedema and haziness, obscuring the view of the intraocular structures. (**b**) Removal of the swollen and hazy corneal epithelium to improve the intraoperative view. (**c**) Manual descemetorrhexis. (**d**) Staining of the pre-stripped DMEK graft with vital blue dye. (**e**) Trephination of the donor central posterior cornea using an 8-mm donor punch. (**f**) Removal of the peripheral DM strip from the central DMEK graft. (**g**) Marking of the DMEK graft orientation using an asymmetrical cut. (**h**) Preparation of the DMEK graft in a tri-folded, endothelium-in fashion. (**i, j**) Loading of the DMEK graft into the DMEK Endoglide. (**k**) Insertion of the DMEK graft into the anterior chamber. (**l**) Complete graft unfolding while securing the DMEK graft with a curved forceps, followed by a complete air or gas tamponade

Innovative DMEK Techniques

Splitting of graft to address shortage of donor corneas

Currently, there is a global shortage of donor corneal tissues in both developed and developing countries [63]. Despite many initiatives have been introduced to increase the eye donation rate and the utilisation of the donor corneas [63–66], such issue remains a persistent barrier to corneal transplantation. In the current standard practice of DMEK surgery, one donor cornea is utilised for only one recipient. To increase the utilisation of the donor corneas, other variants of DMEK such as hemi-DMEK and quarter-DMEK have also been proposed to increase the use of one donor cornea for two and four patients, respectively [67, 68]. The technique is similar to a DMEK but only differs in the size and shape of the graft. Three-quarter DMEK technique has also been described in eyes with glaucoma drainage device to avoid secondary graft failure [69]. Both hemi-DMEK and quarter-DMEK have demonstrated comparable results to DMEK up to 2 years in terms of visual outcome (with 40–60% eyes achieving a corrected-distance-visual-acuity of 6/6 or better), albeit the central endothelial cell density was shown to be lower than DMEK. Further studies are required to confirm the long-term clinical outcomes in a larger patient sample size. It is also noteworthy to mention that all these DMEK variants have only been performed in a single centre; therefore, the generalisability of this technique remains to be elucidated.

Descemetorrhexis

Studies showed that having a descemetorrhexis larger than the graft size (to avoid peripheral host DM-graft overlap) is associated with a lower risk of postoperative graft detachment [70]. In standard DMEK, descemetorrhexis is often performed manually using various types of DM scorers and strippers, which may sometimes lead to inconsistency in the size and shape of the descemetorrhexis, or incomplete tear/flap of the host DM at the periphery, which may interfere with the attachment of the DMEK graft.

In the past decade, femtosecond laser (FSL) has gained popularity in a number of ophthalmic surgical procedures, including cataract surgery [71, 72], refractive surgery [73], penetrating keratoplasty [74], DALK [75], pterygium surgery [76] and removal of conjunctival neoplasia [77]. Pilger et al. [78] previously explored the feasibility of FSL in performing descemetorrhexis and found that FSL was able to achieve highly consistent size and shape of descemetorrhexis. Recently, Sorkin et al. [79] reported the 5-year outcome of a novel FSL-assisted technique in performing descemetorrhexis in DMEK (known as F-DMEK). Comparing with the manual descemetorrhexis technique, F-DMEK was shown to result in substantially lower rates of graft detachment (33.3% vs. 6.3%)

and endothelial cell loss at 5 years (13.6% difference at 5 years). The low rate of graft detachment observed in FSL-assisted DMEK surgery is likely attributed to the precise sizing and cutting of the descemetorrhexis, which helps reduce the overlapping of the DMEK graft and host peripheral DM and minimise the area of denuded stroma uncovered by the DMEK graft (which can lead to bullous keratopathy) [70, 78, 79].

Use of Intraoperative Optical Coherence Tomography (iOCT)

The advent of optical coherence tomography (OCT) has significantly revolutionised the clinical diagnosis and management of many ophthalmic conditions [80, 81]. Recently, there has been an emerging interest of employing intraoperative OCT (iOCT) for assisting ophthalmic surgeries, including both anterior and posterior segments surgeries [82, 83]. Ehlers et al. [82] previously conducted the DISCOVER study examining the feasibility and utility of iOCT during ophthalmic surgeries. They demonstrated that iOCT was able to assist and augment the decision-making process during lamellar keratoplasty by ~40%. In addition, iOCT has been shown to be a useful tool in facilitating various steps during DMEK surgery, including graft preparation, orientation, graft–host apposition, and tissue interface fluid dynamics [84].

Based on our personal experience, we have found iOCT to be particularly useful in eyes with difficult view (secondary to significant corneal haze/oedema) as it facilitates the visualisation of the Descemet membrane during descemetorrhexis, graft unfolding and attachment (Fig. 29.4a–f) (Video 29.2), and the presence of any graft–host interface fluid (Fig. 29.5). Additional measure such as intraoperative retroillumination using a light pipe could also help improve the visualisation of the DMEK graft in eyes with difficult view.

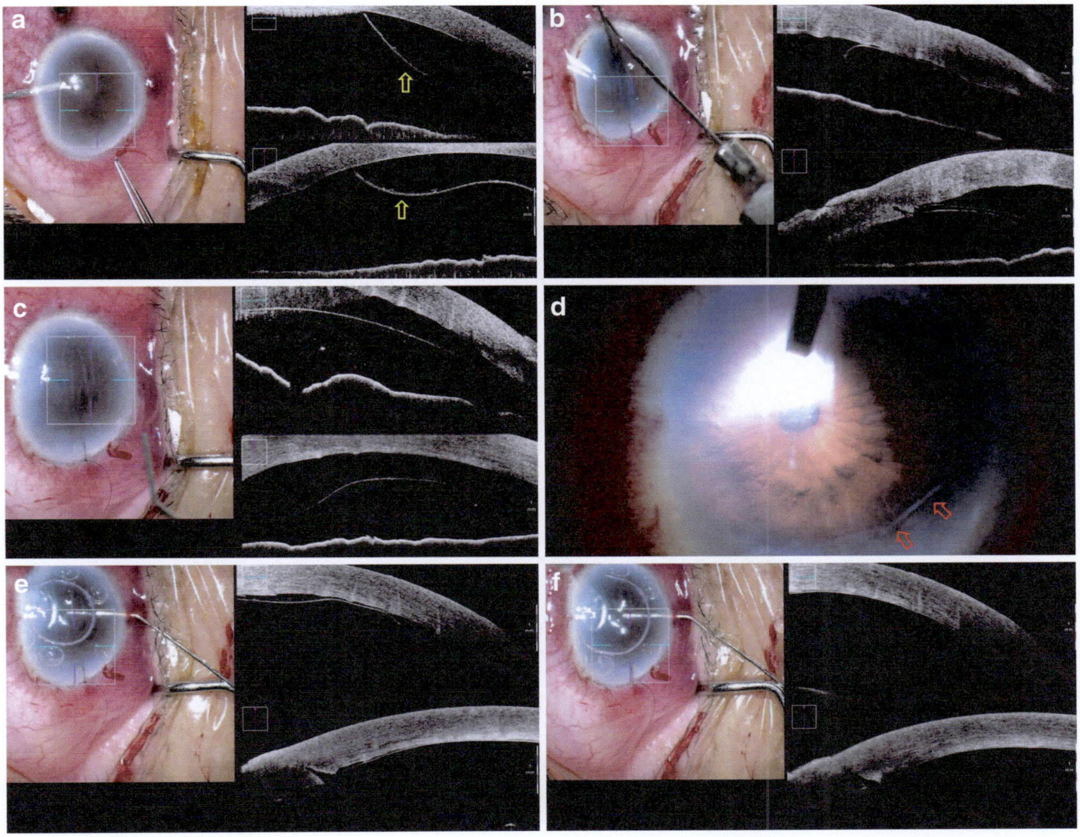

Fig. 29.4 The use of intraoperative optical coherence tomography (iOCT) in Descemet membrane endothelial keratoplasty in an eye with difficult view. (**a**) Visualisation of the Descemet membrane (DM; yellow arrows) during the descemetorrhexis. (**b**) Demonstration of DMEK graft in a tight scroll with endothelium-out. (**c**) Confirmation of a complete unfolding of the DMEK graft. (**d**) The use of an illuminating light pipe demonstrating the position of DMEK graft (the edge of graft is highlighted by the "red arrows"). (**e**, **f**) Intracameral injection of air/gas to achieve complete tamponade of the graft against the recipient's posterior cornea

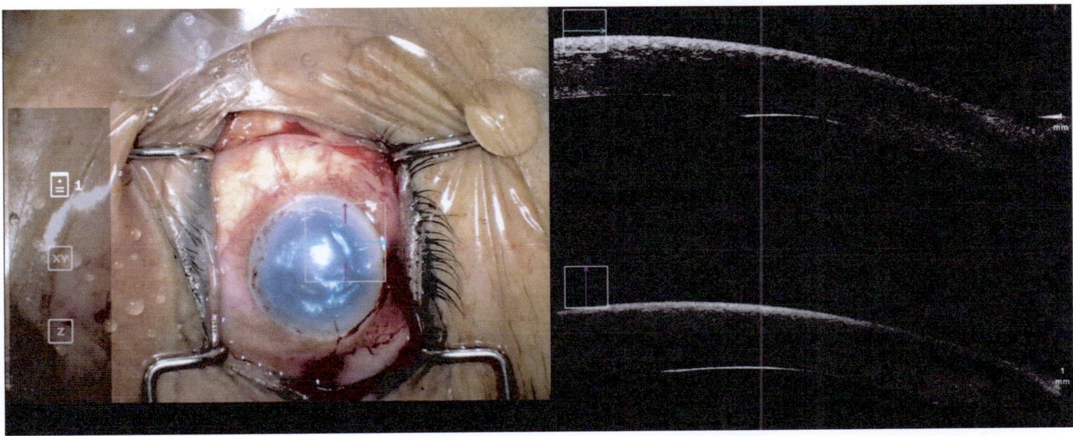

Fig. 29.5 The use of intraoperative optical coherence tomography (iOCT) in Descemet membrane endothelial keratoplasty in visualising the graft-host interface. The iOCT demonstrates an incomplete attachment of the DMEK graft to the recipient's corneal stroma. In view of this intraoperative finding, further manoeuvres such as tapping of the cornea and venting incision were performed to facilitate a complete attachment of the DMEK graft

Techniques in complex eyes or patients

In certain cases, DMEK techniques may require modifications or adjunctive steps in order to improve the outcomes or reduce potential complications. With the increasing experience in DMEK, many surgeons have started performing combined DMEK-cataract surgery (or "triple DMEK") in eyes with co-existing cataract and corneal endothelial disease. However, there has been concern that combined cataract surgery and DMEK may lead to increased risk of postoperative complications, particularly graft detachment requiring re-bubbling [23, 85, 86]. In a recent meta-analysis of 11,401 eyes, Tey et al. [87] demonstrated that staged DMEK-cataract surgery and combined DMEK-cataract surgery achieve similar clinical outcomes and safety, including corrected-distance-visual-acuity, postoperative re-bubbling rate, endothelial cell loss, graft failure and cystoid macular oedema. However, there are several scenarios that increase the complexity of combining DMEK with cataract surgery and/or anterior segment surgery:

Eyes with Angle Closure

Eyes with angle closure commonly seen in Asian eyes can pose considerable challenges to performing a successful DMEK [88, 89]. Angle closure eyes may have floppy iris, iris damage from previous iridotomy or iridoplasty, and high vitreous pressures—all of which can cause difficulty during graft insertion and unfolding. In view of these potential issues, Hayashi et al. [88] described an innovative preoperative strategy to increase the success of DMEK in Asian eyes with angle closure, using a combination of preoperative diuretic (e.g., mannitol or acetazolamide) and core vitrectomy (to reduce positive vitreous pressure). Comparing with the standard technique, a similar optimised DMEK technique for Asian eyes was shown to reduce the surgical time (by 7 min) and corneal endothelial cell loss at 6 months (by 14%) [89].

Eyes with Aphakia or Iris Defects

Performing DMEK in eyes with aphakia or significant iris defects can be particularly challenging during donor insertion, donor unfolding and achieving an effective air/gas tamponade. Recently, several innovative adjunctive techniques have been described to overcome this.

Safety-Net Suture

Berger et al. [90] recently described a low-cost, accessible "safety-net suture" method to create a temporary, partial barrier between the anterior and posterior chambers, which enables an effective air tamponade and reducing the risk of posterior graft dislocation in DMEK for eyes with aphakia and large iris defects. The safety-net suture is performed using a continuous 10–0 polypropylene suture placed across the anterior chamber in a cat's-cradle pattern anterior to the trabecular meshwork. The suture is left in placed during the air tamponade of the DMEK graft intraoperatively and is removed at the conclusion of the surgery after a period of air tamponade.

Phakic IOL Implantation

Shweikh et al. [91] described another inventive technique of using an implantable collamer phakic IOL (ICL) to temporarily create an anterior and posterior chamber to enable the DMEK in an aphakic eye with fixed and dilated pupil. In this technique, an ICL is inserted into the eye, unfolded over the iris and supported over the anterior chamber angle. The DMEK graft is then inserted into the anterior chamber and unfolded. The anterior chamber is then filled with 100% air for 5 min at a supraphysiological IOP. After 5 min of air tamponade, the air is partially removed and the anterior chamber is filled with cohesive viscoelastic, followed by removal of the ICL with a pair of forceps. The viscoelastic is gradually removed using low-pressure irrigation and aspiration with a Simcoe cannula, alternating with air injection to ensure attachment of the DMEK graft. The surgery is then concluded with an intracameral air injection to achieve a firm physiological IOP.

Artificial Iris Implantation

Customised artificial iris implant serves as a useful device in managing congenital and acquired iris defects [92]. Recently, Ang and Tan [93] described a staged anterior segment reconstruction technique to facilitate DMEK in complex eyes, including those with significant iris abnormalities [e.g., fixed-dilated pupil, significant peripheral anterior synechiae (PAS), and partial to near-total aniridia]. The surgery involves a 4-step approach, starting with synechiolysis of PAS and excision of iris remnants (to widen the anterior chamber angle), ensuring a stable and well-positioned posterior chamber IOL, and implantation of a CustomFlex Artificial Iris (CAI; HumanOptics, Erlangen, Germany). The CAI is first trephined to 1 mm less than the corneal white-to-white diameter. After inserting and unfolding the CAI in the anterior chamber, the edge of the CAI is secured to the anterior sclera via four pre-placed mattress sutures. Following the recovery from the initial anterior segment reconstruction (usually around 2 months), the DMEK is then performed.

Difficulty in Supine Posturing

Traditionally with EK, the patient is instructed to lie in a supine position during the immediate postoperative period to maximise the air tamponade of the graft against the posterior aspect of the host cornea [86, 94]. However, two recent studies [95, 96] have highlighted the possibility of achieving good DMEK graft attachment and outcomes without the need for supine posturing intraoperatively or postoperatively. These patients' eyes were filled with 99–100% air or SF6 gas intraoperatively, and an inferior PI is performed to reduce the risk of pupillary block. Clinically significant graft detachment (>30% area) was observed in only 4–22%, with 5–6% cases requiring regrafting due to primary graft failure or persistent graft detachment. Furthermore, one of the studies demonstrated a similar graft detachment rate when compared to a historical cohort of patients who underwent 48 h of postoperative supine posturing [96]. These findings suggest that patients who have difficulty in maintaining supine posturing can now benefit from the surgery. In addition, this will reduce patient's inconvenience (as it obviates the need for 48 h of postoperative supine posturing) and will place less demand on the limited hospital space and resources as the patients do not need to a hospital bed postoperatively to perform supine posturing.

Summary

Since its inception, various innovative modifications or adjunctive techniques have been described in an attempt to improve outcomes and reduce complications in DMEK. The development of various DMEK devices has facilitated both endothelium-out and endothelium-in donor insertion. In addition, eyes that were once thought to be less suitable, including those with angle closure or aphakia with iris defects can now undergo DMEK using modified surgical technique. Advances in imaging such as iOCT may be useful in enhancing intraoperative visualisation during graft unfolding and attachment during DMEK surgery, especially in eyes with advanced cornea decompensation. Finally, pre-stripped and preloaded DMEK donors prepared by eye banks may help to reduce intraoperative surgical time and lessen risk of donor preparation failure, which may improve uptake and practice of DMEK surgeries.

Take Home Notes

- Both endothelium-out and endothelium-in techniques serve as effective and safe DMEK techniques.
- Various recent innovations have helped refine the original DMEK technique, leading to better clinical outcome, improved graft survival rate, and lower risk of complications such as graft detachment and pupillary block.
- With suitable modifications to the original technique, DMEK can lead to good clinical outcomes in difficult eyes.
- Pre-stripped and pre-loaded DMEK graft has been shown to reduce intraoperative surgical

time and risk of graft harvesting failure, though long-term outcomes remain to be determined.

Funding/Support   None.

Conflict of Interest   None.

References

1. Park CY, Lee JK, Gore PK, Lim CY, Chuck RS. Keratoplasty in the United States: a 10-year review from 2005 through 2014. Ophthalmology. 2015;122(12):2432–42.
2. Tan DT, Dart JK, Holland EJ, Kinoshita S. Corneal transplantation. Lancet. 2012;379(9827):1749–61.
3. Soh YQ, Mehta JS. Regenerative therapy for Fuchs endothelial corneal dystrophy. Cornea. 2018;37(4):523–7.
4. Ting DS, Sau CY, Srinivasan S, Ramaesh K, Mantry S, Roberts F. Changing trends in keratoplasty in the west of scotland: a 10-year review. Br J Ophthalmol. 2012;96(3):405–8.
5. Ang M, Soh Y, Htoon HM, Mehta JS, Tan D. Five-year graft survival comparing Descemet stripping automated endothelial keratoplasty and penetrating keratoplasty. Ophthalmology. 2016;123(8):1646–52.
6. Ang M, Mehta JS, Lim F, Bose S, Htoon HM, Tan D. Endothelial cell loss and graft survival after Descemet's stripping automated endothelial kerato-plasty and penetrating keratoplasty. Ophthalmology. 2012;119(11):2239–44.
7. Ting DSJ, Deshmukh R, Ting DSW, Ang M. Big data in corneal diseases and cataract: Current applications and future directions. Front Big Data. 2023;6:1017420.
8. Ong HS, Ang M, Mehta J. Evolution of therapies for the corneal endothelium: past, present and future approaches. Br J Ophthalmol. 2021;105(4):454–67.
9. Ang M, Wilkins MR, Mehta JS, Tan D. Descemet membrane endothelial keratoplasty. Br J Ophthalmol. 2016;100(1):15–21.
10. Woo JH, Ang M, Htoon HM, Tan D. Descemet membrane endothelial keratoplasty versus Descemet stripping automated endothelial keratoplasty and penetrating keratoplasty. Am J Ophthalmol. 2019;207:288–303.
11. Ang M, Mehta JS, Anshu A, Wong HK, Htoon HM, Tan D. Endothelial cell counts after Descemet's stripping automated endothelial keratoplasty versus penetrating keratoplasty in Asian eyes. Clin Ophthalmol. 2012;6:537–44.
12. Bose S, Ang M, Mehta JS, Tan DT, Finkelstein E. Cost-effectiveness of Descemet's stripping endo-thelial keratoplasty versus penetrating keratoplasty. Ophthalmology. 2013;120(3):464–70.
13. Ang M, Saroj L, Htoon HM, Kiew S, Mehta JS, Tan D. Comparison of a donor insertion device to sheets glide in Descemet stripping endothelial keratoplasty: 3-year outcomes. Am J Ophthalmol. 2014;157(6):1163–9 e3.
14. Marques RE, Guerra PS, Sousa DC, Gonçalves AI, Quintas AM, Rodrigues W. DMEK versus DSAEK for Fuchs' endothelial dystrophy: a meta-analysis. Eur J Ophthalmol. 2019;29(1):15–22.
15. Ang M, Lim F, Htoon HM, Tan D, Mehta JS. Visual acuity and contrast sensitivity following Descemet stripping automated endothelial keratoplasty. Br J Ophthalmol. 2016;100(3):307–11.
16. Fuest M, Ang M, Htoon HM, Tan D, Mehta JS. Long-term visual outcomes comparing Descemet stripping automated endothelial keratoplasty and penetrating keratoplasty. Am J Ophthalmol. 2017;182:62–71.
17. Melles GRJ, Ong TS, Ververs B, van der Wees J. Descemet membrane endothelial keratoplasty (DMEK). Cornea. 2006;25(8):987–90.
18. Deng SX, Lee WB, Hammersmith KM, Kuo AN, Li JY, Shen JF, et al. Descemet membrane endo-thelial keratoplasty: safety and outcomes: a report by the American academy of ophthalmology. Ophthalmology. 2018;125(2):295–310.
19. Stuart AJ, Romano V, Virgili G, Shortt AJ. Descemet's membrane endothelial keratoplasty (DMEK) versus Descemet's stripping automated endothelial kera-toplasty (DSAEK) for corneal endothelial failure. Cochrane Database Syst Rev. 2018;6(6):CD012097.
20. Ang M, Sng CCA. Descemet membrane endothelial keratoplasty and glaucoma. Curr Opin Ophthalmol. 2018;29(2):178–84.
21. Heinzelmann S, Maier P, Böhringer D, Hüther S, Eberwein P, Reinhard T. Cystoid macular oedema fol-lowing Descemet membrane endothelial keratoplasty. Br J Ophthalmol. 2015;99(1):98–102.
22. Myerscough J, Roberts HW, Yu AC, Mimouni M, Furiosi L, Mandrioli M, et al. Factors predictive of cystoid macular oedema following endothelial kera-toplasty: a single-centre review of 2233 cases. Br J Ophthalmol. 2021;107(1):24–9.
23. Deshmukh R, Nair S, Ting DSJ, Agarwal T, Beltz J, Vajpayee RB. Graft detachments in endothelial kera-toplasty. Br J Ophthalmol. 2022;106(1):1–13.
24. Muraine M. Techniques for graft preparation in DMEK. Acta Ophthalmol. 2019;97:S263.
25. Solley KD, Berges A, Diaz C, Ostrander BT, Ding AS, Larson SA, et al. Evaluation of efficacy, efficiency, and cell viability of a novel Descemet membrane endothelial keratoplasty graft preparation device, DescePrep, in nondiabetic and diabetic human donor corneas. Cornea. 2022;41(4):505–11.
26. Bhogal M, Balda MS, Matter K, Allan BD. Global cell-by-cell evaluation of endothelial viability after two methods of graft preparation in Descemet mem-brane endothelial keratoplasty. Br J Ophthalmol. 2016;100(4):572–8.

27. Tan TE, Devarajan K, Seah XY, Lin SJ, Peh GSL, Cajucom-Uy HY, et al. Lamellar dissection technique for Descemet membrane endothelial keratoplasty graft preparation. Cornea. 2020;39(1):23–9.

28. McKee HD, Jhanji V. Femtosecond laser-assisted graft preparation for Descemet membrane endothelial keratoplasty. Cornea. 2018;37(10):1342–4.

29. Rodríguez-Calvo-de-Mora M, Quilendrino R, Ham L, Liarakos VS, van Dijk K, Baydoun L, et al. Clinical outcome of 500 consecutive cases undergoing Descemet's membrane endothelial keratoplasty. Ophthalmology. 2015;122(3):464–70.

30. Hayashi T, Yuda K, Oyakawa I, Kato N. Use of brilliant blue G in Descemet's membrane endothelial keratoplasty. Biomed Res Int. 2017;2017:9720389.

31. Maharana PK, Sahay P, Singhal D, Sharma N, Titiyal JS. Donor preparation in descemet membrane endothelial keratoplasty. New Front Ophthalmol. 2019;5:2–6.

32. Price MO, Giebel AW, Fairchild KM, Price FW Jr. Descemet's membrane endothelial keratoplasty: prospective multicenter study of visual and refractive outcomes and endothelial survival. Ophthalmology. 2009;116(12):2361–8.

33. Schlötzer-Schrehardt U, Bachmann BO, Tourtas T, Cursiefen C, Zenkel M, Rössler K, et al. Reproducibility of graft preparations in Descemet's membrane endothelial keratoplasty. Ophthalmology. 2013;120(9):1769–77.

34. Veldman PB, Dye PK, Holiman JD, Mayko ZM, Sáles CS, Straiko MD, et al. The S-stamp in Descemet membrane endothelial keratoplasty safely eliminates upside-down graft implantation. Ophthalmology. 2016;123(1):161–4.

35. Bardan AS, Goweida MB, El Goweini HF, Liu CS. Management of upside-down Descemet membrane endothelial keratoplasty: a case series. J Curr Ophthalmol. 2020;32(2):142–8.

36. Narayanan N, Dubey A. Resource maximization during COVID-19 crunch—a novel graft marking technique to use one cornea for two recipients for either Descemet membrane endothelial keratoplasty or deep anterior lamellar keratoplasty. Indian J Ophthalmol. 2022;70(3):1037–41.

37. Veldman PB, Dye PK, Holiman JD, Mayko ZM, Sáles CS, Straiko MD, et al. Stamping an S on DMEK donor tissue to prevent upside-down grafts: laboratory validation and detailed preparation technique description. Cornea. 2015;34(9):1175–8.

38. Or L, Krakauer Y, Sorkin N, Knyazer B, Ashkenazy Z, Gushansky K, et al. A novel marking technique for Descemet membrane endothelial graft using an ophthalmic viscoelastic device. Cornea. 2021;40(4):529–32.

39. Basak SK, Basak S. Marking DMEK grafts using bandage contact lens Interface technique: doubling the utilization during the acute shortage of donor corneas. Cornea. 2022;41(4):512–7.

40. Ang M, Moriyama A, Colby K, Sutton G, Liang L, Sharma N, et al. Corneal transplantation in the aftermath of the COVID-19 pandemic: an international perspective. Br J Ophthalmol. 2020;104(11):1477–81.

41. Parekh M, Romano V, Hassanin K, Testa V, Wongvisavavit R, Ferrari S, et al. Delivering endothelial keratoplasty grafts: modern day transplant devices. Curr Eye Res. 2022;47(4):493.

42. Chen C, Solar SJ, Lohmeier J, Terrin S, Baliga S, Wiener BG, et al. Viability of preloaded Descemet membrane endothelial keratoplasty grafts with 96-hour shipment. BMJ Open Ophthalmol. 2021;6(1):e000679.

43. Parekh M, Pedrotti E, Viola P, Leon P, Neri E, Bosio L, et al. Factors affecting the success rate of pre-loaded DMEK with endothelium-inwards technique: a multicentre clinical study. Am J Ophthalmol. 2022;241:272. https://doi.org/10.1016/j.ajo.2022.03.009.

44. Birbal RS, Ni Dhubhghaill S, Bourgonje VJA, Hanko J, Ham L, Jager MJ, et al. Five-year graft survival and clinical outcomes of 500 consecutive cases after Descemet membrane endothelial keratoplasty. Cornea. 2020;39(3):290–7.

45. Tan TE, Devarajan K, Seah XY, Lin SJ, Peh GSL, Cajucom-Uy HY, et al. Descemet membrane endothelial keratoplasty with a pull-through insertion device: surgical technique, endothelial cell loss, and early clinical results. Cornea. 2020;39(5):558–65.

46. Mohammed I, Ross AR, Britton JO, Said DG, Dua HS. Elastin content and distribution in endothelial keratoplasty tissue determines direction of scrolling. Am J Ophthalmol. 2018;194:16–25.

47. Bennett A, Mahmoud S, Drury D, Cavanagh HD, McCulley JP, Petroll WM, et al. Impact of donor age on corneal endothelium-Descemet membrane layer scroll formation. Eye Contact Lens. 2015;41(4):236–9.

48. Romano V, Kazaili A, Pagano L, Gadhvi KA, Titley M, Steger B, et al. Eye bank versus surgeon prepared DMEK tissues: influence on adhesion and re-bubbling rate. Br J Ophthalmol. 2022;106(2):177–83.

49. Kim EC, Bonfadini G, Todd L, Zhu A, Jun AS. Simple, inexpensive, and effective injector for descemet membrane endothelial keratoplasty. Cornea. 2014;33(6):649–52.

50. Arnalich-Montiel F, Muñoz-Negrete FJ, De Miguel MP. Double port injector device to reduce endothelial damage in DMEK. Eye (Lond). 2014;28(6):748–51.

51. Ang M, Mehta JS, Newman SD, Han SB, Chai J, Tan D. Descemet membrane endothelial keratoplasty: preliminary results of a donor insertion pull-through technique using a donor mat device. Am J Ophthalmol. 2016;171:27–34.

52. Shen E, Fox A, Johnson B, Farid M. Comparing the effect of three Descemet membrane endothelial keratoplasty injectors on endothelial damage of grafts. Indian J Ophthalmol. 2020;68(6):1040–3.

53. Droutsas K, Lazaridis A, Kymionis GD, Chatzistefanou K, Moschos MM, Koutsandrea C, et al. Comparison of endothelial cell loss and complications following DMEK with the use

of three different graft injectors. Eye (Lond). 2018;32(1):19–25.

54. Vasquez-Perez A, Phylactou M, Din N, Liu C. "The spinning technique" for unfolding tightly scrolled DMEK grafts. Cornea. 2022;41(1):130–4.

55. Liarakos VS, Dapena I, Ham L, van Dijk K, Melles GR. Intraocular graft unfolding techniques in descemet membrane endothelial keratoplasty. JAMA Ophthalmol. 2013;131(1):29–35.

56. Hayashi T, Kobayashi A. Double-bubble technique in Descemet membrane endothelial keratoplasty for vitrectomized eyes: a case series. Cornea. 2018;37(9):1185–8.

57. Parker JS, Parker JS, Melles GRJ. "Double-bubble" Descemet membrane endothelial keratoplasty unfolding in eyes with deep anterior chambers and anterior chamber intraocular lenses. Cornea. 2020;39(7):919–23.

58. Saad A, Awwad ST, El Salloukh NA, Panthier C, Bashur Z, Gatinel D. C-press technique to facilitate Descemet membrane endothelial keratoplasty surgery in vitrectomized patients: a case series. Cornea. 2019;38(9):1198–201.

59. Kobayashi A, Yokogawa H, Mori N, Masaki T, Sugiyama K. Development of a donor tissue holding technique for Descemet's membrane endothelial keratoplasty using a 25-gauge graft manipulator. Case Rep Ophthalmol. 2018;9(3):431–8.

60. Sorkin N, Einan-Lifshitz A, Ashkenazy Z, Boutin T, Showail M, Borovik A, et al. Enhancing Descemet membrane endothelial keratoplasty in postvitrectomy eyes with the use of pars plana infusion. Cornea. 2017;36(3):280–3.

61. Busin M, Leon P, D'Angelo S, Ruzza A, Ferrari S, Ponzin D, et al. Clinical outcomes of preloaded Descemet membrane endothelial keratoplasty grafts with endothelium tri-folded inwards. Am J Ophthalmol. 2018;193:106–13.

62. Woo JH, Htoon HM, Tan D. Hybrid Descemet membrane endothelial keratoplasty (H-DMEK): results of a donor insertion pull-through technique using donor stroma as carrier. Br J Ophthalmol. 2020;104(10):1358–62.

63. Gain P, Jullienne R, He Z, Aldossary M, Acquart S, Cognasse F, et al. Global survey of corneal transplantation and eye banking. JAMA Ophthalmol. 2016;134(2):167–73.

64. Gupta N, Vashist P, Ganger A, Tandon R, Gupta SK. Eye donation and eye banking in India. Natl Med J India. 2018;31(5):283–6.

65. Ting DS, Potts J, Jones M, Lawther T, Armitage WJ, Figueiredo FC. Changing trend in the utilisation rate of donated corneas for keratoplasty in the UK: the North East England study. Eye (Lond). 2016;30(11):1475–80.

66. Ting DS, Potts J, Jones M, Lawther T, Armitage WJ, Figueiredo FC. Impact of telephone consent and potential for eye donation in the UK: the newcastle eye centre study. Eye (Lond). 2016;30(3):342–8.

67. Birbal RS, Hsien S, Zygoura V, Parker JS, Ham L, van Dijk K, et al. Outcomes of hemi-Descemet membrane endothelial keratoplasty for Fuchs endothelial corneal dystrophy. Cornea. 2018;37(7):854–8.

68. Birbal RS, Ni Dhubhghaill S, Baydoun L, Ham L, Bourgonje VJA, Dapena I, et al. Quarter-Descemet membrane endothelial keratoplasty: one- to two-year clinical outcomes. Cornea. 2020;39(3):277–82.

69. Oganesyan O, Makarov P, Grdikanyan A, Oganesyan C, Getadaryan V, Melles GRJ. Three-quarter DMEK in eyes with glaucoma draining devices to avoid secondary graft failure. Acta Ophthalmol. 2021;99(5):569–74.

70. Tourtas T, Schlomberg J, Wessel JM, Bachmann BO, Schlötzer-Schrehardt U, Kruse FE. Graft adhesion in descemet membrane endothelial keratoplasty dependent on size of removal of host's descemet membrane. JAMA Ophthalmol. 2014;132(2):155–61.

71. Schweitzer C, Brezin A, Cochener B, Monnet D, Germain C, Roseng S, et al. Femtosecond laser-assisted versus phacoemulsification cataract surgery (FEMCAT): a multicentre participant-masked randomised superiority and cost-effectiveness trial. Lancet. 2020;395(10219):212–24.

72. Liu YC, Setiawan M, Chin JY, Wu B, Ong HS, Lamoureux E, et al. Randomized controlled trial comparing 1-year outcomes of low-energy femtosecond laser-assisted cataract surgery versus conventional phacoemulsification. Front Med (Lausanne). 2021;8:811093.

73. Ang M, Farook M, Htoon HM, Mehta JS. Randomized clinical trial comparing femtosecond LASIK and small-incision lenticule extraction. Ophthalmology. 2020;127(6):724–30.

74. Wade M, Muniz Castro H, Garg S, Kedhar S, Aggarwal S, Shumway C, et al. Long-term results of femtosecond laser-enabled keratoplasty with zig-zag trephination. Cornea. 2019;38(1):42–9.

75. Gerten G, Oberheide U, Thiée P. Clear cornea femto DALK: a novel technique for performing deep anterior lamellar keratoplasty. Graefes Arch Clin Exp Ophthalmol. 2022;260(9):2941–8.

76. Ting DSJ, Liu YC, Lee YF, Ji AJS, Tan TE, Htoon HM, et al. Cosmetic outcome of femtosecond laser-assisted pterygium surgery. Eye Vis (Lond). 2021;8(1):7.

77. Dimacali VG, Liu YC, Ong HS, Ting DSJ, Mehta JS. Femtosecond laser-assisted excision of conjunctival melanocytic lesions: cosmetic and long-term outcomes. Clin Exp Ophthalmol. 2021;49(3):312–5.

78. Pilger D, von Sonnleithner C, Bertelmann E, Joussen AM, Torun N. Femtosecond laser-assisted Descemetorhexis: a novel technique in Descemet membrane endothelial keratoplasty. Cornea. 2016;35(10):1274–8.

79. Sorkin N, Gouvea L, Din N, Mimouni M, Alshaker S, Weill Y, et al. Five-year safety and efficacy of femtosecond laser-assisted Descemet membrane endothelial keratoplasty. Cornea. 2022;42:145. https://doi.org/10.1097/ICO.0000000000003019.

80. Huang D, Swanson EA, Lin CP, Schuman JS, Stinson WG, Chang W, et al. Optical coherence tomography. Science. 1991;254(5035):1178–81.
81. Ang M, Ting DSJ, Sng CCA, Schmetterer L. Anterior segment OCT: angiography. In: Alió JL, Alio del Barrio JL, editors. Atlas of anterior segment optical coherence tomography essentials in ophthalmology. Cham: Springer; 2021. p. 159–69.
82. Ehlers JP, Goshe J, Dupps WJ, Kaiser PK, Singh RP, Gans R, et al. Determination of feasibility and utility of microscope-integrated optical coherence tomography during ophthalmic surgery: the DISCOVER study RESCAN results. JAMA Ophthalmol. 2015;133(10):1124–32.
83. Ang M, Baskaran M, Werkmeister RM, Chua J, Schmidl D, Aranha Dos Santos V, et al. Anterior segment optical coherence tomography. Prog Retin Eye Res. 2018;66:132–56.
84. Cost B, Goshe JM, Srivastava S, Ehlers JP. Intraoperative optical coherence tomography-assisted descemet membrane endothelial keratoplasty in the DISCOVER study. Am J Ophthalmol. 2015;160(3):430–7.
85. Röck D, Bartz-Schmidt KU, Röck T, Yoeruek E. Air bubble-induced high intraocular pressure after Descemet membrane endothelial keratoplasty. Cornea. 2016;35(8):1035–9.
86. Leon P, Parekh M, Nahum Y, Mimouni M, Giannaccare G, Sapigni L, et al. Factors associated with early graft detachment in primary Descemet membrane endothelial keratoplasty. Am J Ophthalmol. 2018;187:117–24.
87. Tey KY, Tan SY, Ting DSJ, Mehta JS, Ang M. Effects of combined cataract surgery on outcomes of Descemet's membrane endothelial keratoplasty: a systematic review and meta-analysis. Front Med. 2022;9:857200.
88. Hayashi T, Oyakawa I, Kato N. Techniques for learning Descemet membrane endothelial keratoplasty for eyes of Asian patients with shallow anterior chamber. Cornea. 2017;36(3):390–3.
89. Ang M, Ting DSJ, Kumar A, May KO, Htoon HM, Mehta JS. Descemet membrane endothelial keratoplasty in Asian eyes: intraoperative and postoperative complications. Cornea. 2020;39(8):940–5.
90. Berger O, Kriman J, Vasquez-Perez A, Allan BD. Safety-net suture for Aphakic Descemet membrane endothelial keratoplasty. Cornea. 2022;41(6):789–91.
91. Shweikh Y, Vasquez-Perez A, Allan BD. Phakic intraocular lens as a temporary barrier in aphakic Descemet's membrane endothelial keratoplasty. Eur J Ophthalmol. 2019;29(5):566–70.
92. Srinivasan S, Ting DS, Snyder ME, Prasad S, Koch HR. Prosthetic iris devices. Can J Ophthalmol. 2014;49(1):6–17.
93. Ang M, Tan D. Anterior segment reconstruction with artificial iris and Descemet membrane endothelial keratoplasty: a staged surgical approach. Br J Ophthalmol. 2022;106(7):908–13.
94. Marques RE, Guerra PS, Sousa DC, Ferreira NP, Gonçalves AI, Quintas AM, et al. Sulfur hexafluoride 20% versus air 100% for anterior chamber tamponade in DMEK: a meta-analysis. Cornea. 2018;37(6):691–7.
95. Roberts HW, Kit V, Phylactou M, Din N, Wilkins MR. 'Posture-less' DMEK: is posturing after Descemet membrane endothelial keratoplasty actually necessary? Am J Ophthalmol. 2022;240:23–9.
96. Parker JS, Parker JS, Tate H, Melles GRJ. DMEK without postoperative supine posturing. Cornea. 2022;42:32. https://doi.org/10.1097/ICO.0000000000003000.

Maryam Eslami and Greg Moloney

Key Points

- The history of the Descemet stripping-only procedure is outlined in this chapter.
- The suspected mechanism of corneal clearance and the role of Rho Kinase inhibitors in this procedure is explained.
- The importance of patient selection and other predictors of successful outcomes are described in detail.
- Surgical steps for a successful corneal clearance are summarized, and common pitfalls are highlighted.

Fuchs' endothelial corneal dystrophy (FECD) is the most common posterior corneal dystrophy [1]. It is characterized by progressive endothelial cell loss and Descemet membrane (DM) excrescences called guttae, which may lead to gradual and fluctuating decreased vision and contrast

sensitivity [2]. In the late stages, vision loss becomes constant as corneal oedema worsens, and the patient may experience intermittent pain from ruptured bullae and epithelial defects [2].

Prior to the advent of endothelial keratoplasty (EK), penetrating keratoplasty (PK) was the only surgical option to treat FECD [3]. With the refinement of the surgical technique in the preparation of both the host and donor cornea in the past two decades, EK has become the gold standard surgical treatment of FECD and has outnumbered PK in the United States since 2012 [3]. The two commonly utilized techniques of EK are Descemet stripping automated endothelial keratoplasty (DSAEK) and Descemet membrane endothelial keratoplasty (DMEK).

Posterior lamellar keratoplasty was first performed by Tillett in 1956 using lamellar posterior dissection and suture fixation of donor cornea to the recipient [4]. Melles et al. outlined the posterior surgical approach to EK in 1998 [5] and further refined it in 2004 [6] using descemetorhexis to prepare the host cornea. Additional surgical

Supplementary Information The online version contains supplementary material available at https://doi.org/10.1007/978-3-031-32408-6_30.

M. Eslami
Ophthalmology and Visual Sciences, University of British Columbia, Vancouver, BC, Canada
e-mail: maryam.eslami@alumni.ubc.ca

G. Moloney (✉)
University of British Columbia,
Vancouver, BC, Canada

Sydney Eye Hospital, Sydney University,
Sydney, Australia

advancements, including the use of an automated microkeratome to prepare donor lenticule [6], gave rise to the DSAEK technique utilized today. In 2006, Melles et al. introduced DMEK, which, unlike DSAEK, involved selective transplantation of donor DM and endothelial layer only [7]. In both techniques, the donor cornea is approximated to the host stroma using air or gas bubbles [8].

The most common early postoperative complication of DSAEK and DMEK is partial or complete graft detachment [8]. Interestingly, multiple cases were reported on spontaneous clearance of cornea and repopulation of endothelial cells following complete graft detachment [9–16]. Additionally, multiple authors noted similar findings after inadvertent central descemetorhexis during cataract surgery [16, 17]. These findings prompted experimentation with descemetorhexis only as the primary intervention for corneal endothelial disease. This technique was first proposed as an intervention decades earlier by Paufique, who described this surgery, with accompanying illustration in 1955 [18]. The first modern case report of intentional stripping without graft placement was in 2012. Shah et al. reported on the intentional Descemet stripping procedure after the fellow eye's "unusual pattern of healing" following DSAEK graft detachment [19]. In 2013, Bleyen et al. reported on 8 eyes with phacoemulsification combined with 8 mm DSO [20]. They observed some corneal clearing in 3/8 eyes with 7/8 eyes requiring grafting within 18 months [20]. Subsequently, Arbelaez et al. tried smaller 6–6.5 mm DSOs in 3 eyes but with variable and disappointing results [21].

In a report of a successful corneal clearance on 2/2 eyes using a 4 mm descemetorhexis in 2015, Moloney et al. emphasized the importance of patient selection, hypothesized higher success with smaller descemetorhexis and recommended the procedure for patients with dense central guttae but adequate peripheral endothelial reserve [16]. Borkar et al. [21], Malyugin et al. [22] and Iovieno et al. [23] also reported a higher success rate at clearing cornea using 4 mm descemetorhexis. However, the variability of response rate and time to resolution remained a challenge in all reported studies. Iovieno et al. also remarked on the induced postoperative astigmatism from posterior elevation in the patients who achieved complete corneal clarity; these results were possibly affected by posterior stromal trauma, the significance of which has become better understood over time [23].

Early in this surgical journey, the mechanism of spontaneous corneal clearance after DMEK/DSAEK graft detachment was debated [24]. Some authors hypothesized that the repopulation of endothelial cells is a result of the migration of transplanted donor endothelial cells from the attached donor–host area in a partially detached graft or from the anterior chamber in a completely detached graft [25]. This procedure was therefore named DMET, Descemet membrane endothelial transfer. However, it is now believed that the repopulated endothelial cells originate from the stimulated host endothelium [24, 26, 27]. Prior studies have shown that endothelial cells have mitotic regeneration capabilities in vitro, which are arrested in vivo in the G1 phase of the cell cycle [3, 28]. This mitotic quiescence is thought to be secondary to TGF-β inhibition in aqueous humour, lack of effective growth factor stimulation and cell–cell contact inhibition [28]. It is hypothesized that the loss of cell–cell contact inhibition in DSO promotes peripheral endothelial cells to migrate and possibly proliferate in the denuded area of descemetorhexis [24, 27]. A study of cell counts over time demonstrating a reduction in overall counts post-DSO would suggest that without additive stimulation of mitosis, corneas achieve clearance post-DSO primarily via migration of existing cells [29]. This hypothesis along with other medical treatments for in-vivo reactivation of regenerative capabilities of endothelial cells is currently the subject of intense research. Notable among these is the use of Rho-Kinase (ROCK) inhibitors in corneal endothelial disease.

ROCK is a serine/threonine protein kinase with two isoforms, ROCK1 and ROCK2, that phosphorylate several targets with multiple downstream cellular effects but primarily result in alteration of the internal cell cytoskeleton [30, 31]. This results in altered cellular adhesion, membrane permeability, motility, proliferation, differentiation, apoptosis and extracellular matrix dynamics [30, 31]. In ophthalmology, two ROCK inhibitors, netarsudil and ripasudil, are under investigation for their potential use in lowering intraocular pressure in glaucoma, intravitreal injection for diabetic retinopathy and endothelial wound healing in cornea [30]. Ripasudil 0.4% (Glanatec; Kowa Co. Ltd., Tokyo, Japan) was approved in Japan in 2014 for glaucoma [32]. Netarsudil 0.02% is a ROCK inhibitor with added norepinephrine transport inhibition, marketed as Rhopressa (Aerie Pharmaceuticals, Bedminster, NJ), which was approved by the United States Food and Drug Administration in 2017 for similar indication [33]. Currently, their use in corneal endothelial disease is considered off-label.

ROCK inhibitors promote corneal wound healing through three mechanisms: inhibiting apoptosis, promoting migration and increasing intercellular adhesions [30]. Stimulation of proliferation is also postulated. Extensive work done by Okumura, Kinoshita and Koizumi et al. in this area has demonstrated a high safety profile and has shown promise in an array of corneal endothelial cell diseases including FECD [34–38].

Moloney et al. were the first to use ROCK inhibitors as a salvage treatment for non-clearing corneas after DSO [39]. They reported rapid and complete clearance of residual corneal edema within 2 weeks from initiation of ripasudil in 3 eyes that failed to clear initially. In a comparative study of patients undergoing DSO with or without ripasudil, Macsai and Shiloch report higher endothelial cell count and faster resolution of symptoms and visual rehabilitation in the group treated with ROCK inhibitors [40]. In a recent systematic review and meta-analysis in 2021 including 127 eyes, the overall rate of DSO failure was reported at 17% [41]. This figure included patients with or without ROCK inhibitors and all descemetorhexis sizes and decreased to 4% with a descemetorhexis size of 4 mm. In their study published in 2020, Moloney et al. reported a similar failure rate of 4.3% (1/23) and an average resolution time of 4.1 weeks in their cohort of 23 patients who were all treated with 4 mm descemetorhexis and started on ripasudil from the first

postoperative day [42]. They also reported the best spectacle-corrected visual acuity gain of 0.16 LogMAR post-DSO that was statistically significant [42].

The true impact of DSO on visual acuity and refractive change is currently unclear in the literature owing to some reports being combined with cataract surgery confounding the results. The systematic review and meta-analysis mentioned above found statistically significant improvement in visual acuity in both DSO only and DSO combined with cataract surgery [41]. Some authors have postulated that the observed induced posterior astigmatism mentioned earlier may be due to stromal fibrosis resulting from stromal scoring intraoperatively [43]. Interestingly, in their 5-year follow-up report, Iovieno et al. observed an improvement in their previously reported posterior stromal opacities and irregular astigmatism [44]. In a comparative cohort study of DSO versus DMEK, Huang et al. reported similar visual outcomes in mild to moderate FECD with a higher rate of adverse events in the DMEK group [45]. However, similar to other studies of DSO, the authors emphasized the importance of patient selection to achieve their reported outcomes.

Due to its reliance on an existing cell population to migrate, Descemet stripping only is not suitable in cases of pseudophakic bullous keratopathy or other endothelial cell diseases with a more diffuse endotheliopathy as reported by multiple authors [3, 25, 34]. However, it can be considered the primary procedure of choice for FECD in isolation or in combination with cataract surgery in patients with more central guttata affecting visual acuity who have a higher endothelial cell reserve peripherally. For instance, Moloney et al. only included patients with a superior cell density of 1000 or higher in their study mentioned above [42]. However, no correlation has yet been found between peripheral cell count and the rate or speed of corneal clearance. Age was also not a contributing factor in patient selection [39, 46]. Nevertheless, the healing response was reported to be strikingly similar between the two eyes of the same patient, implying that there are patient factors beyond age and cell count that are yet to be uncovered [43, 46].

Local aqueous factors or underlying patient genetics arise as areas of future study.

On the other hand, the surgical technique and the size of descemetorhexis were found to be important factors [42, 43, 46]. Davies et al. reported 3 surgical techniques to remove the central 4 mm Descemet membrane in their cohort of 17 eyes [46]. They had 3 eyes that failed to clear; in all 3 eyes, the Descemet membrane was removed using a reverse Sinskey hook to score the posterior cornea 360° followed by Descemet membrane stripping. The remainder of the eyes that successfully cleared within 3 months had their Descemet membrane removed with only 2 clock hours scored or with a descemetorhexis technique instead [46]. The scoring may also lead to posterior stromal scarring, even in cases that did clear eventually [43, 46]. This abnormal healing response may even result in posterior stromal nodules, as illustrated by Garcerant et al. [43]. There is also evidence that endothelial cell migration is improved if the endothelial layer alone is stripped, leaving the Descemet membrane behind [38]. These findings suggest that bare or roughened stroma may not be the most suitable bed for endothelial cell migration, and care must be taken to leave the stroma undisturbed intraoperatively [43]. Figures 30.1 and 30.2 demonstrate the corneal clarity and expected descemetorhexis appearance at postoperative year 2.

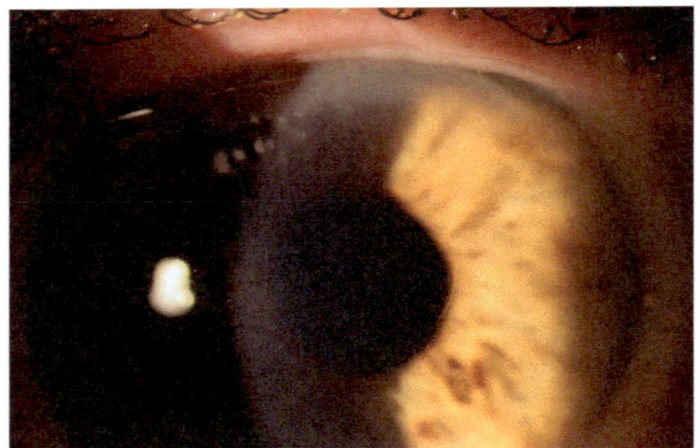

Fig. 30.2 16x magnification slit lamp image of DSO at year 2

To this end, Garcerant et al. outline their proposed surgical technique; after creating a 2 mm wound and instillation of cohesive viscoelastic, they propose creating a small Descemet membrane tag via small side-to-side movements using a reverse Sinskey at the edge of the 4 mm central circle. This tag can then be peeled in a circular fashion using grasping forceps [43]. Care is advised not to leave any Descemet tags behind. This technique is highlighted by the supplemental Video 30.1 attached.

In summary, DSO is a safe and effective intervention in the treatment of select cases of FECD, especially if supplemented with ripasudil or possibly other ROCKi. It is more accessible, quicker, and easier to perform than alternatives such as DMEK, which requires a donor graft placement. Careful patient selection is key to success, as highlighted in this review. The long-term outcomes of this operation still must be reported to ensure that this is a viable surgical option for patients in the medium to long term.

Take Home Notes
- DSO is slowly transitioning from an experimental procedure to an acceptable surgical option for select patients with Fuchs' Dystrophy.
- It remains suitable only for patients with central guttae but adequate peripheral endothelial reserve.
- Surgical factors of importance include limiting the size of the descemetorhexis to 4.5 mm

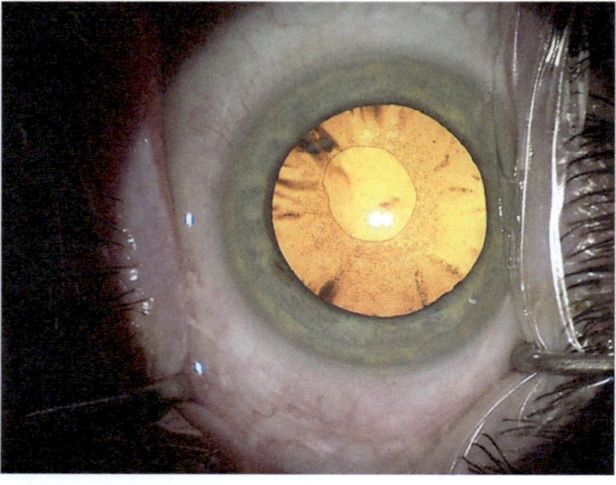

Fig. 30.1 Intraoperative view of DSO at year 2, return to theatre for phacoemulsification

or less and avoiding stromal injury with a peeling technique.

- A failure rate still exists with conversion to DMEK required in some patients, but success rates are improved with emerging supplemental medical therapies.

References

1. Franceschino A, Dutheil F, Pereira B, Watson S, Chiambaretta F, Navel V. Descemetorhexis without endothelial keratoplasty in Fuchs endothelial corneal dystrophy. Cornea. 2021;41(7):815.
2. Elhalis H, Azizi B, Jurkunas UV. Fuchs endothelial corneal dystrophy. Ocul Surf. 2010;8(4):173–84. https://doi.org/10.1016/s1542-0124(12)70232-x.
3. Blitzer AL, Colby KA. Update on the surgical management of Fuchs endothelial corneal dystrophy. Ophthalmol Ther. 2020;9:757–65.
4. Melles GR, Eggink FA, Lander F, Pels E, Rietveld FJ, Beekhuis WH, et al. A surgical technique for posterior lamellar keratoplasty. Cornea. 1998;17:618–26.
5. Melles GR, Wijdh RH, Nieuwendaal CP. A technique to excise the descemet membrane from a recipient cornea (descemetorhexis). Cornea. 2004;23:286–8.
6. Gorovoy MS. Descemet-stripping automated endothelial keratoplasty. Cornea. 2006;25:886–9.
7. Melles GRJ, Ong TS, Ververs B, van der Wees J. Descemet membrane endothelial keratoplasty (DMEK). Cornea. 2006;25:987–90.
8. Price MO, Gupta P, Lass J, Price FW. EK (DLEK, DSEK, DMEK): new frontier in cornea surgery. Annu Rev Vis Sci. 2017;3:69–90.
9. Watson SL, Abiad G, Coroneo MT. Spontaneous resolution of corneal oedema following Descemet's detachment. Clin Experiment Ophthalmol. 2006;34:797–9.
10. Balachandran C, Ham L, Verschoor CA, et al. Spontaneous corneal clearance despite graft detachment in Descemet membrane endothelial keratoplasty. Am J Ophthalmol. 2009;148:227–34.
11. Zafirakis P, Kymionis GD, Grentzelos MA, et al. Corneal graft detachment without corneal edema after Descemet stripping automated endothelial keratoplasty. Cornea. 2010;29:456–8.
12. Ziaei M, Barsam A, Mearza AA. Spontaneous corneal clearance despite graft removal in Descemet stripping endothelial keratoplasty in Fuchs endothelial dystrophy. Cornea. 2013;32:e164–6.
13. Braunstein RE, Airiani S, Chang MA, et al. Corneal edema resolution after "descemetorhexis". J Cataract Refract Surg. 2003;29:1436–9.
14. Patel DV, Phang KL, Grupcheva CN, et al. Surgical detachment of Descemet's membrane and endothelium imaged over time by in vivo confocal microscopy. Clin Experiment Ophthalmol. 2004;32:539–42.
15. Choo SY, Zahidin AZ, Then KY. Re: spontaneous corneal clearance despite graft detachment in Descemet endothelial keratoplasty. Am J Ophthamol. 2010;149:531.
16. Moloney G, Chan UT, Hamilton A, et al. Descemetorhexis for Fuchs' dystrophy. Can J Ophthalmol. 2015;50:68–72.
17. Pan JC, Au Eong KG. Spontaneous resolution of corneal oedema after inadvertent "descemetorhexis" during cataract surgery. Clin Experiment Ophthalmol. 2006;34:896–7.
18. Paufique. Lamellar keratoplasty. In: Rycroft BW, editor. Corneal grafts. London: Butterworth and Co; 1955. p. 132–3.
19. Shah RD, Randleman JB, Grossniklaus HE. Spontaneous corneal clearing after Descemet's stripping without endothelial replacement. Ophthalmology. 2012;119:256–60.
20. Bleyen I, Saelens I, Van Dooren B, et al. Spontaneous corneal clearing after Descemet's stripping. Ophthalmology. 2013;120:215.
21. Borkar DS, Veldman P, Colby KA. Treatment of Fuchs endothelial dystrophy by descemet stripping without endothelial keratoplasty. Cornea. 2016;35:1267–73.
22. Malyugin BE, Izmaylova SB, Malyutina EA, et al. Clinical and functional results of one-step phaco surgery and central descemetorhexis for cataract and Fuchs primary endothelial corneal dystrophy. Vestn Oftalmol. 2017;133:16–22.
23. Iovieno A, Neri A, Soldani AM, et al. Descemetorhexis without graft placement for the treatment of Fuchs endothelial dystrophy: preliminary results and review of the literature. Cornea. 2017;36:637–41.
24. Dirisamer M, Yeh RY, van Dijk K, et al. Recipient endothelium mayrelate to corneal clearance in Descemet membrane endothelial transfer. Am J Ophthalmol. 2012;154:290–6.
25. Dirisamer M, Ham L, Dapena I, et al. Descemet membrane endothelial transfer: "free-floating" donor Descemet implantation as a potential alternative to "keratoplasty". Cornea. 2012;31:194–7.
26. Birbal R, Parker J, Dirisamer M, et al. Descemet membrane endothelial transfer: ultimate outcome. Cornea. 2018;37(2):141–4. https://doi.org/10.1097/ICO.0000000000001395.
27. Anitha V, Swarup R, Ravindran M. Descemet membrane endothelial transfer (DMET) in pseudophakic bullous keratopathy after DSEK—a case report and review of literature. Cornea. 2002;41:1179. https://doi.org/10.1097/ICO.0000000000002942; Publish Ahead of Print.
28. Joyce NC, Harris DL, Mello DM. Mechanisms of mitotic inhibition in corneal endothelium: contact inhibition and TGF-beta2. Invest Ophthalmol Vis Sci. 2002;43:2152–9.
29. Artaechevarria Artieda J, Wells M, Devasahayam RN, Moloney G. 5-year outcomes of Descemet stripping

only in Fuchs dystrophy. Cornea. 2020;39(8):1048–51. https://doi.org/10.1097/ICO.0000000000002270.

30. Syed ZA, Rapuano CJ. Rho kinase (ROCK) inhibitors in the management of corneal endothelial disease. Curr Opin Ophthalmol. 2021;32:268–74.

31. Meekins LC, Rosado-Adames N, Maddala R, Zhao JJ, Rao PV, Afshari NA. Corneal endothelial cell migration and proliferation enhanced by rho kinase (ROCK) inhibitors in in vitro and in vivo models. Invest Ophthalmol Vis Sci. 2016;57(15):6731–8. https://doi.org/10.1167/iovs.16-20414.

32. Garnock-Jones KP. Ripasudil: first global approval. Drugs. 2014;74:2211–5.

33. Hoy SM. Netarsudil ophthalmic solution 0.02%: first global approval. Drugs. 2018;78:389–96.

34. Okumura N, Koizumi N, Kay EP, et al. The ROCK inhibitor eye drop accelerates corneal endothelium wound healing. Invest Ophthalmol Vis Sci. 2013;54(4):2493–502.

35. Okumura N, Inoue R, Okazaki Y, et al. Effect of the rho kinase inhibitor Y-27632 on corneal endothelial wound healing. Invest Ophthalmol Vis Sci. 2015;56(10):6067–74.

36. Okumura N, Okazaki Y, Inoue R, et al. Effect of the Rhoassociated kinase inhibitor eye drop (ripasudil) on corneal endothelial wound healing. Invest Ophthalmol Vis Sci. 2016;57(3):1284–92.

37. Koizumi N, Okumura N, Ueno M, Nakagawa H, Hamuro J, Kinoshita S. Rho-associated kinase inhibitor eye drop treatment as a possible medical treatment for Fuchs corneal dystrophy. Cornea. 2013;32(8):1167–70.

38. Okumura N, Matsumoto D, Fukui Y, et al. Feasibility of cell-based therapy combined with descemetorhexis

for treating Fuchs endothelial corneal dystrophy in rabbit model. PloS One. 2018;13:e0191306.

39. Moloney G, Petsoglou C, Ball M, et al. Descemetorhexis without grafting for Fuchs endothelial dystrophy—supplementation with topical ripasudil. Cornea. 2017;36:642–8.

40. Macsai MS, Shiloach M. Use of topical rho kinase inhibitors in the treatment of Fuchs dystrophy after Descemet stripping only. Cornea. 2019;38:529–34.

41. Franceschino A, Dutheil F, Pereira B, Watson SL, Chiambaretta F, Navel V. Descemetorhexis without endothelial keratoplasty in Fuchs endothelial corneal dystrophy: a systematic review and meta-analysis. Cornea. 2021;41(7):815; Publish Ahead of Print.

42. Moloney G, Garcerant Congote D, Hirnschall N, et al. Descemet stripping only supplemented with topical ripasudil for Fuchs endothelial dystrophy 12-month outcomes of the sydney eye hospital study. Cornea. 2020;2021(40):320–6.

43. Garcerant D, Hirnschall N, Toalster N, Zhu M, Wen L, Moloney G. Descemet's stripping without endothelial keratoplasty. Curr Opin Ophthalmol. 2019;30:275–85.

44. Iovieno A, Moramarco A, Fontana L. Descemet stripping only in Fuchs' endothelial dystrophy without use of topical rho-kinase inhibitors: 5-year follow-up. Can J Ophthalmol. 2021;57(6):402.

45. Huang MJ, Kane S, Dhaliwal DK. Descemetorhexis without endothelial keratoplasty versus DMEK for treatment of Fuchs endothelial corneal dystrophy. Cornea. 2018;37:1479–83.

46. Davies E, Jurkunas U, Pineda R. Predictive factors for corneal clearance after Descemetorhexis without endothelial keratoplasty. Cornea. 2018;37:137–40.

Pre-Descemets Endothelial Keratoplasty (PDEK): Science and Surgery

31

Harminder Singh Dua

Key Points

- DSAEK, DMEK and PDEK are examples of endothelial keratopathy.
- DMEK is a true like-for-like replacement of diseased Descemet's membrane (DM) and endothelial cells (EC) with healthy donor DM and EC.
- PDEK involves the transplantation of the pre-Descemet's layer (Dua's layer), DM and EC.
- PDEK tissue can be obtained by separating the layers from the stroma with air or viscoelastic.
- PDEK tissue is easier to handle and unscroll in the eye as it scrolls less. A big advantage is that it can be obtained from very young donors as well.
- PDEK gives similar visual outcomes as DMEK without any induced refractive change.

Introduction

For more than 100 years after the first successful corneal transplant was performed in the human eye, penetrating keratoplasty (PK) remained the gold standard. Then occurred a paradigm shift making selective lamellar keratoplasty the accepted norm replacing penetrating keratoplasty for many indications [1–3]. For all conditions affecting the corneal stroma, like dystrophies, degenerations, scars and ectasias; deep anterior lamellar keratoplasty (DALK), wherein the host endothelium is retained, became the preferred option [4]. For endothelial diseases causing persistent corneal edema, endothelial keratoplasty (EK), wherein the host endothelial cells are replaced, is the first choice procedure [5]. In DALK, the risk of graft failure due to endothelial rejection is eliminated, and in EK, avoidance of induced astigmatism and other suture-related problems and rapid visual recovery are distinct advantages over PK. Descemet's stripping automated endothelial keratoplasty (DSAEK) and Descemet's membrane endothelial keratoplasty (DMEK) are EK procedures, to which Pre-Descemet's endothelial keratoplasty (PDEK) is the later addition [4, 6].

The Science Behind PDEK Surgery

Though improved patient outcome was the major benefit of selective lamellar keratoplasty, another significant consequential benefit was our improved understanding of corneal anatomy, of concepts in lamellar corneal surgery and corneal pathology. DALK was shown to be not a Descemet's baring procedure in most cases but

H. S. Dua (✉)
Professor of Ophthalmology, University of Nottingham, Nottingham, UK

Consultant Ophthalmologist, Eye ENT Centre, Queens Medical Centre, University Hospitals NHS Trust, Nottingham, UK

© The Author(s), under exclusive license to Springer Nature Switzerland AG 2023
J. L. Alió, J. L. A. del Barrio (eds.), *Modern Keratoplasty*, Essentials in Ophthalmology,
https://doi.org/10.1007/978-3-031-32408-6_31

rather that the plane of cleavage was between the posterior stroma and the anterior surface of the pre-Descemet's layer (PDL) (Dua's layer) [7]. Ex vivo simulation of DALK by pneumo-dissection in human sclero-corneal discs provided insights into posterior corneal anatomy that inform our concepts on corneal surgery today. Three types of big bubbles (BB) can form; Type 1, where the posterior wall of the BB is made of the PDL, Descemet's membrane (DM) and endothelium; Type 2 where the posterior wall of the BB is formed by the DM and endothelium; and Mixed BB (also referred to as type 3), where both types 1 and 2 occur together and each may be partial or complete [7]. A type 2 BB usually starts at the periphery and spreads across the posterior surface of the cornea, though at times, especially in advanced keratoconus eyes, it can start centrally and remain localised. Examination of the periphery of the PDL at the point of commencement of a type 2 BB after reflecting the DM revealed tiny fenestrations in the PDL, which is essentially impervious to air. There are 15–20 such fenestrations with an average size of 20 microns present singly or in clusters, and distributed randomly along the circumference of the periphery of the PDL [8]. When these fenestrations are located

central to the termination of the DM, air escaping through them accesses the plane between the posterior surface of the PDL and anterior surface of the DM and lifts the DM off to form a type 2 BB. When the fenestrations are located peripheral to the termination of the DM, air escaping through them enters the anterior chamber, as is often seen in DALK [8] (Fig. 31.1).

Characterization of the PDL has demonstrated that it is made of 5 to 11 lamellae of compact type 1 and long spacing collagen; the lamellae are thinner than corresponding layers of the posterior corneal stroma and are essentially devoid of keratocytes. The PDL has the highest concentration of elastin fibres relative to the rest of the cornea [7, 9] (Fig. 31.2). At the periphery, the fibres of the PDL separate and fan out to continue as the core of the trabecular beams of the trabecular meshwork [10, 11]. The fenestrations described above are located in this part of the PDL. The compactness and arrangement of the lamellae, the proteoglycan content and the lack of keratocyte spaces could explain why it is impervious to air. There is anecdotal evidence to suggest that air passes along the keratocyte spaces in the stroma to fill the stroma and reach the plane anterior to the PDL, where its progress is arrested, and it

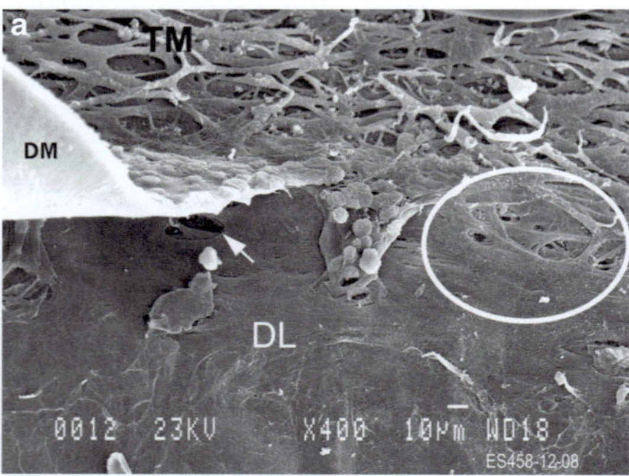

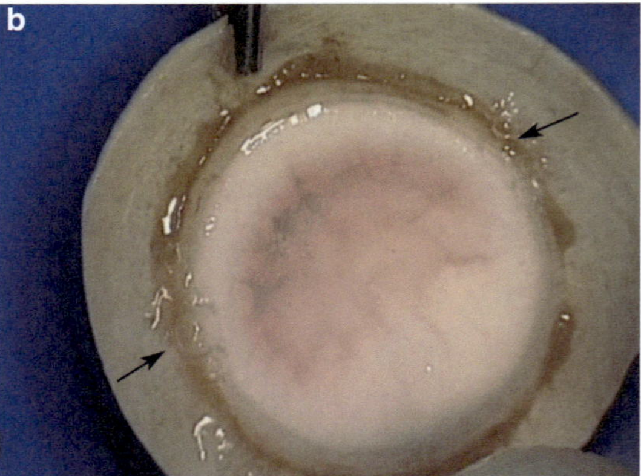

Fig. 31.1 Features of the periphery of the pre-Descemet's layer (Dua's Layer. DL). (**a**) The Descemet's membrane (DM) has been peeled off the periphery of DL to reveal a fenestration (white arrow). Air escaping through this fenestration will access the plane between DM and DL and create a type 2 big bubble. The area enclosed in the white circle shows the periphery of the DL fanning out as the

beams of the trabecular meshwork (TM). Some fenestrations are also seen. (**b**) The black arrows point to escaping bubbles or air at the periphery. These are emerging peripheral to the attachment of the DM; hence, in vivo during deep anterior lamellar keratoplasty they enter the anterior chamber

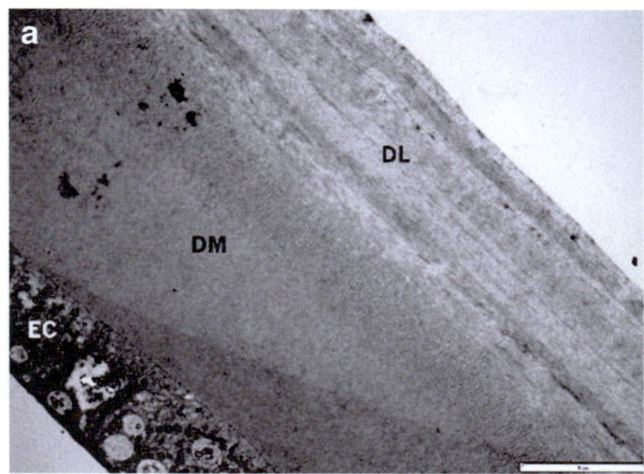
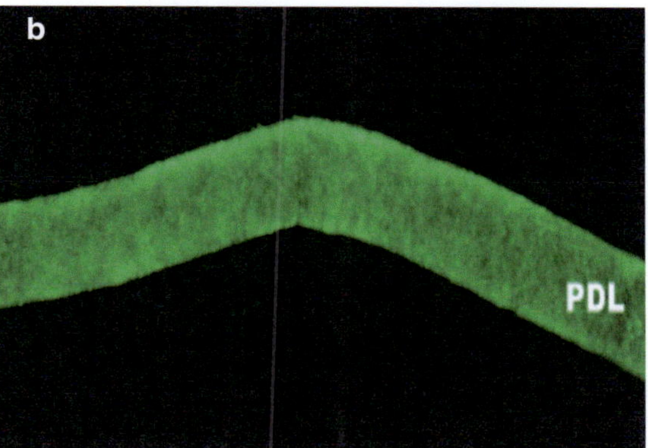

Fig. 31.2 Histology and elastin staining of the pre-Descemet's layer (Dua's layer, DL). (**a**) The pre-Descemet's layer (PDL/DL) is seen anterior to the Descemet's membrane (DM). This is made of thin and compact lamellae of collagen. (**b**) Immunostaining of the PDL for elastin (green). The entire thickness of the PDL is staining positive for elastin

accumulates to build enough pressure to spread along the cleavage plane anterior to the PDL. The imperviousness of the PDL to air is a key feature that enables the PDL to be lifted off the deep stroma when air reaches the plane between it and the posterior surface of the deep stroma. It has been shown that if the DM is stripped off the PDL, air injection can still produce a type 1 BB [7]. However, if the PDL is ablated by excimer laser treatment, a type 1 BB can never be formed [12]. There are therefore several features that illustrate the uniqueness of the PDL, which bear on lamellar corneal surgery, including DALK and PDEK and corneal pathology.

In PDEK, the posterior wall of a type 1 BB, made of the PDL, DM and endothelium, is excised, and the composite (PDEK tissue) (Fig. 31.3) is transplanted in the host eye to restore endothelial cell function. PDEK was first proposed by Dua et al. [7, 13] PDEK tissue, like DMEK tissue (DM and endothelium only), scrolls with the endothelial cells on the outside of the scroll. The scrolling, however, is less tight compared to DMEK tissue (Fig. 31.4), making unscrolling in the eye easier [14]. Hence, compared to DMEK, endothelial cell loss related to manoeuvres performed to open the scroll in the host anterior chamber should be less. Endothelial cell loss using pneumodissection to create PDEK and DMEK tissue is similar, if not slightly less for PDEK tissue compared to DEMK tissue [15–

17]. The PDL on it own scrolls the least when compared to DMEK tissue and PDEK tissue. This relates to the distribution of elastin in the components of the respective tissues. In the PDL, elastin is distributed uniformly across its entire thickness, unlike in the DM, where it is concentrated as a band on the anterior surface, most likely corresponding to the banded layer [18, 19]. (Fig. 31.3). The PDL therefore can stretch and return to its original shape and position without much, if any scrolling. The anterior concentration of elastin on the DM on the other hand, forces the isolated DM to form a scroll with the posterior (endothelial) surface on the outside of the scroll. Experimental data has confirmed that when isolated scrolled DM is treated with elastase enzyme, the scroll spontaneously unscrolls, and the DM disc becomes flat. Histology of the DM so treated shows the degradation of the anterior elastin band [15]. In PDEK tissue where the two components are together, the PDL splints the DM to reduce its scrolling effect, and conversely, almost all the scrolling of PDEK tissue can be attributed to the DM [14].

When air is injected in the corneal stroma to create a type 1 BB, to harvest PDEK tissue, a fairly consistent pattern of movement of air is observed [8]. Upon emerging from the tip of the needle, depending on the state of hydration of the donor stroma, the air may spread diffusely or as fine lines like cracks in glass. It then almost

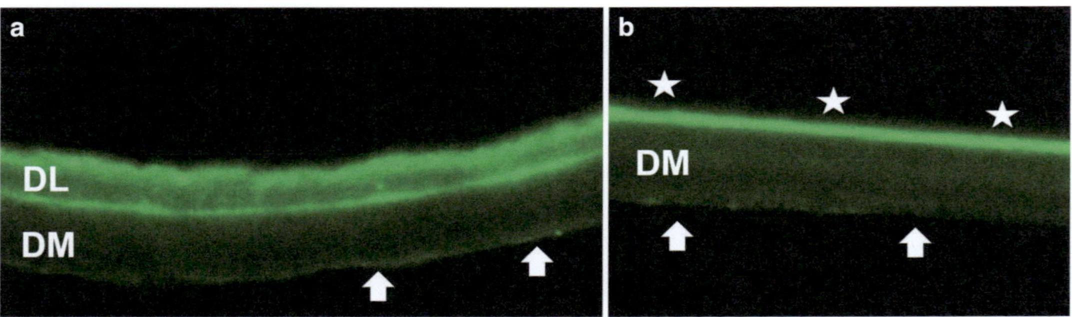

Fig. 31.3 Distribution of elastin in pre-Descemet's endothelial keratoplasty (PDEK) tissue and in Descemet's membrane (DM) shown by immunofluorescent staining. Elastin stains green. (**a**) PDEK tissue shows the anterior layer made of Dua's layer (DL) with diffuse elastin staining. The DM shows elastin only on its anterior surface. The white arrows point to the endothelial surface of DM. (**b**) The DM shows a distinct anterior band of elastin (stars) with the rest of the DM showing no elastin stain

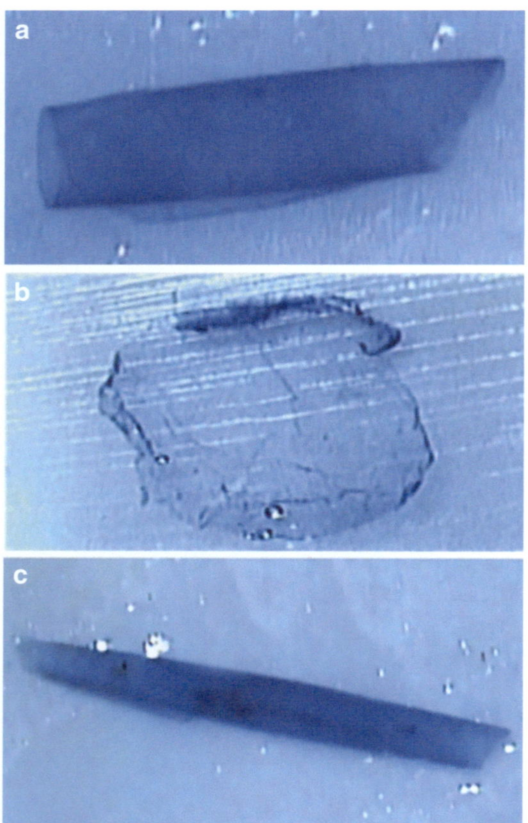

Fig. 31.4 Scrolling characteristics of pre-Descemet's endothelial keratoplasty (PDEK) tissue and its component layers. (**a**) PDEK tissue shows a grade 2 scroll. The pre-Descemet's layer/Dua's layer (PDL/DL) were peeled apart from the tissue in 'A'. (**b**) The PDL/DL shows minimal scrolling. (**c**) The Descemet's membrane shows a grade 4 scroll. Almost all the scrolling of PDEK tissue is conferred by the attached DM

always, tracks towards the limbus as radial streaks. Upon reaching the limbus, it moves circumferentially in a clockwise and counterclockwise direction, as narrow white bands of 1.5 to 2 mm, until the two bands meet. Air then moves centripetally filling the stroma. The aerated stroma of the circumferential bands is thicker than the central aerated stroma. As air is continually injected, multiple small pockets of air appear in the central cornea, lifting the PDL. These coalesce to form a type 1 BB that expands centrifugally to reach a maximum diameter of around 8.5 mm [8]. During this process, several points of air leakage can be seen along the circumference of the sclero-corneal disc. For a type 1 BB to form, a critical intra tissue pressure of air has to be created to force air along the cleavage plane anterior to the PDL. If air leakage at the periphery is excessive, more air has to be injected with greater force to compensate for the leaking air and attain the critical pressure required. This process is difficult to control and balance. If the critical intratissue pressure is not attained, a type 1 BB will not form, and conversely, if too much force is used, a type 1 BB could form very rapidly and burst with a popping sound [8].

In a series of experiments, we [20] demonstrated that the maximum pressure reached to create a type 1 BB was 96.25+/−21.61 kpa, and the mean bursting pressure for a type 1 BB was 66.65+/−18.65 kpa. The pressure in the type 1 BB measured 10.16+/−3.65 kpa, and the volume of a type 1 BB was 0.1 mL. In these experiments, a clamp (see below) was used to prevent any peripheral escape of air. The mean volume of air required to create type1 BB was 0.54 mL, but this can be variable as the injected air does not always follow the course of radial, circumferential and centripetal movement. At any point during the injection, most likely depending on the depth of the needle in the stroma, air can access the cleavage plane and create a type 1 BB. The sooner this happens, the less is the amount of air required to create the BB.

The formation of a type 2 BB during the production of PDEK tissue is an undesirable event. A type 2 BB would generate tissue suitable for DMEK but not for PDEK. To avoid this the PDEK clamp [21] was developed by exploiting the knowledge of the peripheral fenestrations in the PDL (Fig. 31.5). The PDEK clamp is manufactured by *e. Janach* of Italy. The clamp is made of two opposing rings of 1 mm width and 9 mm in diameter. The sclerocorneal disc is clamped in this instrument, which compresses the peripheral tissue occluding the fenestrations. There is a

side-port in the lower ring through which the needle, attached to an air-filled syringe, is inserted in the corneal stroma to inject air (Fig. 31.5). Occluding the fenestrations prevents any escape of injected air and stops air reaching the plane between DL and DM avoiding a type 2 BB. Injected air is retained in the stroma and eventually makes its way to the plane along the anterior surface of the PDL creating a type-1 BB, which can be created in donor discs of all ages, hence even young donor eyes with higher endothelial cell counts can be used for PDEK [21, 22].

Another strategy to avoid the formation of a type 2 BB is adopted in the scoring technique [23, 24]. Here, the extreme periphery of the DM along the entire circumference is scored by a reverse Sinski hook. Any air that reaches the plane between the PDL and DM escapes through the cut edge of the DM without lifting it off as a type 2 BB. In this technique, however, the difficulty in maintaining a balance between escaping air and attainment of the critical intra-tissue pres-

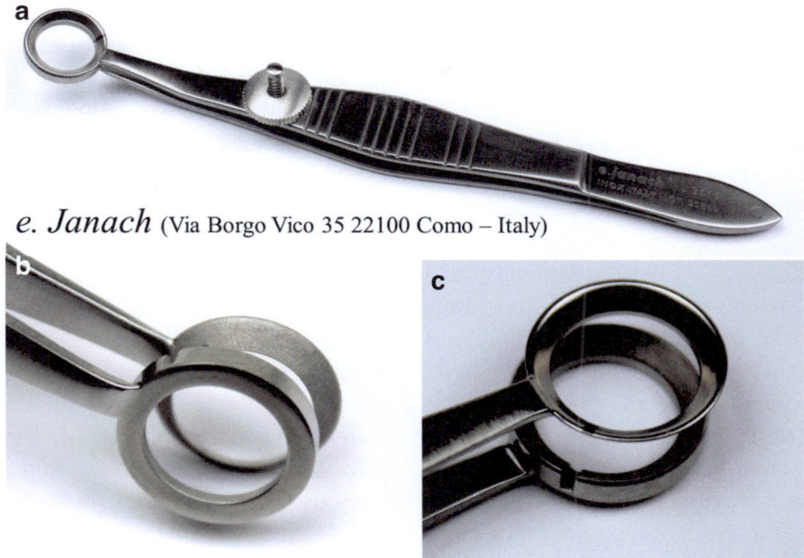

Fig. 31.5 The Pre-Descemet's endothelial keratoplasty (PDEK) clamp. (**a**) The PDEK-clamp is made of two arms with a 9 mm ring attached at the end of each. The two arms can be tightened by rotating the screw. (**b**) The contour of the rims of the two apposing rings conform to the periphery of the cornea and are roughened to allow a firm grip. (**c**) The lower ring has a notch for inserting the needle for injecting air in the stroma, on the right of the handles (or on the left for left handed individuals). The position of the notch is indicated by a mark on the upper ring

sure to create a type 1 BB remains, with the potential consequences mentioned above.

It is evident from the above account that the new scientific knowledge on posterior corneal anatomy gained with the advent of lamellar keratoplasty has enabled the development of adaptations, modifications and innovations in instrumentation and surgical steps, including the innovation of PDEK itself. As stated above, it has also considerably enhanced our understanding of corneal pathology, challenging concepts that were held as gospel for almost a century.

It is now clearly understood that Descemet's membrane detachment (DMD) is not a detachment of the DM alone. Often, the PDL is also detached. In fact, DMD follows the exact same patterns as three types of BB and has been classified as type 1 DMD, wherein the PDL and DM are detached together and on optical coherence tomography (OCT) appear as a straight line, like the cord of a circle; type 2 DMD, which represents a detachment of the DM alone appearing as a fine double contour wavy line on OCT; and Mixed DMD (type 3) where both the PDL and DM are detached and also separated from each other, with the anteriorly located PDL detachment appearing as a straight line and the posteriorly located DM detachment as a wavy line [25].

Acute hydrops in keratoconus, hitherto considered to be due to a tear in the DM, is due to a tear in the DM and the PDL in the background of the abnormal collagen and proteoglycans of a keratoconus cornea. DM detachment and tear in keratoconus eyes do not result in acute hydrops unless associated with a tear in the PDL as well. Furthermore, loss or degradation of elastin in the PDL has been implicated in the pathogenesis of keratoconus [8, 10, 26–28].

Descemetoceles too are of type 1, protrusion of the DM covered with the PDL; or type 2, protrusion of the DM alone; or type 3 a protrusion of the DM covered with the PDL and a variable amount of deep corneal stroma [8, 10, 29]. Intracorneal hypopyon is due to the accumulation of inflammatory debris (pus) in the plane between a detached PDL and posterior stroma. The spread of infecting microbes, especially fungi, has been shown to preferentially occur along the pre-

Descemet's plane [30]. The PDL is also implicated in macular corneal dystrophy and in Lewis syndrome, where there is a biclonal gammopathy with paraproteinemic keratopathy manifesting in the form of a central discoid yellow-brownish discoloration in the PDL [31]. A thickened opaque PDL that could be peeled off was noted during DSEK [32].

Lamellar corneal surgery thus revealed novel anatomical features that in turn informed and improved our understanding of corneal pathology and corneal surgery, leading to the innovation of three procedures, namely suture management of acute hydrops, DALK-Triple and PDEK.

PDEK: Surgical Principles

Tissue Harvesting

PDEK tissue is usually obtained by pneumo-dissection. Fresh or preserved donor sclero-corneal discs can be used. Corneal stromal swelling postmortem, or induced by storage in different media for up to 4 weeks, may be an advantage as it would make it easier to insert the needle or canula in the stroma with reduced risk of perforation and also allow intrastromal dispersion of air. The principle of air injection and excising PDEK tissue is the same with the use of the PDEK clamp, scoring technique or direct injection [21, 23, 24] (Figs. 31.6 and 31.7). For reasons explained above (under 'science behind PDEK surgery'), the use of the clamp is recommended. Under an operating microscope, the sclero-corneal disc, endothelial side up, is mounted on the lower ring with the clamp in the fully open position (Fig. 31.7). The disc is carefully centered on the lower ring and clamped into position by tightening the screw on the handle. During this manoeuvre, the disc can slip and become decentered. Centering is important as an eccentrically clamped donor disc may leave some peripheral fenestrations unoccluded, resulting in the escape of air and/or the formation of a type 2 BB. One strategy to ensure centration is to place four ink marks on the epithelial surface at 12, 3, 6, and 9 o'clock

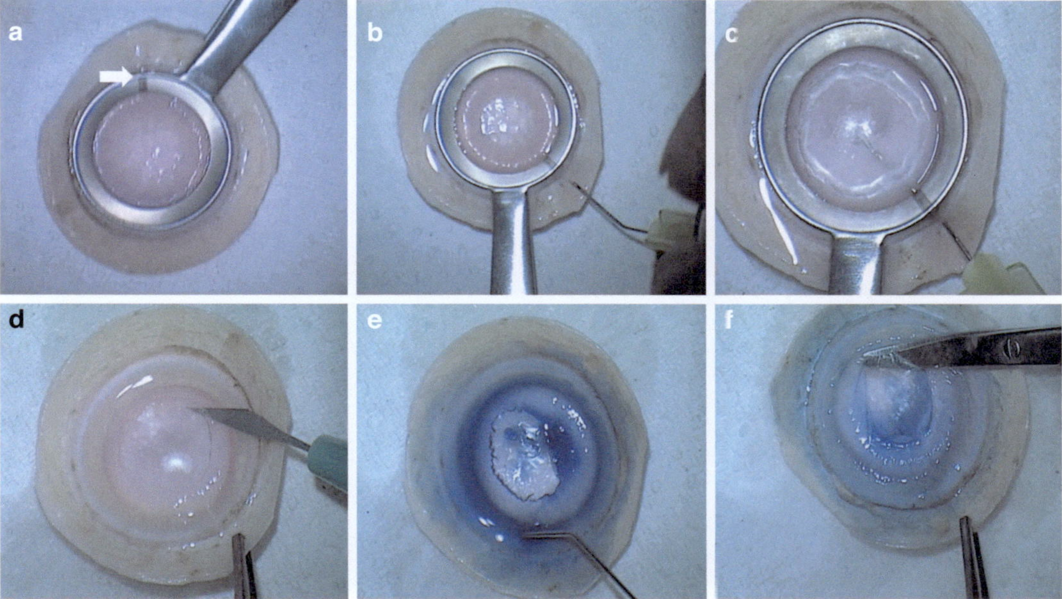

Fig. 31.6 Harvesting Pre-Descemet's endothelial keratoplasty (PDEK) tissue. (**a**) Air is injected into a sclero-corneal disc stained with vision blue. (**b**) A type 1 big bubble (BB), has formed. (**c**) The needle tip is advanced into the cavity of the BB, and air is aspirated to collapse the BB. (**d**) A trephine of appropriate size is placed on the area of the collapsed BB and the PDEK-tissue is trephined. (**e**) The cut PDEK tissue is gently peeled off. (**f**) The PDEK tissue shows only mild to moderate scrolling giving the tissue a triangular shape

Fig. 31.7 Preparing pre-Descemet's keratoplasty (PDEK) tissue using the PDEK clamp. (**a**) The clamp is centred on a sclero-corneal disc, endothelial side up, and screwed tight. The white arrow points to the mark on the upper ring that indicates the position of the notch in the inferior ring. (**b**) A 30 gauge needle, bent to 135 degrees with the bevel up, attached to a 5 mL luer lock syringe filled with air, is inserted in the scleral rim corresponding to the mark, and advanced in the posterior stroma, towards the centre of the cornea. (**c**) Air is injected to fill the stroma and create a type 1 big bubble (BB). (**d**) The clamp is removed and the wall of the BB is incised at the edge. (**e**) Vision blue dye is injected into the BB to delineate circumference. (**f**) PDEK tissue is excised by cutting the attachment of the BB to the stroma

positions, 1.5 mm inside the limbus. During the tightening of the clamp, the sclero-corneal disc is held such that all four ink marks are visible within the diameter of the clamp ring [33].

A 30 gauge needle, bent to approximately 135° bevel up, is mounted on a 5 mL luer lock syringe filled with air. It helps to move the plunger back and forth a few times to ensure ease of movement. Most plastic syringes present considerable resistance before the plunger starts to move. This can build up a high-pressure head and risk rapid formation and bursting of the BB. The needle is inserted into the mid-corneal stroma through the side-port of the clamp, starting in the rim of sclera around the cornea (Fig. 31.7). A black metal plate is provided with the clamp and can be used as a background to improve contrast and enhance depth perception while inserting and advancing the needle. A guiding principle is that the tip of the needle should be positioned close to the endothelial surface without risking perforation. When the tip is advanced to the centre of the disc, air is slowly and firmly injected in a continuous manner until a type 1 BB is formed. The tip of the needle can

then be gently advanced into the cavity of the BB, and a little more air is injected to enlarge the BB further. Once a BB is obtained, it can be collapsed by sucking the air out before removing the needle, or it can be left inflated. The needle is withdrawn, the clamp is opened and the tissue removed. PDEK tissue is then either cut with an appropriate size trephine, or the edge of the BB punctured with a lance blade. Vision Blue® is injected in the cavity of the BB to enhance visualization of the circumference of the BB and the PDEK tissue is excised with a pair of scissors. It is left on the stromal bed, covered with balanced salt solution (BSS) or culture medium until ready for insertion in the recipient eye.

Recipient Bed Preparation

The recipient eye is prepared in a manner similar to any EK procedure. A corneal or sclero-corneal main entry tunnel and side ports are created. The area from which the recipient DM is to be removed, usually larger than the size of the PDEK tissue, is marked and the DM stripped (Fig. 31.8).

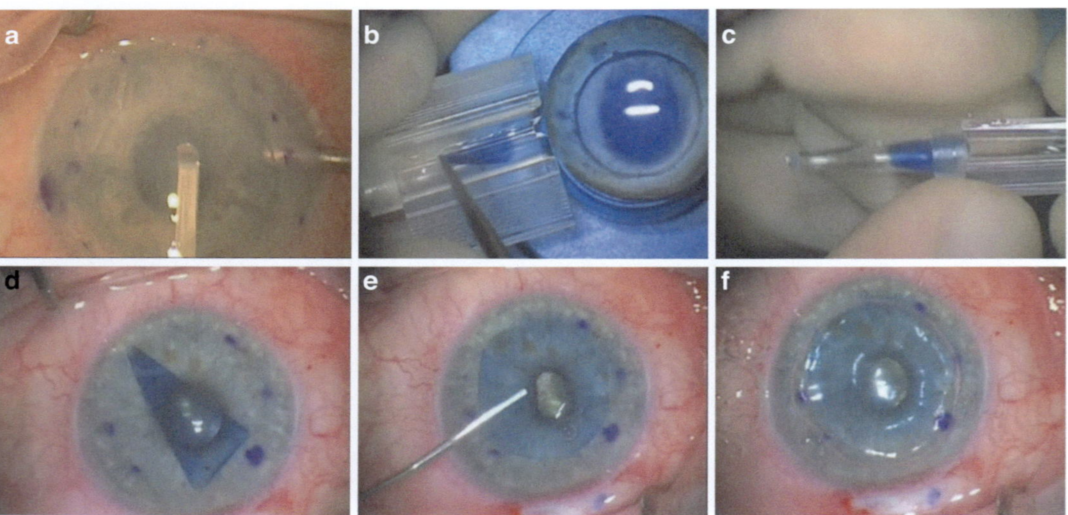

Fig. 31.8 Pre-Descemet's endothelial keratoplasty (PDEK). (**a**) The host diseased Descemet's membrane (DM) is scored and stripped. (**b**) The prepared PDEK tissue is stained with vision blue and loaded in an injector cartridge. (**c**) The scrolled PDEK tissue, endothelial cells outside, is nudged into the nozzle of the injector. (**d**) The tissue is injected into the anterior chamber (AC) where it lies with the scrolls up. (**e**) The scrolls are gently tapped to an open position, endothelial cells down, and centred. (**f**) Air is injected between the iris and the endothelial surface of the PDEK tissue to fill the AC

PDEK Tissue Preparation and Insertion

PDEK tissue can be inserted by injecting the scroll in the recipient eye or by the pull-through technique. The former is the preferred option. The PDEK tissue, whether excised with scissors or trephined is carefully lifted off the stromal bed. At this point, some attachments along the circumference or fine strands extending between the anterior surface of the PDEK tissue and the stromal bed may be noted. These are cut to release the PDEK tissue. The tissue can be folded with the endothelium inside, the PDL dried with a surgical sponge and an 'F' or 'S' mark placed if required. The tissue is then covered with BSS and allowed to form a scroll. It is then stained with Vision Blue® or Membrane Blue® for 1–3 min and washed. A standard lens injector or glass pipette is used to introduce the tissue in the recipient's anterior chamber. The injector cartridge is filled with BSS, the scroll of PDEK tissue is placed in the groove and gently nudged into the nozzle. The cartridge is mounted on a 2 mL syringe filled with BSS, and the scroll is inspected and the syringe is rotated such that the overlapping edges of the scroll are anteriorly located (facing up). The nozzle is inserted in the anterior chamber regardless of the direction of the bevel, keeping the scroll facing up (Fig. 31.8). Alternatively, a fine forceps can be inserted through a paracentesis wound opposite to the main entry incision, advanced to the tip of the nozzle and the PDEK tissue grasped in the nozzle and pulled in (pull through technique).

Before loading, PDEK tissue can alternatively be folded, whilst lying on the stromal bed, with the endothelium inside and the PDL outside, in three one-thirds parts. This is then loaded into the cartridge as described, but the overlapping edges of the fold should be facing down (not up) before injecting. Once in the anterior chamber, the natural tendency of the tissue to scroll with the endothelium outside causes the folded tissue to open, with the endothelium facing the iris and the PDL facing the cornea, which is the correct orientation.

Maneuvers in the Anterior Chamber (AC)

Once in the AC, the aim is to unfold the tissue, ensure correct orientation, centre it on the pupil and appose it to the posterior surface of the cornea from which the DM has been stripped. Key principles here are (a) to move the scroll and unscrolled tissue into the desired position, there should be some fluid in the AC; (b) to ascertain orientation, the rolls of the scroll should be facing the cornea or the 'F'/'S' marks should read correctly; and (c) to unscroll the tissue, the AC should be kept shallow during the tapping maneuvers. As the tissue unscrolls, the narrow space and contact with iris and cornea keeps the tissue from re-scrolling. Once in the correct position, orientation and fully open, air or 20% SF6 gas is injected under the tissue. The canula is inserted through one of the side ports and advanced along the iris plane to the centre of the tissue before commencing injection. If air is injected at one edge, the bubble can displace the tissue and cause decentration. Once the tissue is attached to the back of the cornea, ensure that the marks, if used, are correct. The 'F'/'S' marks are best seen when the tissue is attached to the cornea. Air fill is then completed and maintained for 10 min during which the entry sites are secured if needed (Fig. 31.8). Antibiotic, steroid and mydriatic either by subconjunctival injection or topically are administered. Some air/gas is released to maintain normal pressure whilst retaining a full fill.

Post-operative Management

Post-operative management with topical steroids, antibiotics and mydriatic drops is continued. Pupil block glaucoma is an issue whenever air is left in the AC. The patient is rested in a supine position and the pressure checked approximately 1 h later. High pressure, depending on the measurement, is managed with pupil dilation, air release, oral or intravenous acetazolamide or intravenous mannitol injection. An inferior peripheral iridectomy (PI) is very useful in mitigating the risk of post operative high pressure. The timing of the PI is important. It can be done preoperatively with a YAG laser or intraoperatively. The latter has a major risk of inducing bleeding or fibrin release in the AC. If this were to happen, it can seriously comprise the procedure as the fibrin traps the PDEK tissue and prevents it from unscrolling. Intraoperative PI should always be followed by careful observation for any blood or fibrin and this cleared by washing, aspiration or viscoelastic tamponade, before inserting the tissue.

Once the graft attaches to the host bed, clearing starts within a couple of days and any epithelial bull® settle with complete stromal clearing and visual improvement occurring between 1 and 3 weeks (Fig. 31.9).

Discussion

When Dua et al. demonstrated the presence of the PDL they also were the first to expound the concept of using what is now termed "PDEK-tissue" in endothelial keratoplasty thus: "Knowledge of the existence of this layer and its characteristics will influence corneal surgery; for example, the plane between the DL and stroma can be exploited in generating tissue for endothelial transplant, allowing easier handling and insertion of the tissue because it does not tend to scroll as much as the DM, with the DL splinting the DM [14]. This concept was realized in collaboration with Dr. Amar Agarwal, and the first report on PDEK was published in 2014 [13].

PDEK has several advantages as an EK procedure. The thickness of the tissue is around thirty microns, which allows visual acuity improvement to a normal level as with DMEK. The tissue is easier to handle, insert and unscroll in the eye. This is partly related to the splinting of the DM

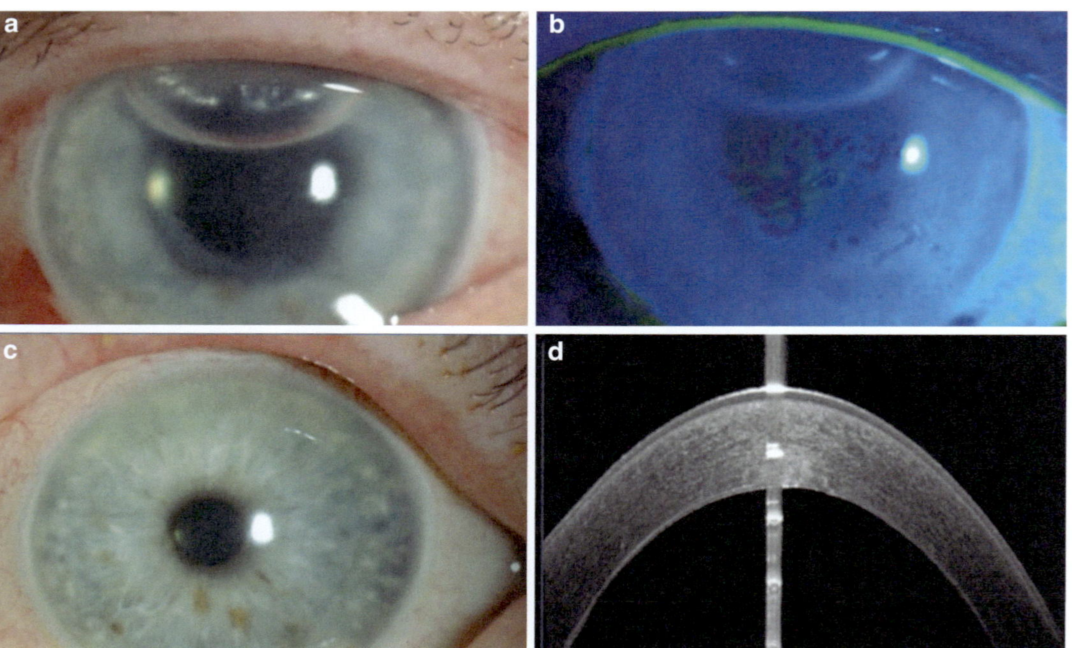

Fig. 31.9 Post-operative outcome after pre-Descemet's endothelial keratoplasty (PDEK). (**a**) Day one post-operative. A small residual bubble of air is visible in the anterior chamber. (**b**) With fluorescein stain, the epithelial bullae are clearly visible. (**c**) At 4 weeks post-operative the cornea has completely cleared. (**d**) Optical coherence tomography at 4 weeks post-operative showing the epithelium, stroma and the attached PDEK tissue

by the PDL, which restricts the amount of scrolling, which in turn makes it easier to unscroll in the eye, reducing endothelial cell loss from tissue handling. Donors of any age can be used, especially young donors, as a type 1 BB can be created in corneas of all ages, even in infants [22]. Younger donors come with higher endothelial cell counts. This contrasts with DMEK tissue which become more difficult to obtain, the younger the donor due to the stronger attachment of the DM with the overlying PDL. Young DM is thinner and scrolls tightly, requiring greater manipulation inside the AC. The PDL in PDEK tissue contributes to the ease of handling, as it can be stroked with a blunt spatula when centering the PDL in the AC. Experience has shown that when younger donors are used, corneas with gross edema and opacification clear remarkably well [22]. On the other hand, the maximum diameter of PDEK is usually less than 8 mm, which is the commonest diameter of DMEK tissue used. This disadvantage is more than offset by the advantages described.

EK procedures have a steep learning curve related to both the preparation of tissue and transplantation. Once the techniques are mastered both are relatively simple but invariably some tissue loss does occur in the process. Pre-prepared DMEK and PDEK tissues are provided by eye banks. PDEK can be a good procedure for beginners to gain confidence and refine skills, which are transferrable to DMEK. Details of the technique and surgical tips for successful PDEK have been variously published [3, 21, 33–38].

Though publications on PDEK are comparatively few, good outcomes comparable to other EK procedures have been reported [39, 40]. PDEK is compatible with other simultaneous surgical interventions performed to maximize outcomes. Combined PDEK and cataract extraction, pupilloplasty and glued-on lens implantation have been reported [31, 41, 42] and also offers some advantage in phakic eyes, especially in younger patients preserving accommodation [43]. As PDEK becomes more acceptable and experience with it grows, more data on outcomes will emerge. It is anticipated that the long-term outcomes of PDEK might surpass those of DMEK on account of the ability to use younger donor tissue and the accompanying high endothelial cell density coupled with less loss of cells related to preparation techniques and the limited intraocular manipulations required.

Take Home Notes

- Pre-Descemet's endothelial keratoplasty (PDEK) is a viable option for endothelial keratoplasty.
- PDEK tissue is made of the endothelium, Descemet's membrane and the pre-Descemet's layer (Dua's layer).
- PDEK tissue is obtained by injecting air into the donor tissue and creating a type 1 big bubble.
- The PDEK clamp can be used for the controlled creation of a type 1 BB.
- PDEK tissue can be obtained from donor eyes of any age, including infant eyes.
- Support provided by the PDL/DL limits the scrolling of PDEK tissue.
- PDEK tissue is easier to unscroll, centre and attach, in the recipient eye.

References

1. Moffatt SL, Cartwright VA, Stumpf TH. Centennial review of corneal transplantation. Clin Experiment Ophthalmol. 2005;33(6):642–57.
2. Terry MA. The evolution of lamellar grafting techniques over twenty-five years. Cornea. 2000;19(5):611–6.
3. Singh NP, Said DG, Dua HS. Lamellar keratoplasty techniques. Indian J Ophthalmol. 2018;66(9):1239–50.
4. Dua HS, Said DG. Deep anterior lamellar keratoplasty (DALK) science and surgery. In: Albert DM, et al., editors. Albert and Jakobiec's principles and practice of ophthalmology. Switzerland: Springer Nature; 2021. https://doi.org/10.1007/978-3-319-90495-5_218-1.
5. Anshu A, Price MO, Tan DT, Price FW Jr. Endothelial keratoplasty: a revolution in evolution. Surv Ophthalmol. 2012;57(3):236–52.
6. Lee WB, Jacobs DS, Musch DC, et al. Descemet's stripping endothelial keratoplasty: safety and outcomes: a report by the American academy of ophthalmology. Ophthalmology. 2009;116:18–30.

7. Dua HS, Faraj LA, Said DG, et al. Human corneal anatomy redefined: a novel pre-Descemet's layer (Dua's layer). Ophthalmology. 2013;120:1778–85.

8. Dua HS, Faraj LA, Kenawy MB, AlTaan S, Elalfy MS, Katamish T, Said DG. Dynamics of big bubble formation in deep anterior lamellar keratoplasty by the big bubble technique: in vitro studies. Acta Ophthalmol. 2018;96(1):69–76.

9. Bizheva K, Haines L, Mason E, MacLellan B, Tan B, Hileeto D, Sorbara L. In vivo imaging and morphometry of the human pre-Descemet's layer and endothelium with ultrahigh-resolution optical coherence tomography. Invest Ophthalmol Vis Sci. 2016;57(6):2782–7.

10. Dua HS, Faraj LA, Said DG. Dua's layer: discovery, characteristics, clinical applications, controversy and potential relevance to glaucoma. Expert Rev Ophthalmol. 2015;10:531–47.

11. Dua HS, Faraj LA, Branch MJ, et al. The collagen matrix of the human trabecular meshwork is an extension of the novel pre-Descemet's layer (Dua's layer). Br J Ophthalmol. 2014;98:691–7.

12. Dua HS, Mastropasqua L, Faraj L, et al. Big bubble deep anterior lamellar keratoplasty: the collagen layer in the wall of the big bubble is unique. Acta Ophthalmol. 2015;93:427–30.

13. Agarwal A, Dua HS, Narang P, et al. Pre-Descemet's endothelial keratoplasty (PDEK). Br J Ophthalmol. 2014;98:1181–5.

14. Dua HS, Termote K, Kenawy MB, et al. Scrolling characteristics of pre-Descemet endothelial keratoplasty tissue: an ex vivo study. Am J Ophthalmol. 2016;166:84–90.

15. Altaan SL, Gupta A, Sidney LE, at al. Endothelial cell loss following tissue harvesting by pneumodissection for endothelial keratoplasty: an ex vivo study. Br J Ophthalmol. 2015;99:710–3.

16. Gamal El Din SA, Salama MM, El Shazly MI. Seven-day storage of pneumatically dissected Descemet's endothelial grafts with and without Dua's layer. Acta Ophthalmol. 2016;94:e130–4. Characterization of Endothelial, 94, e130.

17. Bedard P, Hou JH. Cell loss in pre-Descemet endothelial keratoplasty graft preparation. Cornea. 2021;40(3):364–9.

18. Mohammed I, Ross AR, Britton JO, Said DG, Dua HS. Elastin content and distribution in endothelial keratoplasty tissue determines direction of scrolling. Am J Ophthalmol. 2018;194:16–25.

19. Lewis PN, White TL, Young RD, Bell JS, Winlove CP, Meek KM. Three-dimensional arrangement of elastic fibers in the human corneal stroma. Exp Eye Res. 2015;146:43–53.

20. AlTaan SL, Mohammed I, Said DG, Dua HS. Air pressure changes in the creation and bursting of the type-1 big bubble in deep anterior lamellar keratoplasty: an ex vivo study. Eye (Lond). 2018;32(1):146–51.

21. Dua HS, Said DG. Pre-Descemets endothelial keratoplasty: the PDEK clamp for successful PDEK. Eye (Lond). 2017;31(7):1106–10.

22. Agarwal A, Agarwal A, Narang P, et al. Pre-Descemet endothelial keratoplasty with infant donor corneas: a prospective analysis. Cornea. 2015;34:859–65.

23. Pereira NC, Forseto ADS, Maluf RCP, Dua HS. Pre-Descemet's endothelial keratoplasty: a simple, Descemet's membrane scoring technique for successful graft preparation. Br J Ophthalmol. 2022;106(6):786–9.

24. Saint-Jean A, Soper M, Den Beste K, Iverson S, Price MO, Price FW. Technique for ensuring type I bubble formation for pre-Descemet endothelial keratoplasty preparation. Cornea. 2019;38(10):1336–8.

25. Dua HS, Sinha R, D'Souza S, Potgieter F, Ross A, Kenawy M, Scott I, Said DG. "Descemet membrane detachment": a novel concept in diagnosis and classification. Am J Ophthalmol. 2020;218:84–98.

26. Parker J, Birbal RS, van Dijk K, Oellerich S, Dapena I, Melles GRJ. Are Descemet membrane ruptures the root cause of corneal hydrops in keratoconic eyes? Am J Ophthalmol. 2019;205:204–5.

27. Ting DSJ, Said DG, Dua HS. Are Descemet membrane ruptures the root cause of corneal hydrops in keratoconic eyes? Am J Ophthalmol. 2019;205:204.

28. Parker JS, Birbal RS, van Dijk K, Oellerich S, Dapena I, Melles GRJ. Are Descemet membrane ruptures the root cause of corneal hydrops in keratoconic eyes? Am J Ophthalmol. 2019;205:147–52.

29. Narang P, Agarwal A, Kumar DA. Predescemetocele: a distinct clinical entity. Indian J Ophthalmol. 2017;65(11):1224–6.

30. Liu Z, Zhang P, Liu C, Zhang W, Hong J, Wang W. Split of Descemet's membrane and pre-Descemet's layer in fungal keratitis: new definition of corneal anatomy incorporating new knowledge of fungal infection. Histopathology. 2015;66(7):1046–9.

31. Lisch W, Vossmerbaeumer U. Corneal opacity and copper levels of the Lewis syndrome after systemic chemotherapy. Am J Ophthalmol Case Rep. 2020;20:100926; eCollection 2020 Dec.

32. Sharma VK, Sinha R, Sati A, Agarwal M. Was it thickened Dua's layer? clinical, tomographical, and histopathological correlation: a case report. Eur J Ophthalmol. 2020:1120672120974271.

33. Ross AR, Said DG, Colabelli Gisoldi RAM, Nubile M, El-Amin A, Gabr AF, Abd Ed-Moniem M, Mencucci R, Pocobelli A, Mastropasqua L, Dua HS. Optimising pre-Descemet endothelial keratoplasty technique. J Cataract Refract Surg. 2020;46(5):667–74.

34. Jacob S. Use of pressurized air infusion for pre Descemet's endothelial keratoplasty (PDEK)—the air pump assisted PDEK technique. Open Ophthalmol J. 2018;12:175–80.

35. Agarwal A. PDEK in 15 steps. Ophthalmol. 2017. https://theophthalmologist.com/subspecialties/pdek-in-15-steps.

36. Tsatsos M, Mironidou M, Jacob S, Ziakas N. Factors influencing corneal predescemetic endothelial keratoplasty (PDEK) graft creation: it's all in a bubble. Hell J Nucl Med. 2019;22(Suppl 2):42–6.

37. Jacob S, Narasimhan S, Agarwal A, Agarwal A, A I S. Air pump-assisted graft centration, graft edge unfolding, and graft uncreasing in young donor graft pre-Descemet endothelial keratoplasty. Cornea. 2017;36(8):1009–13.

38. Studeny P, Netukova M, Hlozanek M, Bednar J, Jirsova K, Krizova D. Frequency of complications during preparation of corneal lamellae used in posterior lamellar keratoplasty using the pneumodissection technique (big bubble). Cornea. 2018;37(7):904–8.

39. Huang T, Jiang L, Zhan J, Ouyang C. Pre-descement membrane endothelial keratoplasty for treatment of patients with corneal endothelial decompensation. Zhonghua Yan Ke Za Zhi. 2018;54(2):105–10.

40. Kumar DA, Dua HS, Agarwal A, Jacob S. Postoperative spectral-domain optical coherence tomography evaluation of pre-Descemet endothelial keratoplasty grafts. J Cataract Refract Surg. 2015;41:1535–6.

41. Narang P, Mehta K, Agarwal A. Phacoemulsification with single-pass four-throw pupilloplasty and pre-Descemet's endothelial keratoplasty for management of cosmetic iris implant complication. Indian J Ophthalmol. 2018;66(6):841–4.

42. Narang P, Agarwal A, Kumar DA. Single-pass 4-throw pupilloplasty for pre-Descemet endothelial keratoplasty. Cornea. 2017;36(12):1580–3.

43. Dítě J, Netuková M, Klimešová KD, Studený P. Results of posterior lamellar keratoplasties in phakic eyes. Cesk Slov Oftalmol. 2022;78(1):20–3.

Pre-Descemet's Endothelial Keratoplasty (Pdek): Clinical Considerations and Surgical Details

Priya Narang and Amar Agarwal

Key Points

- The PDEK graft comprises of Pre-Descemet's layer (Dua's layer) along with Descemet's membrane and endothelium.
- Type-1 bubble is formed for performing PDEK surgery.
- The PDEK graft is less flimsy than the DMEK graft due to the additional splinting effect of Pre-Descemet's layer.
- Young donor grafts can be used for PDEK surgery.

Take Home Notes

The essential for performing a PDEK surgery is the creation of Type-1 bubble. The graft can then be harvested, and endothelial keratoplasty can be performed.

Supplementary Information The online version contains supplementary material available at https://doi.org/10.1007/978-3-031-32408-6_32.

P. Narang
Narang Eye Care and Laser Centre,
Ahmedabad, India

A. Agarwal (✉)
Dr. Agarwal's Eye Hospital and Research Centre,
Chennai, India

Introduction

Posterior lamellar keratoplasty (PLK) has revolutionized the management of corneal endothelial disorders. The widespread adoption of PLK techniques has led to better visual outcomes and enhanced globe stability due to closed chamber manipulation, unlike penetrating keratoplasty that leads to refractive instability and delayed recovery.

Dua et al. [1] discovered and described a novel, well-defined, acellular layer known as Pre-Descemet's layer (PDL; Dua's layer)—a distinct layer that is considered to have considerable impact on posterior corneal surgery. PDL is documented to be an acellular layer composed of 5–8 lamellae of predominantly type-1 collagen bundle that measured approximately 10.15 ± 3.6 microns [1]. Pre-Descemet's endothelial keratoplasty (PDEK) [2] originated after the description of PDL in 2013. Type-1 bubble achieved in PDEK is a well-circumscribed, central dome-shaped elevation up to 8.5 mm in diameter. The

PDEK graft involves implanting a graft that involves a PDL with an endothelial layer. The first PDEK surgery was performed by Dr. Amar Agarwal in 2013.

Technique

Donor Graft Preparation

An air-filled 5 mL syringe attached to a 30 G needle is introduced in a bevel-up position, with the endothelial side up, from the rim of the corneo-scleral junction. The needle is introduced up to the mid-periphery and the air is injected. This forms a Type-1 bubble that is characterized by a dome-shaped elevation, is around 7–8 mm in diameter and typically spreads from the center to the periphery with a distinct edge all around. Trypan blue is injected inside the bubble with a 26 G needle introduced from the edge of the bubble. A corneo-scleral scissor is used to cut the graft all around the edges of the bubble, and the graft is harvested and stored in the McCarey Kaufman tissue culture media (Fig. 32.1).

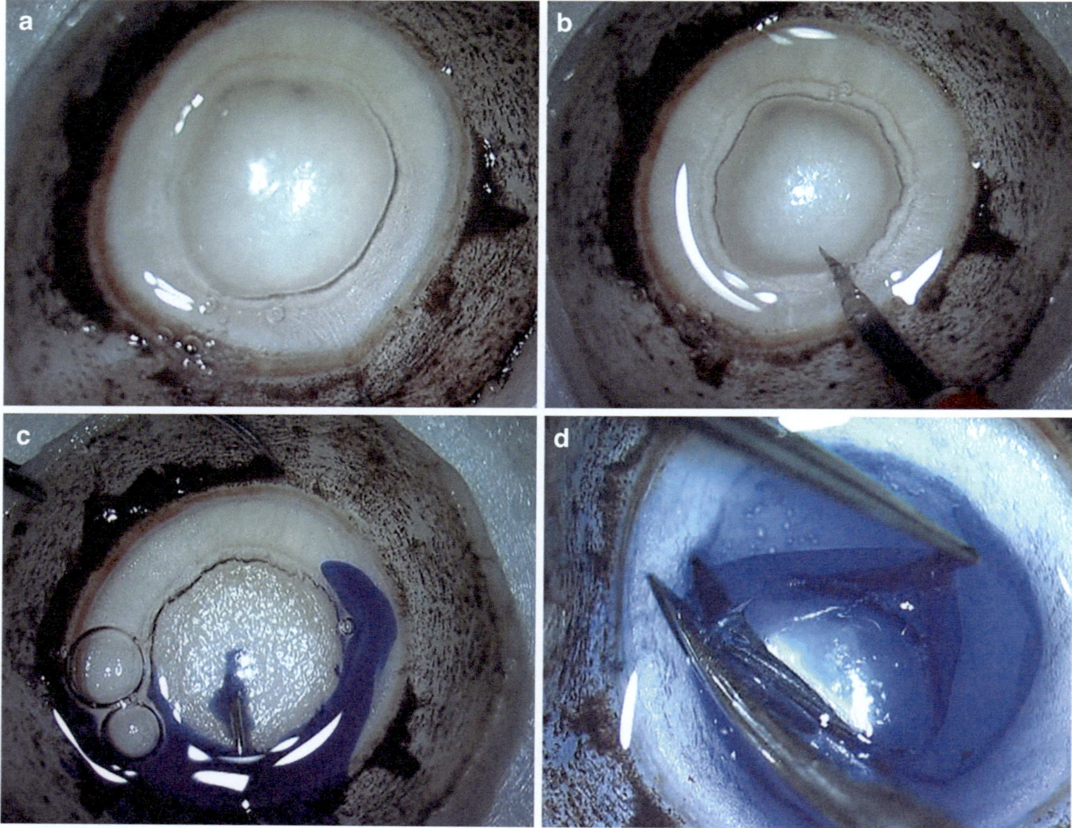

Fig. 32.1 Donor graft preparation. (**a**) An air-filled 30G needle is introduced from the corneo-scleral rim up to the mid-periphery, and air is injected to create a type-1 big bubble (bb). (**b**) The bb is punctured at the extreme periphery with the help of a side port blade. (**c**) Trypan blue is injected to stain the bb. (**d**) The graft is cut along the peripheral edge of the bb with the corneo-scleral scissor

Recipient Bed Preparation

This step is essentially the same as in DMEK. Descemetorhexis is performed, and the scored edges of DM are grasped with non-toothed forceps and slowly stripped away from the stroma (Fig. 32.2).

Graft Insertion

The harvested donor graft is loaded onto the injector of a foldable IOL. As described by Price et al. [3], the spring of the injector is removed to prevent any damage to the graft. The graft is slowly injected inside the eye, centered and oriented, with the rolls of the scroll facing upward. It is gradually unrolled using air and fluidics. In cases of extremely hazy cornea, an endoilluminator can be used to direct the light obliquely on the cornea so as to check the correct orientation of the graft [4]. Once the graft is uncurled, the air is injected beneath the graft to enhance the adherence to the posterior corneal stroma of the recipient tissue (Fig. 32.3, Video 32.1).

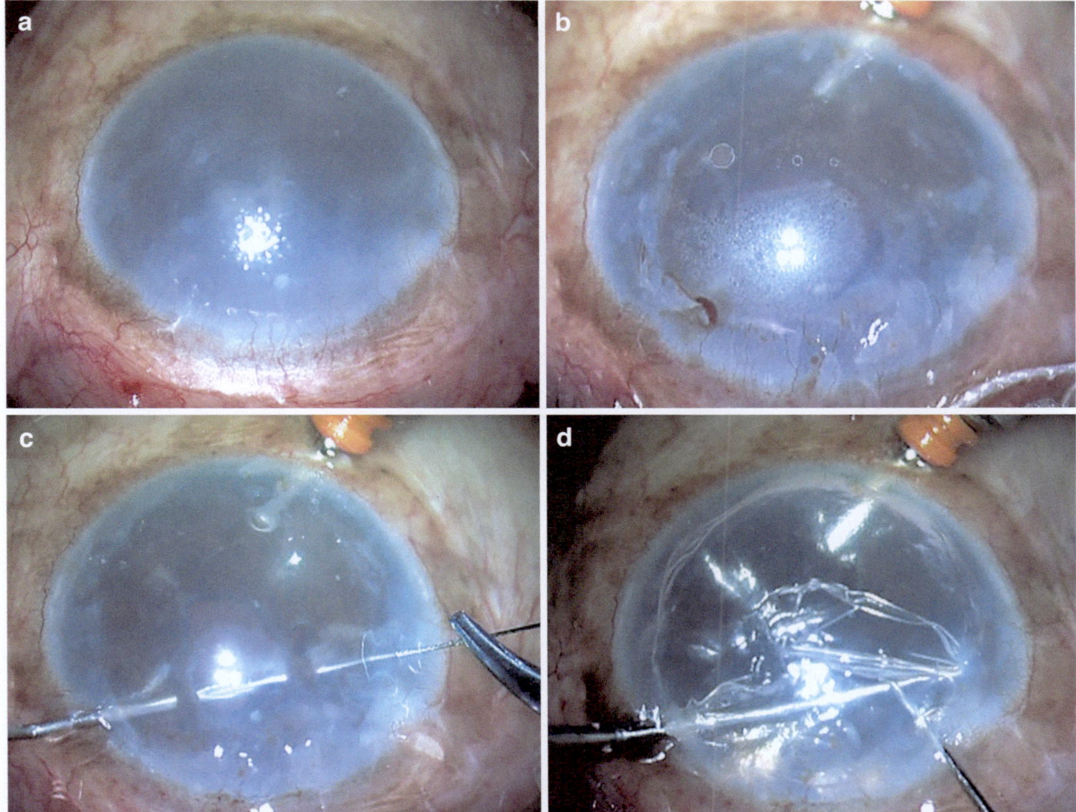

Fig. 32.2 Pseudophakic bullous keraopathy (one-eyed patient) with silicone oil in the eye- Part 1. (**a**) Pseudophakic bullous keratopathy. (**b**) Silicone oil removal—note the trocar AC maintainer. (**c**) Single pass 4 throw pupilloplasty. (**d**) Continuous air infusion and descemtorhexis

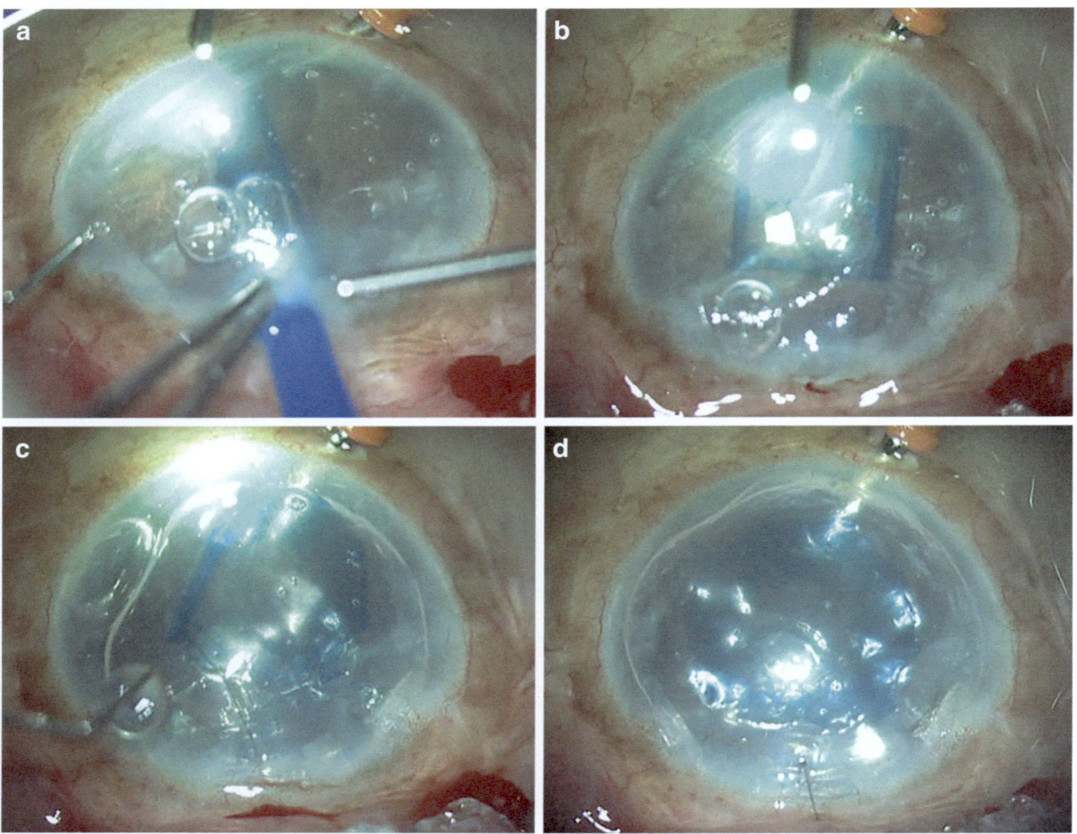

Fig. 32.3 Pseudophakic bullous keraopathy (one-eyed patient) with silicone oil in the eye—Part 2. (**a–d**) PDEK graft injected inside the Ac, unrolled and fixed

Post-op Regimen

The patient is advised to lie supine for the most part during the first postoperative day. The standard postoperative protocol includes the application of moxifloxacin eye drops (4 times a day) and prednisolone acetate 1% (6 times a day) for the initial 2 weeks, 4 times daily for 1 month, twice daily for 2 months and once daily thereafter for 3 months (Fig. 32.4).

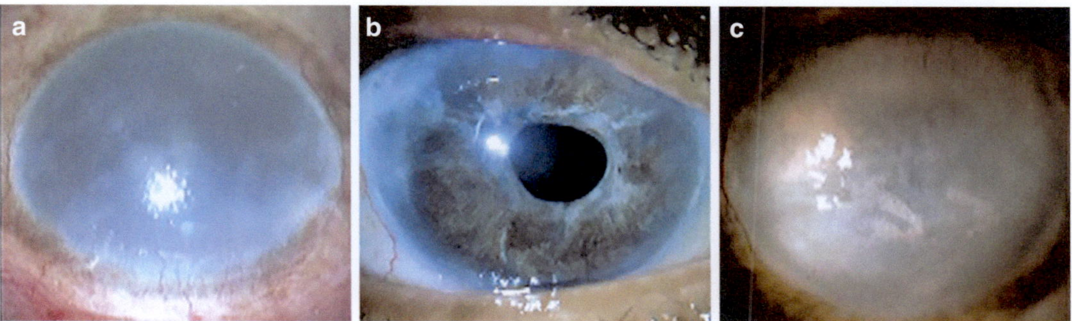

Fig. 32.4 Pseudophakic bullous keraopathy (one-eyed patient) with silicone oil in the eye. Preop on the left and post op on the middle and fellow eye on the right. (**a**) Preoperative image of a case with silicon oil in the eye and pseudophakic bullous keratopathy. (**b**) Postoperative image of the case, (**c**) Dense keraopathy in the other eye of the case.

Donor Tissue

Donor graft characteristics form a crucial part of tissue selection for endothelial keratoplasty procedure. Harvesting a donor graft for the DMEK procedure from individuals less than 40 years of age is difficult as the tissue gets rolled and curls up against itself. Surgeons therefore prefer to use tissue from older donors. This situation does not seem to be a limitation for the PDEK procedure as the graft is comparatively thicker, and the additional layer of PDL provides a splinting effect to the tissue.

The authors have a wide experience with the usage of young donor corneas for the PDEK procedure. In a prospective study, the application and usage of infant donor corneas where the donor age ranged from 9 months to 1 year have also been documented [5, 6].

In a young donor, strong adhesions are present between the DM and the PDL. Therefore, it is easy to create a Type-1 bubble as compared to type-2 bubble, which is a pre-requisite for DMEK. These adhesions therefore facilitate achieving a graft for the PDEK procedure than a DMEK procedure.

Importance of Performing an Iris Repair for Endothelial Keratoplasty Procedure in Complicated Cases

In cases with traumatic/iatrogenic iris defects, the importance of iris reconstruction with pupilloplasty method cannot be undermined [7, 8]. An inadvertent opening in the iris can act as a potential source of air leakage into the retroiridial space or the vitreous cavity depending upon the clinical situation. This eventually decreases the air-tamponade effect on the donor lenticule and may contribute to decreased graft adhesion to the host interface, eventually leading to graft detachment.

The authors usually perform Single pass 4-throw (SFT) pupilloplasty [9] procedure for iris repair in cases associated with dislocated/subluxated IOL with endothelial decompensation (Figs. 32.5, 32.6, 32.7 and 32.8).

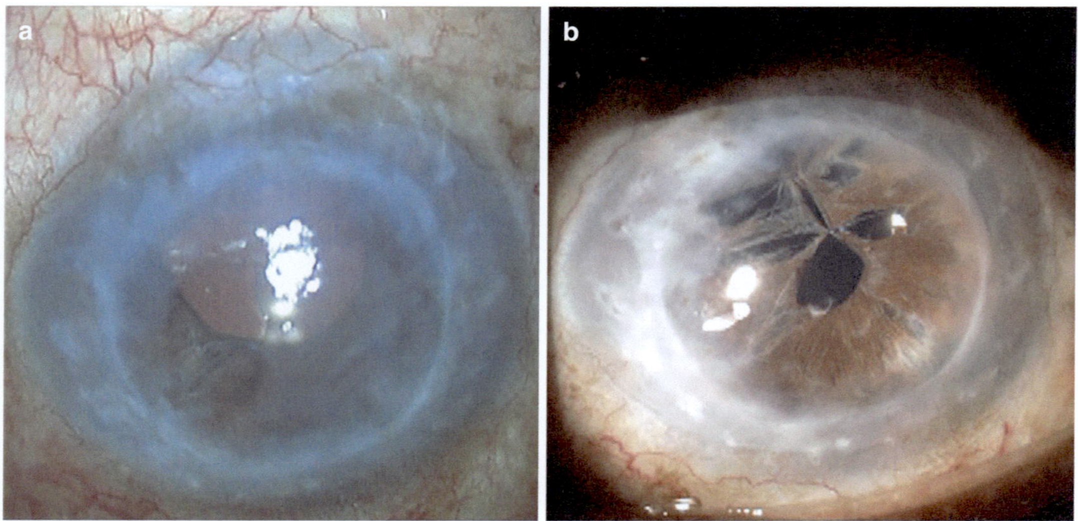

Fig. 32.5 Failed PK case treated with PDEK and single pass 4 throw pupilloplasty. Preop on the left and post op on the right

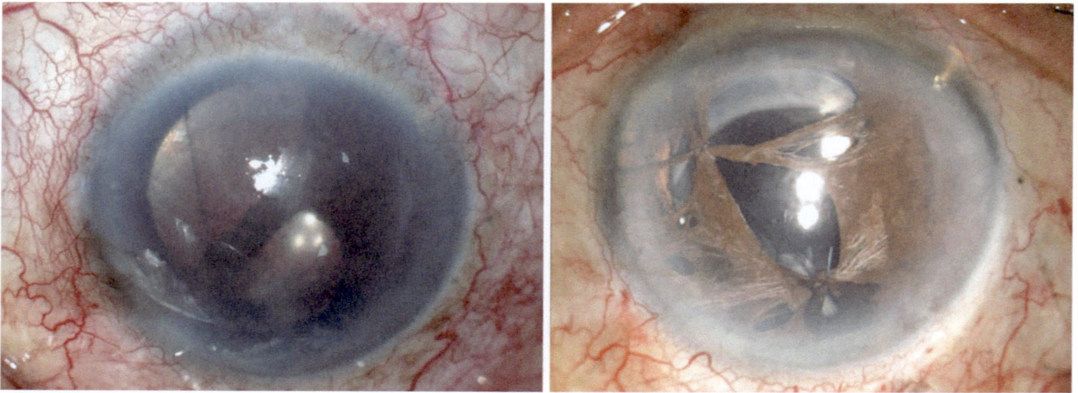

Fig. 32.6 Pseudophakic bullous keratopathy with iridodialysis treated with PDEK and trocar assisted iridodialysis repair and single pass 4 throw pupilloplasty. Preop on the left and post op on the right

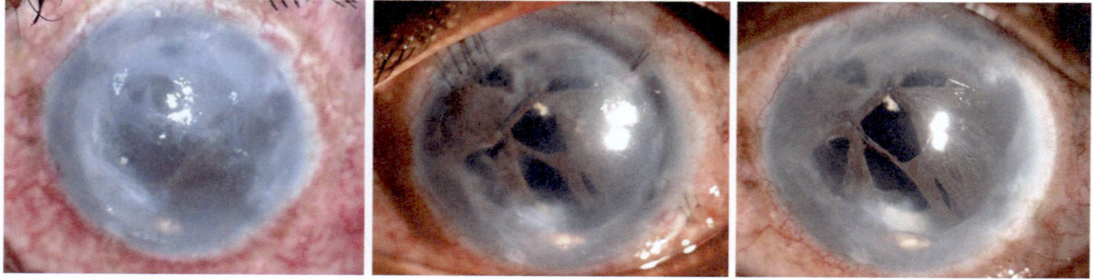

Fig. 32.7 Pseudophakic bullous keratopathy in a one-eyed patient treated with PDEK and single pass 4 throw pupilloplasty

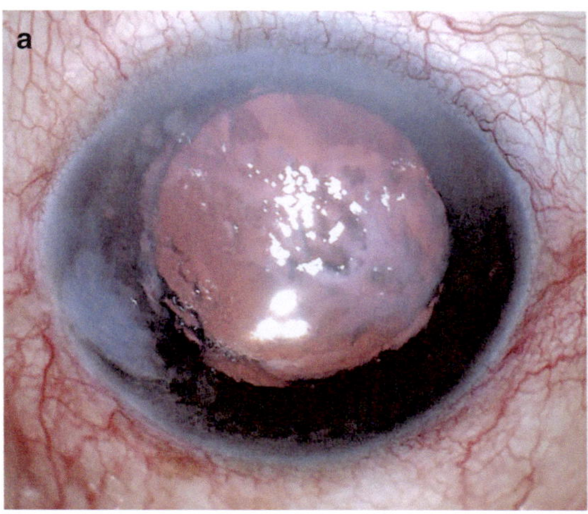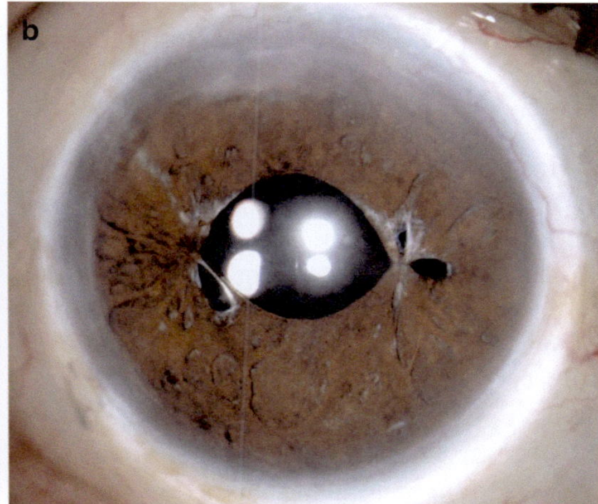

Fig. 32.8 Pseudophakic bullous keratopathy treated with PDEK and single pass 4 throw pupilloplasty. (**a**) Pre-op, (**b**) Post-op

Combined Procedures

Double-Infusion Cannula Technique (DICT)

In double infusion cannula technique (DICT) [10], two infusion cannulas are introduced: Trocar cannula for fluid infusion is introduced at the pars plana site and either an anterior chamber maintainer (ACM) or a trocar ACM (T-ACM) is introduced in the anterior segment for air infusion while performing a combined procedure of glued IOL with an endothelial keratoplasty procedure. Aphakic, prior vitrectomized eyes, and complicated IOL cases pose a definite challenge to graft unfolding and its adherence to the recipient's eye. In the absence of posterior segment infusion, these eyes are more prone to global collapse. This automatically translates into poor outcomes for the EK surgery. The infusion fluid in the vitreous cavity prevents globe collapse and helps to maintain adequate pressure in the posterior segment. This also prevents seepage of air from the anterior to the posterior segment, thereby maintaining an adequate air tamponade anteriorly that facilitates graft adherence intraoperatively as well as in the postoperative period too.

Optimizing PDEK Graft

Microscope-integrated optical coherence tomography (i-OCT) [11] can optimize the PDEK donor graft preparation by providing direct visualization and guiding the surgeon by providing details of the appropriate depth of corneal tissue. I-OCT has been demonstrated to facilitate Type-1 bubble formation, thereby decreasing the chances of donor tissue loss. I-OCT navigates the surgeon through all the stages of PDEK surgery in addition to serving as an indicator for appropriate graft adhesion and wound apposition.

PDEK clamp described by Dua et al. enables appropriate handling of the sclero-corneal donor tissue and allows consistently obtaining a PDEK graft [12, 13]. The clamp prevents the air to escape from the fenestration around the PDL, thereby decreasing the chances of the formation of Type-2 bubble. The mean size of type-1 bubble achieved with the PDEK clamp, as documented in a study, was $7.255 \pm 0.535 \times 6.745 \pm 0.668$ mm, and the volume of air required to obtain type-1 bubble is 0.14–0.37 mL.

PDEK Results and Analyses

In our study [14], we analyzed the postoperative graft thickness, graft configuration and detachment using spectral-domain optical coherence tomography (SD-OCT) at 1, 7, 30 and 90 days postoperatively.

The donor age ranged from 1 to 65 years, and the graft size ranged from 7.5 to 8.0 mm. The mean graft thickness observed at 1 day was 37.3 G3.5 mm (range 32–44 mm), at 7 days, 30 days and 90 days was 35.5 ± 3.4 mm (range 32–40 mm), 33 ± 1.8 mm (range 32–36 mm) and 30.3 ± 2.6 mm (range 28–36 mm), respectively. A statistically significant difference was observed in the graft thickness over the time period. The graft was well attached in all eyes except one eye that had grade 3 detachment. Total graft detachment or lenticular drop was not observed in any case.

Interface haze was minimal (1 eye/12 eyes) that receded over a period of 1 month postoperatively. The 1-day postoperative corneal edema showed significant resolution over 1-week follow-up. A statistically significant improvement in visual acuity from preoperatively to postoperatively. The final corrected distance visual acuity (CDVA) was 0.61 G 0.2. In our analysis, no significant correlation between the graft thickness and the CDVA at 1 day was observed.

As per Busin et al., the mean central graft thickness in the ultrathin DSAEK graft was 78.28 ± 28.89 mm at 3 months postoperatively [15]. The PDEK grafts are thicker than DMEK grafts but thinner than those observed in ultrathin DSAEK.

Raising the pressure in the anterior chamber might be helpful by increasing the intracorneal pressure, as negative imbibition pressure of both the donor and recipient corneal tissues might add to tissue adherence [16].

Summary

To summarize, PDEK is a technique that is reproducible and is easy to perform. It scores over DMEK in ways that it allows the usage of donors of any age group. This can be a huge advantage, especially in situations where there is a shortage of pool of donor corneas.

Dislosures No financial disclosures.

References

1. Dua HS, Faraj LA, Said DG, et al. Human corneal anatomy redefined: a novel pre-Descemet's layer (Dua's layer). Ophthalmology. 2013;120:1778–85.
2. Agarwal A, Dua HS, Narang P, et al. Pre-Descemet's endothelial keratoplasty (PDEK). Br J Ophthalmol. 2014;98:1181–5.
3. Price FW Jr, Price MO. Descemet's stripping with endothelial keratoplasty in 200 eyes: early challenges and technique to enhance donor adherence. J Cataract Refract Surg. 2006;32:411–8.
4. Jacob S, Agarwal A, Agarwal A, et al. Endoilluminator-assisted transcorneal illumination for Descemet membrane endothelial keratoplasty: enhanced intraoperative visualization of the graft in corneal decompensation secondary to pseudophakic bullous keratopathy. J Cataract Refract Surg. 2014;40:1332–6.
5. Agarwal A, Agarwal A, Narang P, Kumar DA, Jacob S. Pre-Descemet endothelial keratoplasty with infant donor corneas: a prospective analysis. Cornea. 2015;34(8):859–65.
6. Agarwal A, Narang P, Kumar DA, Agarwal A. Young donor-graft assisted endothelial keratoplasty (PDEK/DMEK) with epithelial debridement for chronic pseudophakic bullous keratopathy. Can J Ophthalmol. 2017;52(5):519–26.
7. Narang P, Agarwal A. Triple procedure for pseudophakic bullous keratopathy in complicated cataract surgery: glued IOL with single-pass four-throw pupilloplasty with pre-Descemet's endothelial keratoplasty. J Cataract Refract Surg. 2019;45(4):398–403.
8. Narang P, Agarwal A, Kumar DA. Single-pass 4-throw pupilloplasty for pre-Descemet endothelial keratoplasty. Cornea. 2017;36(12):1580–3.

9. Narang P. Agarwal a single-pass four-throw technique for pupilloplasty. Eur J Ophthalmol. 2017;27(4):506–8.
10. Narang P, Agarwal A. Double-infusion cannula technique for glued fixation of intraocular lens with endothelial keratoplasty. Can J Ophthalmol. 2018;53(5):503–9.
11. Sharma N, Devi C, Agarwal R, Bafna RK, Agarwal A. I-PDEK: microscope-integrated OCT-assisted pre-Descemet endothelial keratoplasty. J Cataract Refract Surg. 2021;47(12):e44–8.
12. Dua HS. Said DG pre-Descemets endothelial keratoplasty: the PDEK clamp for successful PDEK. Eye (Lond). 2017;31(7):1106–10.
13. Ross AR, Said DG, Colabelli Gisoldi RAM, Nubile M, El-Amin A, Gabr AF, Abd Ed-Moniem M, Mencucci R, Pocobelli A, Mastropasqua L, Dua HS. Optimizing pre-Descemet endothelial keratoplasty technique. J Cataract Refract Surg. 2020;46(5):667–74.
14. Kumar DA, Dua HS, Agarwal A, Jacob S. Postoperative spectral-domain optical coherence tomography evaluation of pre-Descemet endothelial keratoplasty grafts. J Cataract Refract Surg. 2015;41(7):1535–6. https://doi.org/10.1016/j.jcrs.2015.05.015.
15. Busin M, Madi S, Santorum P, Scoria V, Beltz J. Ultrathin Descemet's stripping automated endothelial keratoplasty with the microkeratome double-pass technique; two-year outcomes. Ophthalmology. 2013;120:1186–94.
16. Dapena I, Ham L, Melles GRJ. Endothelial keratoplasty: DSEK/DSAEK or DMEK—the thinner the better? Curr Opin Ophthalmol. 2009;20:299–307.

Descemet Membrane Transplantation

33

Hon Shing Ong and Jodhbir S. Mehta

Key Points

- Descemet Membrane Transplantation is a form of regenerative therapy.
- It is indicated for patients with localized endothelial dysfunction caused by FECD.
- It requires acellular Descemet Membrane to be used as a scaffold for cellular migration.
- Adjuvant topical Rock Inhibitors are indicated in older patients.

Supplementary Information The online version contains supplementary material available at https://doi.org/10.1007/978-3-031-32408-6_33.

H. S. Ong
Corneal and External Diseases Department,
Singapore National Eye Centre, Singapore, Singapore

Tissue Engineering and Cell Therapy Department,
Singapore Eye Research Institute, Singapore,
Singapore

Ophthalmology and Visual Sciences Academic
Clinical Programme, Duke-NUS Medical School,
Singapore, Singapore
e-mail: ong.hon.shing@singhealth.com.sg

Introduction

The metabolically active corneal endothelium plays an important function in maintaining optimal corneal hydration, which is required to keep the cornea transparent and essential for good vision [1, 2]. In corneal endothelial diseases, there is an accelerated loss of healthy corneal endothelial cells (CEnCs). Below a certain threshold, the corneal endothelium loses its ability to regulate corneal hydration. The cornea becomes oedematous with a consequent loss in its transparency [3–5]. This is corneal endothelial failure, which results in visual impairment.

As human CEnCs are arrested in a dormant, non-proliferative G_1 phase of the cell cycle, their regenerative potential in vivo is thought to be limited [6–9]. The restoration of vision in patients with corneal endothelial failure thus relies on a

J. S. Mehta (✉)
Corneal and External Diseases Department,
Singapore National Eye Centre, Singapore, Singapore

Tissue Engineering and Cell Therapy Department,
Singapore Eye Research Institute, Singapore,
Singapore

Ophthalmology and Visual Sciences Academic
Clinical Programme, Duke-NUS Medical School,
Singapore, Singapore

School of Material Science and Engineering and
School of Mechanical and Aerospace Engineering,
Nanyang Technological University, Singapore,
Singapore

replacement of an exogenous source of donor endothelial cells through corneal transplantation. Corneal transplantation is thus currently the main treatment to restore vision impaired by corneal endothelial diseases.

With significant developments in corneal transplantation surgeries to treat corneal diseases, good outcomes can often be achieved when such advanced techniques are applied. However, limitations do exist with all types of allogenic corneal transplantations. In addition to the need for a considerable level of subspecialised surgical expertise and the cost of surgery, inherent risks of corneal transplantations include allogenic graft rejection and associated graft failure [10–12]. Furthermore, performing donor-reliant corneal transplantations is limited by a shortage of suitable transplantable donor corneal tissues [13]. In a 2012 report, the current donor availability only meets 1.4% of the global requirements for corneal transplantations, with 50% of individuals worldwide without access to suitable donor corneas [13].

Thus, there is an impetus to pursue alternative, less donor-reliant treatment approaches for diseases of the corneal endothelium. One such area approach is regenerative medicine. Regenerative medicine involves the reparation and restoration of diseased cells or the re-distribution of remaining healthy cells to replace lost cells in an attempt to restore physiological function. Various potential regenerative strategies to restore corneal endothelial function have been reported [14]. One approach to corneal endothelial regeneration is the induction of CEnCs to leave the dormant G_1 phase of the cell cycle and enter the proliferative S phase. Pharmacological agents, such as rho-associated protein kinase (ROCK) inhibitors, have been widely reported to promote cell adhesion, inhibit apoptosis and enhance cell proliferation in cultured primate and human CEnCs [15, 16]. Clinical reports have described the recovery of corneal endothelial function following transcorneal freezing of patients with corneal endothelial dysfunction and the administration of ROCK inhibitor drops [17, 18]. Nevertheless, side effects of ROCK inhibitors, such as conjunctival hyperaemia, subconjunctival haemorrhage,

corneal verticillate, ocular surface inflammation and discomfort, and reticular bullous epithelial oedema can occur [19]. Furthermore, by definition, a regenerative approach to the treatment of corneal endothelial disease requires some remaining healthy CEnCs in the patient's cornea. In diseases with widespread damage and loss of CEnCs (e.g. pseudophakic bullous keratopathy), the utility of regenerative medicine will thus be limited. Instead, a cell-based therapeutic approach in these conditions which involves the injection of CEnCs expanded in culture may be more appropriate [20]. In this chapter, we introduce a regenerative therapeutic approach of Descemet membrane transplantation (DMT) as a novel surgical technique to treat corneal endothelial diseases.

The Concept of Centripetal Host Corneal Endothelial Cell Migration

The DMT technique is based on the concept of centripetal host corneal endothelial cell migration. Reports using sex-mismatched transplant tissues have indicated that recipient corneal endothelial cells in the periphery can exhibit centripetal migration across the graft–host junction to populate and integrate with the endothelium of donor tissues [21]. Furthermore, superior graft survival is often observed in transplantations performed for corneal endothelial diseases where the peripheral corneal endothelium is relatively preserved (e.g. Fuchs' Endothelial Corneal Dystrophy), compared to conditions where there is more widespread endothelium damage (e.g. pseudophakic bullous keratopathy) [22]. Such observations suggest that migration of peripheral host corneal endothelial cells to the central cornea contributes towards post-transplantation stability of the corneal endothelium.

Using this concept of centripetal host corneal endothelial cell migration, the first surgical technique introduced to treat patients with Fuchs' Endothelial Corneal Dystrophy (FECD) is 'Descemet Stripping Only' (DSO), previously known as 'Descemet Stripping Without Endothelial Keratoplasty' (DWEK) [23]. In

DSO, the central diseased Descemet membrane of the patient is removed (descemetorhexis) without transplantation, with the anticipation that healthy peripheral corneal endothelial cells will migrate centrally to establish a functional corneal endothelium. Nonetheless, the evidence of DSO is based mostly on non-comparative clinical case series, where varying results have been reported [24–28].

Our group observed that an intact Descemet membrane enhances the migration of endothelial cells and facilitates the formation of a corneal endothelial monolayer [29]. The presence of a Descemet membrane has also been shown to minimize endothelial–mesenchymal transition (EMT) when compared to endothelial cell migration across a bare posterior corneal surface [30]. Based on such observations, a technique of DMT was introduced [31]. In DMT, an acellular Descemet membrane is transferred and made to adhere to the patient's posterior cornea over the central area of descemetorhexis [29, 31]. We observed the restoration of functional integrity of the corneal endothelium through the central migration of peripheral endothelial cells [29, 31]. This technique also allowed us to remove a larger area of diseased central Descemet membrane. In 2018, we reported a first-in-man clinical trial of using DMT as a regenerative therapeutic approach for FECD [31].

Surgical Technique

Descemet Membrane Graft Preparation

A cadaveric donor cornea of low corneal endothelial cell density, unsuitable for penetrating or endothelial keratoplasty was procured from the eye bank. Corneal endothelial cells were removed from the donor cornea using a double freeze-thaw cycle, followed by denudation with a customized silicone soft-tip cannula (catalogue number: SP-125053, ASICO, USA). (Fig. 33.1a–c) A DMT graft was then harvested using the 'Submerged Cornea Using Backgrounds Away' (SCUBA) technique designed for Descemet membrane endothelial keratoplasty (DMEK) graft harvesting. A small acellular Descemet membrane graft (4–5 mm) was harvested using a free-hand corneal trephine. It was also marked to ensure the correct orientation was maintained during graft insertion.

Descemet Membrane Graft Insertion

The technique of insertion of the acellular Descemet membrane graft was similar to that used for standard DMEK surgery. Figure 33.1d–f illustrate the surgical steps of DMT in a patient who had undergone a DMT procedure. A descemetorhexis was performed to remove the central diseased recipient Descemet membrane and endothelium. The diameter to be stripped was 0.5 mm larger than the size of Descemet's membrane graft that was to be transplanted. The harvested Descemet membrane graft was stained using vital dyes (Membrane Blue Dual®, D.O.R.C, The Netherlands), loaded and injected into the eye using a standard glass injector used for DMEK (Geuder, Heidelberg, Germany) through a 2.8-mm temporal corneal incision. An anterior chamber maintainer was placed to avoid anterior chamber collapse during graft insertion. Within the anterior chamber, the graft was unfolded through various tapping manoeuvers over the corneal surface, whilst maintaining a correct graft orientation. It was then made to adhere to the posterior corneal surface within the area of descemetorhexis using a non-expansile concentration of sulphur hexafluoride gas (SF_6 20%) (Video 33.1).

Post-operatively, patients were instructed to adopt a face-up posture for at least 3 h. They were prescribed topical antibiotics (levofloxacin 0.5%, Santen Pharmaceutical, Osaka, Japan) and steroids (dexamethasone 0.1%, Alcon, TX USA), which were tapered off after 1 month. For patients over 50 years of age, a topical ROCK inhibitor was also prescribed in the post-operative period.

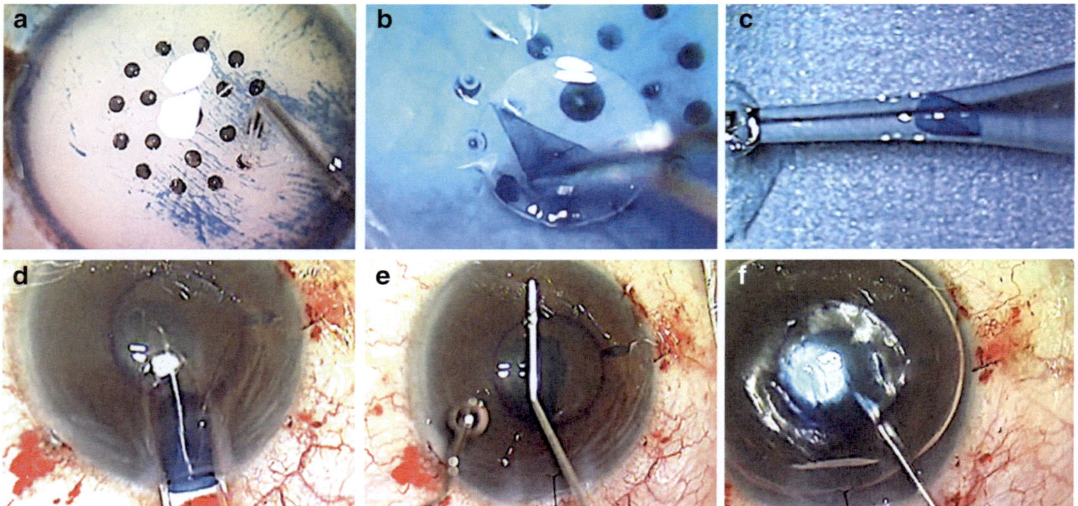

Fig. 33.1 Surgical technique of the Descemet Membrane Transplantation. (**a**) Following a double freeze-thaw cycle, donor Descemet membrane (DM) is scraped with custom-made silicone tip cannula (SP-125053, ASICO, USA) to remove endothelial cells; (**b**) donor DM is scored and peeled and trephined in a similar technique to Descemet Stripping Endothelial Keratoplasty (DMEK); note trypan blue stains the entire posterior surface of the donor DM showing that it is completely acellular; (**c**, **d**) Descemet Membrane graft is loaded into a glass injector (Geuder, Heidelberg, Germany) and inserted into the recipient's anterior chamber; (**e**) the Descemet Membrane graft is unfolded using various tapping techniques on the recipient's corneal surface; (**f**) gas bubble is injected into the anterior chamber to provide tamponade of the Descemet's membrane graft

Case Series

At the time of writing, we have performed a total of seven cases of DMT at the Singapore National Eye Centre (Table 33.1). All patients were recruited under a clinical trial. Ethical approval of the study protocol was granted by the SingHealth Centralized Institutional Review Board (IRB reference number: R1366/52/2016). All surgeries and evaluations were performed in accordance with the tenets of the Declaration of Helsinki.

The diagnosis of all patients was Fuchs' Endothelial Corneal Dystrophy (FECD). The baseline preoperative visual acuities of the patients ranged from 6/12 to 6/21. Preoperative ultrasound measured central corneal thickness ranging from 576 μm to 778 μm (Sonogage Inc., Cleveland, USA). For all patients, the preoperative central corneal endothelial cell densities assessed through specular microscopy were not recordable due to the severity of corneal guttata and oedema (Konan Medical Corp, Hyogo, Japan). All patients had relatively preserved peripheral corneal endothelium, as illustrated in Fig. 33.2.

As all patients had significant lenticular opacities, a combined triple procedure of phacoemulsification with an intraocular lens implant (phaco/IOL) for the management of cataracts and DMT for the management of FECD was offered. Post-operative topical ROCK inhibitor (Netarsudil, Aerie Pharmaceuticals, New Jersey, United States) was administered to five of the patients, starting with a four times daily dosing and tapering over the course of four to 6 months, depending on the clinical course. Two patients experienced conjunctival hyperaemia, and one patient (Case 6) developed a reticular bullous epithelial oedema (Fig. 33.3), thought to be associated with the topical administration of Netarsudil drops.

During the 6 month post-operative period, six out of the seven patients responded favourably

Table 33.1 Demographic data on patients included in the study

Case	Age, Sex, Ethnicity[a]	Diagnosis	Procedure performed	Pre-operative Best corrected visual acuity	Pre-operative CCT (μm)	Resolution of corneal oedema	Best corrected visual acuity[b]	Post-operative CCT (μm)[b]	Post-operative ROCK inhibitor (Netarsudil)
1	56, F, C	FECD	Phaco/IOL/DMT	6/18	603	Yes	6/7.5	483	No
2	37, F, P	FECD	Phaco/IOL/DMT	6/12	673	Yes	6/9	632	No
3	51, M, A	FECD	Phaco/IOL/DMT	6/21	645	Yes	6/12	620	Yes
4	53, F, C	FECD	Phaco/IOL/DMT	6/12	778	Yes	6/12	519	Yes
5	71, F, C	FECD	Phaco/IOL/DMT	6/15	645	Yes	6/15	437	Yes
6[c]	66, M, C	FECD	Phaco/IOL/DMT	6/12	576	No	CF	785	Yes[d]
7	64, F, C	FECD	Phaco/IOL/DMT	6/12	643	Partial	6/18	467	Yes

M Male, *F* Female, *C* Chinese, *P* Filipino *A* Arab, *FECD* fuchs endothelial corneal dystrophy, *Phaco* phacoemulsification, *IOL* intraocular lens implantation, *DMT* descemet membrane transplantation, *CCT* central corneal thickness, *ROCK* rho-associated protein kinase, *NA* not available (data), *CF* counting fingers

[a]Age in years
[b]Outcomes at 6 months
[c]Subsequently underwent a successful Descemet membrane endothelial keratoplasty (DMEK) at month 8
[d]Developed ROCK inhibitor-associated reticular bullous keratopathy

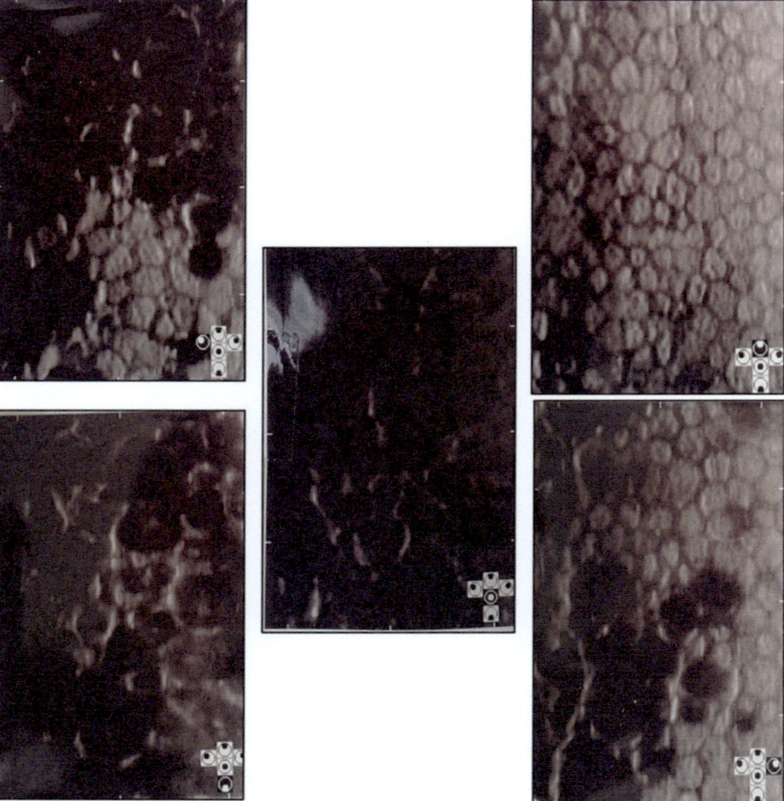

Fig. 33.2 Representative pre-operative specular microscopy (Konan Medical Corp, Hyogo, Japan) images of a patient included in this case series illustrating severe corneal guttata and corneal endothelial cell loss in the central cornea with relatively preserved peripheral corneal endothelium

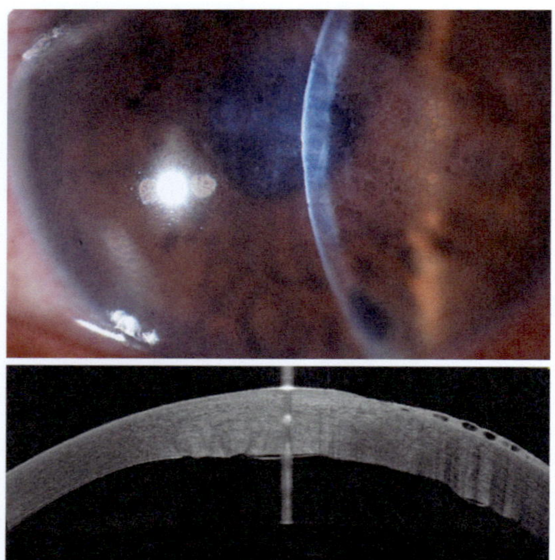

Fig. 33.3 Slit-lamp images and corresponding anterior segment optical coherence tomography (RTVue, Optovue, Fremont, USA) of Case 6 illustrating reticular epithelial bullous oedema associated with the use of rho-associated protein kinase (ROCK) inhibitor

(Fig. 33.4, Table 33.1). There was a progressive resolution of central corneal oedema, with full resolution in five patients and partial resolution of oedema in one patient. All DMT grafts remained attached. Post-operative visual acuities ranged from 6/7.5 to 6/18 in these six patients. By 6 months, all six patients had successfully weaned off all topical medications. One patient's cornea failed to clear following DMT (Case 6). This is the same patient who developed the ROCK inhibitor-associated reticular bullous epithelial oedema, where the drops had to be stopped prematurely. He subsequently underwent a successful DMT removal with Descemet's membrane endothelial keratoplasty at month 8 following his original DMT (Table 33.1).

Time points	POW1	POM6
BCVA	Count Fingers	6/7.5
CCT (μm)	871	570

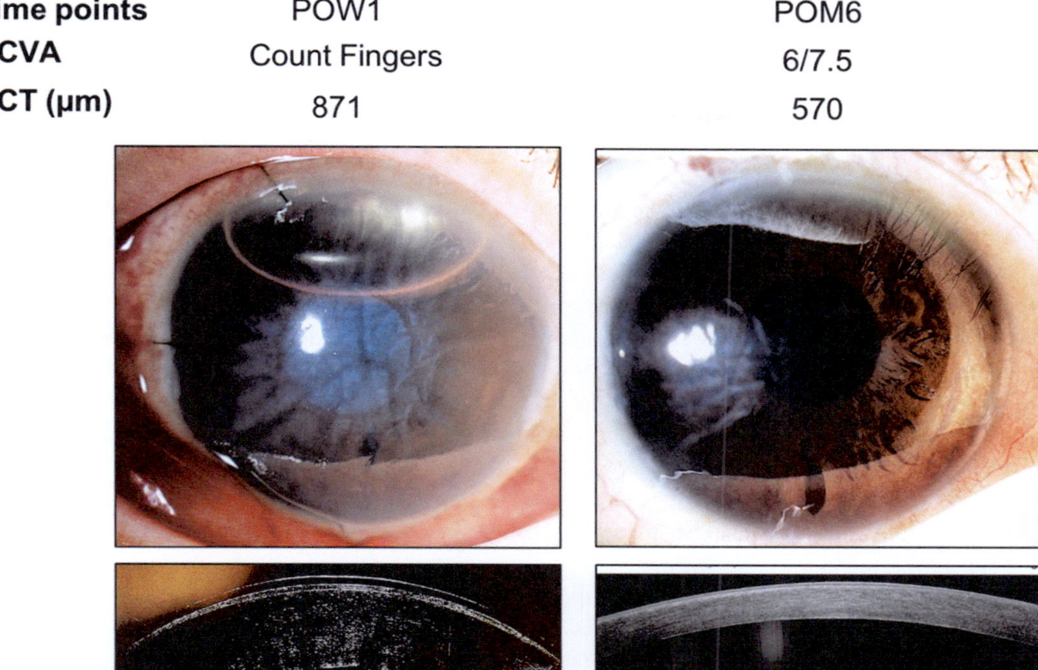

Fig. 33.4 Representative images illustrating the post-operative recovery of a patient who underwent Descemet's Membrane Transplantation. (Top row) Slit lamp images showing progressive resolution of central corneal oedema over 6 months with improved clarity of the cornea. (Bottom row) There is corresponding reduction in corneal thickness as observed on anterior segment optical coherence tomography (RTVue, Optovue, Fremont, USA). *BCVA* best corrected visual acuity, *CCT* central corneal thickness, *POW* post-operative week, *POM* post-operative month

Discussion

Through DMT, we showed that appropriately selected patients with endothelial dysfunction could circumvent the need for allogenic transplantation, thus avoiding the risks of graft rejection and the need for long-term immunosuppressive therapies. Furthermore, a significant proportion of donor corneas harvested worldwide are not utilized due to low corneal endothelial cell densities [13]. Thus, the utilization of acellular tissues allows for the repurposing of donor corneas that are currently not suitable for standard corneal transplantations.

In such a regenerative therapeutic approach, one factor to take into consideration is the population of remaining healthy host CEnCs in the periphery following the central removal of diseased endothelium. It has been shown that a larger population of peripheral CEnCs after Descemet membrane removal contributes to better endothelial stability following centripetal migration and a faster recovery of endothelial function [32]. We thus propose that a small Descemet membrane graft is used (4–5 mm). Given that the size of the Descemet membrane graft is small, multiple grafts can also be harvested from one donor cornea. Indeed, one donor corneal tissue could be potentially used to treat multiple patients with endothelial diseases.

To ensure the success of DMT, the selection of patients is also important. We have previously reported that increasing age is associated with a decline in the migration potential of human corneal endothelial cells [30]. For older patients above the age of 50 years, we propose that corneal endothelial cellular migration should be enhanced with the application of topical ROCK inhibitors (e.g. ripasudil, netarsudil). The role of these agents and the longer term outcomes of DMT requires further evaluation. It is also worth highlighting that in such regenerative therapeutic approaches, the CEnCs that migrate centripetally from the peripheral cornea may be the patient's diseased cells (e.g. FECD). Thus, clinical features such as the presence of guttata may still develop within the migrated cells in the transplanted Descemet membrane graft. Nonetheless, such regenerative approaches would have delayed the timing at which corneal transplantation is needed.

Compared to other regenerative techniques such as DSO, clinical studies assessing DSO for FECDs have reported inconsistent outcomes [24–28]. A recent systematic review of 11 publications indicated that the results of DSO are likely to be more predictable if ≤4 mm of the patient's central diseased Descemet membrane is removed [33]. Other groups have also reported better outcomes of DSO when topical ROCK inhibitors are applied [27, 28]. However, adequately powered randomized controlled studies with sufficient follow-up are still needed to establish the efficacy of DSO as an intervention.

The presence of a Descemet membrane graft in DMT to support CEnC migration appears to reduce the risk of endothelial-to-mesenchymal transition (EMT) compared to CEnC migration across a denuded corneal stroma in DSO [29, 30]. Furthermore, following primary descemetorhexis in DSO may predispose the activation of stromal keratocytes in the posterior cornea to fibroblastic transformation through the exposure of mediators (e.g. TGFß) found in the aqueous humour, which may ultimately lead to fibrosis [34]. The presence of a Descemet membrane graft in DMT may act as a barrier between the aqueous humour and posterior stromal keratocytes to avoid such pro-fibrotic phenotypic transformations. Nevertheless, despite these theoretic advantages of DMT over DSO, further clinical trials with sufficient follow-up are required to determine the longer term safety and efficacies of these novel therapies.

Take Home Notes

- Graft orientation of the acellular membrane is important and must not overlap with the recipient DM.
- DMT allows a larger area of guttata to be removed.
- Membrane adhesion is achieved through the full gas fill.
- Key benefits are the lack of long-term steroid use and the use of otherwise unusable tissue hence increasing the donor pool.
- Early physiological response can be seen by 6 weeks on ASOCT, if there is no response, rescue DMEK can be performed with good outcomes.
- More cases are required for a full evaluation of this technique.

References

1. Bonanno JA. Molecular mechanisms underlying the corneal endothelial pump. Exp Eye Res. 2012;95:2–7. https://doi.org/10.1016/j.exer.2011.06.004.
2. Edelhauser HF. The balance between corneal transparency and edema: the proctor lecture. Invest Ophthalmol Vis Sci. 2006;47:1754–67. https://doi.org/10.1167/iovs.05-1139.
3. Tuft SJ, Coster DJ. The corneal endothelium. Eye. 1990;4(Pt 3):389–424. https://doi.org/10.1038/eye.1990.53.
4. McCartney MD, Wood TO, McLaughlin BJ. Freeze-fracture label of functional and dysfunctional human corneal endothelium. Curr Eye Res. 1987;6:589–97.
5. Mahdy MA, Eid MZ, Mohammed MA, Hafez A, Bhatia JR. elationship between endothelial cell loss and microcoaxial phacoemulsification parameters in noncomplicated cataract surgery. Clinical Ophthalmol. 2012;6:503–10. https://doi.org/10.2147/OPTH.S29865.
6. Joyce NC, Meklir B, Joyce SJ, Zieske JD. Cell cycle protein expression and proliferative status in human corneal cells. Invest Ophthalmol Vis Sci. 1996;37:645–55.
7. Joyce NC, Navon SE, Roy S, Zieske JD. Expression of cell cycle-associated proteins in human and rabbit corneal endothelium in situ. Invest Ophthalmol Vis Sci. 1996;37:1566–75.
8. Murphy C, Alvarado J, Juster R, Maglio M. Prenatal and postnatal cellularity of the human corneal endo-

thelium, a quantitative histologic study. Investig Ophthalmol Vis Sci. 1984;25:312–22.

9. Edelhauser HF. The resiliency of the corneal endothelium to refractive and intraocular surgery. Cornea. 2000;19:263–73.

10. Australian Corneal Graft Registry, C. The Australian graft registry 2018 report. 2018. <https://dspace.flinders.edu.au/xmlui/bitstream/handle/2328/37917/ACGR%202018%20Report.pdf?sequence=3&isAllowed=y>.

11. Ang M, Soh Y, Htoon HM, Mehta JS, Tan D. Five-year graft survival comparing Descemet stripping automated endothelial keratoplasty and penetrating keratoplasty. Ophthalmology. 2016;123:1646–52. https://doi.org/10.1016/j.ophtha.2016.04.049.

12. Woo JH, Ang M, Htoon HM, Tan D. Descemet membrane endothelial keratoplasty versus Descemet stripping automated endothelial keratoplasty and penetrating Keratoplasty. Am J Ophthalmol. 2019;207:288–303. https://doi.org/10.1016/j.ajo.2019.06.012.

13. Gain P, et al. Global survey of corneal transplantation and eye banking. JAMA Ophthalmol. 2016;134:167–73. https://doi.org/10.1001/jamaophthalmol.2015.4776.

14. Kumar A, Yun H, Funderburgh ML, Du Y. Regenerative therapy for the cornea. Prog Retin Eye Res. 2022;87:101011. https://doi.org/10.1016/j.preteyeres.2021.101011.

15. Okumura N, et al. Enhancement on primate corneal endothelial cell survival in vitro by a ROCK inhibitor. Invest Ophthalmol Vis Sci. 2009;50:3680–7. https://doi.org/10.1167/iovs.08-2634.

16. Okumura N, et al. Involvement of cyclin D and p27 in cell proliferation mediated by ROCK inhibitors Y-27632 and Y-39983 during corneal endothelium wound healing. Invest Ophthalmol Vis Sci. 2014;55:318–29. https://doi.org/10.1167/iovs.13-12225.

17. Okumura N, et al. The ROCK inhibitor eye drop accelerates corneal endothelium wound healing. Invest Ophthalmol Vis Sci. 2013;54:2493–502. https://doi.org/10.1167/iovs.12-11320.

18. Koizumi N, et al. Rho-associated kinase inhibitor eye drop treatment as a possible medical treatment for Fuchs corneal dystrophy. Cornea. 2013;32:1167–70. https://doi.org/10.1097/ICO.0b013e318285475d.

19. Syed ZA, Rapuano CJ. Rho kinase (ROCK) inhibitors in the management of corneal endothelial disease. Curr Opin Ophthalmol. 2021;32:268–74. https://doi.org/10.1097/ICU.0000000000000748.

20. Ong HS, Ang M, Mehta J. Evolution of therapies for the corneal endothelium: past, present and future approaches. Br J Ophthalmol. 2021;105:454–67. https://doi.org/10.1136/bjophthalmol-2020-316149.

21. Wollensak G, Green WR. Analysis of sex-mismatched human corneal transplants by fluorescence in situ hybridization of the sex-chromosomes. Exp Eye Res. 1999;68:341–6. https://doi.org/10.1006/exer.1998.0611.

22. Coster DJ, Lowe MT, Keane MC, Williams KA. Australian corneal graft Registry, C. a comparison of lamellar and penetrating keratoplasty outcomes: a registry study. Ophthalmology. 2014;121:979–87. https://doi.org/10.1016/j.ophtha.2013.12.017.

23. Kaufman AR, Nose RM, Pineda R 2nd. Descemetorhexis without endothelial keratoplasty (DWEK): proposal for nomenclature standardization. Cornea. 2018;37:e20–1. https://doi.org/10.1097/ICO.0000000000001528.

24. Borkar DS, Veldman P, Colby KA. Treatment of fuchs endothelial dystrophy by descemet stripping without endothelial keratoplasty. Cornea. 2016;35:1267–73. https://doi.org/10.1097/ICO.0000000000000915.

25. Soh YQ, Peh GS, Mehta JS. Evolving therapies for fuchs' endothelial dystrophy. Regen Med. 2018;13:97–115. https://doi.org/10.2217/rme-2017-0081.

26. Artaechevarria Artieda J, Wells M, Devasahayam RN, Moloney G. 5-year outcomes of descemet stripping only in fuchs dystrophy. Cornea. 2020;38(8):1048. https://doi.org/10.1097/ICO.0000000000002270.

27. Garcerant D, et al. Descemet's stripping without endothelial keratoplasty. Curr Opin Ophthalmol. 2019;30:275–85. https://doi.org/10.1097/ICU.0000000000000579.

28. Macsai MS, Shiloach M. Use of topical rho kinase inhibitors in the treatment of fuchs dystrophy after descemet stripping only. Cornea. 2019;38:529–34. https://doi.org/10.1097/ICO.0000000000001883.

29. Bhogal M, Lwin CN, Seah XY, Peh G, Mehta JS. Allogeneic descemet's membrane transplantation enhances corneal endothelial monolayer formation and restores functional integrity following descemet's stripping. Invest Ophthalmol Vis Sci. 2017;58:4249–60. https://doi.org/10.1167/iovs.17-22106.

30. Soh YQ, et al. Predicative factors for corneal endothelial cell migration. Invest Ophthalmol Vis Sci. 2016;57:338–48. https://doi.org/10.1167/iovs.15-18300.

31. Soh YQ, Mehta JS. Regenerative therapy for fuchs endothelial corneal dystrophy. Cornea. 2018;37:523–7. https://doi.org/10.1097/ICO.0000000000001518.

32. Jullienne R, et al. Corneal endothelium self-healing mathematical model after inadvertent descemetorhexis. J Cataract Refract Surg. 2015;41:2313–8. https://doi.org/10.1016/j.jcrs.2015.10.043.

33. Franceschino A, et al. Descemetorhexis without endothelial keratoplasty in fuchs endothelial corneal dystrophy: a systematic review and meta-analysis. Cornea. 2022;41:815–25. https://doi.org/10.1097/ICO.0000000000002855.

34. Chen J, et al. Descemet's membrane supports corneal endothelial Cell regeneration in rabbits. Sci Rep. 2017;7:6983. https://doi.org/10.1038/s41598-017-07557-2.

Femtosecond Laser-Assisted Deep Lamellar Endothelial Keratoplasty

Jorge L. Alió del Barrio, Verónica Vargas, and Bruce D. Allan

Key Points

- Endothelial keratoplasty is not able to restore the corneal transparency if well-established stromal scars are already present.
- However, if the corneal opacity is limited exclusively to the posterior cornea, the removal of the deeper stromal layers, together with the DM and endothelium, could be a viable alternative to PK, avoiding all well-known drawbacks of full-thickness corneal transplantation.
- Classical deep lamellar endothelial keratoplasty (DLEK) is a challenging and time-consuming surgery as it was initially described.
- In the current chapter, we are showing a simplified DLEK technique that integrates the recent advances in femtosecond laser technology and donor corneal tissue preparation.

Supplementary Information The online version contains supplementary material available at https://doi.org/10.1007/978-3-031-32408-6_34.

J. L. A. del Barrio (✉)
Vissum Miranza, Miguel Hernández University, Alicante, Spain

V. Vargas
Cornea, Cataract and Refractive Surgery Unit, Vissum (Miranza Group), Alicante, Spain

B. D. Allan
Cornea and External Disease Service, Moorfields Eye Hospital, London, UK
e-mail: bruce.allan@ucl.ac.uk

Introduction

Descemet's Stripping Automated Endothelial Keratoplasty (DSAEK) and Descemet's Membrane Endothelial Keratoplasty (DMEK) have become the gold standard treatment for corneal endothelial diseases [1, 2]. In DMEK, the recipient dysfunctional Descemet membrane (DM) and endothelial layers are excised and replaced by a healthy DM-endothelium from a donor cornea (same for DSAEK, but with the exception that the donor lenticule also contains a thin layer of stroma), restoring corneal transparency by a resolution of the pre-existing corneal oedema.

Posterior Lamellar Keratoplasty (PLK) was originally described by Melles in 1998 [3]. The surgery was later modified by Terry in 2001 and was termed Deep Lamellar Endothelial Keratoplasty (DLEK) [4–6]. In DLEK, the failed endothelium, DM and a thin lamella of posterior corneal stroma were replaced by a healthy disc of donor corneal tissue which was positioned in the reciprocal host dissection. Manual host lamellar dissection in DLEK was time-consuming, and the posterior side cut, in particular, was technically challenging. Although femtosecond laser assisted tissue preparation was utilised by a number of investigators to simplify corneal tissue dissection [7, 8], DLEK was largely abandoned in favour of Descemet's stripping techniques which do not require host stromal dissection (DSEK, DSAEK and DMEK), and it is now a largely forgotten endothelial keratoplasty modality.

DMEK and other modalities of endothelial keratoplasty are not able to restore transparency if well-established stromal scars are already present. Penetrating keratoplasty (PK) is the normal elective procedure for such cases. However, if corneal opacity is limited exclusively to the posterior cornea, the removal of the deeper stromal layers together with the DM and endothelium, as in DLEK, would be a viable alternative to PK, avoiding all well-known drawbacks of full-thickness corneal transplantation (long visual rehabilitation, suture-related complications, significant residual ametropia, risk of rejection and glaucoma) [9]. For such cases, with posterior stromal opacity but a normal anterior stroma, we have developed a simplified DLEK technique that integrates the recent advances in femtosecond laser technology and donor corneal tissue preparation [10, 11]. This simplified form of DLEK (Femto-DLEK) combined with conventional DSAEK or DMEK donor preparation and insertion techniques has been safe and effective for treating corneal endothelial diseases associated with posterior stromal opacities [10, 11].

Indications

The main indication for Femto-DLEK is a visual impairment resulting from pathologies involving exclusively the deeper posterior corneal stroma and DM, with or without endothelial failure and corneal oedema (Fig. 34.1). Obviously, for this technique to be successful, it is critical to have a healthy epithelium and anterior/mid stroma.

Alternative indications are as follows:

- Endothelial failure or retained deep scarring after deep anterior lamellar keratoplasty (DALK) (Fig. 34.2).
- Revision of a failed DSAEK in cases of pseudophakic bullous keratopathy with an anterior chamber intraocular lens (AC-IOL). If a pseudophakic AC-IOL is properly placed within the AC, Femto-DLEK can be used to enhance the anterior chamber depth and so increase the distance between the IOL and the new donor tissue, thereby reducing the risk of repeat failure due to endothelial touch (Fig. 34.3c).

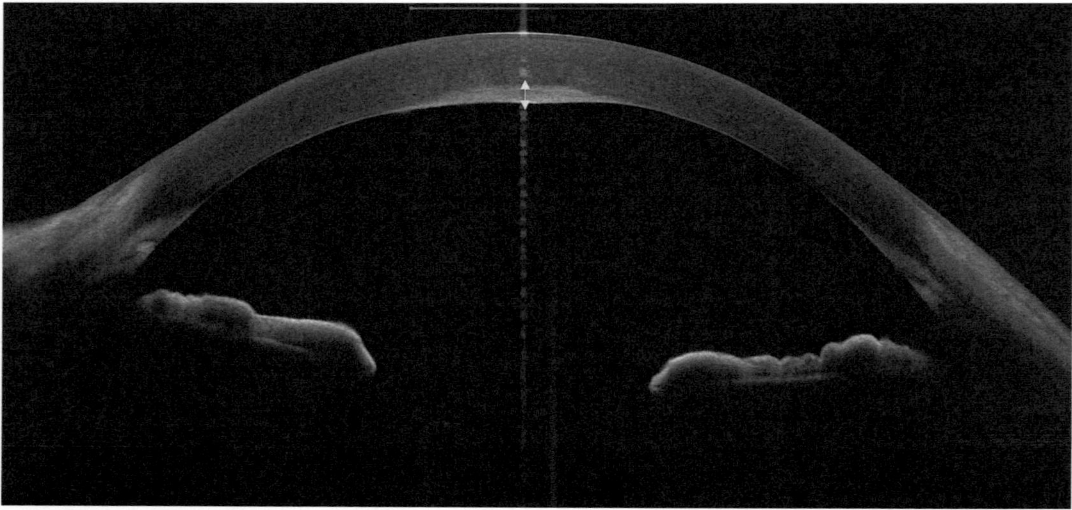

Fig. 34.1 AS-OCT image of a pseudophakic bullous keratopathy associated with a severe deep stromal scar without involving other corneal layers. We can measure the precise depth of the scar (yellow arrows)

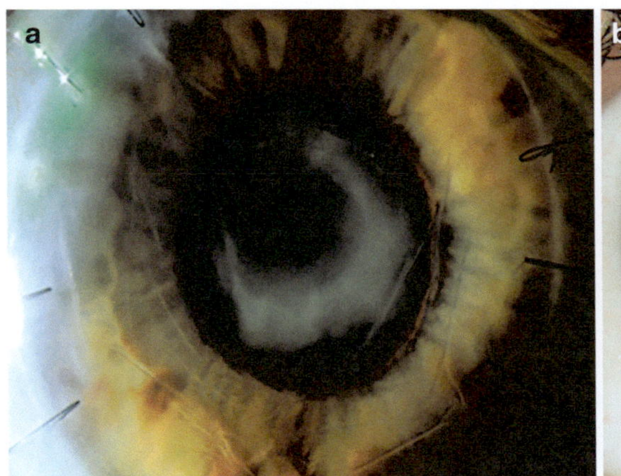
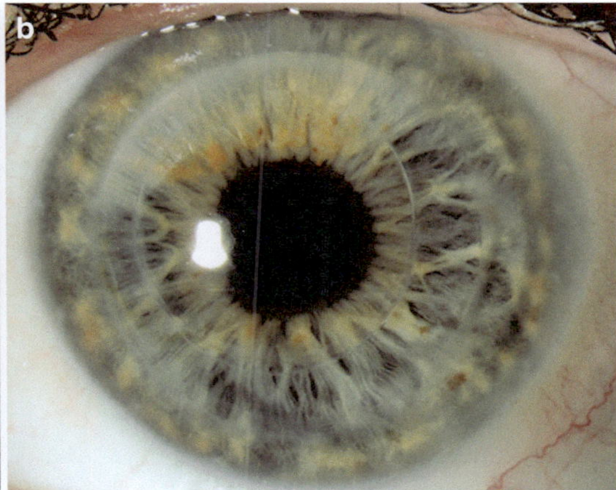

Fig. 34.2 Femto-DLEK (**b**) for retained deep stromal opacity after DALK (**a**)

Preoperative Considerations

Before surgery, the extension and depth of the deep corneal opacity should be identified and measured with anterior segment optical coherence tomography (AS-OCT) (Fig. 34.1).

Surgical Technique

After mapping the extension and depth of the posterior opacification, an overlying manual lamellar dissection plane is created 1 week prior to the endothelial keratoplasty (EK) surgery at approximately 75–85% depth through a 5.0 mm superior scleral incision, using a combination of blunt dissection with the Morlet lamellar dissector (Duckworth & Kent, England) and sharp dissection with a Crescent knife (Alcon, Fort Worth, TX), assisted by an anterior chamber air fill to help judge dissection depth using Melles' air reflection technique. The accuracy of the manually dissected pocket location should be confirmed with AS-OCT prior to the EK surgery (Fig. 34.4).

Then, under local anesthesia with sedation, the IntraLase iFS femtosecond laser (AMO Inc., Irvine, CA) is used to create an intersecting posterior side cut of 7.0–8.5 mm of diameter (depths should be determined by AS-OCT depending on the exact depth of the lamellar dissected plane; femtosecond laser energy settings as previously described) [10]. Subsequently, the dissected posterior recipient disc is removed from the anterior chamber through a 3.2 mm limbal incision placed temporally (Fig. 34.5). A 7.0–8.5 mm DSAEK or DMEK graft is then inserted into the AC and attached to the recipient stroma using a standard DSAEK or DMEK technique (following each surgeon's preference) (Figs. 34.3a, b).

In cases of failure or scarring of the recipient bed after DALK, the posterior side cut is performed without preliminary lamellar dissection, as the deep lamellar plane already exists from the original lamellar surgery, and the unwanted posterior host tissue can simply be peeled away after the posterior side-cut (Video 34.1).

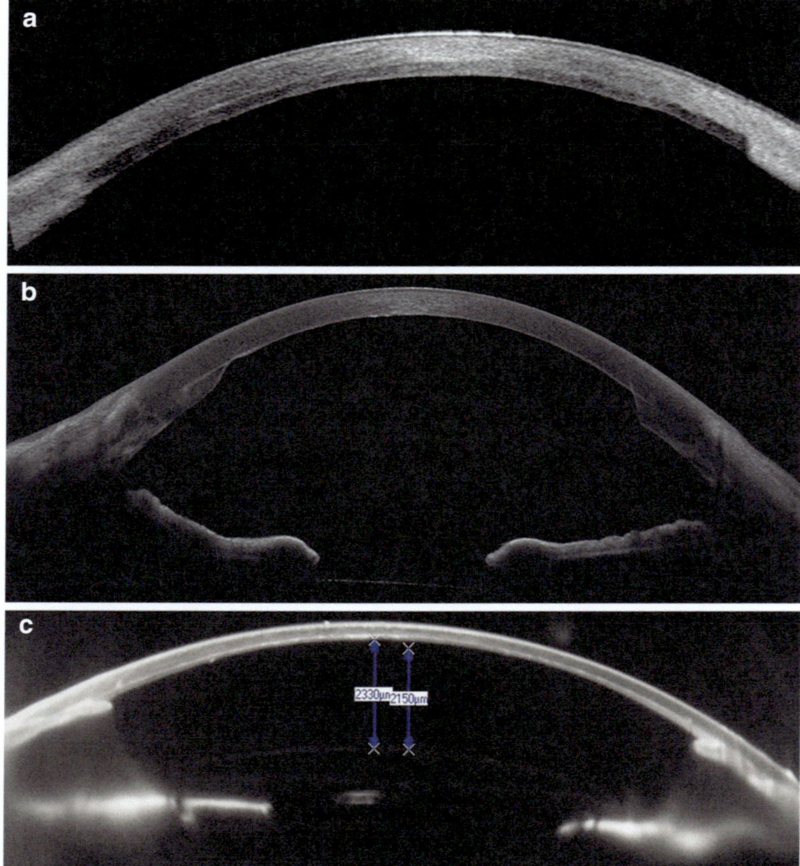

Fig. 34.3 (**a**) AS-OCT image of Femto DL-DSAEK. Observe how the DSAEK lenticule fills the space left after the recipient's posterior cornea removal; (**b**) AS-OCT image of Femto DL-DMEK. Observe how the DMEK lenticule does not fill the space left after the recipient's posterior cornea removal, remaining a step in between the central and peripheral posterior corneal surfaces; (**c**) Scheimpflug image of a Femto DL-DSAEK after previous failed DSAEK providing enhanced clearance between the donor endothelium and the anterior chamber lens in a case of pseudophakic bullous keratopathy

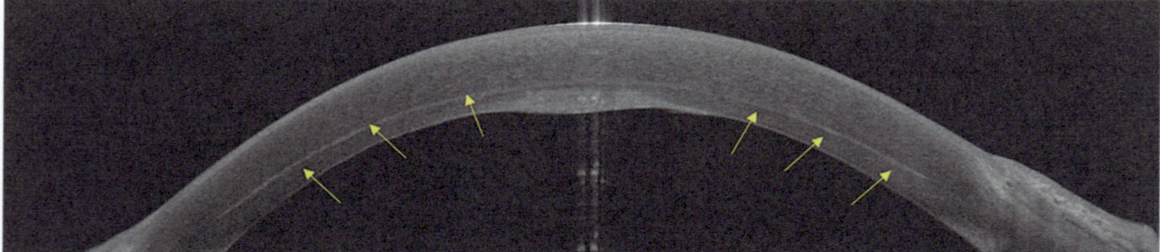

Fig. 34.4 AS-OCT image in which the manually dissected pocket location is confirmed (yellow arrows)

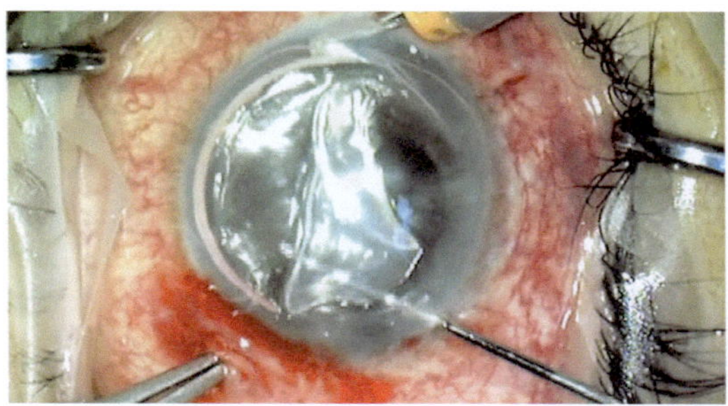

Fig. 34.5 With a reverse sinsky hook, the diseased endothelium-descemet membrane-posterior stroma complex is stripped out from the cornea through a 3.2 mm limbal incision

Postoperative Management

Postoperative care and patient positioning are exactly as for standard DSAEK or DMEK surgery.

Complications

Probably, the most critical step in Femto-DLEK is the manual dissection of the lamellar plane just over the deep stromal opacification (Fig. 34.4). It is not a technically demanding step and its performance is as described for manual DALK by Melles [12]. However, an unsatisfactory dissection plane, either because of a too superficial plane or an incorrect one that leaves a part of the opacity on the anterior cornea in relation to the dissection, will force us to either try a second more accurate lamellar cut (starting from a different pocket) or to abort this technique and to convert into a PK. If available, intraoperative corneal OCT imaging systems could simplify this step by allowing an easy "live" assessment of the correct dissection depth. Alternatively, the femtosecond laser can be used in single pass mode for the recipient posterior corneal lamellar dissection by creating a posterior intrastromal lamellar cut of 7.5–9.0 mm diameter at 400–450 μm depth (depending on the preoperative corneal pachymetry as measured by AS-OCT). However, we recommend manual dissection of this posterior lamellar plane one week in advance as a prepara-

tory step and restricting femtosecond laser assistance to the posterior side cut at the time of DLEK surgery. Our early experience was that posterior stromal femtosecond dissection was incomplete, leaving problematic tissue bridges that were difficult to dissect manually after the posterior side cut. The posterior side cut removes the anchoring counter traction required for easy lamellar dissection, so these tissue bridges usually have to be divided using sharp dissection and counter traction with vitrectomy forceps. This is a challenging manoeuvre that may compromise to host interface smoothness. The reason for this is due to the fact that deep stromal femtosecond laser dissections leave a relatively rougher and more irregular interface compared with the more superficial ones, probably in relation to the scattering of the energy and the anatomical differences between the anterior and the less compacted posterior stromal collagen fibers [13–15].

In Femto-DLEK, after removing the recipient diseased lamellae of the posterior cornea, there will remain a step in between the central and peripheral posterior corneal surfaces, space that will be filled with the endothelial donor tissue (Fig. 34.3a, b). Because of this, correct centration of the DSAEK or DMEK graft into the recipient bed becomes more important than for a standard EK case, as graft decentration may increase the risk for graft detachment.

Outcomes

Existing published evidence ($n = 8$; six cases associated with a DSAEK graft and two associated with a DMEK graft) is insufficient to determine the Femto-DLEK specific rate of other postoperative complications such as rejection, primary failure or graft detachment. Probably, rate of such complications in Femto-DLEK is similar to the observed for standard DSAEK and DMEK surgeries provide the EK graft is well centred within the posterior stromal recipient bed. In our series, two eyes required re-bubbling of the graft for partial detachment 1 week after surgery, and no cases of graft rejection, primary or secondary failure or glaucoma have been observed with more than 1 year follow-up in all cases. Regarding efficacy, aside from two cases with ocular comorbidity affecting the visual outcome, all published eyes achieved a spectacle-corrected distance vision of 6/9 or better.

The use of a DMEK donor graft after Femto-DLEK host dissection (Femto DL-DMEK) may enhance the outcomes by adding the advantages of DMEK over DSAEK (better visual potential, lower rejection rate and faster visual rehabilitation), although a larger sample is still necessary to confirm this statement (Fig. 34.3b) [11, 16].

The potential refractive impact of removing a thick lamella of posterior stroma, particularly when a DMEK donor is used, leaving a countersunk posterior corneal profile (Fig. 34.3a, b) remains uncertain, and further studies will have to explore this. However, considering published evidence and excluding those cases of Femto-DLEK after DALK, no significant impact on the refractive sphere or cylinder has been observed: mean spherical equivalent of +2.85D and mean refractive cylinder of −0.8D ($n = 4$) [10, 11].

Conclusions

DLEK was a technically demanding and challenging surgical technique, but the addition of a femtosecond laser has made the most difficult step – the posterior side cut in host dissection – much easier. Femto DL-DMEK (Fig. 34.3b) or Femto DL-DSAEK (Fig. 34.3a) is a successful and alternative treatment option for treating posterior corneal stromal problems which are causing impaired vision. As far as the anterior and mid stroma are not affected, opacifications of the posterior cornea with or without endothelial dysfunction can benefit from endothelial keratoplasty advantages through a Femto-DLEK procedure, avoiding all well-known drawbacks of PK [9]. The question of whether to exchange AC IOLs for suture-fixated posterior chamber IOLs in cases of pseudophakic bullous keratopathy is unresolved. The goal of exchange for a scleral or iris-fixated posterior chamber IOL, where the existing AC IOL is stable, is to reduce the risk of optic/endothelial touch. Potential complications

of AC IOL exchange include intraoperative haemorrhage, iris trauma, cyclodialysis, pupil distortion, chronic cystoid macular oedema and late failure of fixation with posterior IOL dislocation [17, 18]. Femto-DL-DMEK deepens the anterior chamber and may reduce the risk of graft failure with a stable AC IOL left in situ (Fig. 34.3c).

Take Home Notes

- Femto DL-DMEK or Femto DL-DSAEK is a successful and alternative treatment option for the treatment of posterior corneal stromal problems which are causing impaired vision.
- As far as the anterior and mid-stroma are not affected, opacifications of the posterior cornea with or without endothelial dysfunction can benefit from endothelial keratoplasty advantages through a Femto-DLEK procedure.
- We recommend a manual dissection of the posterior lamellar plane 1 week prior to the transplant as a preparatory step and restricting femtosecond laser assistance to the posterior side cut at the time of DLEK surgery.

Conflict of Interest None of the authors have any conflict of interest to disclose.

References

1. Gorovoy MS. Descemet-stripping automated endothelial keratoplasty. Cornea. 2006;25:886–9.
2. Melles GR, Ong TS, Ververs B, et al. Descemet membrane endothelial Keratoplasty (DMEK). Cornea. 2006;25:987–90.
3. Melles GR, Eggink FA, Lander F, et al. A surgical technique for posterior lamellar keratoplasty. Cornea. 1998;17:618–26.
4. Terry MA, Ousley PJ. Endothelial replacement without surface corneal incisions or sutures: topography of the deep lamellar endothelial keratoplasty procedure. Cornea. 2001;20:14–8.
5. Terry MA. Deep lamellar endothelial keratoplasty (DLEK): pursuing the ideal goals of endothelial replacement. Eye (Lond). 2003;17:982–8.
6. Terry MA, Ousley PJ. Deep lamellar endothelial keratoplasty: visual acuity, astigmatism, and endothelial survival in a large prospective series. Ophthalmology. 2005;112:1541–8.
7. Terry MA, Ousley PJ, Will B. A practical femtosecond laser procedure for DLEK endothelial transplan-

tation: cadaver eye histology and topography. Cornea. 2005;24:453–9.

8. Lee DH, Chung TY, Chung ES, et al. Case report: femtosecond laser-assisted small incision deep lamellar endothelial keratoplasty. Korean J Ophthalmol. 2008;22:43–8.

9. Maier AKB, Gundlach E, Gonnermann J, et al. Fellow eye comparison of descemet membrane endothelial keratoplasty and penetrating keratoplasty. Cornea. 2013;32:1344–8.

10. Alió del Barrio JL, Ziaei M, Bhogal M, Allan BD. Femtosecond laser-assisted deep lamellar endothelial keratoplasty: a new approach to a forgotten technique. Cornea. 2015;34:1369–74.

11. Alió Del Barrio JL, Vargas V. Femtosecond laser-assisted deep lamellar descemet membrane endothelial keratoplasty for the treatment of endothelial dysfunction associated with posterior stromal scarring. Cornea. 2019;38(3):388–91.

12. Melles GR, Lander F, Rietveld FJ, Remeijer L, Beekhuis WH, Binder PS. A new surgical technique for deep stromal, anterior lamellar keratoplasty. Br J Ophthalmol. 1999;83(3):327–33.

13. Rousseau A, Bensalem A, Garnier V, et al. Interface quality of endothelial keratoplasty buttons obtained with optomised FS laser settings. Br J Ophthalmol. 2012;96:122–7.

14. Vetter JM, Butsch C, Faust M, et al. Irregularity of the posterior corneal surface after curved interface femtosecond laser-assisted versus microkeratome-assisted descemet stripping automated endothelial keratoplasty. Cornea. 2012;32:118–24.

15. Phillips PM, Phillips LJ, Saad HA, et al. "Ultrathin" DSAEK tissue prepared with a low-pulse energy, high-frequency femtosecond laser. Cornea. 2013;32:81–6.

16. Goldich Y, Showrail M, Avni-Zauberman N, et al. Contralateral eye comparison of descemet membrane endothelial keratoplasty and descemet stripping automated endothelial keratoplasty. Am J Opthalmol. 2015;159:155–9.

17. Hayashi K, Hirata A, Hayashi H. Possible predisposing factors for in-the-bag and out-of-the-bag intraocular lens dislocation and outcomes of intraocular lens exchange surgery. Ophthalmology. 2007;114:969–75.

18. Gonnermann J, Klamann MK, Maier AK, et al. Visual outcome and complications after posterior iris-claw aphakic intraocular lens implantation. J Cataract Refract Surg. 2012;38:2139–43.

Femtosecond Descemet Membrane Endothelial Keratoplasty

Nir Sorkin, David S. Rootman,
and Michael Mimouni

Key Points

- Despite advances in postoperative DMEK graft detachment, subsequent cell loss is still a matter of concern.
- In femtosecond-assisted DMEK, a femtosecond laser is used to perform the descemetorhexis.
- Femtosecond-assisted DMEK technical parameters and adjustments in technique are reviewed.
- An outline and comparison of femtosecond assisted DMEK compared to manual DMEK outcomes is provided.

Supplementary Information The online version contains supplementary material available at https://doi.org/10.1007/978-3-031-32408-6_35.

N. Sorkin
Department of Ophthalmology, Tel Aviv Medical Center and Sackler Faculty of Medicine, Tel Aviv University, Tel Aviv, Israel

D. S. Rootman
Department of Ophthalmology and Vision Sciences, University of Toronto, Toronto, ON, Canada
e-mail: d.rootman@utoronto.ca

M. Mimouni (✉)
Department of Ophthalmology, Rambam Health Care Campus, Bruce and Ruth Rappaport Faculty of Medicine, Technion-Israel Institute of Technology, Haifa, Israel
e-mail: michael@intername.co.il

Rationale

Descemetorhexis and removal of the recipient's Descemet membrane (DM) from the transplant bed is an important step in Descemet membrane Endothelial Keratoplasty (DMEK). Proper Descemet removal facilitates DMEK graft attachment, thereby reducing rates of graft detachment – the most common complication following DMEK surgery. Graft detachment can affect surgical outcomes and may require a rebubbling procedure (repeat injection of air into the anterior chamber). Graft detachment requiring rebubbling occurs in 12.8% of DMEK cases [1]. Any Descemet tags or islands remaining in the transplant bed can produce spatial interference, which could prevent attachment of the delicate DMEK graft [2–4]. On the other hand, excess removal of the recipient's DM peripheral to the location of the graft is also undesirable since this area may contain viable endothelium (especially in eyes with Fuchs' endothelial dystrophy where the peripheral DM may contain a good number of viable endothelial cells) which will be unnecessarily removed and won't be covered later by the graft. This would necessitate excess migration of endothelial cells of the graft to repopulate the denuded area, thereby reducing the effective endothelial cell density (ECD) [5, 6].

In femtosecond DMEK, a femtosecond laser is used to outline the descemetorhexis [7]. Femtosecond descemetorhexis is accurate in size and shape [5]. Also, in contrast to the mechanical scoring of DM, which inevitably affects DM located peripheral to the descemetorhexis incision, the femtosecond laser performs a nonmechanical incision that does not disturb DM peripheral to the incision site [8]. Further, the femtosecond incision creates a physical barrier that prevents over stripping of DM beyond the planned stripping diameter.

Surgical Technique

Since femtosecond descemetorhexis is precise and does not affect DM beyond the incision site, its diameter can be same-sized (or just slightly oversized) compared to DMEK graft itself [6]. If performed under a failed penetrating keratoplasty (PKP) graft, femtosecond descemetorhexis diameter should be at least 0.25 mm smaller than the PKP graft to avoid the irregularity and opacities around the PKP graft-host interface [9]. In order to determine incision depth settings, pachymetry

can be measured using an ultrasound probe at 8 points along the planned incision location. Pachymetry measurements can be confirmed using either optical coherence tomography (OCT) or Scheimpflug tomography with the consideration that corneal opacities may produce measurement artifacts in optical imaging. The use of femtosecond platforms incorporating intraoperative OCT may obviate the need for preoperative pachymetry measurements.

The iFS IntraLase (J&J Vision, Santa Ana, California, USA) is used with the following cutting parameters: an energy of 2.29 µJ, a spot separation of 3 µm, a layer separation of 2 µm and a sidecut angle of 90°.

The femtosecond laser creates a vertical cylindrical cut whose depth is set from 100 µm below the thickest measured pachymetry (into the anterior chamber) to 100 µm above the thinnest measured pachymetry (into the stroma) (Fig. 35.1). In OCT-guided femtosecond platforms, incision height and location can be determined according to intraoperative OCT imaging. Next, DM is

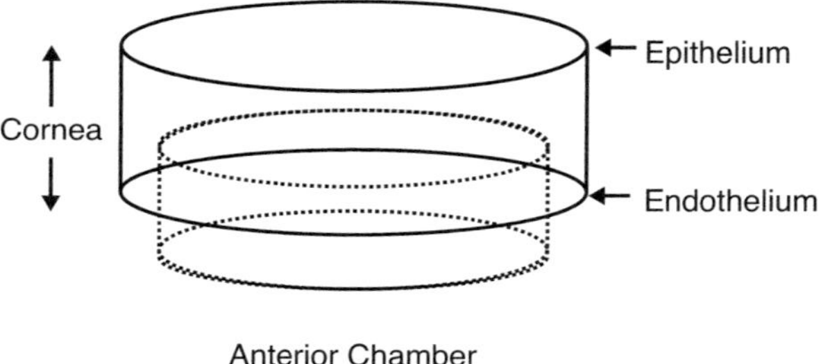

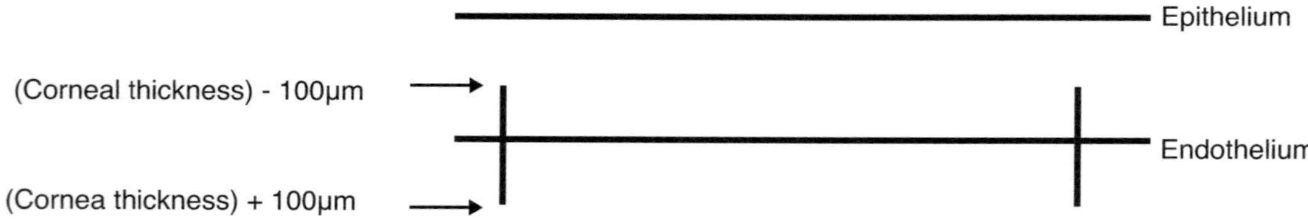

Fig. 35.1 Femtosecond Descemet membrane endothelial keratoplasty incisions: a cylindrical cut at a depth extending from 100 µm below the thickest measured pachymetry to 100 µm above the thinnest measured pachymetry. [Reproduced from: Einan-Lifshitz A, Sorkin N, Boutin T, Showail M, Borovik A, Alobthani M, Chan CC, Rootman DS (2017) Comparison of femtosecond laser-enabled descemetorhexis and manual descemetorhexis in descemet membrane endothelial keratoplasty. Cornea 36:767–770]

stripped using a blunt instrument such as a reverse Sinskey hook. Stripping of DM should not begin at the location of the femtosecond incision itself since the incision extends into the stroma, and therefore, initial separation of DM from the stroma at this location may be difficult due to increased stromal mobility and lack of stromal resistance around the incision. Rather, stripping should be initiated slightly more central to achieve an initial DM flap which can then be normally peeled (Video 35.1). The rest of the DMEK procedure is identical to standard DMEK.

Safety

An ex-vivo study evaluating endothelial vitality and stromal integrity following femtosecond descemetorhexis found a minimal impact of both the laser incision and DM peeling on the vitality of surrounding endothelial cells. A dense amount of vital endothelial cells was seen even very close to the incision edge both after the laser incision and after DM peeling. Phase contrast microscopy and scanning electron microscopy evaluation showed that the laser produced precise, clear-cut edges, leaving no stromal tissue bridges with minimal stromal damage (Fig. 35.2) [8].

The use of a femtosecond laser to create corneal incisions carries the risk of an incomplete cut. In the case of DM incisions, an incomplete incision may lead to radial tears extending to the peripheral DM in a manner similar to an incomplete femtosecond capsulorhexis in femtosecond laser-assisted cataract surgery (FLACS), causing an anterior capsular tear. In contrast to FLACS, where an anterior capsular tear may have serious surgical implications, a radial tear of the recipient's DM, although undesirable, should not be detrimental to the course of the DMEK procedure. There are no reported cases of an incomplete femtosecond descemetorhexis in femtosecond DMEK publications where the cylindrical incision height extended 100 µm into the stroma [6, 7, 10, 11]. Pilger et al. looked at reducing the stromal extension depth of the femtosecond descemetorhexis. They performed femtosecond descemetorhexis incisions with varying stromal extension depths of 100 µm, 75 µm and 60 µm.

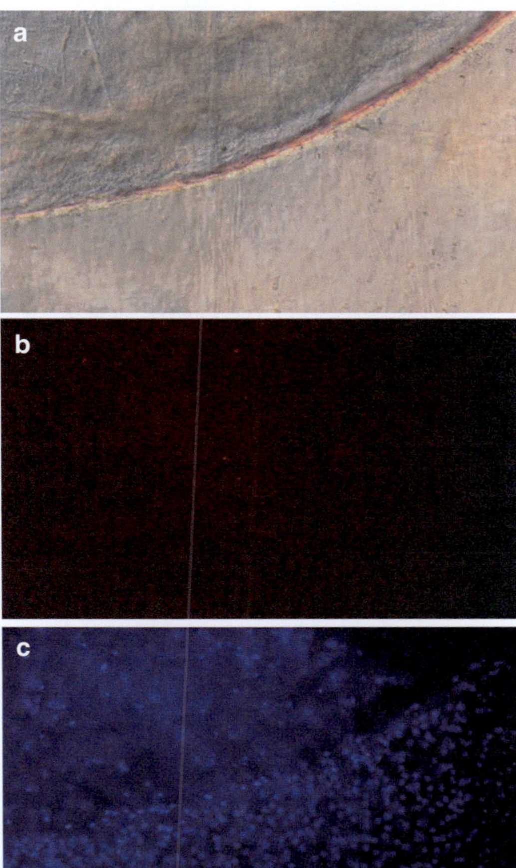

Fig. 35.2 A magnified view of a femtosecond descemetrohexis incision after Descemet stripping. (**a**) Phase contrast imaging showing the exposed corneal stroma following descemet stripping (top part of the image), the continuous laser incision and the area of untouched descemet peripheral to the incision (bottom part of the image). (**b**) Propidium iodide staining shows a minimal amount of devitalized stromal cells (red dots) near the incision and within the exposed stroma. (**c**) Hoechst 33342 staining shows a high density of vital endothelial cells even close to the edge of the cut. (Reproduced from: Feldhaus L, Dirisamer M, Ohlmann A, Luft N, Kassumeh S, Shajari M, Priglinger SG, Mayer WJ (2022) Femtosecond laser-assisted descemetorhexis for Descemet membrane endothelial keratoplasty: cell-based and tissue-based ex vivo analysis of precision and safety. J Cataract Refract Surg 48:89–94)

Their results showed that while incisions extending 100 µm into the posterior stroma yielded a completely separated descemetorhexis cut in all cases, incisions extending only 75 or 60 µm into the stroma were associated with incomplete cut edges, DM bridges over the incision and the occurrence of small radial tears when the DM was removed [5]. This was attributed in part to thickness changes throughout the cornea and corneal positioning in relation to the laser, as well as to the presence of Descemet folds which reduce tissue clarity and deform the posterior surface of the cornea. Therefore, we would recommend keeping the stromal incision depth at 100 μm.

Performing a femtosecond incision that extends 100 μm into the posterior stroma raises the question of its influence on corneal biomechanics, corneal curvature and the refractive stability of the cornea. In a study evaluating 3-year outcomes of femtosecond DMEK, our group found postoperative spherical equivalent to be stable, decreasing by just 0.28 ± 0.54 D (range -0.75 to $+0.75$ D) throughout follow-up.

There are no reported cases of corneal perforation following femtosecond descemetorhexis.

Efficacy

In femtosecond DMEK, the accurate and complete removal of the recipient's DM can improve attachment of the graft and preserve more viable recipient endothelial cells. Pilger et al. have shown that the diameter of a descemetorhexis performed using a femtosecond laser varies in size by just 1% compared with 7–8% size variability of a standard descemetorhexis ($p = 0.001$). They also found that the accuracy of the femtosecond incisions was associated with a smaller area of denuded stroma around the area of planned descemetorhexis and graft location. For example, for a planned 8.0 mm descemetorhexis, they found the surrounding denuded area to be 2.5 mm^2 in femtosecond DMEK and 11.6 mm^2 in standard DMEK – a difference of 9.1 mm^2 ($p < 0.001$) [5]. Considering that an 8.0 mm DMEK graft has a total area of 50.3 mm^2, the addition of 9.1 mm^2 of surrounding denuded stroma in standard DMEK equals roughly 18% of the graft area. The denuded area needs to be repopulated by endothelial cells migrating off the graft, thereby causing a more significant decrease in ECD in manual DMEK.

In Fuchs' dystrophy patients, femtosecond DMEK has been found to have reduced detach-

ment and rebubble rates, as well as reduced endothelial cell loss (ECL) compared with standard DMEK [5, 6, 10]. Rates of ECL following femtosecond DMEK were reduced by 5.8–13.6% compared with standard DMEK over 5 years of follow-up [12]. The reduction in ECL following femtosecond DMEK may extend graft survival by several years.

DMEK performed to replenish a failed PKP graft is associated with high rates of postoperative graft detachment, ranging between 26 and 100% [13–15]. We found that femtosecond DMEK performed under a failed PKP graft has low detachment rates, [11] significantly lower than standard DMEK performed in this setting [9]. Rates of ECL in this setting did not differ between femtosecond and standard DMEK. The advantages of femtosecond DMEK relating to ECL seem not to be realized in eyes with a failed PKP. This may be because the descemetorhexis area is limited by the PKP graft size and therefore, there may not be a big difference in the denuded stromal area between femtosecond and manual descemetorhexis (Fig. 35.3). Additionally, in the setting of graft failure, there are few remaining viable recipient endothelial cells, and therefore, preserving more of the recipient's DM

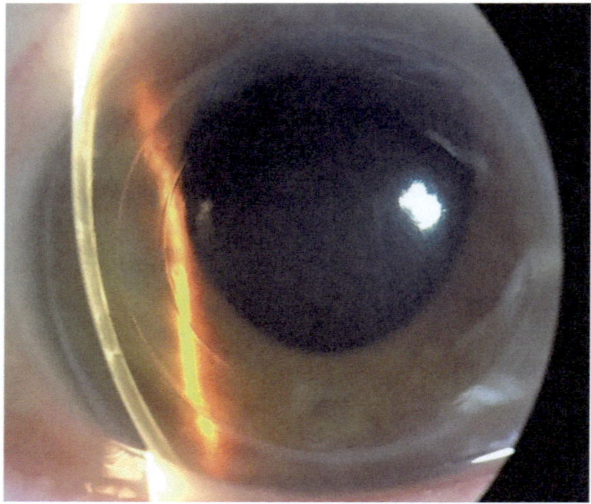

Fig. 35.3 A postoperative slit-lamp photograph of a patient with a femtosecond Descemet membrane endothelial keratoplasty (DMEK) graft performed under a failed penetrating keratoplasty (PKP). The larger circle represents the PKP graft edge, and the smaller circle represents the femtosecond descemetorhexis and DMEK graft diameters which were the same sized in this case. PKP functionality and clarity were restored following femtosecond DMEK

in femtosecond DMEK does not substantially increase the total postoperative endothelial cell count.

Conclusion

Femtosecond DMEK is safe and effective, with the advantages of better graft attachment and improved endothelial cell viability.

Take Home Notes
- Femtosecond-assisted DMEK may be safely and efficiently performed in routine DMEK cases.
- Femtosecond-assisted DMEK has advantages over manual DMEK in patients with a prior failed penetrating keratoplasty.
- Using the provided femtosecond parameters and adjustments in technique transition to femtosecond-assisted DMEK is feasible.

References

1. Deng SX, Lee WB, Hammersmith KM, Kuo AN, Li JY, Shen JF, Weikert MP, Shtein RM. Descemet membrane endothelial keratoplasty: safety and outcomes. Ophthalmology. 2018;125:295–310.
2. Müller TM, Verdijk RM, Lavy I, Bruinsma M, Parker J, Binder PS, Melles GRJ. Histopathologic features of descemet membrane endothelial keratoplasty graft remnants, folds, and detachments. Ophthalmology. 2016;123:2489–97.
3. Baydoun L, Ham L, Borderie V, Dapena I, Hou J, Frank LE, Oellerich S, Melles GRJ. Endothelial survival after descemet membrane endothelial keratoplasty: effect of surgical indication and graft adherence status. JAMA Ophthalmol. 2015;133:1277–85.
4. Dapena I, Ham L, Moutsouris K, Melles GRJ. Incidence of recipient Descemet membrane remnants at the donor-to-stromal interface after descemetorhexis in endothelial keratoplasty. Br J Ophthalmol. 2010;94:1689–90.
5. Pilger D, Von Sonnleithner C, Bertelmann E, Maier AKB, Joussen AM, Torun N. Exploring the precision of femtosecond laser-assisted descemetorhexis in descemet membrane endothelial keratoplasty. BMJ Open Ophthalmol. 2018;3:e000148. https://doi.org/10.1136/BMJOPHTH-2018-000148.
6. Sorkin N, Mednick Z, Einan-Lifshitz A, Trinh T, Santaella G, Telli A, Chan CC, Rootman DS. Three-year outcome comparison between femtosecond laser-assisted and manual Descemet membrane endothelial Keratoplasty. Cornea. 2019;38:812–6.
7. Pilger D, von Sonnleithner C, Bertelmann E, Joussen AM, Torun N. Femtosecond laser-assisted descemetorhexis: a novel technique in descemet membrane endothelial Keratoplasty. Cornea. 2016;35:1274–8.
8. Feldhaus L, Dirisamer M, Ohlmann A, Luft N, Kassumeh S, Shajari M, Priglinger SG, Mayer WJ. Femtosecond laser-assisted descemetorhexis for Descemet membrane endothelial keratoplasty: cell-based and tissue-based ex vivo analysis of precision and safety. J Cataract Refract Surg. 2022;48:89–94.
9. Sorkin N, Mimouni M, Santaella G, Trinh T, Cohen E, Einan-Lifshitz A, Chan CC, Rootman DS. Comparison of manual and femtosecond laser-assisted descemet membrane endothelial keratoplasty for failed penetrating keratoplasty. Am J Ophthalmol. 2020;214:1–8.
10. Einan-Lifshitz A, Sorkin N, Boutin T, Showail M, Borovik A, Alobthani M, Chan CC, Rootman DS. Comparison of femtosecond laser-enabled descemetorhexis and manual descemetorhexis in descemet membrane endothelial keratoplasty. Cornea. 2017;36:767–70.
11. Sorkin N, Trinh T, Einan-Lifshitz A, Mednick Z, Santaella G, Telli A, Belkin A, Chan CC, Rootman DS. Outcomes of femtosecond laser-assisted descemet membrane endothelial keratoplasty for failed penetrating keratoplasty. Can J Ophthalmol. 2019;54:741. https://doi.org/10.1016/j.jcjo.2019.04.003.
12. Sorkin N, Gouvea L, Din N, Mimouni M, Alshaker S, Weill Y, Gendler S, Slomovic AR, Chan CC, Rootman DS. Five-year safety and efficacy of femtosecond laser—assisted descemet membrane endothelial Keratoplasty. Cornea. 2022;42:145–9.
13. Einan-Lifshitz A, Belkin A, Sorkin N, Mednick Z, Boutin T, Gill I, Karimi M, Chan CC, Rootman DS. Descemet membrane endothelial Keratoplasty after penetrating Keratoplasty: features for success. Cornea. 2018;37:1093–7.
14. Pasari A, Price MO, Feng MT, Price FW. Descemet membrane endothelial Keratoplasty for failed penetrating keratoplasty. Cornea. 2019;38:151–6.
15. Kemer ÖE, Karaca EE, Oellerich S, Melles G. Evolving techniques and indications of Descemet membrane endothelial Keratoplasty. Turk J Ophthalmol. 2021;51:381–92.

Cultured Cells for Corneal Endothelial Therapy

M. P. De Miguel, M. Cadenas Martín, A. Moratilla, and F. Arnalich-Montiel

Key Points

- Corneal endothelial therapeutics has been transformed by lamellar endothelial transplants.
- Recent developments in endothelial cell culture techniques make it possible to expand ex vivo the corneal endothelial cells.
- Expanded cells can be delivered subsequently by direct injection into the anterior chamber or in sheet constructs made up of different materials.
- Recent advances have been achieved in differentiation protocols from extraocular cells capable of differentiating into corneal endothelial cells such as embryonic stem cells and adipose-derived mesenchymal stem cells.

Introduction to Corneal Endothelial Transplant

The cornea is a five-layered tissue that provides two-thirds of the total refractive power of the eye, and it is the first barrier protecting the intraocular

M. P. De Miguel (✉) · M. Cadenas Martín
A. Moratilla
Cell Engineering Laboratory, La Paz University
Hospital Health Research Institute, IdiPAZ,
Madrid, Spain

F. Arnalich-Montiel
IRYCIS, Ophthalmology Department, Ramón y Cajal
University Hospital, Madrid, Spain

content. The corneal endothelium, the inner layer, is in charge of maintaining the cornea in a relatively dehydrated state and therefore transparent. The endothelial cell layer failure leads to corneal swelling, loss of transparency, and blindness. In the past, penetrating keratoplasty (PK) had been the gold standard surgical treatment of corneal diseases for any layer, including primary endothelial diseases [1]. Central endothelial cell density (ECD, expressed in cells per mm^2) decreases at an average rate of about 0.6% per year in normal corneas throughout adult life [2]. In a normal individual, this decline in endothelial cells (EC) does not impair corneal transparency, even in centenarians, and only if the density falls below the threshold of 300–500 cells per mm^2, irreversible corneal edema can lead to blindness [3]. This event can occur following intraocular surgeries, traumas, or dystrophies. In fact, blindness due to corneal edema is the indication of corneal grafting of one in every three recipients.

Human corneal endothelium is held in a non-replicative state within the eye [4]. It has been a common belief that in vivo, corneal endothelium has limited wound-healing capacity, mainly by using residual EC which, by enlargement and migration, covers the space left by the lost cells without division [5]. Joyce [6] demonstrated that hCECs are arrested in the G1-phase of the cell cycle in vivo. Mitotic inhibition has been suggested to be due to contact-dependent inhibition and the transforming growth factor beta (TGF-ß) found within the aqueous humor [4]. However, a series of clinical observations suggest the ability of endothelial regeneration in vivo from the human corneal periphery after implanting free floating Descemet membrane in the anterior chamber or in the newly described technique known as Descemet stripping only in selected cases [3, 7, 8].

Currently, the only effective and proven way to restore endothelial function universally is to perform an allogenic graft. Since Melles [9] revolutionized the field in 2004 describing descemetorrhexis, a method to dissect only Descemet Membrane (DM) from the recipient eye, leaving the posterior lamella intact, and after Price [10] and Gorovoy [11] pioneered the procedure known as Descemet stripping endothelial keratoplasty (DSEK) [10], a variety of endothelial keratoplasty techniques have taken over PK as the elective procedure in endothelial keratoplasty. Nowadays, all the different approaches include "descemetorrhexis," and the difference lies in the tissue grafted:

1. In DSAEK, or Descemet stripping automated endothelial keratoplasty, the graft is prepared using a microkeratome and includes not only DM and endothelium but also part of the posterior stroma [11]. It has been widely adopted, and the eye bank produces precut tissue which is used directly by the surgeon [12]. Although the correlation between preoperative graft thickness and clinical outcomes has been disputed [13, 14], there is a tendency to believe that thinner grafts are associated with better visual acuity. Ultra-thin DSAEK is a variant of the technique where grafts are around 100 microns to improve the visual acuity of standard DSAEK [15].
2. In DMEK, or Descemet membrane endothelial keratoplasty, a step forward in the endothelial keratoplasty developed by Melles [16, 17], the graft consists of endothelium and DM without any stroma, around 10–15 microns thick. Compared to DSAEK, DMEK has better visual outcomes, faster recovery time, and

a lower immune rejection rate. It is the gold standard in the treatment of endothelial diseases, although it has not been adopted everywhere yet, due to the higher surgical skills needed. In settings with the scarcity of donor tissue, this technique has evolved to hemi-DMEK [18] or quarter-DMEK [19], allowing one donor to provide tissue for several recipients by dividing the graft into two or four pieces, respectively.

3. In DSO, or Descemet stripping only, there is no grafting, only a descemetorrhexis, and relies on primary healing of the peripheral endothelium [8]. There is a need for longer term comparison studies, but it has several advantages over the other two procedures, it requires only basic skills, it does not need donor tissue, there is no risk of rejection, and there are no early postoperative complications such as DM detachment. On the other hand, a good peripheral endothelial cell count is needed, the disease must be limited to the 5 mm-central part, and although it may provide similar visual outcomes to DMEK, it requires longer periods to achieve transparency with lower endothelial cell counts as a baseline point. The instillation of ROCK inhibitors has been used to speed up recovery and to salvage failing cases [20].

Cultured Corneal Endothelial Cells

Human corneal endothelial cells (hCECs) are arrested at G1 phase of the cell cycle, and do not proliferate in vivo, in part due to contact inhibition but also presumably because of lack of growth factor stimulation even when damage to the endothelial layer occurs [21]. Therefore, the supply of human corneal tissue is limited; therefore, in vitro CEC culture is an option to increase the number of cells for potential therapeutic purposes. However, this is challenging by the very biology of CECs, and it is important to consider several factors:

Donor Factors

Age of Donors

For cell culture of corneal endothelial cells, it is essential to start from a source of viable and proliferating cells, i.e., young human corneal tissue. Most human corneas are used for transplantation, leaving those of old donors with less endothelial cell count for research. It has been shown that in the corneas of young donors (<30 years old), the mean cell density is 3000 cells/mm^2, while in old donors (> 50 years old), it is 2700 cells/mm^2 [22].

There are also differences in cellular morphology within these two groups, young donor endothelial cells show homogeneous hexagonal morphology, while older donor cells were polymorphic. Proliferative capability was maintained from young donor CECs, maintaining their morphology and characteristics until the third passage, while old donor CECs were senescent earlier during the culture [23] hence culturing cells from old donors is more challenging.

Tissue Preservation

The quality of donor corneas also depends on tissue preservation conditions. There are two fundamental methods, maintenance in Optisol-GS and organ culture. Optisol-GS corneal storage medium (Bausch & Lomb, Irvine, California), a hybrid of K-sol and DexSol media containing chondroitin sulfate and dextran, is stored at 2 °C to 8 °C for 14 days [24]. Meanwhile, organ culture maintains the corneas between 31 °C and 37 °C for up to 28 days, using different culture media. Most of these media are supplemented with serum such as CorneaMax, but serum-free media such as Human Endothelial-SFM is also used [25]. Viability comparison studies showed a dead cell percentage of 9.34% ± 4% and 0.46% ± 0.3% in Optisol-GS and organ culture, respectively [26]. Nevertheless, successful cell culture was obtained from tissue preserved in both conditions. Although the viability is higher with organ culture, in both cases proliferation, hexagonal morphology and expression of typical CECs markers are achieved.

Cell Isolation Protocols

Isolation of hCECs is one of the most critical steps for a successful culture. The most commonly used method is the peel-and-digest protocol by Peh's Laboratory [23]. The endothelium along with the Descemet membrane is separated from the rest of the cornea, and this is enzymatically digested by collagenase. This enzyme gently digests the junctions of the endothelial cells to the Descemet membrane (DM), consisting mainly of ECM proteins like collagen IV. The intercellular junctions mediated by ZO-1 are maintained as well as cell-to-basement membrane interactions [23]. Other enzymatic methods have also been tried, such as trypsin, causing complete degradation of the CECs when too aggressive, or separation by EDTA and pipetting, a technique by which the CECs did not maintain viability either [27, 28].

Cell viability is checked routinely in eye banks using Trypan blue positive cell count, using Trypan Blue staining (0.25%), and counting blue stained cells as dead cells. Using this method and a hemocytometer for counting, viability and plating density can also be checked after cell isolation [26].

Coatings

In vivo, endothelial cells adhere to the Descemet membrane via extracellular matrix proteins. The extracellular matrix is composed of different collagens, laminin, and fibronectin among others. With the idea of creating a biomimetic environment, these and other cell adhesion coatings have been evaluated for culturing endothelial cells. Comparison of wells precoated with Fibronectin, Poly-D-Lysine, Collagen I, Fibronectin/Collagen I, or FNC Coating Mix [29] showed that the coating with the higher adhesion with almost 100% of cells attached after rinsing while maintaining cell morphology was FNC Coating Mix, followed by Collagen I and Fibronectin/Collagen I (with 90% of cells attached). On the downside, FNC Coating Mix is a commercially formulated reagent containing bovine fibronectin and bovine collagen I among other components so it is useful for cell culture but not suitable for clinical studies [29, 30]. Other studies have shown collagen IV as an optimal coating for the culture of CECs for tissue engineering as it is part of the endothelial basement membrane [31].

Media

Different culture media have been used for the expansion of CECs, usually with a dual approach, with a proliferation medium followed by a maintenance medium.

For proliferation, combinations of one or two media with external growth factors have been used. The media include DMEM, DMEM/F12, Opti-MEM-I, and Ham's F12/M199, compared by Peh [23]. CECs cultured with DMEM or DMEM/F12 do not go beyond the first or second passage, while using Opti-MEM-I or Ham's F12/M199, the cells start to show typical endothelial markers such as Na^+/K^+ ATPase or ZO-1 from passage 3 [23]. As human CECs do not proliferate, external factors and supplements have been used to overcome the cell cycle arrest such as serum, ascorbic acid, FGF, or insulin [32]. However, hexagonal morphology was not achieved by culturing in proliferation media alone. For the maintenance of CECs five media were compared, including HCEC growth medium (F99), MEM with FCS, and humanized endothelial SFM, the latter being the one with the best results in terms of lower endothelial cell apoptosis [33, 34].

Parekh [35] cultured CECs using only a proliferation medium based on Ham's F12/M199. Other groups used Opti-MEM-I with 8% FBS and supplemented with ROCK inhibitor (Y-27632) [36–38]. One of the most effective protocols is Peh's Laboratory [23], which uses a proliferation media with Ham's F12/M199 with 5% FBS, 20 µg/mL ascorbic acid, 1% ITS, 10 ng/mL FGF2 and 1% antibiotic/antimycotic combined a maintenance media Human endothelial-

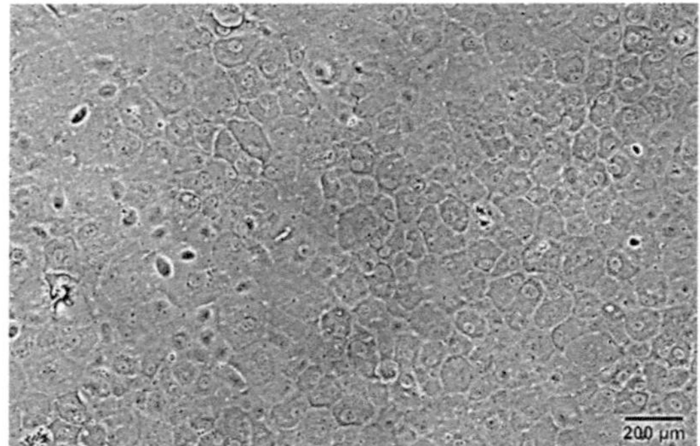

Fig. 36.1 Phase contrast microphotograph of a human CEC culture showing the typical polygonal cell morphology. Bar: 200 µm

SFM 4% FBS, 50 µg/mL gentamicin, and 1% antibiotic/antimycotic (Fig. 36.1).

Carriers for DSAEK and DMEK

Following the isolation of hCECs, the next step is to engineer a scaffold mimicking DM and use it as a graft. This scaffold needs to provide a favorable environment for endothelial cell expansion and maintenance as well as a robust tissue that can be handled easily for transplantation. In recent decades, studies have been carried out using both natural and synthetic materials that can serve as grafts with CECs. Today, in addition to using biomaterials as scaffolds, their use is being studied to increase cell viability and long-term transplantation success [39].

Natural Scaffolds

Natural scaffolds can be obtained from different animal sources, which mimic components of DM, improving biocompatibility, proliferation, and maintaining the phenotype of CECs. However, since they are derived from animals, their composition is not well defined, and the resulting scaffolds show little optical transparency and weak mechanical properties.

Initially, as with coatings, the use of natural polymer from the extracellular matrix such as *collagen* was considered because of its biocompatibility properties, low immunogenicity, and degradability. However, the laminas were not consistent, difficult to handle, and easily degraded by proteases. To solve this, different hardening techniques have been used, such as chemical crosslinking or physical crosslinking by ultraviolet light, rendering suboptimal results [40, 41]. Over time, technologies have appeared that allow for the creation of plastic compressed collagen films, based on Real Architecture for 3D Tissues (RAFT) that allow rapid production of grafts with improved mechanical properties without compromising biosafety; however, transparency is not adequate, and there are no in vivo studies yet [42].

Other natural polymers have been tried such as gelatin or chitosan. *Gelatin* has great porosity, permeability to water, helps cell adhesion, and is widely available [43]. However, gelatin hydrogels do not provide stability as a graft, and there is a risk of carrying bovine spongiform encephalopathy due to the source of gelatin [44]. *Chitosan* is a biomimetic polysaccharide derived from chitin and has great biocompatibility but low strength. To create a hard construct, it was combined with other natural materials, and a graft consisting of hydroxyethyl chitosan, gelatin, and chondroitin sulfate was created and tested on CECs, showing promising results but causing in vivo inflammation in animal models [45].

An approach using *silk fibroin* precoated with collagen type IV, has also been evaluated for human CEC culture [46]. Silk fibroin a natural fibrin derived from silk has low immunogenicity and good transparency but on its own cannot maintain a CEC culture, lacks elasticity and mechanical strength, and can cause hypersensitivity. Using non-mulberry silk combined with other materials shows better biocompatibility, but further studies need to be done [47].

Other biologically derived scaffolds are membranes such as amniotic membrane, decellularized cornea, and human anterior lens capsule. In both, the high dependency on the human donor is a limitation.

The human *amniotic membrane* is a collagen-based scaffold that can be used intact, decellularized or lyophilized and possesses anti-inflammatory, anti-fibrosis, and anti-angiogenic properties that reduce potential graft rejection and have been used in other ocular applications [27]. The main problems are availability and lack of mass manufacturing, suboptimal transparency with a low biodegradation rate in long-term transplantation, and risk of contamination and transmission of infectious diseases [48].

Decellularized corneas provide the perfect substrate for CECs to grow while maintaining optimal transparency and ultrastructure. Decellularization removes native cells and other immunogenic compounds while preserving the structural and functional proteins of the stroma [49]. Different corneal scaffolds have been used, from porcine corneas to human. Due to a low number of donated corneas and a lengthy decellularization process, obtaining various lamellae per cornea with the femtosecond laser method is vital for the usage of this material as a scaffold [30]. There are various studies with clinical applications leading to corneal edema relief [50, 51].

Human *crystalline* lens capsule is composed of collagen IV and sulfated glycosaminoglycans. The anterior lens capsule is a byproduct of cataract surgery and presents biomechanical properties similar to DMEK grafts, can be used decellularized with good biocompatibility and inherent transparency; however, there are limitations due to their small diameter and high dependency on the supply of cadaveric eye donors [52].

In addition, a natural material xenograft using *decellularized fish scales* is being assessed. It presents a collagen I pattern similar to the human cornea and provides a cost-effective available substrate for corneal grafts. CECs adhesion is adequate but can be improved with FNC coating, and proliferation is irregular, but post-modification fish scale scaffolds show some promise due to their inherent transparency being similar to DSAEK grafts [53].

Synthetic Scaffolds

There are interesting materials because their properties such as the structure, shape, chemical composition, mechanical strength, and durability can be customized. Therefore, many authors try to find the best synthetic scaffold-based to regenerate the corneal endothelium.

Kruse [54] compared scaffolds of poly (methyl-methacrylate) (*PMMA*), poly (lactic-co-glycolic acid) (*PLGA*) and polycaprolactone (*PCL*) for the culture of hCECs. PLGA fibers were spun from a solution with a mass concentration of 5 w/v% in 75% chloroform and 25% methanol. PCL fibers were spun from a 14 w/v% solution in 75% CHCl3 and 25% MeOH. PMMA fibers were produced from a 16 w/v% solution of 75% CHCl3 and 25% MeOH. Even using identical production parameters, the three scaffolds differed significantly in terms of viscosity, pore size, thickness, and light transmittance. Then, 40,000 cells/cm^2 of human corneal endothelial cell line (HCEC-12) were seeded onto the scaffolds and cultured for a week. The results revealed that HCEC-12 mainly grew on the surface and retained physiological morphology, but the formation of a uniform monolayer was not evident in PLGA. The PCL scaffold maintained high cell viability, while PMMA showed cytotoxicity. In conclusion, PLGA and PCL electro-spun scaffolds showed similar biocompatibility, but only PLGA maintained the characteristic polygonal shape of hCECs.

Poly (ethylene glycol) (*PEG*)-based hydrogel films containing sebacoyl chloride (SebCl) and 5 w/v% of α, ω-dihydroxy-poly (ε-caprolactone) (PCL) dissolved in dichloromethane showed similar tensile strengths to human corneal tissue and more than 98% optical transparency activity [55]. In vitro analysis performed with sheep CECs on hydrogel films resulted in 100% confluence with natural morphology after 7 days. In vivo studies revealed that the cell-free hydrogel implanted on the inner surface of ovine corneas for 28 days showed no toxicity or inflammatory response and did not compromise the native CEC function, as the corneas maintained their optical transparency.

Synthetic hydrogels of *poly-ε-lysine* cross-linked 60% with octanedioic-acid to a polymer density of 0.066 g/mL using N-hydroxysulfosuccinimide (NHS) and 1-ethyl-3-(3-dimethylaminopropyl) carbodiimide (EDC), produced a thin, transparent, porous, and robust substrate for corneal endothelial cells culture [56]. Their results demonstrated that functionalization of the poly-ε-lysine hydrogel with arginine-glycine-aspartic acid (RGD) provides a suitable surface for 5-week culture of primary porcine hCECs and facilitates the generation of the confluent monolayer with of ZO-1 and Na$^+$/K$^+$ ATPase expression.

Combination of Natural and Synthetic Materials

Other authors combine natural and synthetic polymers to create a biomaterial with the advantages of both. The mechanical properties of the synthetic scaffolds and the extracellular matrix (ECM) proteins of natural ones.

Kim [57] created the *Col-I-PLGA* scaffold by combining the appropriate mechanical strength of the 5 w/v% PLGA films as a substrate with 5 μg/cm^2 collagen I coating to enhance its biocompatibility. This polymer adequately resembled the required surface properties to facilitate adhesion, migration, and proliferation of primary rabbit corneal endothelial cells, as well as roughness, appropriate hydrophilicity, stability, and water uptake, compared to bare PLGA films. Also, the cultured cells on Col I-PLGA scaffolds showed significant enhancement in the expression of corneal endothelial cell-associated marker genes such as aquaporin and Na$^+$/K$^+$ ATPase, along with well-maintained cell morphology.

Palchesko [58] demonstrated that bovine CECs cultured in vitro on a *polydimethylsiloxane* surface with an elastic modulus of 50 kPa previously coated with collagen IV grew in monolayer with a polygonal morphology and positive staining for the characteristic endothelial marker ZO-1.

Rizwan [59] produced an improved *gelatin methacrylate* hydrogel named GelMA+ and UV crosslinking. GelMA+ showed an eight-fold increase in mechanical strength and slower degradation compared to regular GelMA. In addition, primary human CECs at passage 3 from donor corneas reached confluence in a monolayer with rise ZO-1 expression, higher cell density and cell size homogeneity on GelMA+ carrier compared to GelMA.

Wang [60] hybridized *chitosan and polycaprolactone* (PCL) and cultured bovine corneal endothelial cells on this scaffold and reported that the cells reached confluence on day 11, displayed a normal polygonal morphology and showed ZO-1, Na^+/K^+ ATPase expression after 14 days of incubation on the 25% PCL and 75% chitosan blend membrane.

An alternative method to is cell sheet engineering. Cells were cultured on the surface of a stimuli-sensitive polymer that allows controlled cell adhesion and detachment without using proteolytic enzymes.

Several studies have shown that Poly-N-isopropylacrylamide (*PIPAAm*) is a good temperature-responsive polymer for generating hCEC sheets. Their chains display hydrophobic properties at 37 °C so the cultured cells could adhere and proliferate on the polymer. In contrast, by lowering the culture temperature to 20 °C, the polymer turns into a hydrophilic state with fully extended chains, so the formed cell sheets spontaneously detach from the surface with intact ECM proteins. The harvested hCECs, which exhibit hexagonal morphology with the presence of microvilli and cellular interconnections, were transferred to gelatin disc supports for transplantation into the anterior chamber of rabbit models. After 2 weeks, the hCEC film was attached to the denuded surface of Descemet's membrane with tight junction formation (ZO-1) between cells [61–64]. This approach has not gone clinically forward because cultured corneal endothelial sheets, as

cell monolayers, are highly fragile and technically difficult to transplant into the anterior chamber. To overcome this problem, some researchers have transplanted cultured corneal endothelial sheets with a carrier, but they have adhered only temporarily before eventually detaching, with the exception of corneal stromal laminas, which is a limited source and whose necessity hinders the advantages of transplantation of cultured CEC [65]. However, this thermoresponsive polymer has been used for patient therapy to enable corneal epithelial reconstruction [66].

Stem Cells Induced Differentiation to Human Corneal Endothelial Cells

Since the corneal endothelium was shown to be derived from neural crest [67, 68], most approaches to induce corneal endothelial cell differentiation from stem cells in vitro started mimicking the developmental process. The strategy consisted of a first phase in which stem cells were differentiated into neural crest cells and a second stage in which corneal endothelial cells were further differentiated from these neural crest cells.

Three labs, McCabe [69], Ali [70], and Wagoner [71], independently derived corneal endothelium from pluripotent stem cells under chemically defined conditions with a first step called "dual inhibition" to promote neural crest cell induction, either embryonic stem cells (ESC) or induced pluripotent stem cells (iPSC). McCabe [69] and Ali [70] used 10 µM TGF beta signaling inhibitor SB431542 and 500 ng/mL BMP signaling inhibitor Noggin in a basal medium of DMEM-F12, knock out serum replacement, nonessential AA, and 8 ng/mL fibroblast growth factor 2 (FGF2). However, Wagoner [71] used 3 µM GSK-3 inhibitor CHIR99021 instead of a BMP signaling blocker in a basal medium of DMEM/F12, bovine serum albumin (BSA), 50 µg/ml (+)-sodium L-ascorbate, 10 µg/mL transferrin, 10 ng/mL Heregulin β-1, 200 ng/mL IGF-I, and 8 ng/mL FGF2. After a minimum of 3 days, the

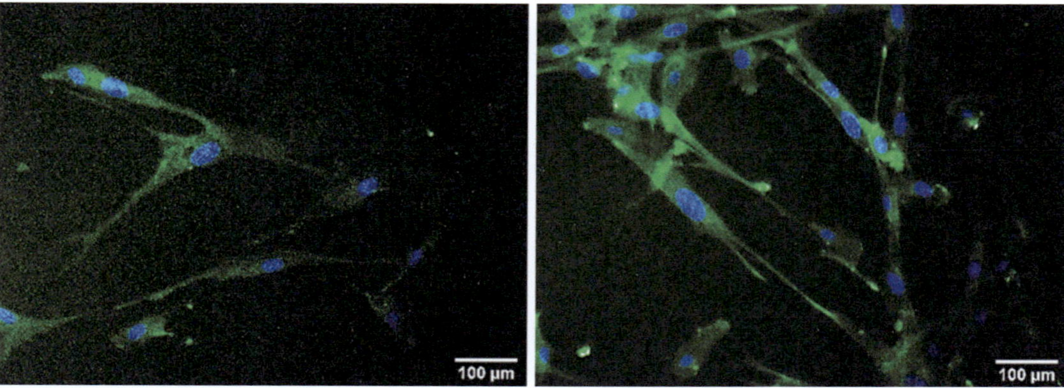

Fig. 36.2 Confocal images of Na⁺/K⁺ ATPase immunofluorescence (in green) in human ADSC-derived CEC using Wagoner et al. (left) or Ali et al. (right) differentiation media. DAPI nuclear staining in blue. Bars: 100 μm.

dual inhibitors were replaced by 10 ng/mL platelet-derived growth factor B (PDGF-BB), 10 ng/mL Dickkopf-related protein 2 (DKK-2), and 0.1 × B27 supplement for at least 7 days to generate hexagonal corneal endothelial-like cells. Their analyses revealed increased expression of corneal endothelial cell-associated markers such as ZO-1 and Na⁺/K⁺ ATPase α1 (ATP1A1) as well as the key Descemet's membrane protein, Collagen type VIII (COL8A1 and COL8A2).

At the same time, Zhao and Afshari [72] used a three-step chemical method. A first dual inhibition step like previous researchers with 5 μM SB431542 and 50 nM BMP signaling inhibitor LDN193189, adding a Wnt inhibitor 1 μM IWP2 to raise eye field stem cell development in a priming medium of DMEM/F12, N2, B27, BSA, nonessential AA for 6 days. Next, they derived neural crest cells from these stem cells using an induction medium of DMEM/F12 50:50, N2, B27, 0.3 mM 2-phospho-L-ascorbic acid supplemented with 3 μM CHIR99021. Lastly, they were able to differentiate neural crest cells into corneal endothelial-like cells, which expressed Na⁺/K⁺ ATPase, ZO-1, and N-cadherin, with human endothelial-SFM, 5% FBS, 0.3 mM 2-phosphate ascorbic acid, 1 μM SB431542, and a 2.5 μM ROCK inhibitor H-1125.

In our opinion, both Ali [70] and Wagoner [71] are better protocols than the others mentioned above because both have been able to achieve the generation of CECs using cells from

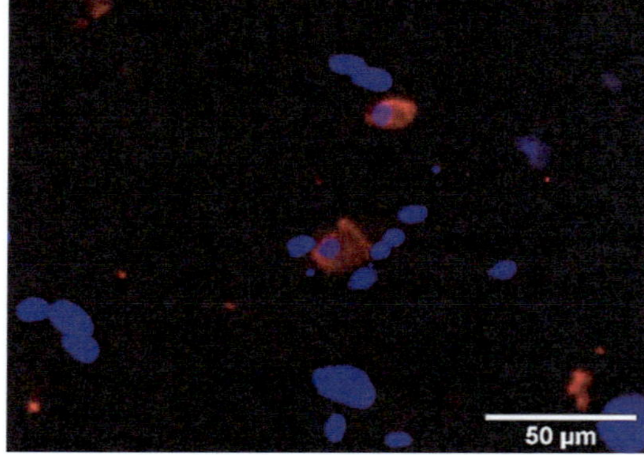

Fig. 36.3 Confocal image of N-Cadherin immunofluorescence in human ADSC-derived CEC using Wagoner et al. differentiation media. DAPI nuclear staining in blue. Bar: 50 μm

adult patients. This would be advantageous because the risk of rejection may be reduced when patient-specific autologous cells are used for the treatment of corneal endothelial disorders. Among them, Ali et al. [70] show the highest advantage because with only 20 days of procedure, they generated CECs with 90.82% proteome similarity to a human corneal endothelium (Figs. 36.2 and 36.3).

On the other hand, three other labs derived corneal endothelial-like cells from stem cells using different cell-conditioned media. Obviously, these approaches with conditioned media are less applicable to clinical practice, as undefined factors and concentrations of the molecules present in the conditioned media prevent their safe and reproducible use:

Zhang [73] derived corneal endothelial-like cells from human ESCs by co-culture for 5 days with human corneal stroma cells in a basal medium contained DMEM/F12 supplemented with 10% FBS, B27, 20 ng/ml EGF and 40 ng/ml bFGF to generate an outgrowth of precursors of neural crest cells which expressed CD73 and FoxC1. Next, the medium was changed to SV-40 transformed human lens epithelial cell-conditioned medium for 14 additional days to obtain a monolayer of corneal endothelial-like cells with positive signals for Na^+/K^+ ATPase, ZO-1, vimentin, and N-cadherin.

Chen [74] promoted neural crest cell differentiation from mouse ESC and mouse iPSC by culturing them in a first stage with embryonic body differentiation medium adding 1 μM all-trans retinoic acid during 4 days. Then, they induced differentiation towards corneal endothelial cells by exposing them for 14–17 days to conditioned medium collected from rabbit lens epithelial cell culture medium. The differentiated cells presented an up-regulation of corneal endothelial cell-associated marker genes as Aquaporin-1, ZO-1, Na^+/K^+ ATPase, N-cadherin, and Collage type VIII compared with undifferentiated cells.

In search for adult stem cells capable of CEC differentiation, Bosch [75] used dental pulp stem cells. They transdifferentiated these stem cells into neural crest stem cells with an induction medium consisting of DMEM-F12 supplemented with 1× B-27, 1× N-2, 20 ng/mL EGF, 20 ng/ml FGF2, 5 ng/mL heparin, and 2 mM L-alanyl-L-glutamine. On day 4, an adequate number of cells showed up-regulation of neural crest stem cells markers such as AP2, Nestin, and p75; therefore, these cells were cultured in the human corneal endothelial conditioned medium for a further 15 days to derive corneal endothelial cells. At the end of the differentiation process, gene expression of typical CEC markers like ZO-1, Na^+/K^+ ATPase pump ATP1A1 and extracellular matrix components COL4A2 and COL8A2 were significantly increased compared to undifferentiated dental pulp stem cells.

Clinical Studies on CEC Transplantation

There are some alternative procedures that are currently evaluated under clinical trials and study the use of carriers and endothelial cells in culture:

1. CECs migrate much more efficiently over intact DM rather than bare corneal stroma in DSO, leading to the idea that for the treatment of FECD, DSO could potentially be improved by increasing the size of the descemetorrhexis to incorporate most of the large guttas, but providing a cell-free Descemet's membrane graft afterwards to complete a descemetorrhexis. This way it acts as a support for endothelial cells favoring their proliferation and centripetal migration. This technique is known as Descemet membrane transfer (DMT) [76]. Unlike endothelial keratoplasty, it has the advantage of using an acellular graft that is widely available and avoiding problems related to postoperative graft rejection due to the absence of allogeneic endothelium. A clinical trial is currently underway to evaluate the efficacy of DMT for the treatment of FECD in a larger cohort of patients and for longer-term monitoring of its safety and efficacy (ClinicalTrials.gov; identifier: NCT03275896).

2. Cell culture techniques make it possible to expand ex vivo the CEC to subsequently inject a cell solution into the anterior chamber [37], or else to manufacture constructs made up of acellular corneal stroma, acellular Descemet membrane or material manufactured by tissue bioengineering [51], and colonized by expanded CEC. These grafts could then be transplanted onto the recipient in the same way as in the previously seen endothelial keratoplasties. In both approaches, a single population of endothelial cells can be amplified many times for distribution to large numbers of patients. Currently, within the framework of a clinical trial that included 11 patients, it has been found that the injection of cells in suspension is capable of effectively treating cor-

neal edema secondary to various conditions, including Fuchs' Dystrophy and pseudophakic bullous keratopathy, in addition to secondary corneal edema, argon laser peripheral iridotomy (LPI) or pseudoexfoliation syndrome [37]. At 2 years after cell injection, corneal thickness was less than 600 μm in 10 eyes, and the cornea was thinner than the baseline measure in all 11 eyes. The same study [37], however, also found a relatively broad range of endothelial counts among trial participants 2 years after treatment (mean CEC density, 1534 cells per square millimeter [95% CI, 1213 to 1855]). Each of the 11 eyes maintained corneal transparency. Regarding the efficacy of tissue bioengineered constructs, there are no human data yet, although a clinical trial is currently underway (ClinicalTrials.gov; identifier: NCT04319848).

Concluding Remarks and Future Perspectives

Nowadays, we are in an outstanding position to develop corneal endothelial cell sheets for endothelial keratoplasty: With respect to culture conditions, reproducible and well-defined culturing methods, and conditions have been achieved in the last decades [23, 33, 34, 36, 77–79].

Regardless of advances in promoting hCEC proliferation, the achieved capacity for expanding human CECs is still highly limited; new sources of CECs are therefore sought. The use of extraocular cells capable of differentiating into corneal endothelial cells is highly desirable. Recent advances have been achieved in differentiation protocols from adipose-derived mesenchymal stem cells (ADSC) from our lab [80]. Our results broaden the type of cells of autologous extraocular origin that could be employed in the clinical setting for corneal endothelial deficiency. In addition, recent in vivo demonstration of the functionality of hESC-derived hCEC together with nicotinamide [81] provides experimental evidence for a potential approach for treating corneal endothelial dysfunction.

Respect to carriers, so far, the most advantageous carrier is a corneal stroma decellularized lamina [30, 51, 82]. However, this carrier still depends on donors; new advances in biomimetic materials and manufacturing protocols such as electrospinning, electrogradient transport, shear flow, nano-lithography, flow-induced crystallization, vitrification, and advances in novel 3D printing techniques such as LIFT, laser-assisted bioprinting, and fused filament fabrication, and other methods of achieving lamellar parallel bundles of collagen, such as molecular crowding and densification to a liquid crystalline state [83–86] will aid in the search for a donor-independent biocompatible carrier.

Further development of these and previous approaches by defining the growth factors, the signaling pathways implicated in directed differentiation, the use of more practical cells to derive hCECs, and the in vivo demonstration of functionality are urgently needed.

Take Home Notes
- Recently, a variety of endothelial keratoplasty techniques to restore endothelial function have taken over the classical allogenic graft. However, there is a scarcity of donors to adequate to high and increasing demand.
- Nowadays, we are in an outstanding position to develop corneal endothelial cell sheets for endothelial keratoplasty: reproducible and well-defined culturing methods and conditions have been achieved in the last decades.
- The use of extraocular cells capable of differentiating into corneal endothelial cells from embryonic stem cells and adipose-derived mesenchymal stem cells is readily available.
- New advances in biomimetic materials and manufacturing protocols such as electrospinning, nanolithography, vitrification, and advances in novel 3D printing techniques and others will aid in the search for a donor-independent biocompatible carrier.

- Further development of these and previous approaches by defining the growth factors, the signaling pathways implicated in directed differentiation, the use of more practical cells to derive hCECs, and the in vivo demonstration of functionality are urgently needed.

References

1. Moshirfar M, Thomson AC, Ronquillo Y. Corneal endothelial transplantation. Treasure Islad, FL: StatPearls Publishing; 2022.
2. Bourne W, Nelson L, Hodge D. Central corneal endothelial cell changes over a ten-year period. Invest Ophthalmol Vis Sci. 1997;38(3):779–82.
3. He Z, Campolmi N, Gain P, Ha Thi BM, Dumollard JM, Duband S, et al. Revisited microanatomy of the corneal endothelial periphery: new evidence for continuous centripetal migration of endothelial cells in humans. Stem Cells. 2012;30(11):2523–34.
4. Joyce NC, Harris DL, Mello DM. Mechanisms of mitotic inhibition in corneal endothelium: contact inhibition and TGF-β2. Investig Ophthalmol Vis Sci. 2002;43(7):2152–9.
5. Sherrard ES. The corneal endothelium in vivo: its response to mild trauma. Exp Eye Res. 1976;22(4):347–57.
6. Joyce NC, Meklir B, Joyce SJ, Zieske JD. Cell cycle protein expression and proliferative status in human corneal cells. Investig Ophthalmol Vis Sci. 1996;37(4):645–55.
7. Dirisamer M, Yeh RY, Van Dijk K, Ham L, Dapena I, Melles GRJ. Recipient endothelium may relate to corneal clearance in descemet membrane endothelial transfer. Am J Ophthalmol. 2012;154(2):290–296.e1.
8. Garcerant D, Hirnschall N, Toalster N, Zhu M, Wen L, Moloney G. Descemet's stripping without endothelial keratoplasty. Curr Opin Ophthalmol. 2019;30(4):275–85.
9. Melles GRJ, Wijdh RHJ, Nieuwendaal CP. A technique to excise the descemet membrane from a recipient cornea (Descemetorhexis). Cornea. 2004;23(3):286–8.
10. Price FW, Price MO. Descemet's stripping with endothelial keratoplasty in 50 eyes: a refractive neutral corneal transplant. J Refract Surg. 2005;21(4):339–45.
11. Gorovoy MS. Descemet-stripping automated endothelial keratoplasty. Cornea. 2006;25(8):886–9.
12. Chen ES, Terry MA, Shamie N, Hoar KL, Friend DJ. Precut tissue in descemet's stripping automated endothelial keratoplasty. Donor characteristics and early postoperative complications. Ophthalmology. 2008;115(3):497–502.
13. Tourabaly M, Chetrit Y, Provost J, Georgeon C, Kallel S, Temstet C, et al. Influence of graft thickness and regularity on vision recovery after endothelial keratoplasty. Br J Ophthalmol. 2020;104(9):1317–23.
14. Perone J-M, Goetz C, Zevering Y, Derumigny A, Bloch F, Vermion J-C, et al. Graft thickness at 6 months postoperatively predicts long-term visual acuity outcomes of descemet stripping automated endothelial keratoplasty for fuchs dystrophy and moderate phakic bullous keratopathy. Cornea. 2021;41(11):1362.
15. Busin M, Madi S, Santorum P, Scorcia V, Beltz J. Ultrathin descemet's stripping automated endothelial keratoplasty with the microkeratome double-pass technique: two-year outcomes. Ophthalmology. 2013;120(6):1186–94.
16. Melles GRJ, Ong TS, Ververs B, van der Wees J. Preliminary clinical results of descemet membrane endothelial keratoplasty. Am J Ophthalmol. 2008;145(2):222.
17. Melles GRJ, Ong TS, Ververs B, van der Wees J. Descemet membrane endothelial keratoplasty (DMEK). Cornea. 2006;25(8):987–90.
18. Lam FC, Baydoun L, Dirisamer M, Lie J, Dapena I, Melles GRJ. Hemi-descemet membrane endothelial keratoplasty transplantation: a potential method for increasing the pool of endothelial graft tissue. JAMA Ophthalmol. 2014;132(12):1469–73.
19. Birbal RS, Ni Dhubhghaill S, Baydoun L, Ham L, Bourgonje VJA, Dapena I, et al. Quarter-descemet membrane endothelial keratoplasty: one- to two-year clinical outcomes. Cornea. 2020;39(3):277–82.
20. Moloney G, Garcerant Congote D, Hirnschall N, Arsiwalla T, Luiza Mylla Boso A, Toalster N, et al. Descemet stripping only supplemented with topical Ripasudil for Fuchs endothelial dystrophy 12-month outcomes of the Sydney eye hospital study. Cornea. 2021;40(3):320–6.
21. Joyce NC. Proliferative capacity of corneal endothelial cells. Exp Eye Res. 2012;95(1):16–23.
22. McGlumphy EJ, Margo JA, Haidara M, Brown CH, Hoover CK, Munir WM. Predictive value of corneal donor demographics on endothelial cell density. Cornea. 2018;37(9):1159–62.
23. Peh GSL, Toh KP, Wu FY, Tan DT, Mehta JS. Cultivation of human corneal endothelial cells isolated from paired donor corneas. PLoS One. 2011;6(12):e28310.
24. Kitazawa K, Inatomi T, Tanioka H, Kawasaki S, Nakagawa H, Hieda O, et al. The existence of dead cells in donor corneal endothelium preserved with storage media. Br J Ophthalmol. 2017;101(12):1725–30.
25. Valtink M, Donath P, Engelmann K, Knels L. Effect of different culture media and deswelling agents on survival of human corneal endothelial and epithelial cells in vitro. Graefes Arch Clin Exp Ophthalmol. 2016;254(2):285–95.
26. Parekh M, Peh G, Mehta JS, Ahmad S, Ponzin D, Ferrari S. Effects of corneal preservation conditions on human corneal endothelial cell culture. Exp Eye Res. 2019;179:93–101.
27. Ishino Y, Sano Y, Nakamura T, Connon CJ, Rigby H, Fullwood NJ, et al. Amniotic membrane as a

carrier for cultivated human corneal endothelial cell transplantation. Investig Ophthalmol Vis Sci. 2004;45(3):800–6.

28. Engelmann K, Bednarz J, Valtink M. Prospects for endothelial transplantation. Exp Eye Res. 2004;78(3):573–8.

29. Engler C, Kelliher C, Speck CL, Jun AS. Assessment of attachment factors for primary cultured human corneal endothelial cells. Cornea. 2009;28(9):1050–4.

30. He Z, Forest F, Bernard A, Gauthier AS, Montard R, Peoc'h M, et al. Cutting and decellularization of multiple corneal stromal lamellae for the bioengineering of endothelial grafts. Investig Ophthalmol Vis Sci. 2016;57(15):6639–51.

31. Zhu YT, Tighe S, Chen SL, John T, Kao WY, Tseng SCG. Engineering of human corneal endothelial grafts. Curr Ophthalmol Rep. 2015;3(3):207–17.

32. Møller-Pedersen T, Hartmann U, Ehlers N, Engelmann K. Evaluation of potential organ culture media for eye banking using a human corneal endothelial cell growth assay. Graefes Arch Clin Exp Ophthalmol. 2001;239(10):778–82.

33. Jäckel T, Knels L, Valtink M, Funk RHW, Engelmann K. Serum-free corneal organ culture medium (SFM) but not conventional minimal essential organ culture medium (MEM) protects human corneal endothelial cells from apoptotic and necrotic cell death. Br J Ophthalmol. 2011;95(1):123–30.

34. Bednarz J, Doubilei V, Wollnik PCM, Engelmann K. Effect of three different media on serum free culture of donor corneas and isolated human corneal endothelial cells. Br J Ophthalmol. 2001;85(12):1416–20.

35. Parekh M, Romano V, Ruzza A, Kaye SB, Ponzin D, Ahmad S, et al. Culturing discarded peripheral human corneal endothelial cells from the tissues deemed for preloaded DMEK transplants. Cornea. 2019;38(9):1175–81.

36. Okumura N, Sakamoto Y, Fujii K, Kitano J, Nakano S, Tsujimoto Y, et al. Rho kinase inhibitor enables cell-based therapy for corneal endothelial dysfunction. Sci Rep. 2016;6(January):1–11.

37. Kinoshita S, Koizumi N, Ueno M, Okumura N, Imai K, Tanaka H, et al. Injection of cultured cells with a ROCK inhibitor for bullous keratopathy. N Engl J Med. 2018;378(11):995–1003.

38. Okumura N, Matsumoto D, Fukui Y, Teramoto M, Imai H, Kurosawa T, et al. Feasibility of cell-based therapy combined with descemetorhexis for treating Fuchs endothelial corneal dystrophy in rabbit model. PLoS One. 2018;13(1):1–14.

39. Parekh M, Romano V, Hassanin K, Testa V, Wongvisavavit R, Ferrari S, et al. Biomaterials for corneal endothelial cell culture and tissue engineering. J Tissue Eng. 2021;12:2041731421990536.

40. Koizumi N, Sakamoto Y, Okumura N, Okahara N, Tsuchiya H, Torii R, et al. Cultivated corneal endothelial cell sheet transplantation in a primate model. Investig Ophthalmol Vis Sci. 2007;48(10):4519–26.

41. Navaratnam J, Utheim T, Rajasekhar V, Shahdadfar A. Substrates for expansion of corneal endothelial cells towards bioengineering of human corneal endothelium. J Funct Biomater. 2015;6(3):917–45.

42. Levis H, Kureshi A, Massie I, Morgan L, Vernon A, Daniels J. Tissue engineering the cornea: the evolution of RAFT. J Funct Biomater. 2015;6(1):50–65.

43. Watanabe R, Hayashi R, Kimura Y, Tanaka Y, Kageyama T, Hara S, et al. A novel gelatin hydrogel carrier sheet for corneal endothelial transplantation. Tissue Eng Part A. 2011;17(17–18):2213–9.

44. Lai JY, Cheng HY, Hui-Kang MD. Investigation of overrun-processed porous hyaluronic acid carriers in corneal endothelial tissue engineering. PLoS One. 2015;10(8):1–20.

45. Liang Y, Liu W, Han B, Yang C, Ma Q, Zhao W, et al. Fabrication and characters of a corneal endothelial cells scaffold based on chitosan. J Mater Sci Mater Med. 2011;22(1):175–83.

46. Madden PW, Lai JNX, George KA, Giovenco T, Harkin DG, Chirila TV. Human corneal endothelial cell growth on a silk fibroin membrane. Biomaterials. 2011;32(17):4076–84.

47. Ramachandran C, Gupta P, Hazra S, Mandal BB. In vitro culture of human corneal endothelium on non-mulberry silk fibroin films for tissue regeneration. Transl Vis Sci Technol. 2020;9(4):1–15.

48. Mimura T, Yamagami S, Amano S. Corneal endothelial regeneration and tissue engineering. Prog Retin Eye Res. 2013;35:1–17.

49. Bayyoud T, Thaler S, Hofmann J, Maurus C, Spitzer MS, Bartz-Schmidt KU, et al. Decellularized bovine corneal posterior lamellae as carrier matrix for cultivated human corneal endothelial cells. Curr Eye Res. 2012;37(3):179–86.

50. Chakraborty J, Roy S, Murab S, Ravani R, Kaur K, Devi S, et al. Modulation of macrophage phenotype, maturation, and graft integration through chondroitin sulfate cross-linking to Decellularized cornea. ACS Biomater Sci Eng. 2019;5(1):165–79.

51. Arnalich-Montiel F, Moratilla A, Fuentes-Julián S, Aparicio V, Martin MC, Peh G, et al. Treatment of corneal endothelial damage in a rabbit model with a bioengineered graft using human decellularized corneal lamina and cultured human corneal endothelium. PLoS One. 2019;14(11):1–16.

52. Yoeruek E, Saygili O, Spitzer MS, Tatar O, Bartz-Schmidt KU. Human anterior lens capsule as carrier matrix for cultivated human corneal endothelial cells. Cornea. 2009;28(4):416–20.

53. Parekh M, Van den Bogerd B, Zakaria N, Ponzin D, Ferrari S. Fish scale-derived scaffolds for culturing human corneal endothelial cells. Stem Cells Int. 2018;2018:8146834.

54. Kruse M, Walter P, Bauer B, Rütten S, Schaefer K, Plange N, et al. Electro-spun membranes as scaffolds for human corneal endothelial cells. Curr Eye Res. 2018;43(1):1–11.

55. Ozcelik B, Brown KD, Blencowe A, Ladewig K, Stevens GW, Scheerlinck JPY, et al. Biodegradable and biocompatible poly(ethylene glycol)-based hydrogel films for the regeneration of corneal endothelium. Adv Healthc Mater. 2014;3(9):1496–507.

56. Kennedy S, Lace R, Carserides C, Gallagher AG, Wellings DA, Williams RL, et al. Poly-ε-lysine based hydrogels as synthetic substrates for the expansion of corneal endothelial cells for transplantation. J Mater Sci Mater Med. 2019;30(9):1–13.

57. Kim EY, Tripathy N, Cho SA, Lee D, Khang G. Collagen type I–PLGA film as an efficient substratum for corneal endothelial cells regeneration. J Tissue Eng Regen Med. 2017;11(9):2471–8.

58. Palchesko RN, Lathrop KL, Funderburgh JL, Feinberg AW. In vitro expansion of corneal endothelial cells on biomimetic substrates. Sci Rep. 2015;5:32–4.

59. Rizwan M, Peh GS, Adnan K, Naso SL, Mendez AR, Mehta JS, et al. In vitro topographical model of Fuchs dystrophy for evaluation of corneal endothelial cell monolayer formation. Adv Healthc Mater. 2016;5(22):2896–910.

60. Wang YH, Young TH, Wang TJ. Investigating the effect of chitosan/ polycaprolactone blends in differentiation of corneal endothelial cells and extracellular matrix compositions. Exp Eye Res. 2019;185:107679.

61. Hsiue GH, Lai JY, Chen KH, Hsu WM. A novel strategy for corneal endothelial reconstruction with a bioengineered cell sheet. Transplantation. 2006;81(3):473–6.

62. Sumide T, Nishida K, Yamato M, Ide T, Hayashida Y, Watanabe K, et al. Functional human corneal endothelial cell sheets harvested from temperature-responsive culture surfaces. FASEB J. 2006;20(2):392–4.

63. Ide T, Nishida K, Yamato M, Sumide T, Utsumi M, Nozaki T, et al. Structural characterization of bioengineered human corneal endothelial cell sheets fabricated on temperature-responsive culture dishes. Biomaterials. 2006;27(4):607–14.

64. Lai JY, Chen KH, Hsiue GH. Tissue-engineered human corneal endothelial cell sheet transplantation in a rabbit model using functional biomaterials. Transplantation. 2007;84(10):1222–32.

65. Okumura N, Koizumi N. Regeneration of the corneal endothelium. Curr Eye Res. 2020;45(3):303–12.

66. Burillon C, Huot L, Justin V, Nataf S, Chapuis F, Decullier E, et al. Cultured autologous oral mucosal epithelial cell sheet (CAOMECS) transplantation for the treatment of corneal limbal epithelial stem cell deficiency. Investig Ophthalmol Vis Sci. 2012;53(3):1325–31.

67. Tuft SJ, Coster DJ. The corneal endothelium. Eye. 1990;4(3):389–424.

68. Zavala J, López Jaime GR, Rodríguez Barrientos CA, Valdez-Garcia J. Corneal endothelium: developmental strategies for regeneration. Eye. 2013;27(5):579–88.

69. McCabe KL, Kunzevitzky NJ, Chiswell BP, Xia X, Goldberg JL, Lanza R. Efficient generation of human embryonic stem cell-derived corneal endothelial cells by directed differentiation. PLoS One. 2015;10(12):1–24.

70. Ali M, Kabir F, Raskar S, Renuse S, Na CH, Delannoy M, et al. Generation and proteome profiling of PBMC-originated, iPSC-derived lentoid bodies. Stem Cell Res. 2020;46:101813.

71. Wagoner MD, Bohrer LR, Aldrich BT, Greiner MA, Mullins RF, Worthington KS, et al. Feeder-free differentiation of cells exhibiting characteristics of corneal endothelium from human induced pluripotent stem cells. Biol Open. 2018;7(5):1–10.

72. Zhao JJ, Afshari NA. Generation of human corneal endothelial cells via in vitro ocular lineage restriction of pluripotent stem cells. Investig Ophthalmol Vis Sci. 2016;57(15):6878–84.

73. Zhang K, Pang K, Wu X. Isolation and transplantation of corneal endothelial cell-like cells derived from in-vitro-differentiated human embryonic stem cells. Stem Cells Dev. 2014;23(12):1340–54.

74. Chen P, Chen JZ, Shao CY, Li CY, Zhang YD, Lu WJ, et al. Treatment with retinoic acid and lens epithelial cell-conditioned medium in vitro directed the differentiation of pluripotent stem cells towards corneal endothelial cell-like cells. Exp Ther Med. 2015;9(2):351–60.

75. Bosch BM, Salero E, Núñez-Toldrà R, Sabater AL, Gil FJ, Perez RA. Discovering the potential of dental pulp stem cells for corneal endothelial cell production: a proof of concept. Front Bioeng Biotechnol. 2021;96:17724.

76. Soh YQ, Mehta JS. Regenerative therapy for fuchs endothelial corneal dystrophy. Cornea. 2018;37(4):523–7.

77. Peh GSL, Chng Z, Ang HP, Cheng TYD, Adnan K, Seah XY, et al. Propagation of human corneal endothelial cells: a novel dual media approach. Cell Transplant. 2015;24(2):287–304.

78. Peh GSL, Ang HP, Lwin CN, Adnan K, George BL, Seah XY, et al. Regulatory compliant tissue-engineered human corneal endothelial grafts restore corneal function of rabbits with bullous keratopathy. Sci Rep. 2017;7(1):1–17.

79. Numa K, Imai K, Ueno M, Kitazawa K, Tanaka H, Bush JD, et al. Five-year follow-up of first 11 patients undergoing injection of cultured corneal endothelial cells for corneal endothelial failure. Ophthalmology. 2021;128(4):504–14.

80. Marta CM, Adrian M, Jorge FD, Francisco AM, De Miguel MP. Improvement of an effective protocol for directed differentiation of human adipose tissue-derived adult mesenchymal stem cells to corneal endothelial cells. Int J Mol Sci. 2021;22(21):11982.

81. Li Z, Duan H, Jia Y, Zhao C, Li W, Wang X, et al. Long-term corneal recovery by simultaneous delivery of hPSC-derived corneal endothelial precursors and nicotinamide. J Clin Invest. 2022;132(1):1–11.

82. Wongvisavavit R, Parekh M, Ahmad S, Daniels JT. Challenges in corneal endothelial cell culture. Regen Med. 2021;16(9):871–91.
83. Brunette I, Roberts CJ, Vidal F, Harissi-Dagher M, Lachaine J, Sheardown H, et al. Alternatives to eye bank native tissue for corneal stromal replacement. Prog Retin Eye Res. 2017;59:97–130.
84. Matthyssen S, Van den Bogerd B, Dhubhghaill SN, Koppen C, Zakaria N. Corneal regeneration: a review of stromal replacements. Acta Biomater. 2018;69:31–41.
85. Lagali N. Corneal stromal regeneration: current status and future therapeutic potential. Curr Eye Res. 2020;45(3):278–90.
86. Alió del Barrio JL, Arnalich-Montiel F, De Miguel MP, El Zarif M, Alió JL. Corneal stroma regeneration: preclinical studies. Exp Eye Res. 2021;202:108314.

What Is New in Keratoprostheses

Saif Bani Oraba and Christopher Liu

Key Points

- Cadaveric Keratoplasty is the preferred option for the treatment of corneal opacity, scarring and deformation but not in cases of end-stage and ocular surface diseases.
- Keratoprosthesis is the last resort for end-stage corneal and ocular surface disease and may, in the future, offer an alternative to cadaveric keratoplasty.
- The main keratoprostheses currently in use are the Boston KPro Type 1 (BKPro1) and the osteo-odonto-keratoprosthesis (OOKP).
- BKPro1 is indicated for wet blinking eyes, while the OOKP is indicated for dry eyes and those with defective or absent blink or lids.
- Although they may be visually devastating, the rate of complications of keratoprostheses has been significantly reduced by improving the design of the devices and the development of prevention and management protocols for the complications.

Introduction

Corneal disease is a major cause of blindness in the world, both in developed and developing countries. The preferred option for treatment of corneal opacity, scarring and deformed cornea is keratoplasty. However, in situations where the ocular surface is keratinised, lids and blinking are defective, or the corneal vascularisation is significant, keratoplasty is not an option anymore, and an alternative to the cornea as an optical system is necessary. The last resort in such end-stage corneal and ocular surface diseases is keratoprostheses. Keratoprosthesis surgery and its long-term management are very complex and require broad and extensive multidisciplinary team involvement. Although several devices have been developed and trialled, very few have had successful long-term results and continue in regular clinical use [1]. The main current keratoprostheses are Boston KPro Type 1 (BKPro1) for wet blinking eyes and the osteo-odonto-keratoprosthesis (OOKP) for dry eyes and those with defective or absent blink or lids.

S. Bani Oraba
Sussex Eye Hospital, Brighton, UK

Ibra Hospital, Ibra, Sultanate of Oman

C. Liu (✉)
Brighton and Sussex Medical School, Brighton, UK

Brighton and Tongdean Eye Clinic, Sussex Eye
Hospital, Hove, UK

Limitations of Keratoplasty

Keratoplasty, both penetrating and lamellar, provides the standard treatment for most corneal opacities that jeopardize vision. It is considered one of the most successful organ transplantations. It provides an excellent outcome and high success rate in low-risk patients. The success rate of keratoplasty depends on the type, indication and the period after the procedure. Outcome analyses for tens of thousands of full-thickness and lamellar corneal transplants have consistently demonstrated that long-term functional graft survival rates are high for recipients of first transplants with non-inflammatory corneal disease such as keratoconus and corneal dystrophies. However, other recipient subgroups experience substantially poorer long-term outcomes. Conditions not amenable to corneal transplant include cases of chronic ocular surface inflammation, extensive corneal vascularisation and multiple graft failure.

The success of keratoplasty is however not fully sustained in the long term. In over one thousand penetrating keratoplasty procedures performed over 20 years, the transplants remained clear in only 55.4% of patients at 10 years, 52% at 15 years and 44% at 20 years post-surgery [2].

Another limitation of keratoplasty is the scarcity of corneal donor tissues due to multiple reasons like cultural, religious, and economic barriers. The availability of donor tissues continues to be a challenge. A recent global survey of eye banking and corneal transplantation quantified the drastic mismatch between the supply and demand of donor corneas worldwide, finding only 1 cornea available for every 70 needed [3]. The unavailability of corneal donor tissues has become even more evident in the post-COVID-19 pandemic.

Limbal stem cell deficiency (LSCD) is an ocular surface disease caused by a decrease in the population and/or function of limbal epithelial stem cells (LSCs), which leads to the inability to sustain the normal homeostasis of the corneal epithelium [4]. This deficiency results in persistent epithelial defects and conjunctivalisation of the corneal surface. In mild cases, LSCD may be treated with debridement of the abnormal epithelial cells, optimizing the ocular surface, use of a scleral contact lens or in advance cases, limbal epithelial transplantation. Although there have been several advances in the field in the last 20–30 years, the management of LSCD remains a challenge. These advances include transplantation of the limbal epithelium (autografts and allografts); cultivated limbal epithelial transplantation (CLET), cultivated oral mucosal epithelial transplantation (COMET) and simple limbal epithelial transplantation (SLET) [5]. Systemic immunosuppression is required to maintain the survival of allotransplanted cells, with attendant side effects.

Some of the aforementioned limitations of keratoplasty and limbal stem cell transplantation can be addressed by keratoprostheses (KPros). KPros are last resort operations and should only be offered to cases not amenable to conventional cadaveric keratoplasty.

History and Development

The first description of a keratoprosthesis is attributed to the French surgeon Guillaume Pellier de Quengsy (1789) [6]. He proposed replacing the opaque cornea with a transparent material to restore vision. This was followed by a number of attempts to develop an ideal keratoprosthesis. Different attempts with various techniques and designs of keratoprostheses were made, all of which failed to have sustainable success. Interest in keratoprostheses faded after the catastrophic complications due to the absence of biotechnology and has been replaced by the introduction of corneal transplantation. The field of keratoplasty continued to develop with the introduction of steroids, fine needles, and suture materials. However, it was eventually realised that corneal transplantation alone is not a permanent solution for all corneal blindness, and keratoprostheses came into consideration again.

Nussbaum described KPro prototypes manufactured from quartz crystal. It was large and rapidly extruded. This was followed by the development of smaller devices that were successfully implanted in animals and tried in humans. These initial KPros had a high failure rate due to infection, leakage, and extrusion of the device [7]. After several years of attempts to develop an ideal KPro, the principle of assembling a device where a central optical cylinder and two plates are assembled into a corneal graft carrier has emerged. This formed the basis to develop the Boston KPro, until the early twentieth century, when Salzer implanted a quartz disc bounded by a platinum ring with prongs into human eyes which lasted a number of years. The next development was to use a lighter, biocompatible material polymethylmethacrylate (PMMA). Multiple further stages of design refinements and developments in the surgical procedure improved outcomes with reduced complications.

BKPro1

The BKPro1, made of polymethylmethacrylate (PMMA) and titanium, is currently a widely used device. It is composed of 2 plates; an anterior 5 mm diameter PMMA plate with a 3.5 mm central optical stem and an 8.5 mm titanium back plate with 16 holes to facilitate access of aqueous humour to the sandwiched corneal graft carrier. The corneal graft carrier is then sutured to the host cornea akin to a full-thickness corneal graft. This KPro device does not eliminate the need of corneal tissue, either fresh or frozen. To help maintain the complex and prevent complications, an extended-wear therapeutic soft contact lens is worn, and daily broad-spectrum antibiotics eye drops are used.

Indications and Pre-operative Assessment

BKPro1 is indicated in cases of multiple graft failure and vascularized corneae, with or without limbal stem cell failure. The device can only be used successfully when there is an intact blink mechanism and adequate tear secretion (so-called "wet blinking eye"). Thus, a detailed ocular history and meticulous eye examination is crucial in the patient selection process. Often the patient has undergone different treatment modalities which failed before considering a BKPro1. The surgeon should acquire details of the underlying diagnosis, current ocular condition, medical systemic and ocular treatment received including use of steroids or immunosuppression, and types and number of any ocular surgical interventions. The initial eye examination aims to identify eyes with good visual potential, with healthy optic nerve function and normal retina. Also, it focuses on the overall health of the ocular surface, the amount of ocular surface scarring and keratinisation and forniceal shortening. Any degree of keratinisation, either bulbar or tarsal, would lead to poor results for the BKPro1. The anatomy and function of the lids, the blinking mechanism and the quality of tear film should be carefully assessed along with the ability to apply and retaining a soft contact lens and the compliance to topical antibiotics. BKPro1 surgery should not be offered for patients in whom keratoplasty carries a good chance of success. Also, it is contraindicated in patients with end-stage glaucoma, retinal or optic nerve pathology, and when there is a seeing fellow eye.

Evaluation of visual potential is necessary before offering the option of keratoprostheses. This can be started by assessing the light perception and projection in all quadrants. Poor accuracy of light projection may be due to media opacity rather than retina or optic nerve pathology. B-scan ultrasonography must be performed to exclude retinal pathology. Electrophysiological tests like electroretinogram and visual-evoked potential could be beneficial in doubtful situations, but they may also not be precise in quantifying the visual potential in the presence of media opacities [8].

Full glaucoma assessment is crucial as it is frequently associated with ocular surface diseases, either as a result of the underlying pathology with damaged trabeculum, anterior chamber angle and episcleral venous drainage, or as a side effect of chronic use of steroids. The diagnosis and management of glaucoma with associated ocular surface diseases may be challenging. A thorough clinical examination should be carried out to identify signs and risk factors, glaucomatous changes and any signs of previous glaucoma surgery. It is difficult to accurately measure the intraocular pressure (IOP) and assess the optic nerve due to poor fundal view. Hence, the surgeon should use available ancillary tests such as anterior segment optical coherence tomography (AS-OCT) or ultrasound biomicroscopy to determine the status of anterior segment structures including irido-corneal angle before planning for surgery. Signs of poor visual prognosis may be part of the underlying disease, for example, nystagmus in case of aniridia. On the other hand, improvement of vision following previous surgical intervention may be considered a good sign of visual potential. Although BKPro1 surgery is offered usually to bilaterally blind patients, only one eye should be operated on, leaving the other as spare, given the inherent instability of the device. The other eye should not be neglected, and care should be taken to treat glaucoma or any other condition to preserve the potential vision.

Before taking the decision to offer the patient or to perform the surgery, it is important to emphasize the need of long-term commitment from both the patient and surgeon. A holistic view should be carried out to understand and address the visual needs, the psychological and general health status. Involvement of a clinical psychologist is recommended to assess the patient's adaptation to the blindness, current lifestyle and coping mechanisms, current employment, and social support in place [9]. The counselling process will provide the patient the required information regarding the preparation for surgery, the surgery itself and its stages, and the post-surgery treatment and follow-up plan. Finally, the team will be able to determine whether the patient is a good candidate for the procedure and to ensure that life-long management plan is sustainable. The candidates should have realistic expectations and full insight of the whole process; this includes continued adherence to long-term treatment plan with regular life-long follow-up with multidisciplinary care. The holistic approach may include multi-specialty team to address the patient's comorbidities, which usually presents, especially if the patient has multi-system involvement condition. This team may consist of anaesthetists, physicians, oculoplastics, vitreoretinal, and glaucoma surgeons. Also, ensuring easy access and clear clinical pathway for patients and health care providers in case of emergency. Patient support groups, leaflets and written information, clear instructions, and education of the patients and carers should form part of the care pathway [9].

Surgical Technique

The BKPro1 complex is assembled by sandwiching a double trephine corneal graft carrier with the front plate and the locking back plate (Fig. 37.1a), prior to host cornea trephination. In more detail, the donor cornea is trephined 0.25 mm to 0.5 mm larger than the back plate diameter, followed by a punch out of a 3 mm central opening using the disposable dermatological trephine supplied. The doughnut-shaped corneal tissue is then placed onto to front plate, which itself is resting upside down on an adhesive tape, with the optical cylinder passing through the central opening. The fenestrated titanium back plate is then placed on top of the donor tissue posteriorly. A titanium locking ring is snapped around the stem portion of the front plate, which protrudes posteriorly through the cornea and the back plate, thus locking the assembly. The latest design of a locking titanium back plate replaces the PMMA back plate and separate titanium locking ring. The recipient bed is then prepared with trephine smaller than the carrier graft by 0.5 to 1 mm. The KPro assembly is then sutured to the recipient bed using 16 interrupted 10–0 nylon sutures (Fig. 37.1b). A hydrophilic therapeutic (bandage) contact lens is placed to keep a certain amount of tear film intact on the KPro and prevent Dellen formation. A concurrent glaucoma tube implant can be implanted if indicated, which could also be done pre- or post-keratoprosthesis surgery. If indicated, pars plana vitreoretinal surgery can be performed after KPro surgery.

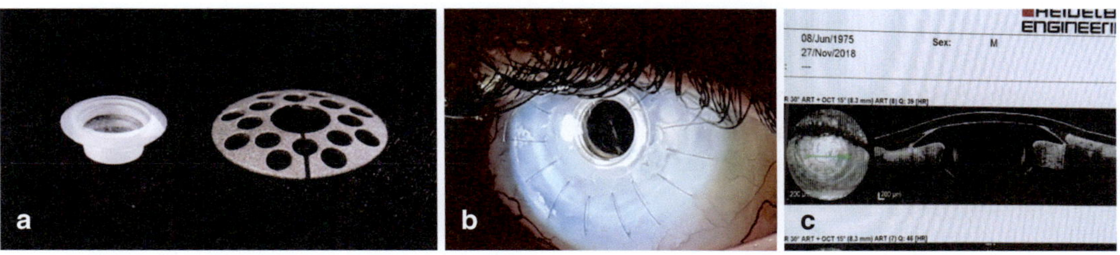

Fig. 37.1 Boston Keratoprosthesis type 1: (**a**) front and back plates, (**b**) *in situ,* (**c**) anterior segment OCT

Results

The majority of short-term (0–2 years follow-up) outcomes of the BKPro1 is favourable [10]. In eyes with successful implants, vision is affected by a number of factors in the postoperative period such as retro-prosthetic membrane (RPM), glaucoma, retinal detachment, endophthalmitis and stromal melts [9]. In one study, the percentage of eyes with post-operative visual acuity (VA) of 20/100 or better was 67% (30/45) of patients at 6 months and 75% (21/28) at 1 year with 90% retention rate at 1 year [11]. In a comparative case study involving various international centres with a cumulative number of 113 procedures, against 110 procedures performed in one of the USA centres, 2% of the patients from the international group and 6% of the patients from the USA group had preoperative visual acuity level of 20/200, whereas six months postoperatively, 70% of the international patients and 69% of the USA patients have regained a VA level of 20/200 [12]. However, the number of patients maintaining the same level of vision gradually declined over 2 years to 59% and 60%, respectively. Interestingly, the percentage of patients with pre- and postoperative VA of less than or equal to light perception did not change significantly in both groups (international: 50% preoperative versus 60% postoperative; USA group: 9% preoperative versus 10% postoperative). A device retention rate of 80% at a mean follow-up period of 14 months in the international group against a similar retention rate of 80% at an average of 24 months in the USA group [12]. In two other studies, retention rates of 100% at 16 months and 95% at an average of 8 months, were reported [13, 14].

There are very few reports on medium-term follow-up (2 to 5 years) and almost none on long-term results (over 5 years). As the lifespan of patients is usually significantly longer than just five years, and there is the possibility of losing visual potential when a device fails, long-term results are very important.

The incidence of an RPM ranges from 25%–65% with the BKPro1s [15]. This proliferation of fibrovascular tissue over the internal surface of the device can occlude the optical portion leading to visual obstruction and make the ocular examination difficult and impossible in some cases. Nearly 45% required treatment with YAG laser or surgical membranectomy [15]. On histological study, it is hypothesized that RPM is derived from corneal stromal downgrowth from the host side due to the gaping of the posterior wound beyond the back plate. Also, metaplastic lens epithelium and native iris stroma contribute to the development of RPM [15]. Risk factors for the development of RPM include anterior segment inflammation, previous keratitis, and simultaneous performance of other intraocular surgery at the time of BKPro1 implantation [16].

BKPro1 implantation is associated with the development of glaucoma and progression of pre-existing glaucoma. Pathophysiology of glaucoma may include distortion of anterior chamber angle structures, occurrence of RPM, and peripheral anterior synechiae [17]. The prevalence of glaucoma ranges from 36% to 76% in BKPro1 patients and de novo glaucoma developed in 2%–28% of the patients after the device implantation [18]. As previously mentioned, glaucoma detection, monitoring and treatment are considered as a significant challenge in BKPro1 patients. The most useful modality to diagnose and monitor glaucoma progression in the BKPro1 patient may be optic disc photography and OCT imaging with OCT or Heidelberg retinal tomography (HRT). Measuring the IOP and conducting a visual field examination may be difficult and less accurate. Treatment options for glaucoma in BKPro1 patients include topical and oral glaucoma medications and glaucoma surgery. Out of 45 eyes after Boston BKPro1 implantation, 17 eyes needed glaucoma drainage tube insertion, with an incidence of 59% of conjunctival erosions following glaucoma tube inserts in BKPro1 patients [19]. 60% of eyes without "glaucoma device-associated conjunctival erosions" retained a VA of 20/200 and only a 25% of the eyes that suffered erosions could retain a VA of 20/200 at 1-year follow-up [19]. The presence of glaucoma is associated with poor visual prognosis but can be ameliorated by prompt pre- and post-operative glaucoma management. Where a glaucoma drainage device is used, the development of erosions and subsequent complications, such as hypotony, endophthalmitis, and choroidal and retinal detachments, may adversely affect the visual potential of the eye [17]. Cyclophotocoagulation can be useful in those who do not respond to drainage tubes [20].

Another complication of BKPro1 is endophthalmitis, with an incidence ranging between 0% and 25% with an estimated prevalence of 5.4% in the last 10 years with BKPro1 [21]. The risk of endophthalmitis is generally considered higher with inflammatory conditions like Stevens-Johnson syndrome (SJS), mucous membrane pemphigoid (MMP), and burns [22]. Although the current standard practice of daily administration of topical vancomycin has reduced the incidence of Gram-positive endophthalmitis, an increased incidence of Gram-negative bacterial and fungal endophthalmitis is observed by some investigators [23]. Should endophthalmitis develops, device explantation followed by vitrectomy and intravitreal injection of broad-spectrum antibiotics is advised in view of the high incidence of posterior segment complications [21]. Posterior segment complications like retinal detachment have been reported in the range of 3–12% [14]. Altered eye anatomy and the presence of a limited field of vision through the optic make vitreoretinal surgery a daunting task.

Despite the existence of various problems, there has been a steady increase (more than three-fold) in the number of BKPro1 implantations performed in the USA and the rest of the world [24]. This may be largely due to the increase in device retention rates and awareness of the procedure.

The current BKPro1 design uses a titanium instead of PMMA back plate (Fig. 37.1). The advantages of using a titanium plate include taking up less space in the anterior chamber, possibly inducing less inflammation, and a larger diameter to stem the migration of keratocytes to form RPM. Moreover, titanium can be coloured by anodisation to improve cosmesis. Also, the newer click-on design replaced the need for a locking ring, making the surgery easier. The Boston KPro team developed another less expensive device, the Lucia. Lucia has a single titanium back plate with radial petaloid-shaped holes and may be anodised to improve the cosmesis.

LVP keratoprosthesis is a modification of BKPro1 implanted under buccal mucosal graft in patients with severely affected ocular surface like Stevens-Johnson syndrome and chemical burns. In this modification, the optical cylinder is elongated to protrude through the buccal mucous membrane. The initial outcomes of its use, including in paediatric patients are promising [25]. Boston KPro2 has been similarly modified to be open through oral mucosal graft instead of upper lid skin. The main changes are an elongated PMMA optical cylinder and titanium sleeve around the cylinder [26].

OOKP

The osteo-odonto keratoprosthesis was first described in 1963 in Italy by Strampelli, who used a donor tooth root and alveolar bone to support a PMMA optical cylinder [27]. Falcinelli improved this design by adding certain modifications such as using a larger biconvex optic and performing cryo-extraction of the lens. This led to the modified technique now known as modified osteo-odonto-keratoprosthesis (MOOKP) [28]. The central optical cylinder is supported by the alveo-dental lamina of a single tooth, usually canine. The complex is covered with a buccal mucosa to provide protection and nourishment.

Indications

The OOKP is indicated in patients with bilateral blindness from severe, end-stage corneal and ocular surface diseases with intact retinal and optic nerve function. Dry eye, keratinisation, and any defective blink or lid preclude success with conventional keratoplasty or ocular surface reconstruction but can be withstood by the OOKP. Examples of these conditions include eyes with severe SJS, severe ocular MMP, severe chemical and thermal burns, and eyes that have unsuccessfully undergone ocular surface or stem cell transplantation. Usually, the procedure is performed only in one eye, with the other eye reserved as a spare in case of procedure failure. OOKP is not suitable in children due to high bone turnover that may lead to complete laminar resorption. It is contraindicated in phthisis bulbi and eyes without light perception. Patients must have intact canine or premolar teeth, minimal gum disease, and, preferably, reasonably good dental hygiene in order to enable a suitable tooth to be harvested [29]. Before the surgery, the patients should be aware of the gravity of their condition, have an insight of the complexity of the surgery and its potential severe complications, and be prepared for life-long follow-up. Also, the issue of altered cosmetic appearance should be discussed adequately with the patients and their relatives before the surgery. Patients should be highly motivated to comply with the long-term management plan. To establish this, a multidisciplinary approach is ideal, and a clinical psychologist should be part of the team. For patients who are psychologically unstable, do not wish or cannot come for follow-up visits and patients with defective light perception possibly due to end-stage glaucoma, OOKP is considered relatively contraindicated [8].

Preoperative Assessment

Preoperative assessment of patients for OOKP is similar to that for BKPro1 (please see above) but there are further specific aims to confirm the suitability of the patient according to the selection criteria, identifying any risk factors that may affect the outcome of OOKP and planning to optimise the eye by managing these risk factors, and to prepare the patient and the family for a mostly irreversible and life-changing decision. The assessment is conducted by a multidisciplinary team comprising of ophthalmologist, oromaxillary surgeon, radiologist, anaesthetist, nurses, and a clinical psychologist.

During the ophthalmic assessment, the underlying pathology and the indication of the surgery is determined, the current status of the eyes is evaluated and any procedure to optimise the eye is performed before the surgery. A patient-centred approach should be followed to choose the eye for the proposed surgery, it is generally offered for bilaterally blind patients and the worse eye is usually selected, except when the visual potential is doubtful.

The oromaxillary surgeon performs a clinical and radiological assessment, usually by way of an orthopantomogram, of the oral cavity and dentition and based on that, selects the tooth. Patients who have poor dental health and oral hygiene are counselled towards improving dental health and to stop smoking if applicable. For patients who are edentulous or do not have any appropriate teeth, related or unrelated tooth donors may be considered and screened as required [9]. Temprano introduced another variation when he used a fragment of the tibia in a patient who lacked teeth. The so-called osteo-keratoprosthesis (OKP) presented comparable anatomical and visual outcomes, although reabsorption of the bone occurred more frequently, resulting in an increased rate of extrusion of the device [30].

The patients' education about the surgery starts as soon as the option of OOKP is discussed with the patients, their family members, and their carers. The clinical psychologist will then assess the patients' perception of the surgery and further investigate their psychological and mental health.

The ability, willingness and motivation for life-long follow up is ensured and stressed on during the psychological session. Patients may need multiple visits to arrive at a decision. Once the decision has been taken the patient is then referred for anaesthetic assessment.

Surgical Technique

OOKP is a multi-staged, complex, and rather invasive surgical programme, which requires highly subspecialised ophthalmic, dental, clinical psychologist and nursing expertise. Details of the OOKP stages and technique are described in the Rome-Vienna protocol [8]. The OOKP procedure is performed in two stages; first preparing the globe, the buccal mucous membrane graft and the osteo-odonto-acrylic lamina, and second implanting the lamina.

Stage 1 OOKP surgery (Fig. 37.2) is further divided into two stages. Initially, the ocular surface is prepared by performing a 360-degree conjunctival peritomy, followed by a superficial keratectomy to remove the corneal scars and epithelium. The eye is then covered with a buccal mucous membrane graft which is sutured to recti insertion sites (deriving a blood supply from the anterior ciliary arteries) and sclera. A single-rooted tooth (usually a canine, alternatives are incisors and premolars) with the largest and straightest root is harvested *en bloc* with the surrounding jawbone. The tooth root and sur-rounding jawbone are shaped into a 3 mm thick and up to 15 mm long rectangular lamina. This is used as a skirt or frame to surround an optical cylinder, which is accommodated in a tight, central and perpendicular tunnel through dentine. Dental cement is used to fill any small gaps between the dentine and optical cylinder; the fit needs to be snug as the cement is a filler and not an adhesive. The PMMA optical cylinder is made up of an anterior stem that ranges in diameter from 3.5 to 4 mm and a posterior section ranging from 4.5 to 5.25 mm in width. The anterior stem protrudes 2–3 mm beyond the alveolar side while the posterior projects into the anterior chamber [31]. The implant is inserted in a submuscular pouch in the orbito-zygomatic area on the contralateral side with the dentine facing the orbit and the bone facing the periorbital muscles. It is kept there for about 3 months to enhance revascularisation of the implant, promote growth of connective tissue and remaining periosteum.

In Stage 2 OOKP surgery (Fig. 37.3), the osteo-odonto-acrylic lamina is retrieved and examined for signs of absorption and infection, and excess fibrovascular and connective tissue is removed. The healthy lamina is then implanted at the anterior surface of the globe under the mucosal membrane. This is achieved by creating a large buccal mucous membrane flap to expose the cornea. A Flieringa ring is used to support the sclera. The centre of the cornea is marked and trephined with the same diameter as the posterior

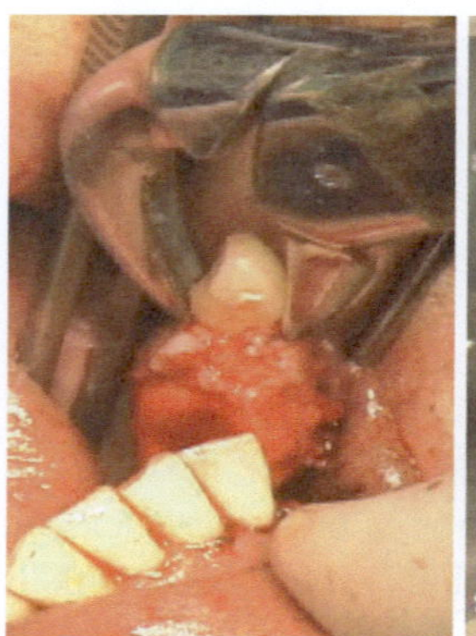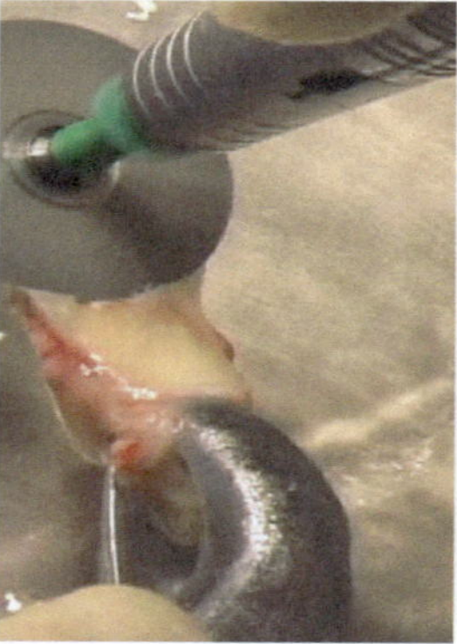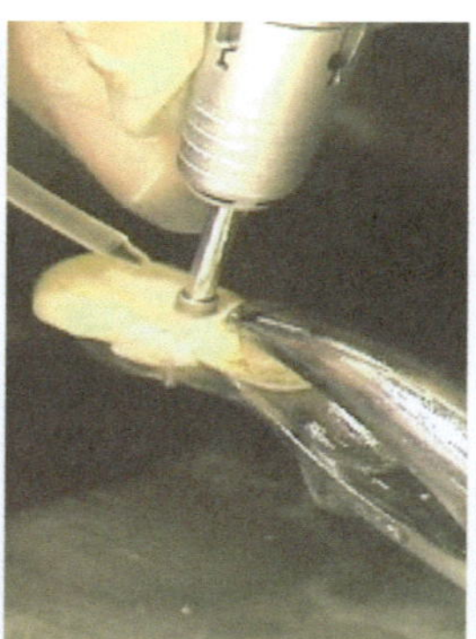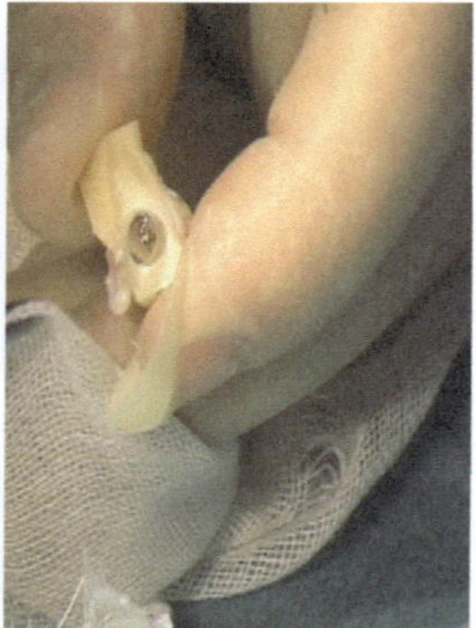

Fig. 37.2 Harvesting the tooth root and surrounding jawbone, and preparation of the lamina

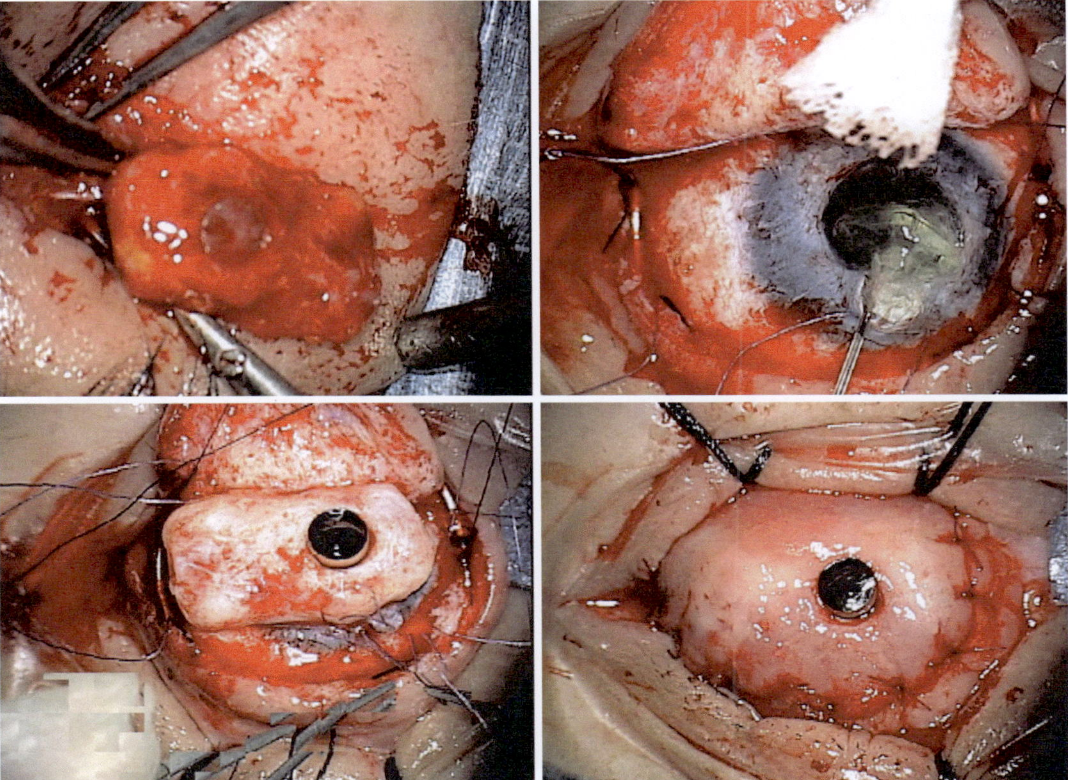

Fig. 37.3 Stage 2 OOKP: retrieval and implantation of the lamina

part of the optical cylinder, avoiding decentration as it may result in visual distortion. Total iridodialysis, cryoextraction of lens and a generous open sky vitrectomy are performed. The lamina is sutured to the sclera and the remaining cornea and is covered by the flap of the oral mucosa. Postoperative treatment includes topical and systemic antibiotics, five days of oral steroids and oral antiglaucoma medications. Topical broad-spectrum antibiotics must be applied for the patient's lifetime with a rotation of antibiotics every few months, whereas oral antibiotics can be stopped after five days. Patients may be advised to wear dark glasses to improve cosmesis and reduce glare, some may wear a hat too to reduce glare. Long-term follow-up requires the OOKP patient to be examined by an OOKP-experienced ophthalmologist every 3 months. The patient is assessed for any signs or symptoms of infection, retinal detachment or high intraocular pressure. The clinical examination aims to evaluate the visual acuity, estimate the intraocular pressure by palpation with a cotton-tip and or fingertip, check the stability and clarity of the optic cylinder and the state of the mucous membrane and the thickness of the lamina, and assess the retina and the optic nerve. A B-scan is carried out as necessary. A CT-scan of the lamina with or without 3-D rendition is done soon after Stage 2 as a baseline and then every few years, as guided by clinical examination, to estimate the bone and dentine.

Results

The visual acuity of patients following OOKP surgery can be as good as 6/4. A systematic review of eight different case studies found VA of $\geq$6/18 in 52% of patients after OOKP [32].

Another study recorded a visual acuity of $\geq$6/12 in 53% of all OOKP patients, and 78% of patients achieved a VA of $\geq$6/60 [33].

Long-term anatomical retention of the OOKP is excellent. The probability of retaining laminar autografts over 5 years is found to be 81% [33]. In 85 patients, the retention of the lamina over a 20-year follow-up was reported to be 98% [34]. 10-year anatomical survival of 145 OOKP and 82 tibial KPro implants was 66% and 47%, respectively [30]. The main factor resulting in anatomical failure was the resorption of the OOKP lamina. Resorption leads to decreased thickness and defects in the lamina, which may in turn lead to optical cylinder tilt, aqueous leak and endophthalmitis. Lamina resorption can be detected even in its early stages by clinical palpation in experienced hands. Radiological studies to detect minor reduction of the laminar dimensions and early laminar resorption may include electron beam tomography (EBT) and CT-scan with or without 3-D rendition. Radiological studies should be correlated with the clinical assessment for a full evaluation of resorption. If progressive or pathological resorption is detected, alendronic acid is prescribed for the patient. Bone morphogenetic protein (BMP) and bone graft can be used independently. However, in severe cases of resorption, they are combined. If the above methods fail, then laminar replacement is required, and in cases of imminent danger of endophthalmitis, the lamina should be explanted and the corneal opening closed with a small full-thickness corneal graft. If another suitable canine is available, a new lamina can be created and exchanged three months later after it has gained soft tissues in a submuscular pocket (as above).

The main complication that affects the visual outcome in anatomically successful OOKP is glaucoma. Glaucoma was observed in 26% of the eyes before OOKP, and in 60% of the eyes after OOKP [1]. Digital (fingertip) estimation is the only usable method for the estimation of IOP, which requires user experience and training. Clinical optic nerve head assessment by fundoscopy, serial photography, optical coherence tomography and periodic visual field testing are useful in glaucoma evaluation and monitoring.

Oral acetazolamide and sublingual timolol eye drops is the mainstay of glaucoma management in OOKP eyes. Surgical treatment is usually by way of drainage tubes. Glaucoma remains a challenging condition to manage in OOKP.

Eyelid and mucosal complications are common after OOKP and make up the bulk of the surgical revisions after each stage of the procedure. Mucosal thinning and ulcerations were common after both Stage 1 and Stage 2 due to inadequate vascularisation and lubrication. This can be managed by mucosal grafting, which itself may create relative eyelids shortening and malposition necessitating surgical repair [35]. On the other hand, mucosal overgrowth concealing the optic cylinder is a common complication that requires excision (Fig. 37.4), with the use of mitomycin-C in case of recurrence [35].

A retroprosthetic membrane (RPM) is a fibrovascular proliferation behind the lamina that can grow across the optic, obscuring vision. A RPM is usually treatable with an Nd-YAG laser, similar to capsulotomy in the early stages. However, it may recur and can be difficult to laser, which may carry risks of optic spoliation and intraocular haemorrhage.

New vitreous haemorrhage long after Stage 2 is a worrying complication. It can denote a retinal tear due to a posterior vitreous detachment. Such eyes must be examined with B-Scan ultrasonography by an experienced operator. Patients must be very closely monitored with serial B-scans in the absence of a retinal detachment. Endoscopic vitrectomy should be performed in case of suspected or confirmed retinal detachment.

Endophthalmitis may develop secondary to laminar resorption or intraocular surgery. It may also result from loose optical cylinder and leakage due to laminar resorption. This is managed by taking samples for culture and sensitivity followed by injection of intravitreal and or systemic antibiotic and or antifungal, and in some cases vitrectomy.

Potential complications during and after Stage 1 may include impending and inadvertent perforation of thin cornea requiring a lamellar or full-thickness graft from a donor cornea and buccal mucosa graft necrosis requiring the additional

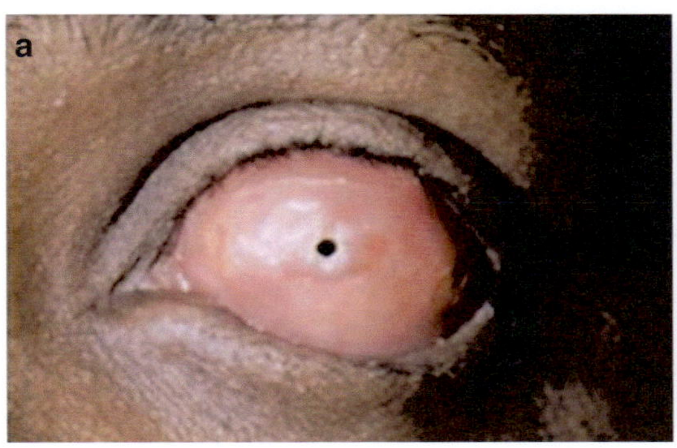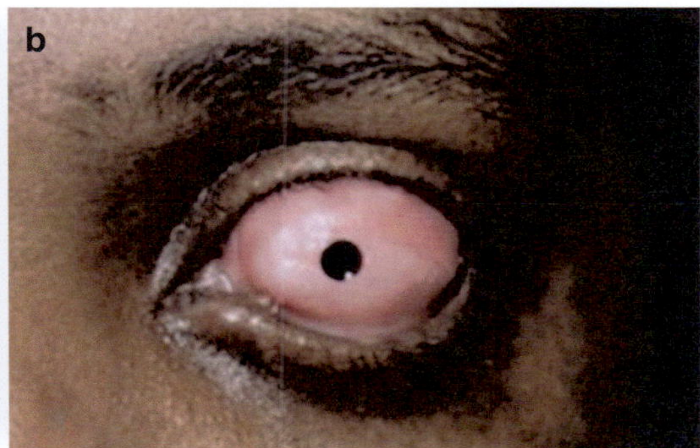

Fig. 37.4 Overgrowth of mucous membrane (**a**) pre- and (**b**) post-surgical excision

grafting procedure. During Stage 1 oromaxillary fistulae, fractures of the mandible, and damage to adjacent teeth may occur. Also, excessive force or overheating during drilling can break the dentine or damage the dentoalveolar ligament. When the implant is in the submuscular pouch, absorption of the dentine, bone infection, or loosening of the optical cylinder can occur.

The rare devastating expulsive suprachoroidal haemorrhage may occur during Stage 2. The risk of this complication may be reduced by controlling high intraocular ocular pressure and blood pressure prior to and during surgery. Positioning the patient in a head-up position, using deep anaesthesia with full paralysis and hyperventilation are some intraoperative strategies to reduce the risk of suprachoroidal haemorrhage. Intravitreous haemorrhage may occur, and it is usually self-limiting. Early postoperative complications include low IOP causing choroidal detachment.

The Future

The BKPro1 needs to be more affordable, especially for developing countries. More attention should be paid to the long-term outcome of this device. This will help guide its use with improvements in retention and prevention, diagnosis, and management of complications. BKPro2 may have reached its end point. It has been modified to be implanted under buccal mucosa rather than that under lid skin [26].

Although the general concept of the surgical technique of OOKP has not changed, certain surgical aspects have been refined. The optical cylinder has been modified to improve the visual field and reduce the glare. Also, the use of bone morphogenetic protein for the augmentation of the resorbed lamina. There is emerging evidence that surgical management of glaucoma, namely tube shunt operations in OOKP patients is more effective than topical and systemic medical treatment. The endoscopic vitrectomy is the modality of choice in repairing retinal detachment.

Future areas of keratoprostheses development, aiming to prolong the survival time of keratoprostheses and improve the quality and field of vision, may include biosynthetic or totally synthetic versions. 3D printing is promising in manufacturing corneal stromal tissue equivalent with embedded human endothelial cells, with the potential of producing full thickness, multilayer corneal model in future. The OOKP procedure will evolve to utilise a lamina made of synthetic materials that would allow the integration of buccal mucous membrane but be more resistant to resorption. Biosynthetic or synthetic OOKP would offer a solution, especially for patients who lack suitable teeth.

On the contrary, advancements in other fields of ophthalmology may decrease the need for any KPro. Community-based prevention implementation will decrease corneal blindness because of infectious keratitis and chemical burn. A better understanding of corneal immunological mechanisms may lead to more effective strategies for increased survival of multiple graft failure and control of immunological eye diseases such as SJS and MMP.

Take Home Notes

- In unilateral corneal blindness, keratoprostheses should not be offered, and in the case of bilateral corneal blindness, only one eye should be rehabilitated, keeping the other eye as spare.
- Keratoprostheses should only be offered by multidisciplinary teams in regional and national centres, which can also provide emergency access 24/7/365.
- While OOKP eliminates the need for any corneal tissue, BKPro requires a full thickness of corneal tissue.
- There has been a steady increase in BKPro1 implantation due to a high device retention rate and awareness of the procedure.
- The visual acuity outcome and the long-term retention rate of OOKP are excellent.

References

1. Gomaa A, Comyn O, Liu C. Keratoprostheses in clinical practice—a review. Clin Exp Ophthalmol. 2010;38:211–24. https://doi.org/10.1111/j.1442-9071.2010.02231.x.
2. Anshu A, Li L, Htoon HM, de Benito-Llopis L, Shuang LS, Singh MJ, et al. Long-term review of penetrating keratoplasty: a 20-year review in Asian eyes. Am J Ophthalmol. 2020;224:254–66. https://doi.org/10.1016/j.ajo.2020.10.014.
3. Gain P, Jullienne R, He Z, et al. Global survey of corneal transplantation and eye banking. JAMA Ophthalmol. 2016;134(2):167–73.
4. Deng SX, Borderie V, Chan CC, et al. And the international Limbal stem cell deficiency working group. Global consensus on definition, classification, diagnosis, and staging of limbal stem cell deficiency. Cornea. 2019;38(3):364–75.
5. Fernandez-Buenaga R, Aiello F, Zaher SS, et al. Twenty years of limbal epithelial therapy: an update on managing limbal stem cell deficiency. BMJ Open Ophthalmol. 2018;3:e000164. https://doi.org/10.1136/bmjophth-2018-000164.
6. de Quengsy GP, Des HD. Pellier de Quengsy Sammlung von Aufsätzen und Wahrnehmungen sowohl über die Fehler der Augen, als der Theile, die sie umgeben Junius. Leipzig: Junius; 1789.
7. Lam FC, Liu C. The future of keratoprostheses (artificial corneae). Br J Ophthalmol. 2011;95:304–5. https://doi.org/10.1136/bjo.2010.188359.
8. Hille K, Grabner G, Liu C, et al. Standards for modified osteo-odonto-keratoprosthesis (OOKP) surgery according to Strampelli and Falcinelli: the Rome-Vienna protocol. Cornea. 2005;24:895–908.
9. Avadhanam VS, Smith HE, Liu C. Keratoprostheses for corneal blindness: a review of contemporary devices. Clin Ophthalmol. 2015;9:697–720. Published 2015 Apr 16. https://doi.org/10.2147/OPTH.S27083.
10. Holland G, Pandit A, Sánchez-Abella L, Haiek A, Loinaz I, Dupin D, Gonzalez M, Larra E, Bidaguren A, Lagali N, Moloney EB, Ritter T. Artificial cornea: past, current, and future directions. Front Med. 2021;8:770780. https://doi.org/10.3389/fmed.2021.770780.
11. Aldave AJ, Kamal KM, Vo RC, Yu F. The Boston type I keratoprosthesis: improving outcomes and expanding indications. Ophthalmology. 2009;116(4):640–51.
12. Aldave AJ, Sangwan VS, Basu S, et al. International results with the Boston type I keratoprosthesis. Ophthalmology. 2012;119(8):1530–8.
13. Chew HF, Ayres BD, Hammersmith KM, et al. Boston keratoprosthesis outcomes and complications. Cornea. 2009;28:989–96.
14. Zerbe BL, Belin MW, Ciolino JB. Boston type 1 keratoprosthesis study group results from the multicenter Boston type 1 keratoprosthesis study. Ophthalmology. 2006;113:1779–84.
15. Stacy RC, Jakobiec FA, Michaud NA, Dohlman CH, Colby KA. Characterization of retrokeratoprosthetic membranes in the Boston type 1 keratoprosthesis. Arch Ophthalmol. 2011;129(3):310–6.
16. Magalhães FP, Sousa LB, Oliveira LA. Boston type I keratoprosthesis: review. Arq Bras Oftalmol. 2012;75(3):218–22.
17. Kamyar R, Weizer JS, de Paula FH, et al. Glaucoma associated with Boston type I keratoprosthesis. Cornea. 2012;31(2):134–9.
18. Banitt M. Evaluation and management of glaucoma after keratoprosthesis. Curr Opin Ophthalmol. 2011;22:133–6.
19. Li JY, Greiner MA, Brandt MC, Lim MC, Mannis MJ. Long-term complications associated with glaucoma drainage devices and Boston keratoprosthesis. Am J Ophthalmol. 2011;152(2):209–18.
20. Rivier D, Paula JS, Kim E, Dohlman CH, Grosskreutz CL. Glaucoma and keratoprosthesis surgery: role of adjunctive cyclophotocoagulation. J Glaucoma. 2009;18:321–4.
21. Robert MC, Moussally K, Harissi-Dagher M. Review of endophthalmitis following Boston keratoprosthesis type 1. Br J Ophthalmol. 2012;96(6):776–80.
22. Nouri M, Terada H, Alfonso EC, Foster CS, Durand ML, Dohlman CH. Endophthalmitis after keratoprosthesis: incidence, bacterial causes, and risk factors. Arch Ophthalmol. 2001;119(4):484–9.
23. Durand ML, Dohlman CH. Successful prevention of bacterial endophthalmitis in eyes with the Boston keratoprosthesis. Cornea. 2009;28(8):896–901.
24. Boston KPro News. Fall. 2011. 8. Accessed 23 Jan 2013. www.masseyeandear.org.
25. Basu S, Nagpal R, Serna-Ojeda JC, Bhalekar S, Bagga B, Sangwan V. LVP keratoprosthesis: ana-

tomical and functional outcomes in bilateral end-stage corneal blindness. Br J Ophthalmol. 2018. pii: bjophthalmol-2017-311649.

26. Mehran Z-G, Liu C. Keratoprosthesis: current choices and future development. Asia Pac J Ophthalmol. 2019;8(6):429–31. https://doi.org/10.1097/APO.0000000000000268.

27. Strampelli B. Keratoprosthesis with osteodontal tissue. Am J Ophthalmol. 1963;89:1029–39.

28. Falcinelli GC. Personal changes and innovations in Strampelli's osteo-odonto-keratoprosthesis. An Inst Barraquer. 1998;28:47–8.

29. Tan A, Tan DT, Tan X-W, Mehta JS, Keratoprosthesis O-o. Systematic review of surgical outcomes and complication rates. Ocul Surf. 2012;10(1):15–25.

30. Michael R, Charoenrook V, de la Paz MF, Hitzl W, Temprano J, Barraquer RI. Long-term functional and anatomical results of osteo- and osteoodonto-keratoprosthesis. Graefes Arch Clin Exp Ophthalmol. 2008;246:1133–7. https://doi.org/10.1007/s00417-008-0850-3.

31. Zarei-Ghanavati M, Avadhanam V, Vasquez Perez A, Liu C. The osteo-odonto-keratoprosthesis. Curr Opin Ophthalmol. 2017;28:397–402.

32. Tan A, Tan DT, Tan XW, Mehta JS. Osteo-odonto keratoprosthesis: systematic review of surgical outcomes and complication rates. Ocul Surf. 2012;10:15–25. https://doi.org/10.1016/j.jtos.2012.01.003.

33. Liu C, Okera S, Tandon R, Herold J, Hull C, Thorp S. Visual rehabilitation in end-stage inflammatory ocular surface disease with the osteo-odontokeratoprosthesis: results from the UK. Br J Ophthalmol. 2008;92:1211–7. https://doi.org/10.1136/bjo.2007.130567.

34. Marchi V, Ricci R, Pecorella I, Ciardi A, Di Tondo U, Osteo-odonto-keratoprosthesis. Description of surgical technique with results in 85 patients. Cornea. 1994;13:125–30.

35. Avadhanam VS, Vasquez-Perez A, Chervenkoff JV, El-Zahab S, Liu C. Mucosal complications in osteo-odonto keratoprosthesis (OOKP) surgery. J EuCornea. 2020;6:13–23. https://doi.org/10.1016/j.xjec.2020.01.001.

Intraoperative OCT in Anterior Segment Surgery

38

Francis W. Price Jr, Anjulie Gang, and Marianne O. Price

Key Points

- Intraoperative OCT allows direct visualization of DMEK graft orientation, eliminating the need for orientation marks on the donor tissue.
- Intraoperative OCT can evaluate graft orientation and placement through cloudy corneas.
- Intraoperative OCT allows direct visualization of the depth and uniformity of a DALK dissection plane.
- In complex DSEK or DMEK cases, Intraoperative OCT allows the surgeon to scan the interface for fluid pockets and loose residual tags of stroma, Descemet membrane, or other tissue.

Introduction

In-office optical coherence tomography (OCT) has dramatically changed the diagnosis and treatment of cataracts and other ocular conditions.

Supplementary Information The online version contains supplementary material available at https://doi.org/10.1007/978-3-031-32408-6_38.

F. W. Price Jr (✉) · A. Gang
Price Vision Group, Indianapolis, IN, USA
e-mail: fprice@pricevisiongroup.net;
anjuliegang@pricevisiongroup.net

M. O. Price
Cornea Research Foundation of America,
Indianapolis, IN, USA
e-mail: mprice@cornea.org

Prior to its introduction, fluorescein angiography was needed to diagnose cystoid macular edema; this was much more invasive than taking an OCT image of the macula. The in-office OCT also allows us to easily screen candidates for multifocal intraocular lenses (IOL) and to rule out epiretinal membrane or other macular pathology, because the OCT shows cellular structures in exquisite detail. Intraoperative OCT has been an important advance because it provides the surgeon with detailed cross-sectional images of ocular structures not well visualized with the coaxial microscope. This chapter will describe the uses of intraoperative OCT in anterior segment surgeries.

We know of three companies that market or have sold intraoperative OCT units with their operating microscopes. Each company's device only works with its own microscope, which limits adoption, because one has to purchase the OCT device plus the operating microscope that is made to utilize it. This limitation has provided a barrier to entry for those who would like to utilize this technology. The three companies that have OCT units in practice are Carl Zeiss Meditec, Leica, and Haag-Streit, but Haag-Streit has discontinued its OCT unit.

There are three ways the OCT images can be viewed in the operating room: on a monitor hooked up to the OCT device, as an inset in the video recording from the operating microscope, and through the oculars of the operating micro-

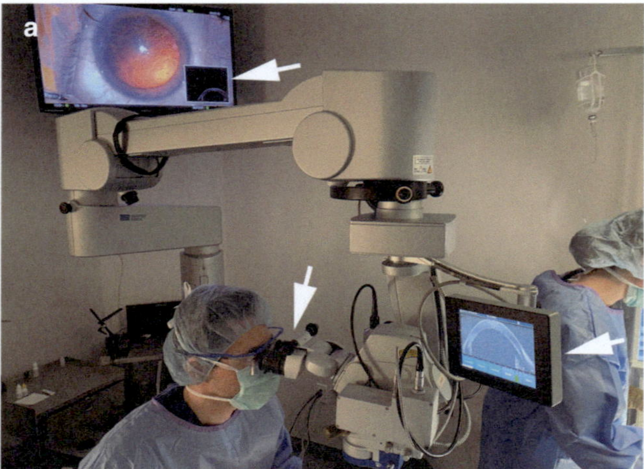
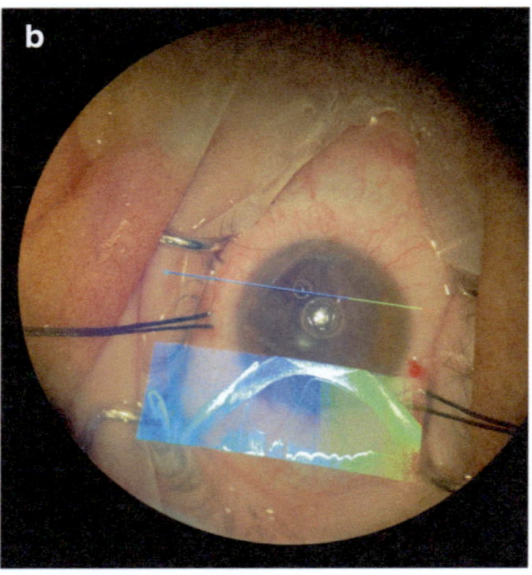

Fig. 38.1 Three ways to view intra-operative OCT images in the operating room. (**a**) With the Haag-Streit iOCT™, the OCT image can be viewed on a television screen as an inset within the surgical video feed (top left; this view is provided by all commercially available intra-operative OCT devices), or it can be viewed on the monitor used to program the OCT which is attached to the microscope (lower right), or it can be viewed by the surgeon through the oculars of the operating microscope (a unique feature of the Haag-Streit device). (**b**) The image seen by the surgeon through the oculars of the operating microscope. This image was captured with an iPhone camera, which made the OCT image appear to be in color, although it is actually in greyscale. The surgeon can use the foot switch of the microscope to turn on or off the OCT image superimposed into the oculars

scope (Fig. 38.1). To our knowledge, only the Haag-Streit device provides a sufficiently high-resolution image superimposed in the oculars to allow the surgeon to operate without having to look away from the surgical field to view a monitor. With the other two devices, the surgeon either has to look away from the surgical field to view the monitor or they could ask someone else in the room to relay to them what is visible on the monitor. These later two devices provide very nice images for teaching and documentation but are not as efficient in surgery as the unit that allows the surgeon to view the image superimposed in the oculars. We have the Haag-Streit device, so our images and discussion are based on experience with that device, the iOCT™.

Intraoperative OCT and EK

The iOCT™ image superimposed in the oculars (Fig. 38.2) can be turned on and off with the foot switch, so the OCT image is only visible when desired by the surgeon. We use the iOCT™ most frequently in DMEK cases for the treatment of Fuchs' dystrophy. In these cases, the cornea is relatively clear, so we turn the OCT image on when the donor tissue is being inserted into the recipient's anterior chamber, and after confirming that the tissue is correctly oriented with the donor endothelium facing the recipient iris, we turn the OCT image off. By using the iOCT™ to determine whether the tissue is correctly oriented, we do not have to place orientation marks on the tissue, which can cause endothelial cell damage. Gentian violet marks on a DMEK graft typically cause about 5% cell loss, and any notches or slits made along the edge of the tissue to show orientation also cause cell loss.

In eyes with more advanced corneal decompensation, which makes it more difficult for the surgeon to visualize the posterior cornea, we use the iOCT™ while stripping the host Descemet membrane (DM) to look for loose strands of DM, stroma, or scar tissue in the anterior chamber or for abnormalities on the back surface of

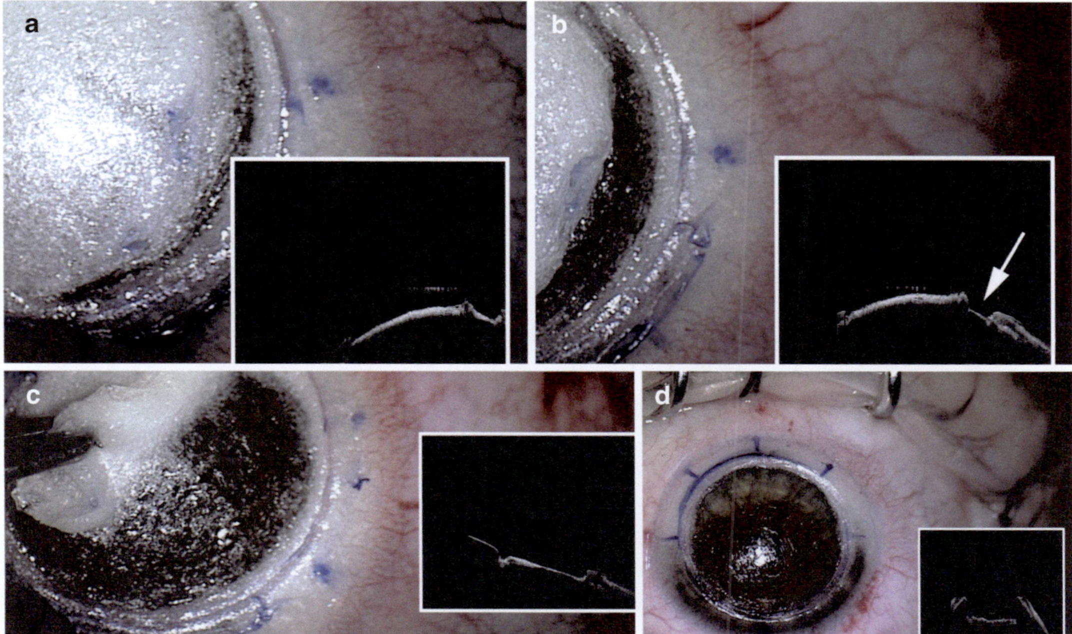

Fig. 38.2 Use of intraoperative OCT with the DALK peeling technique. The intraoperative OCT helps the surgeon visualize the dissection depth and adjust as needed before starting the peel technique. Typically the desired dissection depth is almost down to the Descemet membrane, although a thicker residual bed is safer in cases of previous hydrops or perforation. (**a**)The dissection plane is not deep enough and has not reached the desired depth of the residual bed. (**b**) The appropriate dissection depth is now reached, as indicated by the arrow. (**c**) In this image taken while peeling, the residual bed appears thinner on the right and thicker on the left, but the left still has areas of injected air and stretched stromal fibers indicating that it has not been completely peeled. After peeling is completed, the bed will be uniformly thin. It is important for the surgeon to only grasp one spot on the cornea while pulling the stroma away from the bed. (**d**) In a different case, note the uniform and very thin residual bed achieved with the peeling technique. This residual bed is very similar to that achieved with a Type 1 big bubble

the cornea which could interfere with donor placement or attachment. We can also use the iOCT™ to help center the graft if it is hard to see the graft edges through the recipient cornea. This improved visualization allows us to successfully use thinner DMEK grafts instead of thicker DSEK grafts in cases with very cloudy corneas. Once the EK graft is in place, the OCT allows the surgeon to evaluate the apposition of the donor against the recipient cornea to make sure that there are no areas of detachment or obstructions preventing attachment, such as loose DM, stromal strands, iris, or scar tissue. The chapter entitled Endothelial Keratoplasty: Current State of the Art includes a video demonstrating the use of the iOCT™ while positioning a DMEK graft and confirming its orientation in an eye with a very cloudy cornea.

Intraoperative OCT and DALK

The iOCT™ greatly improved the efficiency of our EK surgery and has been even more impactful with DALK. The big bubble (BB) technique introduced by Anwar was a key DALK advance [1], because it provided a consistent and uniformly thin dissection bed that produced better visual outcomes than manual dissection, which often resulted in inconsistent bed depth and irregularities across the dissection plane. Malbran had earlier introduced manual peeling techniques [2, 3], but determining the dissection and peeling depth was difficult with a coaxial microscope. Melles et al. introduced the use of an air bubble in the anterior chamber to determine dissection depth [4], but it was difficult to keep the manual dissection depth uniform with his technique, and in cases of advanced keratoconus, it was challenging to get the dissecting blade across and over the apex of the large cone. Video 38.1 shows Type 1 and Type 2 big bubbles. Video 38.2 shows an irregular bed produced with manual dissection. In both videos, the ability to scan the bed with the intraoperative OCT is demonstrated.

Because the intraoperative OCT allows direct viewing of the lamellar structures of the cornea and the ability to estimate the depth of dissection, we now have the ability to perform DALK dissections without a BB that postoperatively are indistinguishable from BB cases. This is very helpful for cases where either a BB is difficult to achieve or is not desirable to try. In eyes with previous hydrops, penetrating scars, or previous cataract or anterior segment surgery, it can be difficult to successfully create a BB without rupture of the previous perforations. Our current technique is to make a side cut with a calibrated trephine or femtosecond laser zig-zag incision. After making the side cut, we begin a lamellar dissection inward from the side cut and check the depth of dissection, then gradually deepen the depth until we reach the desired residual bed thickness, which is typically close to a BB depth unless we want a thicker bed because of scarring. Once the desired depth is reached, we dissect centrally for 1–2 mm, 360 ° around the side cut, and then perform a peel as described by Malbran. Figure 38.1 shows the peeling technique with the use of the iOCT™ to guide the depth of the dissection; the residual bed after a successful peel resembles that achieved with a type 1 big bubble.

We have not found any difference in the incidence of stromal rejection episodes between DALK procedures performed with BB vs. peel techniques, but we did find that the rejection episode rate was significantly lower with the use of femtosecond laser zig-zag side cut incisions compared with standard metal trephination [5].

A double anterior chamber can form during DALK cases from perforation during dissection or suturing. Intraoperative OCT is very helpful for identifying when a double anterior chamber has formed. Treatment involves injecting air into the anterior chamber and venting fluid from the interface, and the OCT is helpful for assessing when the double anterior chamber has fully collapsed. It is surprising how much larger and extensive the fluid pockets appear when viewed with the OCT intraoperatively.

As we do more DALK procedures and the patients get older and develop cataracts, we have found that occasionally a double anterior chamber may form between the donor graft and the residual stromal bed when cataract incisions are hydrated to close them at the end of the case. It is difficult to appreciate the extent of the double anterior chamber or its resolution with the coaxial microscope. Video 38.3 shows such a case and demonstrates the use of the iOCT™ to diagnose and treat the separation of a DALK graft from the host residual bed during subsequent cataract surgery.

Intraoperative OCT and Lens Implants

During cataract surgery, the iOCT™ can be used to assess capsular bag anatomy, lens tilt, and placement of the IOL relative to the capsule. Also, we routinely use the iOCT™ to measure the vault of an ICL implant over the crystalline lens. The final vault after the viscoelastic has dissipated often varies from the vault measured intraoperatively, but the intraoperative assessment is helpful for identifying whether the vault is substantially over or under what was planned. We have used the vault measurements to decide whether to rotate a lens with too much vault from a horizontal position to a vertical position or when deciding whether to change the size of the lens for the second eye when doing bilateral simultaneous cases. It is important to perform all measurements at the same magnification.

Retained Nuclear Fragments

Video 38.4 shows the use of the iOCT™ to facilitate the removal of a nuclear fragment. This patient presented to our clinic with inferior corneal decompensation a few months after undergoing uncomplicated cataract surgery with the placement of an intraocular lens. Notes from the patient's surgeon indicated that he had removed a nuclear fragment from the eye several days after the cataract surgery. Upon taking the patient to surgery, the corneal edema and iris color made it difficult to detect a residual nuclear fragment, but we were able to find it and properly direct the phaco tip to remove it with the use of the iOCT™.

Other Uses

Intraoperative OCT can be used, just like in-office OCT, to evaluate the depth of scars in the cornea or lesions on the conjunctiva.

Take Home Notes
- Intraoperative OCT opens up a whole new view of the anatomical structures of the anterior segment and cornea.
- It allows a more efficient assessment of graft orientation with DMEK surgery.
- Irregularities on the posterior corneal surface are easily visualized real-time by surgeons

alerting them to potential problems in DMEK or DSEK.
- The OCT reveals the depth and uniformity of the dissection plane in DALK and shows whether there is a double anterior chamber or separation of the donor and recipient bed.
- IOL placement relative to the bag and residual capsule can be evaluated.
- ICL vault can be measured, allowing the surgeon to identify cases with unusually high or low vaults.

References

1. Anwar M, Teichmann KD. Big-bubble technique to bare Descemet's membrane in anterior lamellar keratoplasty. J Cataract Refract Surg. 2002;28:398–403.
2. Malbran E, Stefani C. Lamellar keratoplasty in corneal ectasias. Ophthalmologica. 1972;164:50–8.
3. Malbran E. Lamellar keratoplasty in keratoconus. Int Ophthalmol Clin. 1966;6:99–109.
4. Melles G, Lander F, Rietveld F, et al. A new surgical technique for deep stromal, anterior lamellar keratoplasty. Br J Ophthalmol. 1999;83:327–33.
5. Price FW Jr, Price MO, Grandin JC, Kwon R. Deep anterior lamellar keratoplasty with femtosecond-laser zigzag incisions. J Cataract Refract Surg. 2009;35:804–8.

Epilogue: Corneal Graft Surgery, a Glance to the Future

39

Jorge L. Alió and Jorge L. Alió del Barrio

Throughout this book, we have witnessed the major evolution that corneal graft surgery has experienced over the last two decades. A better understanding of the corneal anatomy and physiology, technical improvements in the management of corneal bank tissue, improvements in surgical instrumentations (such as the availability of femtosecond laser), new surgical techniques that have emerged and have finally been consolidated as better options to the classical penetrating keratoplasty with better results, medical education and, above all, the skills and the talent of corneal surgeons, have made corneal surgery enter a final stage of development since its early beginnings with the description of PKP by Zirm in 1906 and popularized by Castroviejo in 1936. Over all these years, the evolution has been constant and always in the benefit of better techniques, better results and better solutions to corneal blindness.

However, even though the results have been widely implemented, we have seen in the early chapters of this book how corneal graft still offers a challenge. Anatomical success does not always happen and anatomic failures are relatively frequent, with reported levels of survival from 52% to 98.8% for penetrating keratoplasty at 10 years, from 77% to 99.3% for deep anterior lamellar keratoplasty at 5 years, from 56% to 94.1% for Descemet stripping endothelial keratoplasty at 5 years and from 90% to 97.4% for Descemet membrane endothelial keratoplasty at 5 years [1]. The main pitfalls are immune graft rejection, comorbidities and relapse of the previous disease. In addition, functional failures, not frequently estimated as real ones, happen in a considerable number of patients, especially in PKP (for example, 10% recurrence of the ectatic disease at the host remnant peripheral cornea after 20 years), leading to a lack of adequate gain of visual acuity [2]. Targeting the control and resolution of these problems, especially immune graft rejection, is mandatory and one of the real challenges that the modern corneal graft surgeons face. However, this is not going to be enough, as functional failures still influence the outcomes, and they are not always within the surgeon's control. So, it seems mandatory to move to a totally different model, a paradigm shift. The philosopher Thomas Kuhn defined a *paradigm shift* as needing to happen first in the mind of the decision-makers in that particular topic [3]. This is exactly what has to happen now in corneal surgery; we need a paradigm shift.

The new paradigm will be, instead of tissue replacement, tissue restoration by regeneration. Corneal regeneration has also been targeted in

J. L. Alió (✉) · J. L. A. del Barrio
Vissum Miranza, Miguel Hernández University,
Alicante, Spain
e-mail: jlalio@vissum.com

J. L. Alió, J. L. A. del Barrio (eds.), *Modern Keratoplasty*, Essentials in Ophthalmology,
https://doi.org/10.1007/978-3-031-32408-6_39

this book, and it is still in its early stages. The possibility of restoring the ocular surface has been a highlight. The challenges that are involved are clear and there is still time ahead to achieve this on a consistent and repeatable basis. Translational research in this area is evolving, and in the coming years, it will probably take an important role in our practice once costs associated with it fade, allowing their availability to be more general. Corneal stroma regeneration, according to our recent pioneer clinical studies, seems to be feasible and even more easily applicable with the use of xenogenic tissue (instead of human corneal tissue, that is so scarce and expensive) [4–7]. Corneal endothelial substitution seems to be feasible even though the lack of biological productivity of the corneal endothelium seems to be a limitation during the culture of these cells. Future clinical research, both basic and translational, will likely increase the efficiency and involved costs of such procedures in order to succeed in real clinical practice. We can clearly foresee that it, in the future eye cellular eye banks, containing the best donor lineages for each cell type, will centralize the production and delivery of the different stem cell regenerative products among all clinical centers, making these new procedures cost-effective and available for all ophthalmology clinics, without the need of investing in expensive facilities. These cells and derived tissues may no longer depend on ocular human sources at some point and start coming from human bioengineering extraocular sources or even xenogenic tissues. Stem cells, that contain proven immunomodulatory properties, will unlikely be provided from the same patient, affected by the same genetic imbalance that made the corneal disease to happen initially (except for those abnormalities caused by external aggressions), but rather from considered genetically "optimal" donors in which immortal stem cells constantly proliferating will provide an easy and cheap way to restore the biology of the cornea.

Corneal graft surgery, as it is practiced today, it will never disappear and indeed will continue evolving, but it may be finally largely substituted by corneal regeneration procedures.

We hope that the reader of this book has foreseen the present and the future of corneal surgery, and this book will contribute to the medical education of those corneal surgeons interested in corneal graft surgery and stimulate them to search for new innovative and better solutions for corneal blindness in the benefit of our patients.

References

1. Alio JL, Montesel A, El Sayyad F, Barraquer RI, Arnalich-Montiel F, Alio Del Barrio JL. Corneal graft failure: an update. Br J Ophthalmol. 2021;105(8):1049–58. https://doi.org/10.1136/bjophthalmol-2020-316705.
2. de Toledo JA, de la Paz MF, Barraquer RI, Barraquer J. Long-term progression of astigmatism after penetrating keratoplasty for keratoconus: evidence of late recurrence. Cornea. 2003;22(4):317–23.
3. Kuhn T. The structure of scientific revolutions. 2nd ed. Chicago, IL: University of Chicago Press; 1970. ISBN 978-0-226-45804-5.
4. Alió Del Barrio JL, Arnalich-Montiel F, De Miguel MP, El Zarif M, Alió JL. Corneal stroma regeneration: preclinical studies. Exp Eye Res. 2021;202:108314. https://doi.org/10.1016/j.exer.2020.108314.
5. Zarif ME, Alió del Barrio JL, Arnalich-Montiel F, De Miguel MP, Makdissy N, Alió JL. Corneal stroma regeneration: new approach for the treatment of cornea disease. Asia Pac J Ophthalmol (Phila). 2020;9(6):571–9. https://doi.org/10.1097/APO.0000000000000337.
6. El Zarif M, Alió JL, Alió Del Barrio JL, Abdul Jawad K, Palazón-Bru A, Abdul Jawad Z, De Miguel MP, Makdissy N. Corneal stromal regeneration therapy for advanced keratoconus: long-term outcomes at 3 years. Cornea. 2021;40(6):741–54. https://doi.org/10.1097/ICO.0000000000002646.
7. Alió del Barrio JL, De la Mata A, De Miguel MP, Arnalich-Montiel F, Nieto-Miguel T, El Zarif M, Cadenas-Martín M, López-Paniagua M, Galindo S, Calonge M, Alió JL. Corneal regeneration using adipose-derived mesenchymal stem cells. Cell. 2022;11(16):2549. https://doi.org/10.3390/cells11162549.

Index